Functional Neuroanatomy

FUNCTIONAL NEUROANATOMY
An Interactive Text and Manual

Jeffrey T. Joseph, M.D., Ph.D.
Departments of Neurology and Pathology
Beth Israel Deaconess Medical Center
Boston, Massachusetts

David L. Cardozo, Ph.D.
Department of Neurobiology
Harvard Medical School
Boston, Massachusetts

WILEY-LISS
A John Wiley & Sons, Inc., Publication

Library of Congress Cataloging-in-Publication Data

Joseph, Jeffrey T.
   Functional neuroanatomy : An interactive text and manual /
Jeffrey T. Joseph, David L. Cardozo.
      p.   cm.
   Includes bibliographical references and index.
   ISBN 0-471-44437-5
   1. Neuroanatomy—Programmed instruction.   I. Cardozo, David L.   II. Title.
QM451.J67   2004
611′.8—dc21   2003009969

Printed in the United States of America.
10 9 8 7 6 5 4 3 2 1

Contents

Preface, vii

1. External Anatomy, 1

2. Internal Anatomy, 29

3. Histology, 49

4. Neuroimaging, 77

5. Somatosensory System, 105

6. Craniosensory Systems, 133

7. Vision and Hearing, 161

8. Neuromuscular System (with David Dawson), 187

9. Basal Ganglia, 211

10. Cerebellum, 233

11. Brainstem and Control Systems, 259

12. Cranial Nerves, 289

13. Hypothalamus, 331

14. Limbic System (with Changiz Geula), 355

15. Cortex (with Changiz Geula), 381

16. Development, 413

17. Trauma, 441

18. Review, 457

Appendix I. Normal Neuroimaging, 493

Appendix II. Brain Atlas, 505

Appendix III. Sheep Brain Dissection, 523

Appendix IV. Neuroimaging Principles (with William Copen), 527

Appendix V. Materials List, 549

Key Terms for Self Study, 559

Index, 567

Preface

This book is a guide to a series of laboratory exercises in neuroanatomy. It evolved from several years of teaching neuroanatomy together with neuroscience to Harvard Medical students. It covers the fundamental topics found in a traditional course on neuroanatomy utilizing a series of exercises that we hope will bring the anatomy of the brain to life. The book is intended for use by medical students, dental students, students of the health sciences, graduate students in the biological sciences, as well as professionals in the neurosciences who wish to brush up on their neuroanatomy.

We believe that the key to learning neuroanatomy is by engaging it. With this in mind, our book is highly interactive. Each chapter starts with a short discussion section, which is followed by a series of exercises designed to develop and reinforce the material. The activities are wide ranging, and include identification of structures and pathways, correlations with radiological images, examination of histological tissue, analysis of pathological brains, interpretation of physiological experiments and model building. All of the exercises are accompanied by complete answer sets. We have emphasized three themes throughout the book: clinical correlations, experimental results and radiological approaches. We use clinical correlations to develop the structure/function relationships. Experimental approaches are discussed to introduce the intellectual basis for neuroanatomy. Finally, we supplement the examination of brain specimens with radiological imaging in order to familiarize the reader with the type information that is most commonly utilized.

This manual can be used in several ways. It can best serve as a blueprint for a laboratory course in neuroanatomy that utilizes brain specimens, histological slides and other materials. With this in mind, we have provided a materials list in one of the appendices. Our book can also be used as a stand-alone guide. We have provided high-resolution images of all the necessary anatomical, histological and radiological material, and there is a short atlas located in the appendices. In addition, high resolution, color images are available on the publisher's website. However it is used, it's essential that the reader participate. The key to learning is doing and committing yourself to an answer. Complete the exercises and attempt the questions before consulting the answer keys. You will learn a great deal more by attempting to answer a question (whether you get it right or wrong) than by reading straight through to the answer.

Many fine neuroanatomy textbooks and atlases provide the necessary background for our interactive approach. In the course that we have taught using this manual, we have found John Martin's *Neuroanatomy,* John Nolte's *The Human Brain,* and Woolsey et al.'s *The Brain Atlas,* to be wonderful resources. In addition, there are many fine digitally based neuroanatomy atlases and interactive programs. We are particularly fond of Washington University's *Digital Anatomist,* which is available on the World Wide Web.

ACKNOWLEDGMENTS

We would like to acknowledge several of our colleagues whose efforts were critical to this book. First we thank Richard Sidman, who created the laboratory course from which this book subsequently arose. Richard has been a mentor, a teacher and a friend for many years. Changiz Geula and David Dawson made major contributions to sections of this book, including initial drafts of several chapters, and were extraordinarily generous in providing materials as well as guidance for many of the exercises throughout the manual. Several other people provided significant assistance. Edison Miyawaki helped in the early stages of this project and has given us numerous useful suggestions as we have implemented it. Ellen Grant provided much of the neuroimaging presented in the book. Clifford Saper, Jean-Paul Vonsattel, Christopher Wright, Reisa Sperling, and Tessa Hedley-Whyte also provided us with key materials. Our laboratory manager, Sheila Salomone has been a fabulous support in all of our teaching efforts. She has demonstrated unreasonable tolerance in putting up with some of our unconventional approaches to teaching. Finally, we thank our Harvard Students who have used this text in its embryonic state and have provided many helpful suggestions.

Chapter 1—EXTERNAL ANATOMY

Our nervous system starts life as a groove on the surface of the embryo and rapidly closes to become a tube. To form the central nervous system, this tube kinks in several spots and proliferates to its final form. Crested offshoots from the tube form the peripheral nervous system. Several layers of protection envelop the developing brain. To support its gelatinous substance, the brain floats in water. Our brain connects to the body via a complex system of nerves and receives sustenance from the body by a complex of vessels.

In this first laboratory session you will focus on three main topics: (1) the overall structure and organization of the brain and spinal cord as revealed by their external anatomy, (2) the brain's critically important vascular supply, and (3) the brain's protective coverings. As you work through this lab, concentrate on obtaining an overview of the general structure of the nervous system and avoid worrying too much about the thousands of details that we will be largely ignoring today. We will revisit all of these structures many times throughout the remaining laboratories and will have lots of opportunity to think about them in great depth.

Before beginning these laboratories, it is important to remind you to always wear gloves when handling human nervous tissue. An extremely rare brain disease (we're literally talking one in a million) has been shown to be transmitted by brain tissue. This class of diseases is known by several names, including Prion diseases, spongiform encephalopathies, and Creutzfeldt-Jacob disease (CJD). Popular names for similar animal diseases include "mad cow disease" and scrapie. The "infectious agent" of such afflictions is very hardy, surviving formalin fixation, paraffin embedding, regular autoclaving, and other standard measures. However, transmission has only been documented by direct brain inoculation, or in some cases by ingestion. You probably won't do either. NO EATING IN THE LABORATORY, WEAR GLOVES WHEN HANDLING BRAIN TISSUE, and BE CAUTIOUS WITH THE DISSECTING EQUIPMENT.

LEARNING OBJECTIVES

- Know the main divisions of the brain and their functional relationships.
- Recognize the salient morphological features on the lateral and medial brain surfaces.

Functional Neuroanatomy: An Interactive Text and Manual, by Jeffrey T. Joseph and David L. Cardozo
ISBN 0-471-44437-5 Copyright © 2004 John Wiley & Sons, Inc.

- Identify the main vessels that serve the brain, distinguish their territories, and understand the perfusion of the brain.
- Identify the main features of the brain's coverings and their relationship to the blood vessels.
- Relate the brain specimen to radiological images.
- Relate the spinal cord to the vertebral column and its significance in lumbar puncture.

INTRODUCTION

The goal of this first chapter is to introduce you to the overall structure and organization of the brain and spinal cord, including their vascular supply and protective coverings.

Neuroanatomy is a vast and complex subject. In order to approach it successfully, you need to order your approach. The secret to a successful attack on the discipline is to intellectually divide the nervous system into the largest chunks of information first, followed by successively finer and finer grains of information. For instance, your first major "cut" should establish that the central nervous system consists of the brain and the spinal cord. Next, before you learn any details of a particular region, recognize that the brain consists of a forebrain, midbrain, and hindbrain. Follow this with the next logical subdivisions of forebrain into cortex, basal ganglia, and thalamus; and hindbrain into cerebellum, pons, and medulla. If you maintain this simple approach of acquiring your neuroanatomical sophistication in incremental steps, you'll find that it is a pleasant way to learn the material, it will make more sense to you, and the knowledge will remain with you.

As you are studying neuroanatomy, always keep in mind that the entire nervous system develops from a neural tube that bulges, bends, and kinks in various ways and places to give the brain its characteristic structure. By relating any structure in the adult nervous system to its origin in the neural tube, you will able to see the logic of its position. For instance, the three main divisions of the brain: the forebrain, midbrain, and hindbrain, arise from three primary bulges in the neural tube (see Fig. 1.1). Similarly, the ventricles are simply what is left of the hollow portion of the tube after the contortion act is completed. They are narrowed where developing nervous tissue has bulged inward, and they are

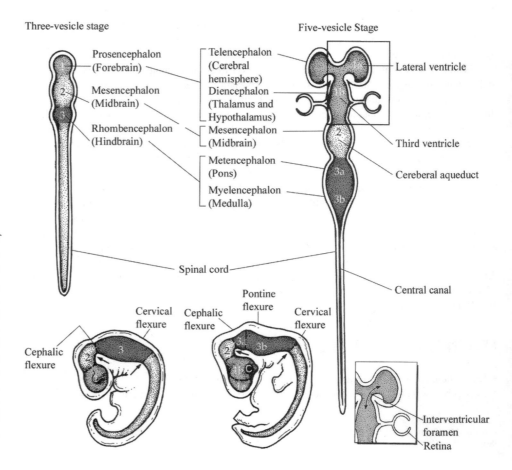

FIGURE 1.1. *Early development of the central nervous system. Early in development, after the neural tube closes, it proliferates in specific regions, which then form bulges or vesicles. While these form, the entire structure undergoes several bends or flexures. It is the vesicles, in part delineated by the flexures, that will form the cerebral hemispheres, thalamus, midbrain, and posterior fossa structures. (Modified from J. H. Martin, Neuroanatomy : Text and Atlas, second edition, © 1996, Appleton & Lange, Stamford, CT, figure 2–3, page 36.)*

bent where the neural tube has grown back on itself. The same holds true for gray matter structures. The caudate nucleus, as an example, arises as an inward bulge at the lateral base of the neural tube. Consequently it will always be found at "bottom" of the lateral ventricles.

TERMINOLOGY

A unified neuroanatomical terminology is used throughout the neurosciences. It is based on an ideal vertebrate whose nervous system is linearly organized like that of the dog shown in Figure 1.2.

Structures are oriented as being:

Rostral (toward the nose) or **caudal** (toward the tail)
Dorsal (toward the back) or **ventral** (toward the belly)
Anterior (toward the front) or **posterior** (toward the rear)
Superior (toward the upper side) or **inferior** (toward the lower side)
Medial (toward the midline) or **lateral** (toward side)

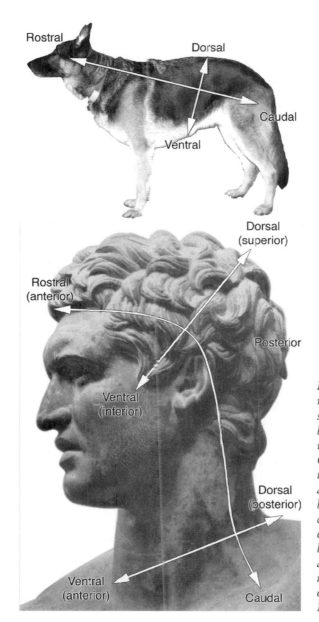

FIGURE 1.2. *Orientation of the nervous system. The terms used in the study of animal nervous systems have been adapted for the human, although we stood up several million years ago. Our modified anatomy is reflected in the terms anterior, posterior, superior, and inferior. While these terms can be used interchangeably in the spinal cord and brainstem with their animal equivalents, they differ in the forebrain. (Figure of Dionysus Soter by an unknown artist, modified from an illustration in G. Bazin, The Loom of Art, ©1962, Simon and Schuster, New York.)*

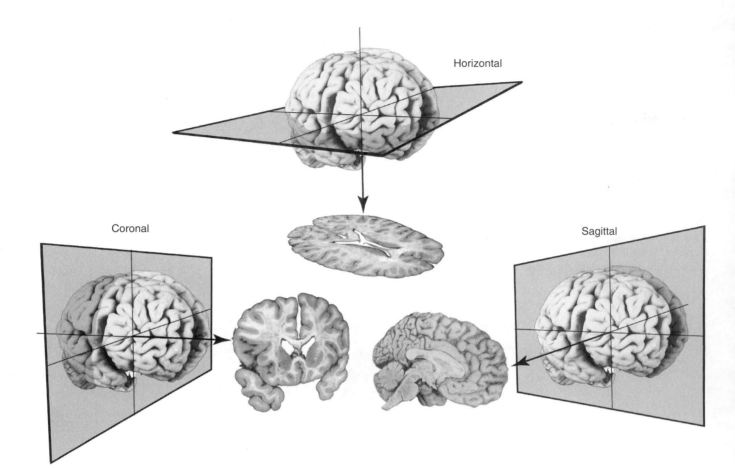

FIGURE 1.3. *Axes of the brain. The brain can be dissected in many planes, both actual specimens and in the MRI. However, the standard planes of dissection are illustrated below. Each plane of dissection has its own utility in illustrating a patient's pathology.*

These terms are applied in slightly different ways to structures in forebrain as opposed to their use in the brainstem and spinal cord. This is because we stood up. The human nervous system bends approximate 90° at the junction between the midbrain and the forebrain (Figure 1.2B). In the spinal cord, dorsal/ventral and anterior/posterior indicate the same relationships. For example, the large tracts of sensory fibers on the dorsal surface of the spinal cord are termed "dorsal columns" as well as "posterior columns." Similarly the site of concentration of motor nerve cells in the spinal cord is known as both the "ventral horn" and the "anterior horn." In the forebrain, anterior/posterior indicates the direction along the axis of the nervous system and is used in the same sense as rostral/caudal in the spinal cord. Dorsal/ventral and medial/lateral have the same meaning in the forebrain as in the spinal cord.

The most frequently used planes of section for the study of brain anatomy are (1) horizontal, (2) coronal, and (3) sagittal (see Fig. 1.3). These terms reflect the approach to dissection. The brain can be cut in parallel horizontal slices from top to bottom, or in anterior-to-posterior transverse sections (coronal), or in medial-to-lateral sections (sagittal). The term *coronal* is primarily used in reference to the cross-sectional plane of the forebrain, while *transverse* is used when referring to cross sections of the brainstem and spinal cord. These approaches to brain cutting are so established in tradition that they are also used in the presentation of standard brain imaging studies.

External Anatomy of the Brain and Spinal Cord

The central nervous system is composed of the spinal cord, contained within the vertebral canal, and the brain (encephalon) located within the skull. The brain itself is divided into the cerebral cortex and its basal ganglia, the thalamus and hypothalamus, the transitional midbrain, and the parts of the brain in the posterior fossa (cerebellum, pons, and medulla). These terms are often grouped together,

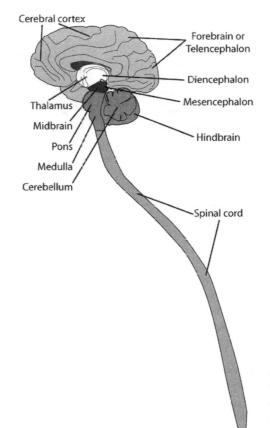

FIGURE 1.4. *Basic layout of the nervous system. Several overlapping terms describe different parts of the nervous system. The "cephalon" terms are occasionally used in clinical practice.*

either in clinical usage or in research. Starting from the midbrain, or mesencephalon, the caudal structures are termed the hindbrain, which includes the cerebellum, pons, and medulla. The diencephalon lies immediately rostral to the mesencephalon and contains the thalamus and hypothalamus. Given our anthropocentric views, the cerebral cortex and its basal ganglia are called the "final brain" or telencephalon. The forebrain (or the less common prosencephalon) groups those brain areas rostral to the mesencephalon. Of the terms used in a classification derived from embryology (the "cephalon" words), the ones most commonly used in adult neurology as adjectives to denote a rostro-caudal "level" are diencephalic and mesencephalic (see Fig. 1.4)

The spinal cord is the caudal continuation of the medulla. It is about 46 cm long and extends from the *atlas* (like the Greek god Atlas holding the world, as this is the bone holding the skull), to approximately L1/L2 where it ends in the conus medullaris. The cord gives off dorsal and ventral nerve roots at each segmental level. The roots pass through an intervertebral foramen and project out to the body. They also send collaterals to the sympathetic chain ganglia that lie outside the vertebral column. The nerve roots exiting below L1/L2 form the cauda equina (horse's tail).

Blood Supply

Specific brain functions are, to a great extent, localized to particular brain areas; these areas, in turn, are perfused by unique arteries. Consequently a malfunction in a given vessel often leads to a specific functional deficit. For example, a small thrombotic occlusion of the posterior cerebral artery can result in unilateral cortical blindness. In this laboratory you will focus on the vascular territories and on the overall path of the circulation.

The main blood supply to the brain comes from two paired sources, the vertebral arteries and the internal carotid arteries. The vertebral arteries ascend on the ventral surface of the medulla and fuse at the level of the pons, where they form the single basilar artery. The left and right internal carotid arteries each run directly into opposite sides of the circle of Willis. Blood supplied by the internal carotid arteries is often referred to as the *anterior circulation,* and that supplied by the vertebral and basilar arteries as the *posterior circulation.* The blood supply to the spinal cord is provided by the anterior spinal and the two posterior spinal arteries that are fed by variable radicular arteries. Blood

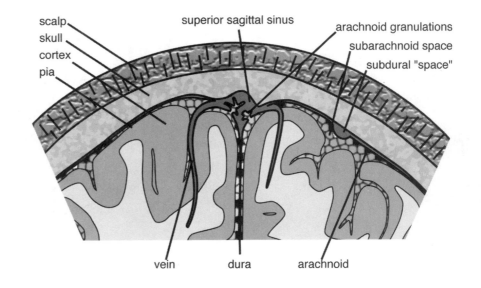

FIGURE 1.5. *Coverings of the brain. Multiple layers of tissue enclose the brain. From outside-in, the main layers are the scalp, skull, dura, arachnoid membrane, and pia mater. Except for the pia, which is really part of the brain, fluids can collect in the "spaces" between these layers in pathologic states. (Note: In this figure the dura is drawn very thick to emphasize its structure. In life it is about the thickness of a piece of thin cardboard.)*

drains from the brain into veins, then into venous sinuses, and leaves the head via the jugular veins and to a much lesser extent, via the vertebral veins. Blood leaves the spinal cord via an intricate venous system.

Brain Coverings

The brain and spinal cord are delicate organs that have a jelly-like consistency. These highly vulnerable structures are protected by the skull and vertebral column, several membrane covers, and by the cerebrospinal fluid (CSF), which provides a cushion against compressive shock. The three membranes covering the brain working from the skull inward, are the dura mater, the arachnoid mater, and the pia mater (see Fig. 1.5). The ***dura*** is a rather tough membrane that can only be torn by hand with some difficulty. It consists of two leaves: an outer periosteal layer that adheres to the inner surface of the skull, and an inner layer. The two dural layers cannot be distinguished from one another except where they depart from the conformation of the skull, and dive into the brain forming the interhemispheric falx and the tentorium overlying the cerebellum, or where they split apart to form the ***venous sinuses.*** The sinuses serve to collect blood from the veins of the brain. At the superior sagittal sinus, CSF is resorbed into the venous system.

The middle membrane, the ***arachnoid,*** has a smooth outer surface and is devoid of vasculature. Like the dura, the arachnoid covers the brain's surface without descending into the individual sulci. Thin, branching filamentous structures extend from its inner surface to the pia mater below giving the arachnoid a weblike appearance. The ***pia***, the thin innermost membrane is closely adherent to the surface of the brain and spinal cord. It follows the brain surface perfectly, covering gyri and sulci alike. Since the arachnoid bridges the sulci and fissures on the surface of the brain and spinal cord, it forms subarachnoid spaces of variable size, containing CSF. The largest spaces are called ***cisterns***.

Because of the continuity of the membranes covering the brain, in certain disease states the region between these membrane may become filled with fluids, blood, air, or tumor. Since these regions are not normally open, they are termed ***potential spaces***. Between the skull (or vertebra) and the dura is a potential space called the ***epidural*** (or extradural) space, containing only blood vessels. Under the meningeal layer of dura, between it and the arachnoid, is a potential space called the subdural space. Head trauma can cause bleeding within this space and lead to a subdural hematoma. The gap between the pia and arachnoid is called the ***subarachnoid*** space. Since these three spaces have different classes of blood vessels associated with them, characteristic types of "bleeds" result from damage to each class of vessel.

Subarachnoid space   The space between the leptomeninges and pia mater. This is a real space and is completely filled with cerebrospinal fluid. The brain essentially floats in the cerebrospinal fluid within the subarachnoid space.

Schedule (2.5 hours)
60   External anatomy
20   Spinal cord
20   Vessels
30   Coverings
20   Case

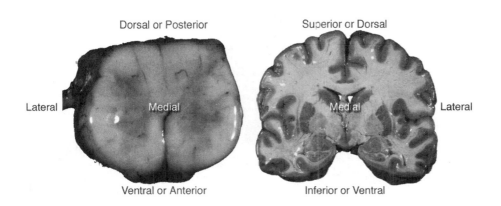

Dorsal or Posterior

Superior or Dorsal

Lateral — Medial — Medial — Lateral

Ventral or Anterior — Inferior or Ventral

FIGURE 1.6. *Transverse section of spinal cord and coronal section of brain.*

EXTERNAL BRAIN

General Orientation of the Brain

INST Examine your whole and half brain specimens and spinal cord. Using Figure 1.2 and 1.6, review the following terms by relating them to the specimens:

- Anterior versus posterior
- Rostral versus caudal
- Ventral versus dorsal
- Lateral versus medial
- Superior versus inferior

INST Using imaginary cuts on your specimens and Figure 1.3, go through the following planes of section:

- Horizontal
- Sagittal
- Parasagittal
- Coronal and transverse

Q1.1. Where do you find transverse sections used?
A1.1. Brainstem and spinal cord.

Major Divisions

INST Using anatomic specimens, identify the four major divisions of the brain: the cerebrum, brainstem, cerebellum, and spinal cord.

Q1.2. What structures lie immediately above and below the junction between the brainstem and cerebrum?
A1.2. The midbrain is the caudal part of this junction, while the thalamus or diencephalon lies rostral to the junction.
Q1.3. What separates the cerebellum from the cerebral hemispheres?
A1.3. The transverse fissure and tentorium.

Cerebral Hemispheres

Q1.4. The cerebral cortex is divided into four major lobes (frontal, parietal, temporal, and occipital) and the smaller insula. In order to determine their boundaries, you have to first recognize the major sulci. Use your whole brain to locate the structures below and label them on Figure 1.7. First locate the longitudinal fissure. Next identify the Sylvian fissure. Then identify the central sulcus. It's not always easy to pick out. The easiest way to locate it is on the medial surface of the half brain. Identify the prominent cingulate sulcus. The next sulcus just anterior is the central sulcus. Follow it along the lateral surface of the brain. The occipital and parietal lobes can easily be distinguished using the half brains. On the medial surface of the half brain, identify the

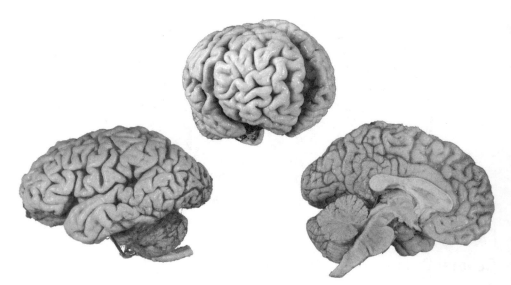

FIGURE 1.7. *External landmarks of the cerebral hemispheres. The left figure is the lateral surface, the right is the medial surface, and the middle figure is an oblique view of the brain.*

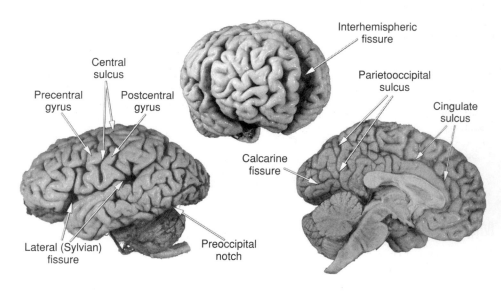

FIGURE 1.8. *External landmarks of the cerebral hemispheres. These major fissures, sulci, and gyri are common to well-formed brains.*

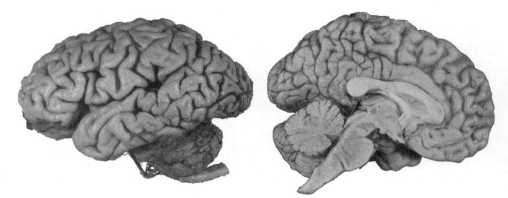

FIGURE 1.9. *Lateral and medial views of the brain.*

parietooccipital sulcus. Note that on the lateral surface about the same distance anterior to the occipital pole you find the preoccipital notch. Label all of these structures in Figure 1.7.

A1.4. *See Figure 1.8.*

Q1.5. Identify the frontal and occipital poles, which are the anterior and posterior tips of the brain. Using the landmarks above, identify on the brain and in Figure 1.9 (shade and label):
- Frontal lobe (FL)
- Temporal lobe (TL)
- Parietal lobe (PL)
- Occipital lobe (OL)
- "Limbic" lobe (LL) (cingulate gyrus)

A1.5. *See Figure 1.10.*

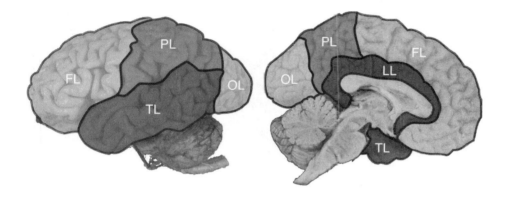

FIGURE 1.10. *Major lobes of the brain.*

INST Finally, gently spread apart the banks of the Sylvian fissure and find the insular cortex buried underneath. Compare what you can see with the dissection in Figure 1.11 of the fully exposed insular cortex.

Q1.6. One of the most striking features of the brain is that many of its morphologically distinct parts have specific functions localized to them. Locate the prominent gyri listed in Table 1.1 and assign a general function in the table.

A1.6. *See Table 1.2.*

INST After you have identified these gyri, compare how consistent they are. Compare the appearance and location of each of these gyri between hemispheres in the same brain and between your brain specimens. How much do they vary?

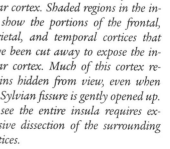

FIGURE 1.11. *Dissection of the insular cortex. Shaded regions in the inset show the portions of the frontal, parietal, and temporal cortices that have been cut away to expose the insular cortex. Much of this cortex remains hidden from view, even when the Sylvian fissure is gently opened up. To see the entire insula requires extensive dissection of the surrounding cortices.*

TABLE 1.1. Gyral Function Worksheet

Gyrus	Function
Precentral	_____
Postcentral	_____
Superior temporal	_____
Calcarine (look at medial face of half brain)	_____
Cingulate	_____

Q1.7. Look at the medial or sagittal aspect of the half brain. Using an atlas for assistance, identify these additional prominent features on the brain and in Figure 1.12:
- Corpus callosum
- Diencephalon/thalamus
- Third ventricle
- Lateral ventricle
- Midbrain
- Pons
- Medulla
- Cerebellum
- Cingulate gyrus
- Cingulate sulcus
- Parietooccipital sulcus
- Calcarine fissure

A1.7. *See Figure 1.13.*

Q1.8. The corpus callosum is the massive white matter tract joining the two hemispheres. To get an excellent perspective on the corpus callosum, examine the dissection in Figure 1.14. From just the photograph, what do you think the fibers interconnect?

A1.8. *The fibers connect the two hemispheres so that they can communicate with each other. When the corpus callosum is surgically transected for certain types of severe epileptic conditions, it results in each cerebral hemisphere functioning more or less autonomously. These are the famous "split brain" cases. When the same information is presented separately to each hemisphere, a visual image for instance, the interpretation varies depending upon whether the left or the right hemisphere is processing the information.*

Base of the Brain

Q1.9. Locate these prominent features on the base of the whole and half brains and label them in Figure 1.15:
- Olfactory bulb and Olfactory tract
- Optic nerve and chiasm
- Mammillary bodies
- Internal carotid artery

TABLE 1.2. Function of Select Gyri

Gyrus	Function
Precentral	Primary motor area
Postcentral	Primary somatosensory area
Superior temporal	Hearing
Calcarine cortex (look at medial face of half brain)	Vision
Cingulate	Emotion and motivation

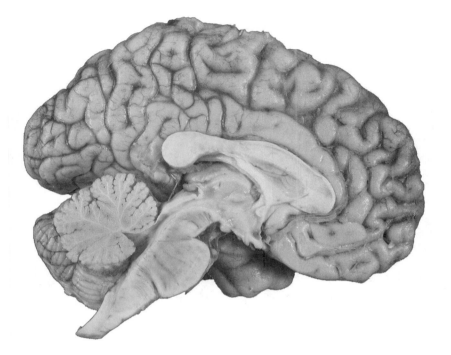

FIGURE 1.12. *Sagittal section of brain.*

- Pituitary (unlikely to remain after the autopsy)
- Cranial nerve III

A1.9. See Figure 1.16.

Brainstem

Q1.10. On both the intact brain and sagittal section, locate these brainstem structures and label them in Figure 1.17:
- Basilar artery
- Midbrain
- Pons
- Cerebellum
- Medulla
- Inferior olive

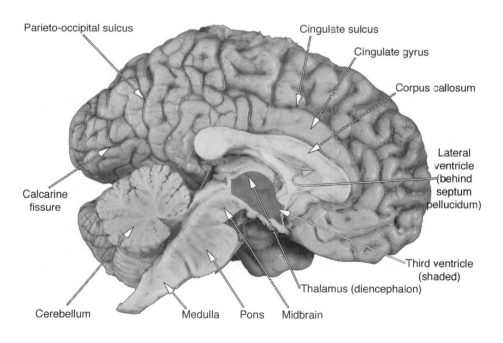

FIGURE 1.13. *Landmarks on the medial brain surface.*

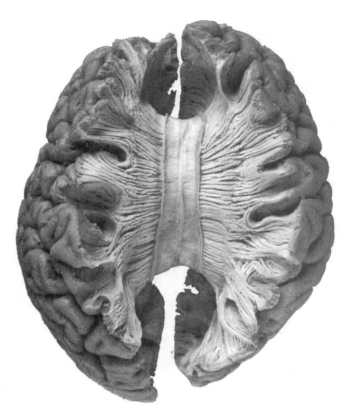

FIGURE 1.14. *Dissection of white matter bundles in the corpus callosum. Special processing of brain will partially separate white matter fibers along major bundles. Gentle dissection and removal of adjacent brain will then reveal major pathways, such as this view of corpus callosum fibers. (Modified from Gluhbegovic and Williams, The Human Brain, a Photographic Guide. © 1980, Harper & Row, figure 5–21, page 141.)*

- Pyramids
- Pyramidal decussation
- Cranial nerve V
- Cerebral aqueduct
- Fourth Ventricle

A1.10. See Figure 1.18.

SPINAL CORD

In this portion of the laboratory you'll examine the external structure of the spinal cord, note its relationship to the spinal column, and examine the implications of the cord being shorter than the spinal column.

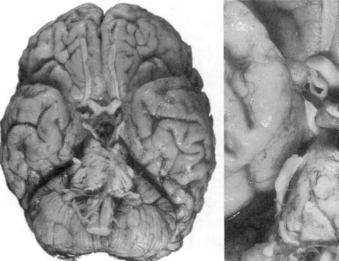
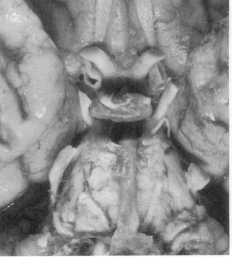

FIGURE 1.15. *Base of brain. In the left specimen, the pituitary was removed at autopsy.*

Olfactory bulb   Olfactory tract   Optic nerve   Optic chiasm

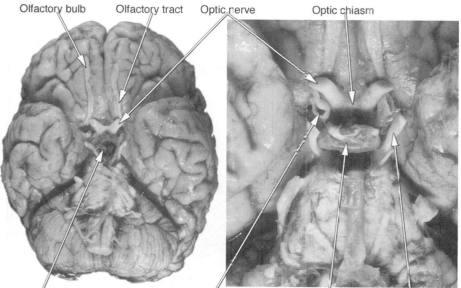

Mammillary bodies   Internal carotid artery   Pituitary   Cranial nerve III

FIGURE 1.16. *Some important structures on the inferior brain surface.*

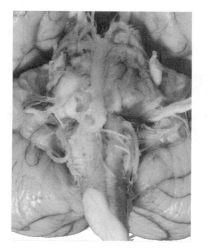

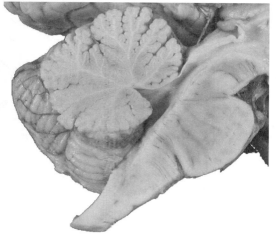

FIGURE 1.17. *Inferior (left) and sagittal (right) views of the brainstem and cerebellum (or hindbrain).*

Basilar artery   Cranial nerve V   Cerebellum   IVth ventricle   Aqueduct

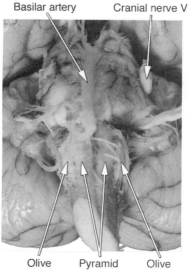

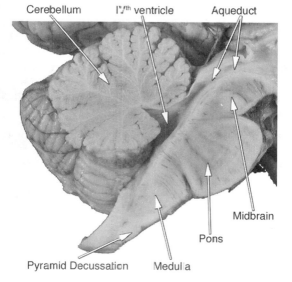

Olive   Pyramid   Olive   Pyramid Decussation   Medulla   Pons   Midbrain

FIGURE 1.18. *Major landmarks on the inferior and medial surfaces of the posterior fossa.*

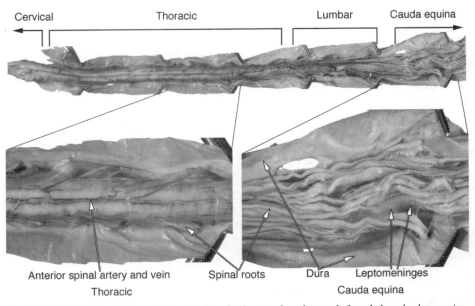

Cervical   Thoracic   Lumbar   Cauda equina

Anterior spinal artery and vein   Spinal roots   Dura   Leptomeninges
Thoracic   Cauda equina

FIGURE 1.19. *Major divisions of the spinal cord. The spinal cord extends from below the decussation of the pyramidal tracts in the medulla to its base or conus medullaris. Extending from the cord at each level are ventral and dorsal spinal roots, which travel caudally to their exits in the longer vertebral column. The rostral and caudal ends of the cord have cervical and lumbar "enlargements" that contain greater amounts of gray matter to control the upper and lower limbs. Below about vertebral level L1–L2 the spinal cord ends, yet its roots continue caudally to their lumbar and sacral exits. This lowest region of the spinal canal contains a plethora of spinal roots resembling a horse's tail or cauda equina. Below the lumbar section of cord lies the short sacral segment, which is not labeled below.*

First determine the rostral and caudal ends of the spinal cord and the general location of each level (cervical, thoracic, lumbar, and sacral). (Many of the cord specimens extend rostrally only to the upper thoracic level.)

Q1.11. Identify the caudal end by means of the ***cauda equina.*** See Figure 1.19. Where is it found in the spinal column and what does this represent?

A1.11. *It is found in the lumbar cistern and represents the collection of dorsal and ventral roots extending caudally toward their respective points of exit.*

Q1.12. Orient the spinal cord with respect to the vertebral column of your skeleton. Do they match? Where does the cord end?

A1.12. *The spinal cord is shorter than the vertebral column. It ends at approximately L1.*

INST   The cerebrospinal fluid (CSF) bathing the cord is sampled by means of a lumbar puncture. A needle is inserted between L4 and L5. Match your cord to the spinal column so that you can visualize the structures that the needle encounters.

INST   Now examine the spinal cord in a bit more detail. Using scissors, carefully cut one side of the dura along the entire length of the cord. DO NOT REMOVE IT, but gently move it to the side so you can visualize the cord. You may want to partially cut up the other side of the dura so you can see both the dorsal and ventral aspects of the cord.

Q1.13. First reorient yourself. How can you tell the rostral from caudal end? How can you identify ventral (anterior) from dorsal (posterior)?

A1.13. *Fortunately, the cord is different along each axis. The caudal end has the cauda equina (horse tail) to distinguish it from the rostral end. The ventral surface has a single central vessel while the dorsal surface has several, irregular, and lateral vessels.*

Q1.14. Note the length of the nerve roots and the angle that they come off of the cord. How does this vary along the length of the cord and what is the explanation for the variation?

A1.14. *In early embryonic life the cord is the same length as the vertebral canal. As it develops, its growth falls behind that of the spinal column. As the cord segments become increasingly displaced*

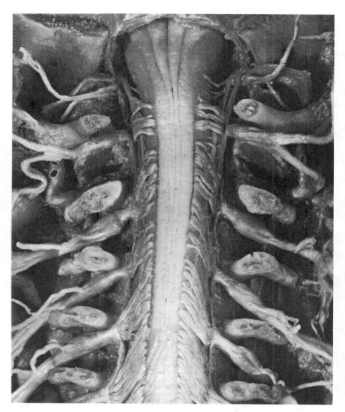

FIGURE 1.20. *Posterior in situ dissection of the spinal cord. The spinous processes and lamina have been removed from the posterior surface to reveal the enclosed spinal cord and its proximal roots with their ganglia. (Modified from Gluhbegovic and Williams, The Human Brain, a Photographic Guide. © 1980, Harper & Row, figure 1–3, page 7.)*

rostrally with respect to the vertebrae, the angle of the roots gradually shifts from a horizontal to a more oblique orientation. The roots also become longer since they have farther to travel to reach their exit foramina.

Q1.15. Examine your specimen and compare it to Figure 1.20. Identify the anterior and posterior aspects of your cord specimen. What features make this possible?

A1.15. The easiest way to distinguish front from back in the cord is to look at its vessels. The anterior has a single median artery and vein, while the posterior has a complex pattern of vessels. The anterior spinal artery lies in the groove of the deep median fissure.

Q1.16. Is the anterior vessel you see an artery or a vein?

A1.16. It is a vein. The artery is a thick-walled muscular structure, which usually contains little blood post-mortem, while the vein is a thin-walled tube filled with blood. It is usually the blood that makes the vein visible. With close inspection, you can see both.

Q1.17. Identify the anterior and posterior roots as well as the cervical and lumbar enlargements. What is the significance of these enlargements?

A1.17. The lumbar and cervical enlargements result from the large number of anterior horn α-motor neurons that are present at these levels to control the muscles of the lower and upper extremities respectively.

Q1.18. Examine a dorsal root ganglion (DRG). Where should you look for them? What type of neurons are contained within it and what is the direction of flow of information? Locate them in Figure 1.20.

*A1.18. The **dorsal root ganglia** are located outside the dura, just after the anterior and posterior roots penetrate this thick tissue. These ganglia contain primary sensory neurons conveying information about touch, pressure, vibration, joint position, pain, and temperature. Information flows from the body surface and muscles, to the DRG neurons, and thence into the spinal cord. In Figure 1.20, the ganglia are located between each pair of cut vertebral arches.*

INST Finally, examine the upper cut end of the cord and observe the relationship of gray matter (predominantly cell bodies) to white matter (predominantly myelinated axons). Note the butterfly or H-shape of the gray matter that surrounds the central canal (see Fig. 1.6). The ends, or horns, of the gray matter are called the posterior (or dorsal) horns (these receive sensory inputs) and the anterior

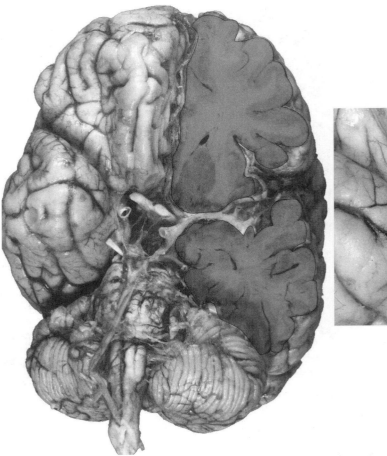
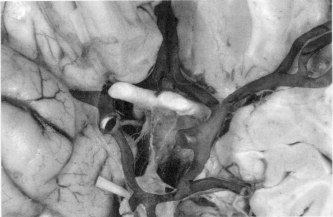

FIGURE 1.21. *Cerebral artery dissection. The inferior surface of the left frontal and temporal lobes has been dissected away to reveal the recessed main cerebral arteries. The dissected surface has been shaded on the left, and the vessels have been darkened in the close-up on the right.*

horns. The anterior horns are the sites of the cell bodies of motor neurons that directly innervate muscles, and form the final common efferent pathway. You'll investigate this relationship some more in the next chapter.

VESSELS

Q1.19. Using the diagrams in the brain atlas, identify the following key structures on the whole brain and in Figure 1.21:
  • Internal carotid artery
  • Circle of Willis
  • Anterior cerebral artery
  • Middle cerebral artery
  • Posterior cerebral artery
  • Vertebral artery
  • Basilar artery.

A1.19. *See Figure 1.22.*

Q1.20. Figure 1.23 is a dissection of the cerebral circulation, showing the circle of Willis in the center. On the figure label the anterior cerebral, middle cerebral, posterior cerebral, internal carotid, basilar, and superior cerebellar arteries.

A1.20. *See Figure 1.24.*

Q1.21. What is the role of the Circle of Willis?

A1.21. *The **circle of Willis** interconnects the major cerebral arteries. If a major vessel becomes occluded either within or proximal to the circle, the communicating arteries permit anastomotic flow,*

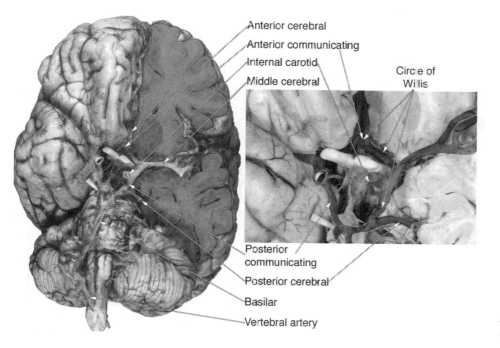

Anterior cerebral
Anterior communicating
Internal carotid
Middle cerebral
Circle of Willis
Posterior communicating
Posterior cerebral
Basilar
Vertebral artery

FIGURE 1.22. *Major arteries of the brain.*

which will maintain perfusion of brain areas. However, don't feel you can now eat cheeseburgers with impunity; by the time you reach adulthood, the anastomotic potential of the circle is greatly diminished. It is useless in acute occlusions and has only a small role in adults, even when the occlusions develop slowly.

It's important to note that there is a great deal of variation in the circle, including large posterior communicating arteries and completely absent vessels. Examine your specimen for abnormalities.

Q1.22. The anterior cerebral artery feeds the sagittal and medial portions of cortex, the posterior cerebral artery distributes to the occipital lobes and inferior temporal lobes, and the middle cerebral artery supplies the lateral cerebrum. On your brain specimens, indicate the territories of these main cerebral arteries. Shade their approximate territories on Figure 1.25.

A1.22. *See Figure 1.26.*

INST Examine the angiograms in Figure 1.27, obtained from postmortem injection of contrast agent into the spinal arteries. Panel *A* shows a mid-sagittal view of the anterior spinal artery at the level of C3. Panel *B* is a microangiogram of a cross section at L2 showing both the anterior and posterior

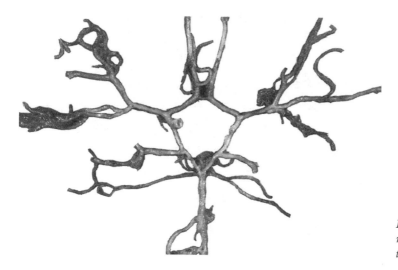

FIGURE 1.23. *Dissection of the main arteries in the cerebral circulation. Rostral is up.*

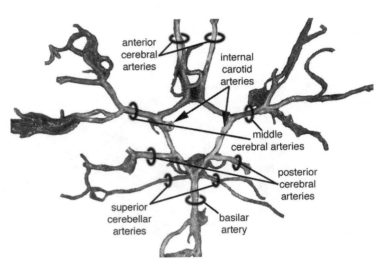

FIGURE 1.24. *Major arteries in a circle of Willis dissection.*

spinal arteries. It is important to correlate the various types of imaging to the actual neuroanatomy learned from your specimens.

Q1.23. Disruption of which spinal artery is more likely to result in lower motor symptoms? Damage the dorsal columns?

A1.23. Anterior. Posterior.

Before moving on, the scanning electron micrograph in Figure 1.28 is to remind you that you've been studying the major vessels only. All nervous tissue is richly invested with vasculature. All neurons are within a few cell diameters of a vessel. The image was made by injection of the vessels with plastic, followed by digesting away of the remaining tissue. Note the amazing complexity of the capillary bed. Changes in blood dynamics at capillary level correlate with local changes in brain activity. This is the basis for functional brain imaging techniques in which local changes in brain activity can be correlated to specific functional tasks.

INST The blood exits the brain via the sinus system. The superficial veins and the CSF empty into the superior sagittal sinus and the deep veins empty into the straight sinus. Examine your specimens including the sheep brain, to see where these sinuses run. Then look at Figure 1.29, which cartoons the organization of the sinuses in the cranium.

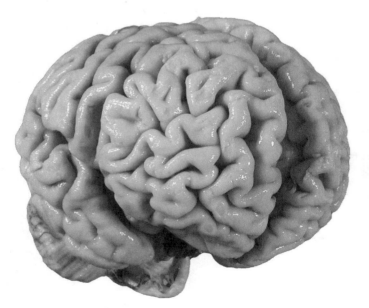

FIGURE 1.25. *Vascular territory worksheet.*

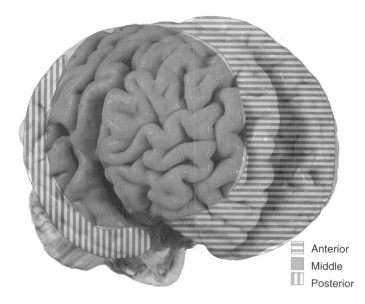

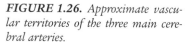
Anterior
Middle
Posterior

FIGURE 1.26. Approximate vascular territories of the three main cerebral arteries.

Q1.24. Look at Figure 1.30, which is an MRI venogram. Using Figure 1.29, identify the numbered structures 1–5. Add arrows to indicate the direction of flow.

1.24.1. _____

1.24.2. _____

1.24.3. _____

1.24.4. _____

1.24.5. _____

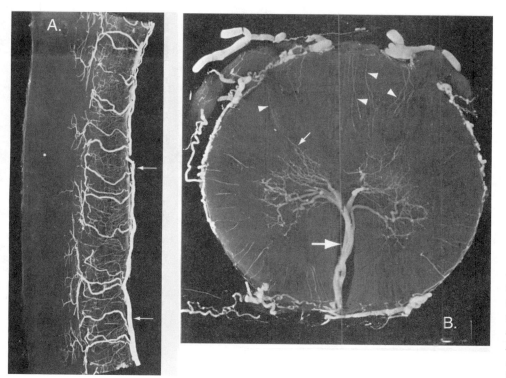

FIGURE 1.27. Spinal arteries after contrast injection into anterior spinal artery. The injection was done postmortem, and then X-rayed after fixation and dissection. (Modified from Nolte, The Human Brain, 4th ed., © 1999, Mosby, St. Louis, figure 10-28, page 249.)

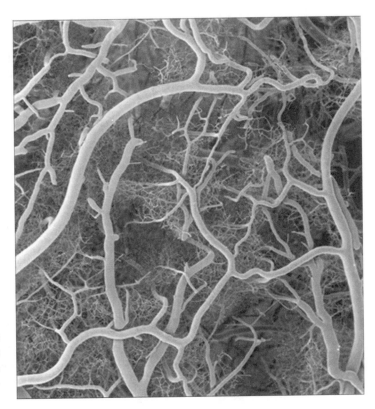

FIGURE 1.28. *Scanning electron micrograph of the capillary network in the temporal lobe of a chincilla. (Modified from Harrison et al., 2002. Cerebral Cortex, 12:225–233.)*

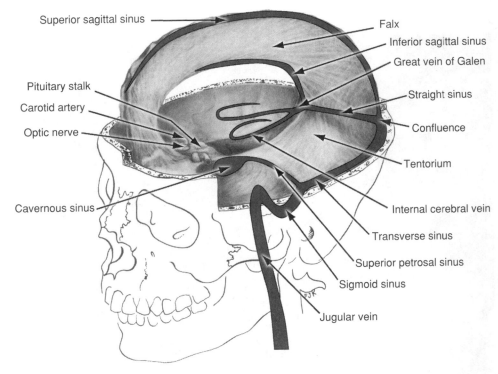

FIGURE 1.29. *Dural folds and sinuses. (Adapted from The Human Brain and Spinal Cord: Functional Neuroanatomy and Dissection Guide by Lennart Heimer, © 1983, Springer-Verlag, New York, figure 24, page 39.)*

Superior sagittal sinus

Falx

Inferior sagittal sinus

Great vein of Galen

Pituitary stalk

Straight sinus

Carotid artery

Confluence

Optic nerve

Tentorium

Internal cerebral vein

Cavernous sinus

Transverse sinus

Superior petrosal sinus

Sigmoid sinus

Jugular vein

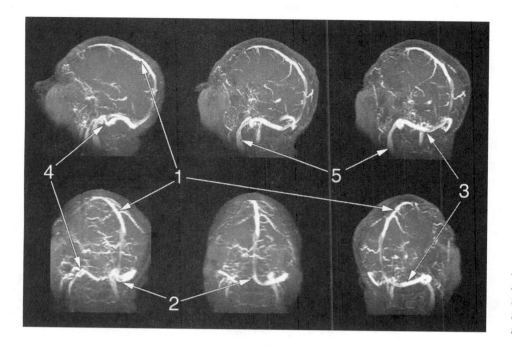

FIGURE 1.30. MRI venogram at select rotations. These scans label protons in one position and then identify those that have moved after a short time interval.

A1.24.   1.24.1. *Superior sagittal sinus*
         1.24.2. *Confluence of the sinuses*
         1.24.3. *Transverse sinus*
         1.24.4. *Sigmoid sinus*
         1.24.5. *Jugular vein*

THE BRAIN'S COVERINGS

Q1.25. Working from the outside in, the brain is covered by the scalp, the skull, the dura mater, and the meninges. These tissues can be distinguished in patients using an MRI scan (magnetic resonance image). Compare the images in Figure 1.31 of a routine MRI scan and a coronal section from the Visible Human Project. Identify the major coverings on the MRI image.

A1.25. *From outside-in on the MRI: The bright material is the scalp, which can be seen as a continuation of the cheeks. Deep to the scalp is a fuzzy irregular layer of masseter muscle and beneath this is the bone (black on MRI). Beneath the bone is a line of dura, well-seen where it descends in the*

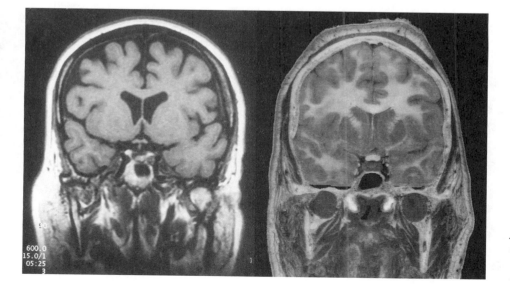

FIGURE 1.31. Comparison of T1-weighted MRI and coronal section through anatomic specimen. The MRI scan was from an elderly patient with a long history of dementia, while the anatomic specimen was from the middle-aged woman in the Visible Human Project. (Right panel adapted from an image created by the Head Browser developed by the University of Michigan, Visible Human Project, National Library of Medicine.)

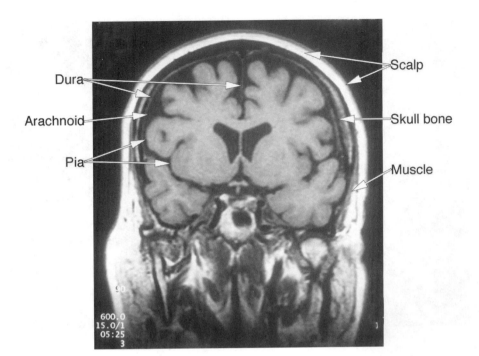

Dura

Arachnoid

Pia

Scalp

Skull bone

Muscle

FIGURE 1.32. *Coverings of the brain on MRI scan.*

midline as the falx. Beneath the dura is the gray matter and the black CSF. The dura cannot easily be distinguished from its closely adherent arachnoid in nonpathologic states. In this case, some separation may be seen on the left side of the image. The pia is really just the surface of the brain; it is not a distinct layer on MRI scans or on a gross brain specimen. See Figure 1.32.

Q1.26. In order to get a true sense for how the brain sits in its coverings, examine Figure 1.33. Try to identify the dura and arachnoid membrane. Where might they be separated?

A1.26. *See Figure 1.34. Only around surface vessels do the dura and arachnoid normally separate from each other. However, this potential space can become a real space in pathologic states, producing a subdural hemorrhage. In contrast, the delicate arachnoid remains slightly separated from the underlying cortex, producing a space that bathes the brain in cerebrospinal fluid.*

Skull

Q1.27. Examine a skull, and a skull-brain model. Identify the following landmarks on the skull and label them in Figure 1.35: foramen magnum, temporal bone, acoustic meatus, cribriform plate, optic canal and superior orbital fissure.

A1.27. *See Figure 1.36.*

FIGURE 1.33. *Close-up, in situ, horizontal view of the brain in the skull. The head in this individual was specially prepared to accurately preserve its anatomic relationships. It was then serially sliced and photographed. (Image courtesy of Peter Ratiu and Berend Hillen, Visible Human Project, National Library of Medicine.)*

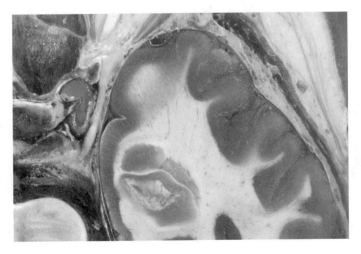

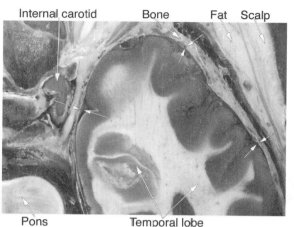

Internal carotid   Bone   Fat   Scalp

Pons   Temporal lobe

FIGURE 1.34. *Membranes on brain surface. Unlabeled white arrows point the dura on the exterior and arachnoid next to the brain surface at the point where surface vessels run.*

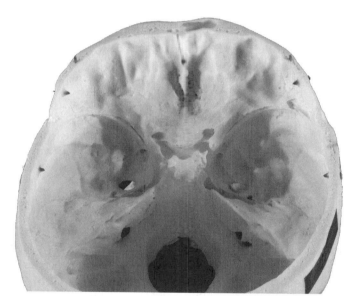

FIGURE 1.35. *Human skull base, view from posterior-superior.*

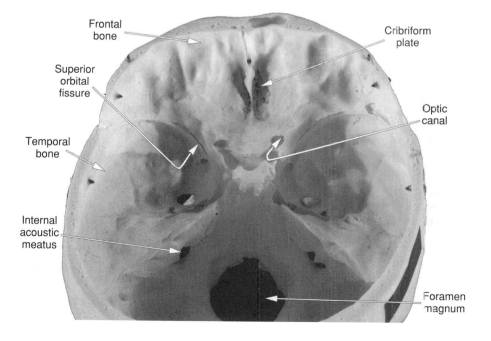

Frontal bone

Cribriform plate

Superior orbital fissure

Optic canal

Temporal bone

Internal acoustic meatus

Foramen magnum

FIGURE 1.36. *Several important structures on the interior skull base.*

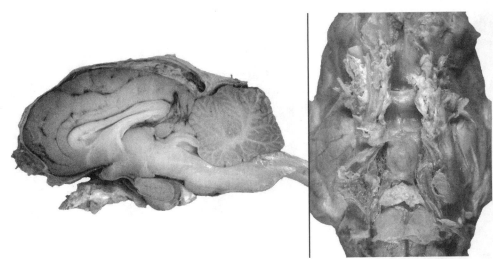

FIGURE 1.37. *Sheep's brain with the dura attached, medial and inferior view.*

Q1.28. Orient the brain with respect to the skull. Where does the cerebellum sit? Locate the positions occupied by the four lobes of the brain. Where is the skull smooth? Where is it sharp? When the brain strikes a massive hard object as with a serious fall, the brain glides over the surface of the skull. Which surfaces are most likely to damage the brain?

A1.28. *The skull is smoothest over the superior convexity and roughest over the eyes (orbitofrontal area) and in the anterior temporal fossa. Head injuries, especially those when the brain and skull are moving together as in a motor vehicle accident, typically produce the greatest injury over the roughest areas of the skull. A fall to the back of the head frequently produces a contusion on the inferior frontal surface of the brain ("**contrecoup**" injury).*

Soft Tissue Coverings

Q1.29. Examine the sheep brain (see Fig. 1.37). Identify cranial nerves I and V. How do they differ from those of humans? Is cranial nerve V extradural or intradural? Dissect one of the sheep brains along the sagittal plain, leaving the dura intact. Compare it with an intact sheep brain. Identify the pituitary gland and the pineal gland. What is their relationship to the dura? Any differences with the human sagittal section?

A1.29. *The olfactory nerve in a sheep is huge compared to the diminutive version in humans. Because the brain has the entire dura intact, you can now see the relationship of the trigeminal ganglion to the brain. It is the paired ragged area off the midline in the right image of Figure 1.37. In the human specimens this ganglion usually remains in the skull, beneath the dura. Remember, the dorsal root ganglia (or its equivalent, the trigeminal or gasserian ganglion) are outside the dural sheath. The pituitary looks huge relative to that in the human (see the base of brain picture in Figure 1.15); most of this is an illusion, since it is the sheep's brain that is so much smaller than ours. Good thing, since we don't want sheep to eat us. The pituitary lies in its own little dural cavity. The dura inserts around the pineal gland, which, like the pituitary, is relatively large in a sheep.*

INST Make a small incision coronally into the top of the dura and identify the superior sagittal sinus. Dissect off the entire dura from sheep's brain being careful to preserve its overall structure. See Figure 1.38. Try to tear it with your hands. You now know why it is called "dura." Note that the brain comes off the dura with great ease, and also has its own, separate vasculature.

Q1.30. Compare the dissected sheep's dura in Figure 1.38 to the human illustration in Figure 1.39. Identify the falx and tentorium. Note the bridging veins extending from cortex to the superior sagittal sinus. Identify the arachnoid granulations on the human and sheep brains. Why are they important?

A1.30. *The CSF passes from the subarachnoid space into the sinus via these granulations, which pierce the otherwise impenetrable dura mater.*

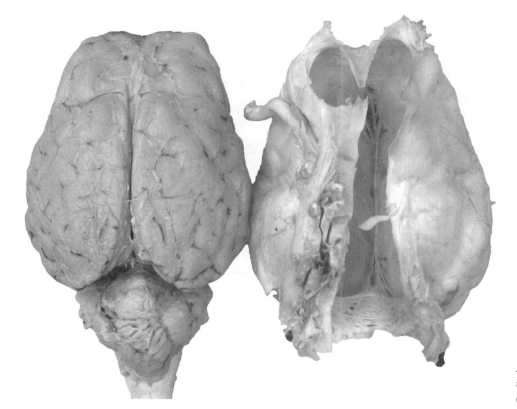

FIGURE 1.38. Dura (right, *inferior view*) dissected from a sheep's brain (left, *superior view*).

Q1.31. Figure 1.40 shows a cross section of the dissected dura from a human brain. What brain structures are apposed to the numbered sites? Name numbers 2 and 3.

1.31.1 _____   1.31.3 _____

1.31.2 _____

A1.31 1.31.1. *Cerebral hemispheres*
 1.31.2. *Medial surface of the hemispheres; falx*
 1.31.3. *Cerebellum below and occipital lobe above; tentorium*

INST Using your specimens and Figure 1.5 of the brain coverings, note the relationship between the meninges and the blood vessels. Determine where the main arteries, venous sinuses, and veins are located.

Q1.32. Examine the arachnoid mater on the brain specimens. While the arachnoid is relatively closely apposed to the brain, it doesn't descend into the sulci or the deep spaces surrounding the brain. This results in the formation of cisterns in the cranial vault that are occupied by the CSF. Look at the sagittal MRI in Figure 1.41. In this image the cerebral spinal fluid appears black (along with bone, but for different reasons).

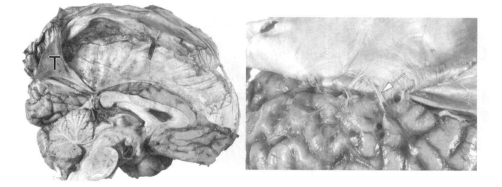

FIGURE 1.39. Dura attached to brain. The left figure shows its insertion onto brain ("T"—tentorium). The right photograph is a close-up of the dura reflected off the cortical surface, illustrating the bridging veins (arrow).

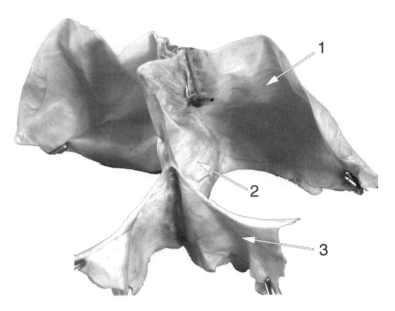

FIGURE 1.40. *Cross-section of human dura, dissected off brain.*

You can see several cisterns outside the brain and ventricular reservoirs within the brain. Identify on Figure 1.41:
• Cisterna magna
• Prepontine cistern
• Interpeduncular cistern
• Quadrigeminal cistern
Should a spinal tap not be possible, which cistern would be the best to choose if you needed to sample the CSF?

A1.32. *See Figure 1.42. The cisterna magna is the easiest and largest of the cisterns, and is typically the one sampled when fluid cannot be gotten from the back.*

CLINICAL CASE: HEMORRHAGE

The patient was a 73-year-old man who had an acute onset of a new, severe headache, nausea, and vomiting. A head CT was performed.

FIGURE 1.41. *Normal sagittal T1 MRI. The CSF is black on T1 images, since water is free to move about and release its proton-labels distant from where they were applied. Bone is also black, but only because it contains little water. The image shows both cisterns and the ventricular system as either black or gray.*

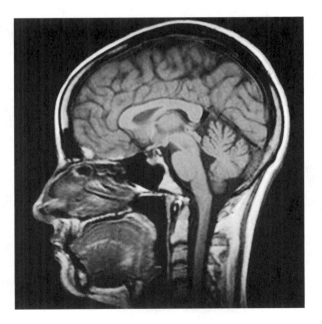

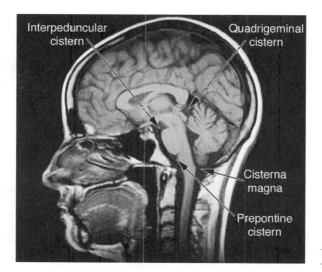

FIGURE 1.42. *Major cisterns in a sagittal T1 MRI.*

Q1.33. Examine the CT scans on the patient in Figure 1.43, and compare it with the normal CT in Figure 1.44. On a CT scan, bone is very opaque to X-rays and hence is white, blood is less opaque, brain even less, and CSF is the most transparent to this radiation. What do you see? Where is the lesion? How can you tell? Is it inside or outside the brain?

A1.33. The "lesion" is a diffuse density around most of the brain surface, which is not present in the normal control. This is blood on a CT scan. You can tell this is sub-arachnoid hemorrhage, since it dives into the depths of the sulci and spreads over much of the brain surface, without "obeying" the boundaries of the dura. The hemorrhage is not present in the ventricular system, hence the blood did not originate in or near the ventricles (a relatively common presentation in middle age and in prematurity). This indicates the most likely source is a vessel between the leptomeninges and the brain.

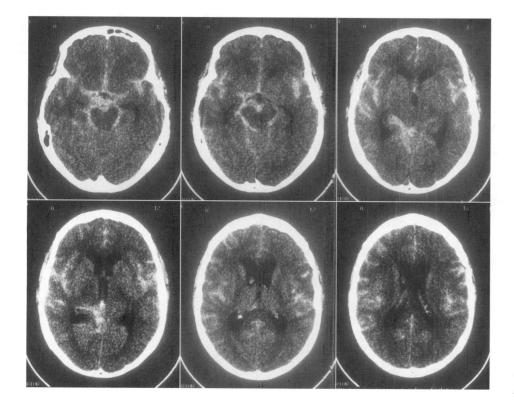

FIGURE 1.43. *Head CT scan from patient.*

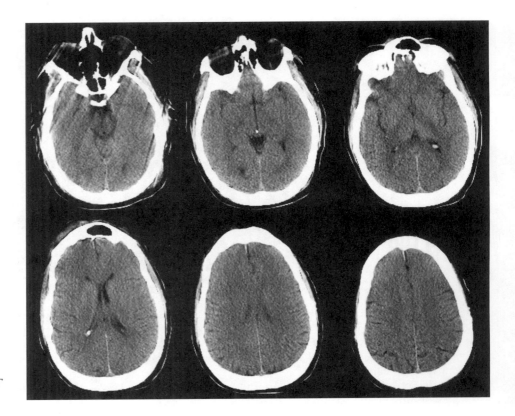

FIGURE 1.44. *Normal head CT scan.*

Q1.34. The patient was found to have an arteriovenous malformation in the cerebellum that had ruptured. Although this malformation was surgically removed, the patient continued to do poorly, and eventually expired. Examine the image of his brain in Figure 1.45. How can you tell in which space the blood resides? How could blood from the cerebellum reach the frontal poles?

A1.34. *The blood is subarachnoid; it lies underneath the glistening surface of the meninges. Unlike subdural blood, this hemorrhage has access to the pain receptors in the meninges, and produces a severe headache. Since the subarachnoid space is a continuous space of cerebrospinal fluid, once the blood reaches the ventricular system, it can spread along the pathways of this fluid. Blood generally does not track back into the brain, since the flow is from the choroid plexus outward.*

In any patient with a sudden onset of a severe new headache, you are obligated to look for blood, either by a head scan or by a spinal tap. Ruptured aneurysms and vascular malformations are the most common suspects, especially in younger patients.

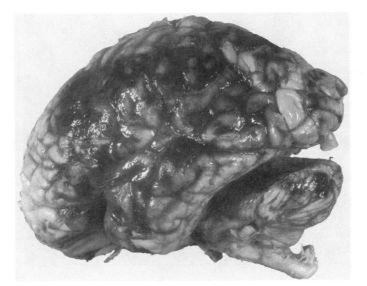

FIGURE 1.45. *Gross brain specimen, showing extensive subarachnoid hemorrhage.*

Chapter 2—INTERNAL ANATOMY

In this laboratory, you will enter the brain.

You may examine a brain in many ways. In this laboratory, you will slice it coronally. In another, you will dissect it horizontally. Brain imaging, to be formally introduced a bit later, will hopefully be the main way you look at your patients' brains. However, the real tissue will always be the fundamental reference, and you should go back to it throughout the laboratories. This may be your only opportunity to get a true sense of its nature. It is only by handling the brain that you will gain the fullest appreciation for its size and structure.

Humans have been scientifically studying the brain for at least two centuries; don't expect to have mastered all of the material by the end of the laboratory. However, these exercises represent an introduction to the brain's interior, on which we will build the remainder of the text. Learning the fundamental layout of the brain and spinal cord, including main nuclei and tracts, should be your goal by the end of the fourth chapter. It is on this database that you will build knowledge of the nervous system.

LEARNING OBJECTIVES

- General elements of the spinal cord, including the gray and white matter. Describe its circulation.
- Major internal structures of the brainstem, cerebellum, and cerebrum and their relationships to the ventricles.
- Flow of cerebrospinal fluid.
- Different types of cortical fiber tracts: association, commissural, and long.
- Corticospinal tract.

INTRODUCTION

Colloquial speech occasionally mentions that someone has a lot of or is missing "gray matter." And indeed in this laboratory you will see a lot of gray matter. This substance really gets it name in

Functional Neuroanatomy: An Interactive Text and Manual, by Jeffrey T. Joseph and David L. Cardozo
ISBN 0-471-44437-5 Copyright © 2004 John Wiley & Sons, Inc.

comparison with white matter. Gray matter is where most neurons live and where most synapses are made, while white matter is a dense collection of myelinated axons. In an early fetus, before myelin has formed, the brain lacks a clear distinction between gray and white. These terms derive from the unaided eye view of the brain. Microscopically (next laboratory) it becomes clear that some neurons are present in white matter and myelinated axons are present in gray matter.

The gray matter of cortex represents a mantle of neurons encasing most of the brain. While some areas are a bit thicker and other areas have some visible substructure, the cortical ribbon overall is quite uniform. This contrasts with the distinct divisions that are present in the deeper nuclei. As you work through this book, you will master some of the essence of these deep nuclei; for this exercise, you will want to master their names.

As you will find out later, neuroanatomists have divided the brain up into ever smaller parcels. The term *nucleus* has meaning at many levels. For example, in this laboratory you will find the "thalamic nucleus." But in later exercises you will learn that the thalamus has multiple subdivisions that may also be considered "nuclei." Generally, the term is used for both functional and anatomic subdivisions of the brain. During your study of neuroanatomy, you will encounter several different "wiring" diagrams that are intended to summarize the connections between brain structures and that link separate nuclei with positive and negative arrows. These diagrams may represent either the results of scientific experiments or the findings in specific diseases. Although such figures are conceptually useful, the brain itself does not recognize such simplifications; no "nucleus" contains a pure population of neurons with projections that can be fully delineated by a single arrow.

On gross inspection and on neuroimaging, the brain has several distinct *white matter bundles.* Such bundles typically contain a plethora of fiber types traveling some distance together. Parts of some bundles, such as the corpus callosum and internal capsule, have distinct boundaries, while others, like the centrum semiovale, are less discrete. Later in an appendix at the book's end, you can examine some of the bundling properties of white matter by dissecting a sheep's brain along these pathways.

As indicated previously, these fiber systems are white because of their fatty myelin. In some projections, such as the *stria terminalis,* the axons are thinly myelinated and hence do not form a grossly evident tract. Within the cerebrum, fiber systems may connect close regions of cortex (*association fibers*), connect cortices in different hemispheres (*callosal fibers*), or connect to more distant regions of the brain (*projection fibers*). Several distinct fiber systems are so noteworthy that they retain their own name. By the end of your studies, you should dream about the corticospinal tract.

Early in development the brain is a tube that later folds in a sequential manner to form the mature brain. The remnants of that tube are the ventricular system. External infoldings of vessels and epithelial cells into the ventricular system form the *choroid plexus,* which produces the *cerebrospinal fluid* (CSF). While the tubular cavity originally spans the entire distance of the central nervous system, it later involutes in the spinal cord, leaving only its original lining *ependymal cells.* Within the rest of the brain, the system acts as a channel for CSF, flowing from the choroid plexus, through the different ventricles, around the outside of the brain beneath the meninges, where it is finally dumped into the venous circulation at the *arachnoid granulations.* You will trace this pathway in the laboratory.

INSTRUCTOR NOTES

The main goal of the first four laboratories is to introduce the students to the brain and to implant the basic vocabulary necessary to further study the brain in detail. To this end, one goal early on is to drill in the boring basics of what named structure is where: What is this gray matter structure? Caudate nucleus! Where is the substantia nigra? Here! While this activity does not require extensive higher order cognitive activity, it will be very useful for the remainder of the course. The only way for the students to master these basics is for them to drill themselves, for example, using an atlas or a computer program (there are many available on- and offline), or to be drilled by you or their classmates.

This laboratory should be fun, since the students will get to slice into the brain. While many instructors may be more proficient than the students at slicing brain (perhaps you worked in a delicatessen), let them handle and cut the tissue. It is often best to select one or two individuals to do this (e.g., one on spinal cord, the other on brain), with the remainder helping out by organizing the slices.

It will be nearly impossible for the students to distinguish anything in the cord. In well-preserved specimens that aren't too mangled and not fixed too long, they may be able to differentiate gray from white matter and see the main columns. These are better fresh, but....

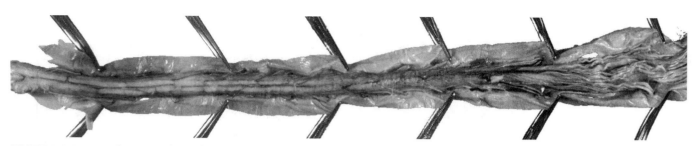

FIGURE 2.1. *Gross dissection of spinal cord. The dura has been cut on one side and retracted with hemostats. A portion of the cervical cord is missing.*

If students feel a bit lost looking at the various scans, remind them to use logic and landmarks when figuring out the MRIs. Orient to the plane of section with respect to the ventricular profile, the presence or absence of gross structures like brainstem and cerebellum. Students should determine the shade of the bone and how the ventricles change on imaging.

Schedule (2.5 hours)
75   Dissection
15   MRI comparison
20   Ventricles
20   Trip through pyramidal tract
20   Case study

SPINAL CORD

INST Examine again the spinal cord specimen you opened in the first laboratory and Figure 2.1. Note how the thickness of the cord changes at different levels. Because of the technical difficulties of removing the cervical cord at the time of autopsy, some of your specimens may lack this region (think about what you would do to remove it).

Q2.1. What do the regions of swelling represent?
A2.1. *The swellings, in essence, represent the greater amount of gray matter (neurons and their synapses) necessary to control your limbs than your "axial" muscles. After all, you don't play the piano with your ribs. The cervical enlargement controls your arms and hands, while the lumbar swelling controls your legs.*

INST Now make several transverse cuts (e.g., one every inch or so) through the spinal cord (BUT NOT THE DURA; this keeps the pieces together) at the different levels. Compare the thinner thoracic sections with the thicker lumbar (and maybe cervical) enlargements. With some imagination, you may be able to distinguish gray matter from white (see Fig. 2.2). This would be much easier to see on fresh spinal cord (see Fig. 2.4).

Q2.2. Using your atlas, try to distinguish the dorsal columns, lateral columns, and central gray matter in either your spinal cord sample or Figure 2.2. How do these change in the different levels of the spinal cord? You know that the brain arose from a tube. Where is this tube in the spinal cord?
A2.2. *See Figure 2.3, which outlines the approximate location of some major ascending and descending tracts in the spinal cord. The former spinal tube with its central canal has collapsed, leaving only*

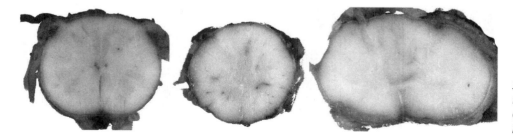

FIGURE 2.2. *Transverse section through a fixed spinal cord, at lumbar* (left), *thoracic, and cervical* (right) *levels.*

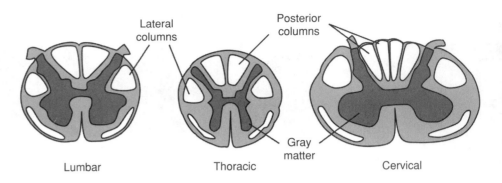

FIGURE 2.3. *Diagram showing approximate location of major tracts and gray matter in corresponding levels of the spinal cord.*

the wall. Microscopically, remnants of the original ependymal lining cells of the neural tube remain, but in most people, no canal has survived. Cerebrospinal fluid bathes the exterior of the cord but does not travel inside.

Trying to distinguish anything in a fixed spinal cord is difficult. Figure 2.4 shows two cross sections of a fresh spinal cord. The gray-white distinction is much better; you should be able to pick out the H-pattern of the central gray matter. Different neuroanatomic structures got their names when they were viewed in freshly dissected brain and spinal cord.

Q2.3. In Figure 2.5 is a slice through an adult female, around the level of the shoulders. On the right the central portion is enlarged to show the vertebral column. Ventral is up in this image (as if she is laying on her back). Label the numbered structures.

2.3.1 _____

2.3.2 _____

2.3.3 _____

2.3.4 _____

2.3.5 _____

2.3.6 _____

2.3.7 _____

A2.3. 2.3.1 *Vertebral artery*
2.3.2 *Dorsal root ganglion*
2.3.3 *Spinal root*
2.3.4 *Vertebral body*
2.3.5 *Ventral horn*
2.3.6 *Dorsal horn*
2.3.7 *Dorsal spinous process*

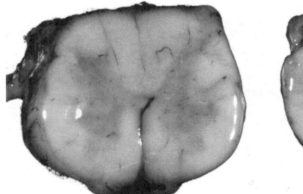
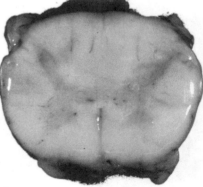

FIGURE 2.4. *Two levels of a fresh spinal cord, lumbar region.*

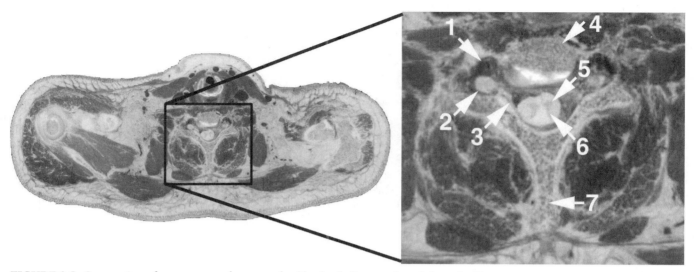

FIGURE 2.5. *Cross-section of a woman at the upper shoulder level. (Image adapted from the Visible Human Project at the National Library of Medicine (http://www.nlm.nih.gov/research/visible/ visible_human.html) using the Head Browser designed at the University of Michigan.)*

Q2.4. We think of the spinal cord as being posterior. Where is it in Figure 2.5? Explain.
A2.4. *At this level the cord is nearly centered in the body. Just above this level, the cord and spine enter the neck, which is placed above the center of our bodies.*

CORONAL SECTIONS OF HALF BRAIN

Now for the fun part. In this section you will dissect the brain. Since you will be coming back to these same sections in future laboratories, it behooves you to be as neat and orderly as possible.

INST With your sharpened anatomic skills, on the "half" brain, carefully identify the "precentral" or "motor" gyrus, with the help of your atlas and laboratory instructor. (Recall the method for locating it from laboratory 1.) Apply India ink along the entire length of this gyrus (see Fig. 2.6). This will enable you to identify it later, after you cut it. You will want to dry the ink in place, since otherwise it will go everywhere. Use a paper towel to first dry the brain surface, and after applying the ink, to dry any remaining ink. India ink has a long history of staining clothing.

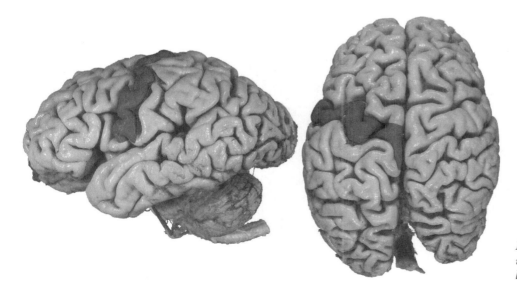

FIGURE 2.6. *Lateral and superior view of brain with motor strip highlighted.*

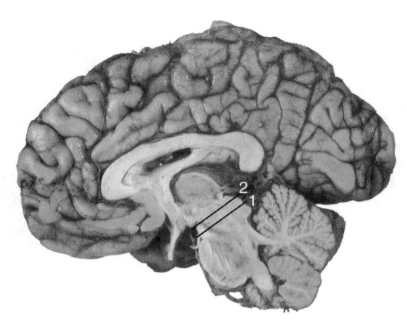

FIGURE 2.7. *Lateral view of brain showing where to dissect the hindbrain from the forebrain.*

INST Lay the half brain on its lateral surface on the cutting board, so you are facing the medial surface. Make sure you can identify the following structures (refer to laboratory 1):

- Corpus callosum
- Cingulate gyrus
- Mammillary body
- Thalamus
- Brainstem, including midbrain, pons, and medulla
- Cerebellum

INST Remove the brainstem from the cerebrum by making a first cut with your scalpel through the inferior colliculus and lower part of the midbrain (lower slice in Fig. 2.7). Take one more higher section of midbrain. Keep these sections moist while you work on the remaining dissection.

INST After removing the brainstem, you will make three coronal cuts through the brain. Note: Dissecting knives should be sharp, so BE CAREFUL. Choose the person in your group who cuts the best slices of bread. Keeping your knife perpendicular to the base of the temporal lobes, make the three cuts as shown in Figure 2.8:

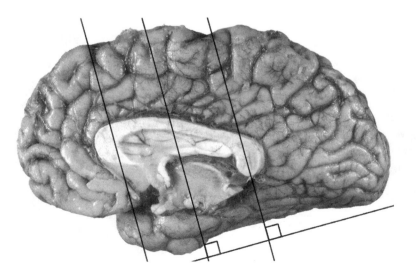

FIGURE 2.8. *Lateral view of brain after removal of the brainstem, showing where to dissect the cerebrum.*

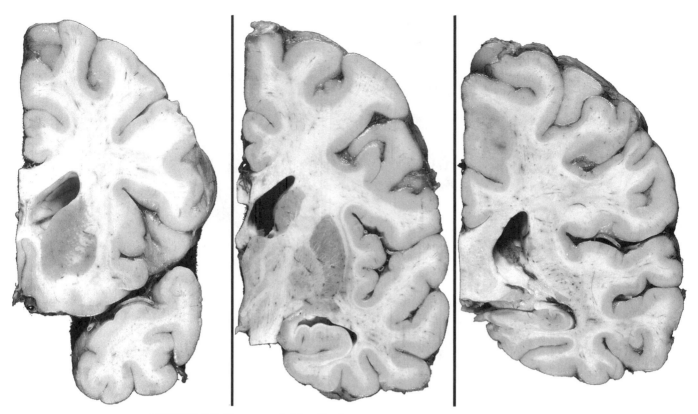

FIGURE 2.9. *First coronal slabs of brain.*

- At posterior end of corpus callosum genu
- Through mammillary body
- Through middle of corpus callosum splenium

INST Make the cuts as evenly as possible. You will be looking at these slabs in subsequent laboratories, so keep the sections as even and uniform as possible. Lay them out in a sequential order, from front to back, as in Figure 2.9.

Q2.5. Compare the gray matter with the white matter. Where does the white matter reach the surface of the brain? Carefully examine the cortical ribbon. Is it of uniform thickness, or does the thickness vary in different regions? (Beware of "plane of section" artifacts.) Try to locate the precentral gyrus. You now know why you applied the ink! Does this differ from the nearby cortex? How does the white matter change from just beneath the cortical surface to its crossing in the corpus callosum? Can you determine the direction of the millions of myelinated axons in the white matter?

A2.5. *Almost all of the white matter in the brain is covered by gray matter. In the cerebrum only the corpus callosum is on the surface. The brainstem has other surface white matter tracts. Overall the cortical ribbon has a uniform appearance, although in careful perpendicular cuts you may be able to see some differences in thickness. In particular, the precentral motor gyrus is significantly thicker than the postcentral sensory gyrus. You may be able to see this using the inked cortex. Looking for gross changes in the white matter is mostly an unrewarding experience. It is made up of many fibers traveling in many directions, which imparts a monotonous macroscopic appearance. However, as fibers approach the corpus callosum, they line up into visible striations. If you can't appreciate this, pull a little of the callosal fibers apart. The other site to look for parallel white matter tracts is in the optic radiation skirting along the edge of the ventricle in the occipital lobes. They stand out because they are perpendicular to most of their surrounding brethren.*

Q2.6. Now locate all aspects of the lateral ventricle: frontal horn, occipital horn, and temporal horn. Notice the fuzzy material lining some of the ventricles in the brain. What is this material? What function does it serve? Where do you find it?

A2.6. *The fuzzy material inside the ventricles is **choroid plexus,** which make the cerebrospinal fluid. It lies along the lateral ventricle, but does not extend into the frontal or occipital horns.*

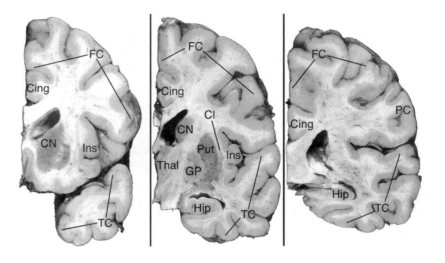

FIGURE 2.10. *Salient structures on coronal sections.*

Q2.7. Using your atlas, identify the following gray matter structures on the brain slabs and label the corresponding sections in Figure 2.9 (you may use the adjacent abbreviations):
- Frontal cortex (FC)
- Temporal cortex (TC)
- Parietal cortex (PC)
- Occipital cortex (present only if posterior cuts are made) (OC)
- Insular cortex (Ins)
- Cingulate gyrus (Cing)
- Hippocampus (Hip)
- Caudate nucleus (CN)
- Putamen (Put)
- Globus pallidus (note its subdivisions) (GP)
- Thalamus (Thal)
- Claustrum (Cl)

A2.7. *See Figure 2.10.*

Q2.8. Follow the caudate nucleus from its head in the frontal lobes backward. How far back does it go? What is its relationship to the ventricles? Describe its overall shape.

A2.8. *During development, as our big brain stretched out, it curled up inside its confined skull. As a result the cerebrum has a C-shape. Structures that follow this pattern include the caudate nucleus and the ventricles (as well as several others). As a consequence the caudate nucleus travels backward from its head and then its tail travels forward into the temporal lobe. It always lies along the surface of the lateral ventricle.*

Q2.9. Using your atlas, identify these white matter structures in the brain slabs and in Figure 2.11:
- Internal capsule
- Corpus callosum
- Anterior commissure (may not be visible in your slabs)
- External capsule
- Extreme capsule

A2.9. *See Figure 2.12.*

Q2.10. What is the functional distinction between the corpus callosum and the internal capsule?

A2.10. *White matter fibers in the corpus callosum extend from hemisphere to hemisphere and are hence called **commissure fibers.** This contrasts with the projections through the internal capsule, which contains long fibers connecting the cortex to distant sites (**projection fibers**) including thalamus, deep brain nuclei, brainstem, and spinal cord.*

INST Leave your cerebral slices on the tray, but cover them with a damp paper towel.

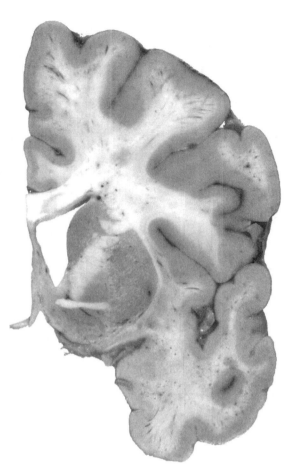

FIGURE 2.11. Coronal slice through cerebrum at the level of the anterior commissure.

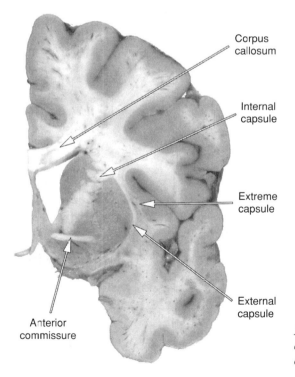

Corpus
callosum

Internal
capsule

Extreme
capsule

External
capsule

Anterior
commissure

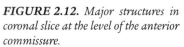

FIGURE 2.12. Major structures in coronal slice at the level of the anterior commissure.

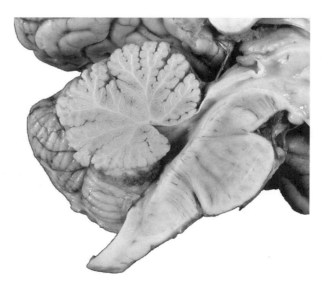

FIGURE 2.13. *Close-up sagittal view of the posterior fossa contents.*

BRAINSTEM AND CEREBELLUM TRANSVERSE SECTIONS

Q2.11. Examine the half of the brainstem and cerebellum you removed earlier. Using your atlas of gross anatomy, identify the divisions of the posterior fossa on the specimen and in Figure 2.13:
- Cerebellum
- Midbrain
- Pons
- Medulla
- Fourth ventricle and the cerebral aqueduct

A2.11. *See Figure 2.14.*

Q2.12. How do the peduncles connect the brainstem to the cerebellum? Identify the three peduncles in the intact brainstem and in Figure 2.15. In the figure on the left, the inferior and middle peduncles are adjacent to each other; try to distinguish them.

A2.12. *See Figure 2.16. As you will see in a subsequent laboratory, the cerebellum connects to the brainstem through three peduncles. The **inferior peduncle** connects the medulla, the **middle peduncle** the pons, and the **superior peduncle** the midbrain. On gross inspection these are not easily distinguishable. However, if you remember that the inferior peduncle extends upward into the cerebellum from the medulla, that the middle peduncle occupies most of the ventral face of the pons, and that the superior peduncle arises from deep within the cerebellum, you may be able to better appreciate these structures.*

Q2.13. Lay the brainstem on its medial surface, and then cut perfect 5 mm transverse sections perpendicular to its axis. Since the brainstem curves slightly, your slices will have to be slightly wedged. Lay these out sequentially on a tray, being careful to maintain the original order. Using your atlases, identify the level of each slice. Find the indicated structures on the slices and in Figure 2.17:
- Midbrain, including the peduncles, aqueduct, red nucleus, and substantia nigra
- Pons, including the base with its perpendicular descending and crossing fibers and the gray matter cover (tegmentum)
- Medulla, including the inferior olivary nucleus, cranial nerve fibers (XII), pyramid, and its decussation
- Cerebellum, specifically the cerebellar folia and dentate nucleus (see middle slice in Figure 2.15)

A2.13. *See Figure 2.18.*

Q2.14. Compare the gray and white matter of the brainstem. Are white matter tracts easier or harder to identify, compared to the cerebrum? How well can you distinguish gray matter nuclei in the brainstem?

A2.14. *Compared to the cerebrum, the brainstem is much more compact. It contains many nuclei (a fraction of which will be discussed in subsequent chapters) and multiple white matter tracts.*

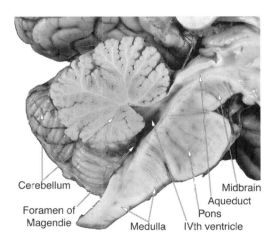

Cerebellum

Foramen of
Magendie

Medulla

IVth ventricle

Pons

Aqueduct

Midbrain

FIGURE 2.14. Posterior fossa land-marks.

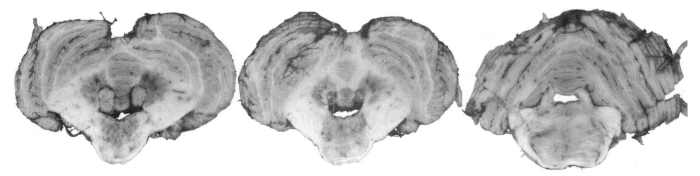

FIGURE 2.15. Transverse sectionsthrough the brainstem and cerebellum.

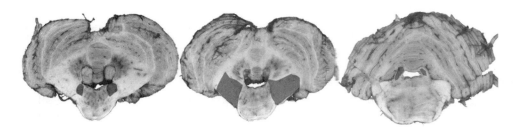

FIGURE 2.16. Inferior (left), middle (middle), and superior cerebellar (right) peduncles on transverse sections.

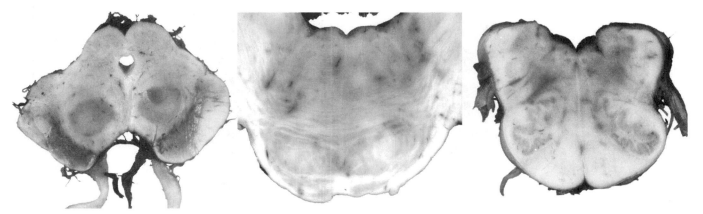

FIGURE 2.17. Close-up views of three brainstem transverse slices.

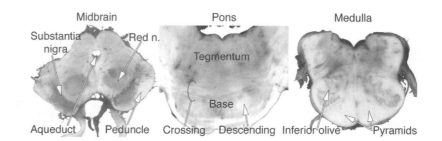

FIGURE 2.18. *Major anatomic landmarks in the brainstem.*

*The cerebral peduncle in the midbrain itself contains several **descending tracts,** including the corticospinal tract to the cord as well as corticobulbar tracts that will end up in the pons. Generally, the tracts are a bit better distinguished grossly than in the cerebrum, since they are more compact and in larger bundles. Nevertheless, they are still very difficult to see and really require a microscope to fully appreciate their anatomical organization. Gray matter nuclei, with some exceptions, are only distinguished microscopically.*

MRI COMPARISON

You will have an entire laboratory devoted to neuroimaging. However, it is useful now to compare the coronal MRI with the coronally dissected brain.

Q2.15. Examine the coronal T1 MRI images of a relatively "normal" brain in Figure 2.19. A contrast agent has been administered, so vascular structures are bright. What shade is gray matter? White matter? How do the ventricles appear? What is the bright material in the ventricle?

A2.15. *Gray matter is a bit darker than the white matter on T1 scans. These distinctions will be greater in the T2 MRI scans. The ventricles are black on T1 scans. The bright material in the ventricle is choroid plexus. It is highly vascular, so it enhances with the contrast agent.*

Q2.16. Now compare the MRI images with the coronal sections you made earlier. Try to match your slices with those produced by the MRI. Do they match exactly? Using your brain slices and atlases as guides, identify the following structures in Figure 2.19:
- Corpus callosum (CC)
- Lateral ventricle (LV)

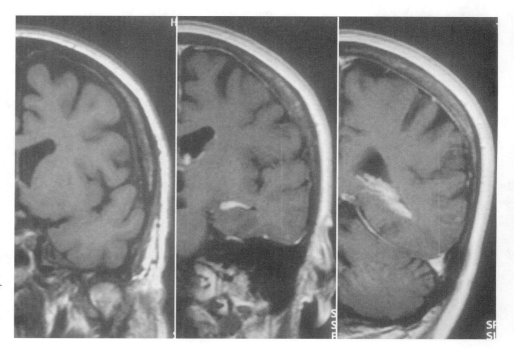

FIGURE 2.19. *Enhanced coronal T1 MRI. The three levels approximately correspond to the slabs of brain cut earlier. Note that in routine MRI examinations, the entire brain is examined, not just three half-sections.*

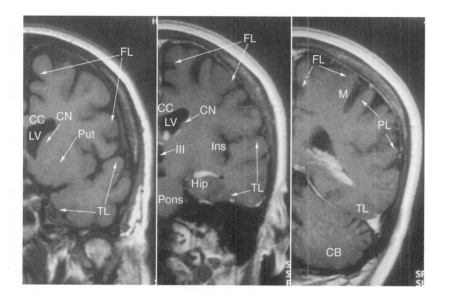

FIGURE 2.20. *A few salient structures on a coronal T1-weighted MRI.*

- Third ventricle (III)
- Frontal lobe (FL)
- Temporal lobe (TL)
- Parietal lobe (PL)
- Insula (Ins)
- Hippocampus (Hip)
- Caudate nucleus (CN)
- Putamen (Put)
- Cerebellum (CB)
- Pons
- Precentral motor gyrus (M) (remember the ink!)

A2.16. See Figure 2.20. The **primary motor cortex** really looks much like any other cortex, especially on scans. However, its adjacent and immediately posterior central sulcus is among the deepest in the brain, which allows for its identification in scans.

Q2.17. Now examine the midsagittal MRI scan in Figure 2.21 and compare it with your sagittal brain. Compared to the coronal view, which structures can you better visualize? Again identify some major structures:
- Frontal lobe (FL)
- Parietal lobe (PL)
- Occipital lobe (OL)
- Corpus callosum (CC)
- Thalamus (Thal)
- Midbrain (Mid)
- Pons
- Medulla (Med)
- Cerebellum (CB)
- Cingulate gyrus (CG)
- Lateral ventricle (LV)
- Fourth ventricle (IV)
- Colliculi (Col) (superior and inferior)
- Pituitary fossa (Pit) (sella turcica)
- Calcarine sulcus (Cal)
- Dura (D)

A2.17. See Figure 2.22.

Q2.18. Finally, compare the more-or-less equivalent sagittal images of the MRI with the cut brain in Figure 2.23. Note the detail present on the dissected brain that is lacking on the MRI. However, the MRI gives information that is not available on the cut brain; describe this. The two images come from different patients. How do the two brains compare? Can you suggest a disease category for either case?

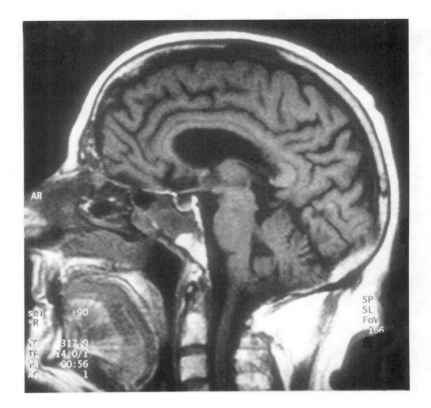

FIGURE 2.21. *Sagittal T1 MRI.*

A2.18. *The MRI is of a living patient, an obvious advantage when you're treating your patient. But in addition, the MRI shows the brain's context with the surrounding tissues. You now visualize the pituitary fossa; the pituitary was lost from the brain during dissection. You can also see the dura and the spaces created by the brain coverings (sinuses and subdural space). You will see in a later laboratory the MRI scans can show many additional features easily, which only a trained eye might see in the actual brain tissue. The brain on the left was from a patient without significant neurologic disease, while the atrophic brain MRI image was of a demented patient. Notice how thin the corpus callosum is on the right, compared to the left brain.*

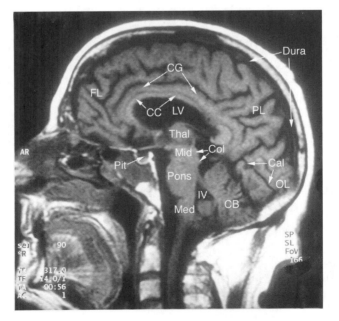

FIGURE 2.22. *Salient structures on sagittal T1 MRI.*

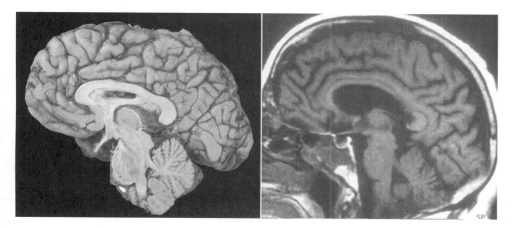

FIGURE 2.23. *Comparison of sagittal brain and T1 MRI images.*

VENTRICLES

Q2.19. Examine a model of the ventricles and Figure 2.24. Identify the key features:
   • Lateral ventricles and their horns (frontal, occipital, temporal; where is the parietal?)
   • Foramen of Monroe
   • Third ventricle
   • Aqueduct
   • Fourth ventricle
   • Exits out of fourth ventricle (foramen of Luschka is lateral and Magendie is medial)
A2.19. *See Figure 2.25. The foramen of Monro is hidden in this view, but connects the lateral to the third ventricles.*

INST Now examine the whole and half brain specimens. On the side of the fourth ventricle is a foramen where cerebrospinal fluid exits the brain. Gently identify this (lateral) foramen of Luschka with a probe (a firm probe can make a foramen anywhere). Another foramen is located at the base of the cerebellum, above the medulla. This is called the (medial) foramen of Magendie. Trace the pathway of the cerebrospinal fluid from the aqueduct through the posterior fossa foramina (see Fig. 2.26).

Q2.20. Look on the top of the brain (see Fig. 2.27). Notice the fuzzy white fibrous tissue near the sagittal crest of each hemisphere. What is this called, and what is its significance?
A2.20. *The arachnoid granulations are arachnoid peninsulas that have drilled into the dural venous sinuses. They are the site where cerebrospinal fluid is reabsorbed into the venous system.*
Q2.21. Try to take each coronal brain slice and determine its equivalent plane of section through the ventricular model. Where is the choroid plexus in the brain and on the model? Examine the ventricles in the coronal MRI images in appendix I. Locate the

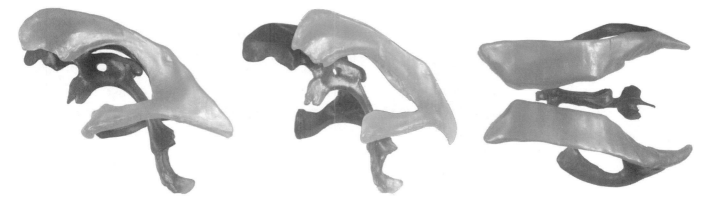

FIGURE 2.24. *Cast of the ventricular system. The left image is a lateral view, the right, superior, and the middle is an oblique lateral view.*

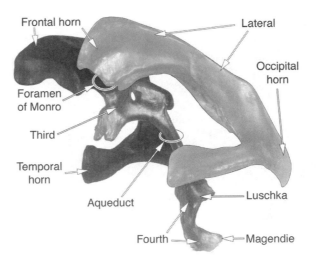

Frontal horn

Lateral

Occipital horn

Foramen of Monro

Third

Temporal horn

Aqueduct

Luschka

Fourth

Magendie

FIGURE 2.25. *Key elements of the ventricular system.*

corresponding brain coronal sections that you have cut. Orient these relative to the ventricular model. In which sections does the slice and/or image cut through the ventricular system more than once? How many times do such sections slice through the flow of cerebrospinal fluid.

A2.21. *The entire brain is bathed in cerebrospinal fluid. If you attend an autopsy and actually see a fresh brain, you'll understand why. Basically your brain has the consistency of a very thick pudding. If left on the table, it will collapse under its own weight. To avoid having a flat brain in your skull, the brain is suspended in the CSF fluid medium. Some coronal sections you may have found cut the lateral ventricle in two sites, and also may slice through either the aqueduct or fourth ventricle. But also remember that the entire outside of the brain is also bathed in CSF, which flows toward the arachnoid granulations. As you can see, the CSF pervades the entire brain structure.*

Q2.22. Using the model and the whole brain (and perhaps dura from the first lab sheep brain), trace the CSF circulation from the choroid plexus in the lateral ventricle through the ventricular system, the cisternae, and back into the venous system. From the size of these structures that you have observed, estimate how much CSF is in the brain.

A2.22. *The brain contains several hundred milliliters of CSF (depending on the atrophy of your brain), which is completely replaced several times a day.*

Q2.23. Figure 2.28 shows a brain superimposed over a cast of the ventricular system. Indicate where you would find choroid plexus. Then draw a curve to show the path of the cerebrospinal fluid from the choroid plexus to the arachnoid granulations.

A2.23. *See Figure 2.29. The choroid plexus has been accentuated, and would not be this voluminous. Also note that the flow has only been shown exiting one lateral foramen of Luschka; it would normally flow from all three posterior fossa exits.*

FIGURE 2.26. *Flow of cerebrospinal fluid in posterior fossa. The left figure has an arrow traveling through the lateral foramen of Luschka, while the right shows the flow of cerebrospinal fluid through the fourth ventricle and exiting through both the lateral and medial (Magendie) foramina.*

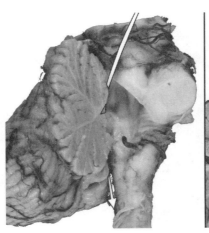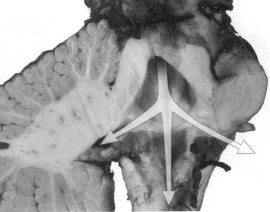

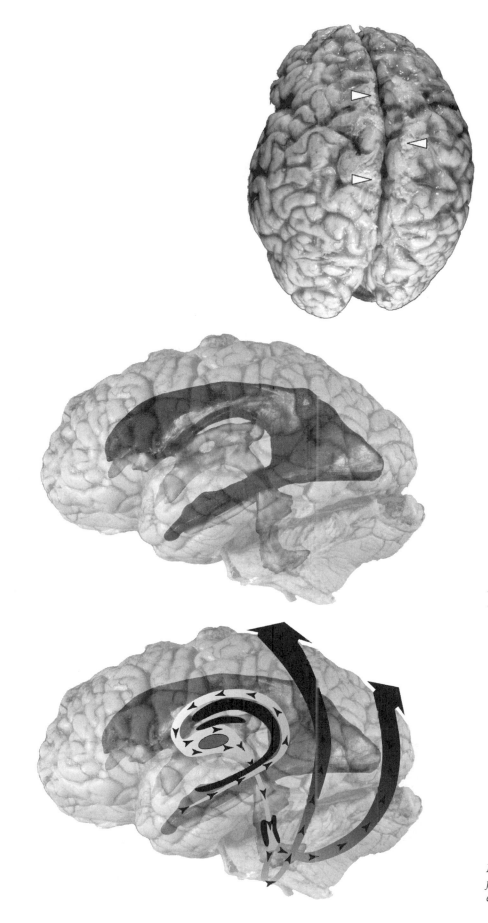

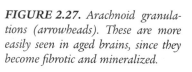

FIGURE 2.27. *Arachnoid granulations (arrowheads). These are more easily seen in aged brains, since they become fibrotic and mineralized.*

FIGURE 2.28. *Ventricular system superimposed on brain.*

FIGURE 2.29. *Ventricular flow from choroid plexus (black) to superior sagittal sinus.*

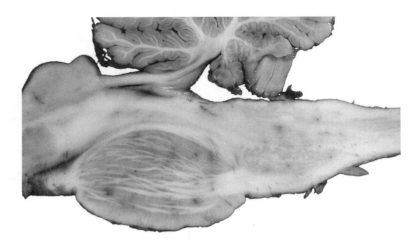

FIGURE 2.30. *Parasagittal view of pyramidal tract coursing through the pons.*

PYRAMIDAL TRACT

Wallerian degeneration. The term used for stereotypical degeneration of an axon distal to the site of a lesion. Multiple types of axonal injury, including infarction, trauma, and in some cases demyelination, prevent nutrients, proteins, and trophic factors from being transported to the axonal segment distal to the injury. When not supported by its cell body, an axon will degenerate. Because Schwann cells and oligodendrocytes require signals from the axon to produce myelin, axonal degeneration also leads to myelin degeneration. The leftover debris from these cellular fragments will slowly be engulfed and digested by the brain's resident sanitation engineer, the macrophage. Astrocytes also undergo changes that support the remaining cells. All of these features together produce Wallerian degeneration. When the involved tracts are large enough, the changes may be seen on macroscopic inspection.

In the next set of questions, you will trace the pyramidal tracts through the nervous system by examining the brain from a patient who had suffered a stroke in this pathway. The axon fibers below the infarct have degenerated on one side, which is visible on the gross anatomic specimens. You will also encounter this type of axonal pathology, termed "Wallerian degeneration," in later labs.

Q2.24. In Figure 2.30 label the pyramidal tract and the medial lemniscus as they travel through the pons.

A2.24. *The pyramidal tract breaks into thick bundles in the pons, but reforms a compact tract in the medulla. The posterior columns start parasagittal, and hence are visible in this section. The medial lemniscus disappears in the medulla, since it is medial, but then appears and disappears in the pons as it moves more laterally, immediately dorsal to the base of the pons. See Figure 2.31.*

Q2.25. Figure 2.32 shows the site of the lesion and Figure 2.33 shows the distal Wallerian degeneration. The patient had a large hemorrhage inside his brain about a year prior to his death. Much of the blood has been resorbed, although the adjacent loss of tissue remains. Right is on right. (Note: Neuropathologists have been displaying brains as left on left and right on right for over a hundred years. The neuroimaging convention of reversing this has its roots in how the CT scan was displayed, about 25 years ago. Radiologists look at people from their feet while Neuropathologists look at them from behind their head. Strictly a matter of convention and your view of human kind.) As best as you can, describe the location of the lesion. What happened to the corpus callosum? Internal capsule? How? From a distance, what would you notice about this patient? Describe how this patient's clinical manifestations arose from the lesion.

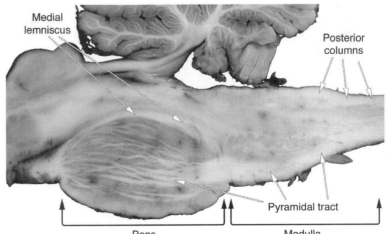

Medial lemniscus

Posterior columns

Pyramidal tract

Pons   Medulla

FIGURE 2.31. *Pyramidal tract and medial lemniscus in pons.*

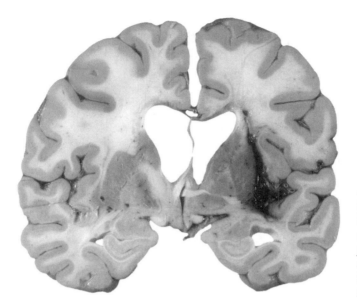

FIGURE 2.32. *Coronal dissection of brain in a patient who suffered a large hemorrhage a year prior to death. The blood has been nearly completely resorbed, leaving only the indigestible blood breakdown product hemosiderin and the subsequent tissue loss. Right is on right.*

A2.25. *The lesion extends along the outer edge of the right putamen up into the cerebral white matter. Damage has occurred in the centrum semi-ovale and coronal radiata, since the corpus callosum is paper-thin and the internal capsule is shrunken. When axons are cut off from their cell body, they involute by a process termed Wallerian degeneration. Axons in the corpus callosum and internal capsule have been destroyed by the hemorrhage, and these structures have degenerated. From a distance, the patient would have a dense LEFT hemiplegia. Although the patient's motor neurons in the precentral motor gyrus are intact, their axonal connections have been severed by the hemorrhage, leading to the hemiparesis.*

Q2.26. Now examine the other accompanying images in Figure 2.33. Specifically identify the anatomic location of the pathology in each section of brainstem and spinal cord. What happens to the tract in the lowest section of the medulla (lower right tissue section)? Outline the pathway of these fibers, from their cell body in the premotor cortex. You have now traced the corticospinal tract throughout the cerebral axis.

A2.26. *In the midbrain (clearly accentuated by the substantia nigra), the right cerebral peduncle is shrunken and discolored, compared to the left. In the center of this peduncle lie the corticospinal fibers. In the medulla in the upper right (highlighted by the inferior olivary nucleus), the "pyramid" is white and shrunken on the right side at the ventral surface. This tract crosses over or decussates from right to left at the lowest medulla levels and then travels primarily in the left lateral corticospinal tract in the spinal cord, which is why the hemiplegia was on the left.*

Corticospinal tract pathway.
Precentral gyrus motor neurons (Betz cells; you'll encounter them in a later laboratory), coronal radiata, internal capsule, cerebral peduncles, base of pons, pyramid of medulla, decussate to contralateral lateral corticospinal tract in spinal cord. Know this tract!

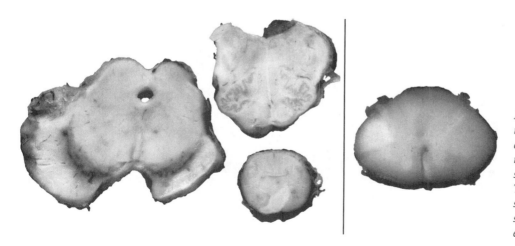

FIGURE 2.33. *Transverse sections through the brainstem and spinal cord, showing the Wallerian degeneration of the pyramidal tract. The third section is from the lowest medulla. The section on the right is through the spinal cord and has been enlarged somewhat. The degeneration has been enhanced.*

CASE: VASCULAR TERRITORY PARTIAL INFARCTION, MOTOR PLUS SENSORY

This 60-year-old woman suffered an embolic infarct with sudden onset hemiparesis, and partial clearing over the course of several days. When examined a year later, she had normal visual fields, a mild left facial weakness, a marked weakness of the left hand and arm, which was held semiflexed against her trunk, with very slow movements of wrist and fingers, although she could generate fair to good power around the elbow and shoulder. The left leg was spastic, but she had good strength and her gait was nearly normal. She had a multimodal sensory loss of the arm and hand only. Figure 2.34 is a CT scan of her head, taken a year later.

Q2.27. Examine her scan. You can see a low density area in the right side laterally (left on the image). Find the closest corresponding slices of brain from the laboratory. Then map the location of her infarct onto the surface of the whole brain. Using the atlas, identify which gyri you think were affected. Which vessel was occluded? Knowing the stroke was embolic, list the possible sources for this embolus. Why was the left hand affected? Hypothesize why her hand was more involved than her foot.

A2.27. *This is a typical embolic infarct, representing an occlusion a middle cerebral artery branch. It is primarily cortical, wedge-shaped, and well defined. The gyri involved are probably the hand and face areas of pre- and postcentral gyri. Most likely the angular, supramarginal, and possibly first temporal gyri are involved too.*

The most likely sources for the embolus begin at the heart and work their way toward the brain. These include a mural thrombus in a patient with atrial fibrillation, an atherosclerotic plaque from the ascending aorta, and an internal carotid plaque at the carotid bifurcation.

As demonstrated previously, the pyramidal tract decussates at the lower medulla as it enters the spinal cord. Left-sided lesions above the decussation will produce right-sided deficits below. You probably have guessed by now that the motor strip is further subdivided into leg (medial surface), arm, hand, and face regions (moving more laterally). This woman's stroke was more lateral, and thus more greatly affected the hand area than the leg. You'll return to cortex in a later chapter.

Note that predicting the patient's deficits from knowledge of the area affected is tough, since we have lots of compensatory mechanisms. A notable example is Broca's aphasia, which often must involve more than back of the inferior frontal lobule (Broca's areas) to produce lasting deficits.

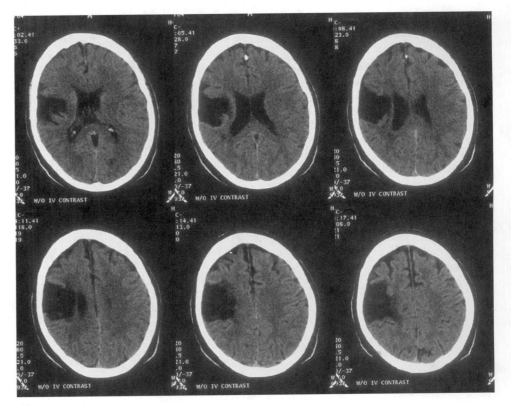

FIGURE 2.34. CT scan of a woman who suffered an embolic infarct a year earlier. Unlike MRI examinations, CT scans utilize the penetration of X-rays through tissue. Tissues with the same X-ray penetration will appear the same intensity. Remember, radiology convention has left on the right.

Chapter 3—HISTOLOGY

The nervous system, like all tissues, is made of cells bound together by a matrix. While this system only contains a handful of different cell types, they can take on a myriad of different morphologies and activities. Unlike elsewhere in the body, the nervous system has incredibly extended cells. The nerve twig governing your toe is operated by a cell body over a meter away in the spinal cord. Even astrocytes and oligodendrocytes have extended processes that bridge many cell diameters. Understanding these cells will help you comprehend the functioning of the nervous system.

Also unlike other tissues in the body, the anatomy where a cell lives determines its action. A liver cell pretty much does the same thing, whether it lies just under the edge of the diaphragm or at the liver's caudal tip. A neuron in the cortex has a completely different function from one in the cerebellum. And even in a particular site like the cerebellar cortex, one neuron type is excitatory and projects distally, while its neighbor is inhibitory and projects centrally.

This chapter is an introduction to the histology of the nervous system. You will travel from the periphery to the central nervous system, first looking at muscle then nerve, before finally digging into the spinal cord and other parts of the brain. The emphasis here is on the cells that run the nervous system. In later chapters you will step back from the cellular level and examine these structures from a neurological systems view.

LEARNING OBJECTIVES

- Distinguish among different major cell types in the nervous system.
- Identify how different cellular structures convey different functions to the cells.
- Understand the basic tenets of the "neuron doctrine" and that neurons show extensive functional specialization.
- Identify what defines neuroanatomic structures, including "nuclei" and "tracts." Appreciate that these can be examined at multiple levels of detail.
- Understand how different techniques of analysis are used to understand the function of cells in the nervous system, including special stains, immunoperoxidase stains, histochemistry, and in situ mRNA expression hybridization.
- Identify cells involved in a central nervous system infection and recognize that selective cellular elements may be affected by disease.

Functional Neuroanatomy: An Interactive Text and Manual, by Jeffrey T. Joseph and David L. Cardozo
ISBN 0-471-44437-5 Copyright © 2004 John Wiley & Sons, Inc.

INTRODUCTION

Several distinctly different tissues and multiple cell types comprise the nervous system. A set of peripheral sensory cells encodes environmental data into biologic signals. Nerve cell *axons* then transfer these signals from the sensory cells to other neurons in the central nervous system. Axons receive several types of support from their accompanying *glial cells.* The brain itself is the ultimate neural net, having excitatory, inhibitory, and modulating neurons in, we hope, the best network around. After various degrees of processing in the central nervous system, control signals are sent out to activate peripheral effector cells, including skeletal muscle and smooth muscle.

Our study of these multiple cell types depends on selected techniques. For the pathologist, the standard hematoxylin and eosin stain (H&E for short) serves as the workhorse. The purple-blue hematoxylin dye stains basic proteins (hence the term basophilic for hematoxylin-staining material), while the eosin dye stains acidic proteins (you guessed it, acidophilic). But further study of the nervous system requires a panel of special techniques. For example, in the study of Alzheimer's disease, certain silver stains greatly enhance our ability to identify the amyloid plaques and neurofibrillary tangles characteristic of this disease. Yet another silver stain, the Golgi, selectively but nearly completely fills single cells with silver, yet leaves adjacent cells unstained. Ramón y Cajal did much of his elegant work using the still poorly understood Golgi stain. Today, with the development of antibody techniques, we look for expression of specific proteins within cells. As an example, antibodies prepared against glial fibrillary acidic protein (GFAP for short), an intermediate filament protein expressed only in glial cells, have both research and clinical utility. Probes hybridizing with specific RNAs, when applied to tissue, demonstrate where a gene is active. Finally, electron microscopy allows us to visualize cells at an ultrastructural level. Throughout the course you will be using most of these techniques to examine the nervous system.

Skeletal muscle is the main effector tissue for the nervous system, provides a substantial fraction of our body mass, and may act as a reservoir of protein to the body or to carnivores. Actin and myosin protein filaments make up the fundamental contractile elements. However, to control, transmit, and sustain the force they generate requires an intricate muscle architecture. Multiple proteins, including dystrophin and its associated set of proteins, make up the architecture that transmits the generated forces from their origin in the sliding filaments to the surface and beyond. During development, individual muscle cells (or *myocytes*) fuse to form more mature muscles, termed *myofibers.* In the adult a normal "muscle cell" is a fused composite of thousands of myocytes, with their corresponding nuclei and mitochondria intact. This concept becomes important when trying to analyze diseases of muscle. For example, an inherited disease of mitochondria may only involve a portion of a given muscle fiber, which contributes to the variable expression of these illnesses. On histologic sections you only examine a sliver of tissue a few micrometers thick from a cell that is actually many centimeters long. Sites like the motor end-plate would be unusual to see in any given section of a fiber. Depending on how the muscle is cut, you may view it in cross section, longitudinally, or in an oblique plane.

Peripheral nerves connect the brain with the body. For the most part these are transmission lines that don't process the information they carry. The main players in the nerve are the axons and the Schwann cell. Each of these is intimately associated with the other; death of axons eventually leads to regression of the Schwann cell, and death of the Schwann cell will lead to axonal dysfunction and eventually death. While axons may branch as they extend, they remain isolated from other axons. Within the nerve are several types of fibers, including those transmitting information very rapidly and those following a more leisurely pace. The former would include sensory fibers conveying limb position and motor fibers to help you escape the saber tooth tiger, while the latter contain some pain sensory fibers and autonomic motor fibers. Larger diameter axons increase the speed of transmission, as does the thickness of the surrounding myelin sheath. In peripheral nerves, the largest axons have the thickest myelin, while tiny axons are unmyelinated. Along a myelinated axon is a chain of Schwann cells, with each cell associated with only one axon. This contrasts with unmyelinated axons, in which a single Schwann cell envelops multiple small axons. The Schwann cells wrap the axon in their specialized membrane containing specific proteins and lipids. Myelin itself is about half water. Excluding the water, it is about three-quarters lipid (phospholipids, glycolipids, and cholesterol) and one-quarter protein (including P0, P1, P2 glycoproteins, peripheral myelin protein or PMP-22, and myelin-associated glycoprotein or MAG). The junctions between Schwann cells are termed *nodes of Ranvier.* The cellular contents of a peripheral nerve, termed the *endoneurium,* are set in an extracellular matrix that includes collagen, fibroblasts, and blood vessels, as well as occasional mast cells, all delimited by the perineurium. This boundary is a fundamental constituent of the "blood-nerve barrier." Finally, the space external to the perineurium is termed the *epineurium.* This space contains fibroblasts, collagen, capillaries, arteries, veins, and fat.

The fundamental unit of the nervous system is the *neuron.* It is this cell that integrates disparate information and decides whether or not to pass it on. Neurons come in many flavors. The massive *dorsal root ganglion* neurons sustain long sensory fibers, including their peripheral and central extensions. The gigantic *Betz cells* in the precentral gyrus project up to a third of your body length to lower motor neurons in the spinal cord and are essential for our control of movements. However, the nervous system is populated by a much larger number of less glamorous cells, including lowly interneurons and minimalist internal granular cerebellar neurons. You will encounter several types of neurons in this laboratory. The generic neuron is a metabolically active cell that must both control neurotransmission and supply its axon and dendrites with a continuous supply of proteins. The protein production is so copious that the ribosomes of the rough endoplasmic reticulum accumulate within the neuron body to form *Nissl substance.* Neuron are cells, just like plasma cells, only more elegant. This generic neuron has many dendrites and a single axon, which are best visualized with special staining techniques.

The central equivalent to the peripheral Schwann cell is the *oligodendrocyte.* This glial cell (glia is a general term for both oligodendrocytes and astrocytes) produces a myelin with different properties from peripheral myelin, which is why diseases of central myelin usually do not affect peripheral nerves. While oligodendroglia get their name from having few processes, more sophisticated techniques clearly demonstrate that they have ramifying appendages and can wrap multiple axons. On routine stains, as you will see, this cell looks just like a floating nucleus, yet all of the myelin around axons in the brain and spinal cord derives from these cells.

Astrocytes fall into the "jack of many trades" category of cell. In normal brain they remain inconspicuous. Yet they enhance axonal conduction, regulate the blood-brain barrier, and provide "support" for their neuronal prodigy. Recent work has shown that astrocytes modify neuronal connections and alter the synaptic milieu. It is in disease that astrocytes come into their own glory, producing an abundant intermediate filament known as glial fibrillary acidic protein (GFAP), which they use like Herculean arms to contain damaged brain. Because astrocytes have many abilities, including the ability to migrate through the brain's extracellular matrix, tumors derived from these cells are devastating in their infiltration and slow destruction of normal brain.

Cells of the brain need nutrients and oxygen, and as you have seen, the brain has an intricate vascular network. In the histologic sections you will see many capillaries, although these remain small and unobtrusive. Arterioles, some larger arteries, and veins also lie within brain tissue. Around larger vessels is a potential space that is topologically connected to the brain surface. This region is termed the *Virchow-Robin space,* which plays an important role in some diseases.

In addition to the usual nervous system constituents are a population of inconspicuous inflammatory cells, ready to destroy invaders or inadvertently injure the brain. These cells include resident microglia normally present in small numbers within the brain, macrophages in the blood that may be recruited during an injury, and lymphocytes that regulate the immune response. The *neutrophil,* which so dominates acute lesions in peripheral organs, becomes important in common bacterial diseases and in acute brain injury.

INSTRUCTOR NOTES

Unless you push glass a lot, instructors may feel intimidated at a microscope. You may get that ill-feeling you once had when faced with a piece of glass containing an incomprehensible sliver of tissue. Any instructor who is facile with microscopic slides should review them with each student or group during the laboratory.

Special Things to Note with the Microscopes

- If your image is dark and unclear, your condenser (that piece of glass just underneath the glass slide) may be off. Try raising it up or lowering it down and see if the image clears.
- If it appears that you are looking at the tissue through a tunnel, the aperture at the bottom may be closed up. Open the lower iris.
- If you want to view the slide at a very low power, and the microscope has only a 4× objective, try putting the slide directly on top of the light aperture below the condenser. Adjust the condenser and focus to get a decent picture.

While this textbook will not make neuropathologists out of medical students, they should end up with a sense about how the form of the cells relates to their function. It is not the histology per se that is important, it is the relationships among the different components of the nervous system. For example, although Schwann cells and oligodendrocytes both myelinate axons, they are different cells and have different properties. Hence patients may have a disease of one or the other cell type, each with its own clinical manifestations and healing potentials.

Make sure students LOOK through their microscopes. They should become familiar with these instruments. Looking just at pictures, even those in this chapter, will not produce lasting memories; suffering with glass slides may. Pain is good.

The most salient points about muscle histology are:

- Muscle cells or myofibers are very long, from insertion to insertion, and disease in one part may incapacitate the entire fiber.
- The muscle fiber type (slow or fast) is determined mostly by the neural input.
- Transmission of force requires that all elements of the muscle be connected and work in concert.

The salient points about peripheral nerve histology are:

- One myelinating Schwann cell myelinates only one axon; a nonmyelinating Schwann cell, however, wraps many unmyelinated axons.
- One axon will be wrapped by many Schwann cells during its course.

While inflammatory cells are not normally considered part of the brain, they do contribute to its diseases. A few wandering lymphocytes are present in normal brain, predominantly around vessels. Neutrophils circulate constantly through the blood and may be recruited by selective agents, including bacterial toxins and necrotic vessels.

Remember, students always have trouble finding anything through a microscope.

Schedule (2.5 hours)
20　Skeletal muscle (H&E, EM, photographs)
20　Peripheral nerve (EM, photographs)
20　Spinal cord (LFB/H&E)
20　Neurons
10　Glia (oligodendrocytes and astrocytes)
10　Inflammatory cells (macrophages/microglia, lymphocytes)
20　Case: AIDS PML
30　In laboratory review at a microscope

SKELETAL MUSCLE

This chapter starts at the periphery, examining muscle and nerve. It then delves into the central nervous system cells, including neurons and glia.

INST　Examine the microscopic slide of normal skeletal muscle (Figs. 3.1 and 3.2). In order to properly orient the tissue and perform histochemical staining (staining of actual muscle enzyme activity), the tissue has been rapidly frozen and then cut on cross section and stained with the pathology workhorse H&E. Look at the shape of the fibers, where the nuclei are located, and the size of the fibers. Search for any vessels.

Q3.1.　What is the overall shape of the "cells" or myofibers? How many nuclei are present in each myofiber? Where are they located? How are the myosin and actin fibrils oriented when looking at the skeletal muscle cross section? What are the slightly darker blobs and lines within each fiber? Identify the vasculature to the muscle. Where are the larger and smaller vessels?

A3.1.　*Muscle "cells" are not like other cells in the body, since they are really a combination of thousands individual cells (or myocytes) into a syncytium. To recognize this fact, these conglomerates are termed* **myofibers** *rather than cells. As the myocytes fuse to form a syncytium, their nuclei become confined to the periphery. Although in the microscopic cross section each myofiber has only a handful of nuclei, it is important to remember that the slice is only a few micrometers thick, and that the myofiber may extend many centimeters between insertion sites. Since the slide is a cross section through a muscle, the actin and myosin filaments are perpendicular to*

Myofiber　*Skeletal muscle starts its life as many single muscle cells or myocytes. During development, these cells fuse to form long tubes (myotubes). As the fetus matures, the myotubes produce the adult muscle proteins, such as actin and myosin, and fill out to form mature myofibers. It is the myofiber, a syncytium of many myocytes extending from insertion point to insertion point, that forms the functional "cell" in a mature muscle.*

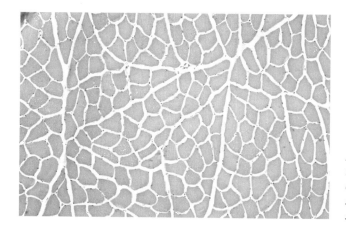

FIGURE 3.1. Low-power cross-sectional view of skeletal muscle. The muscle was snap-frozen, cross-sectional slices were cut on a cryostat and then stained with H&E.

photographs; they are coming directly out at you. Interspersed between bundles of filaments are lines of mitochondria and components of the endoplasmic reticulum (called the sarcoplasmic reticulum). These really lie below the resolution of the light microscope.

Normal myofibers fill the space in the muscle, which gives them a polygonal shape. Rounded fibers often indicate some form of muscle injury. Among the myofibers is an extensive capillary network. Each capillary is a small circle of endothelial cells. Larger vessels feeding the capillary bed are predominantly located in between the bundles of myofibers, rather than among the myofibers themselves.

Q3.2. Now examine the photomicrograph in Figure 3.3 of a longitudinal section of skeletal muscle. Notice the repetitive units within the muscle. How do the units line up? Where are the nuclei in longitudinal sections? How are the contractile elements of the myofiber connected to the surface, and how are they anchored to the extracellular milieu?

A3.2. *In normal muscle the different bands in the muscle generally line up in register, allowing us to perceive the repetitive sarcomeric structure. The heavier bands contain thick filaments of myosin and its regulatory proteins, partially interdigitated with actin, while the lighter bands are the actin thin filaments. Between the actin filaments is a thin, dark Z-band composed of α-actinin. As in the cross sections, the nuclei remain at the periphery, near the sarcolemma (myofiber equivalent of the cell membrane).*

*To transmit force from the primary contractile elements to the anchors in the extracellular matrix, the myofiber has a complex of proteins that links the actin/myosin units to the surface. The main link is dystrophin, while its cell membrane connections are via the dystrophin-related proteins, including the sarcoglycans and dystroglycans. Finally, these connect to the extracellular matrix via a muscle-specific form of laminin termed **merosin**. Many of these structural proteins have been linked to different types of muscular dystrophy.*

Q3.3. The photomicrograph in Figure 3.4 has been prepared by preincubating the snap-frozen muscle at a specific pH, then incubating the tissue with ATP analogues to reveal the muscle filament's intrinsic ATPase enzymatic activity (Figure 3.4). Only myosin ATPase is active; the mitochondrial enzyme is poisoned with specific ions. This technique distinguishes type I slow twitch fibers (light staining at this pH) from type II fast twitch fibers (dark staining). (Don't worry too much about how this works.)

Sarcomere *The fundamental contractile unit in skeletal muscle. It extends from Z-band to Z-band and consists of overlapping actin and myosin rods. The actin filaments are tethered to the Z-bands. During muscle contraction, the two sides of the sarcomere are pulled toward the central myosin chains (sliding filament model) in a process requiring breakdown of ATP.*

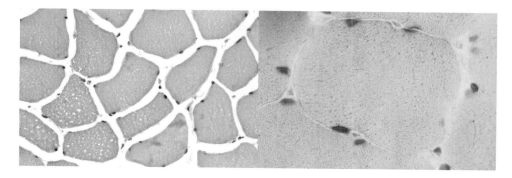

FIGURE 3.2. Intermediate and high power cross sections of normal skeletal muscle, stained with H&E. The spaces between the myofibers in the left figure result from a processing artifact.

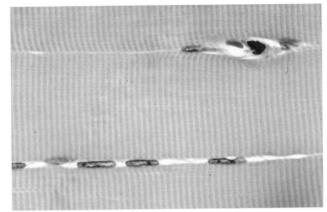

FIGURE 3.3. *Oil-immersion photomicrograph of a longitudinal section through skeletal muscle. The contrast has been increased in this H&E-stained section.*

How are the different fiber types distributed? Groups of one type and groups of another, or in a checkerboard? Are the fibers all about the same size, or do they differ? Knowing that a given motor neuron innervates multiple fibers, but only one fiber type, what does the pattern of staining tell you about the pattern of muscle innervation?

A3.3. *In health, the ATPase stains demonstrate an inexact checkerboard. Generally, one fiber type is not completely surrounded by other similar fibers. This reflects how the axons terminate, splitting into many terminals that branch out into the muscle rather than remaining clumped together. In normal muscle, the two fiber types are about the same size. Variations from the checkerboard pattern or the monotony of myofiber size usually indicate disease.*

For those so inclined, the easy way to remember what fiber type does what, think of "one slow red ox"; type I fibers are slow twitch, red (like the red meat in the wing of a migrating duck), and oxidative. These differences reflect a fundamental distinction between the two types of muscles. The type I slow twitch fibers can be used repeatedly. To maintain their supply of energy, they require the much more efficient respiration-driven generation of ATP by mitochondria. The greater quantity of these heme-containing organelles impart a red color to these muscles. In contrast, fast twitch fibers need a rapid, but not necessarily sustained source of ATP, as is generated by anaerobic respiration. The fewer mitochondria, the less red the fibers. These are the type II myofibers. Most muscles are a mixture of type I and II muscle fibers, whose ratio varies depending on the needs of the muscle.

Q3.4. Finally, examine the electron micrograph of the longitudinal muscle in Figure 3.5. Notice the cross-striations. Locate the actin and myosin filaments. Are the mitochondria at the periphery of the cell or dispersed throughout? How about the glycogen granules?

A3.4. *The section has bundles of filaments (myofibrils) generally aligned in register. The wide dark bands (labeled "A") contain myosin, its regulatory proteins, and portions of the thinner actin filaments. The lighter bands having a dark stripe contain the thin actin filaments anchored to the Z-bands. Mitochondria (large elongated blobs) and glycogen granules (small dark dots) are dispersed around the myofibrils. The close proximity of the energy source to the contractile elements limits the diffusion time for ATP.*

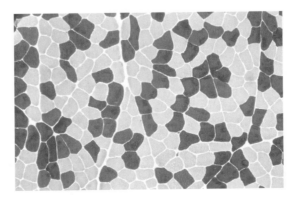

FIGURE 3.4. *ATPase stain of snap-frozen muscle. At this basic pH, the dark fibers are type II.*

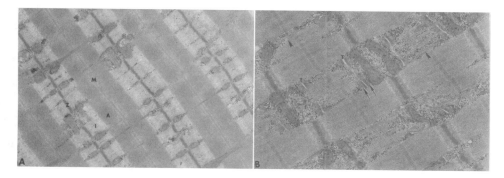

FIGURE 3.5. *Electron microscopy of a longitudinal section of skeletal muscle. (Modified from Ultrastructural Changes in Diseased Muscle by A. G. Engel and B. Q. Banker, in Myology, edited by Andrew G. Engel and Clara Franzini-Armstrong, © 1994, McGraw-Hill, New York, figure 36-1, page 890.)*

PERIPHERAL NERVE (AXONS AND SCHWANN CELLS)

INST Examine a microscopic section of the spinal cord (see Fig. 3.6). The cord in the figure has been stained with Luxol fast blue, which stains myelin blue, in addition to hematoxylin and eosin (the old pathology workhorses). Clustered on the exterior of some segments are groups of blue-staining myelinated fibers. These represent the spinal roots, which are part of the peripheral nervous system.

Q3.5. Examine the roots at higher power (see Fig. 3.7). Describe the shape of the staining. Can you see any detail within the smallest blue structures? What do the structures represent?

A3.5. *The roots are bundles of many myelinated axons. In the H&E/LFB preparation, the myelin sheaths are like tiny dark donuts, and the axons are even smaller pink dots within the donut holes (more difficult to see in black and white: the myelin sheaths are dark-gray donuts while the axon each envelops is a light gray). Because of many different artifacts, not every myelin donut may have an axon in the slide, but these would have axons in life. This arrangement of myelin sheaths surrounding axons is typical both in nerves and within the central nervous system.*

In all histologic sections, artifacts are introduced during processing and staining. While the myelin sheaths may look fairly beat-up in your slides, in life they are really fine envelopes.

Q3.6. Examine a slide containing a peripheral nerve stained with Masson trichrome (see Fig. 3.8). This stain colors the myelin orange-red and collagen green. Identify the endoneurium, perineurium, and epineurium on the cross section of the nerve.

A3.6. *See Figure 3.9. On this type of section, in which the tissue has been put through formalin fixation, complete dehydration in alcohol, and embedded in hot paraffin, much of the fine nerve structure has been lost. In particular, the beautiful, finely wrapped myelin sheath has been reduced to spokes and slivers. You can nevertheless make out the major division of the nerve and get an idea of the number of large, myelinated fibers.*

Q3.7. On your slide and in Figure 3.10, notice the number of large myelinated fibers in the nerve. How well do you visualize the other types of axons? Compare the size of the vessels in the epineurium with those in the endoneurium. Where do you see collagen? On the longitudinal sections and in Figure 3.10, try to distinguish the myelin sheath around an axon from the axon itself. The myelin sheath is extremely vacuolated, since in life it is filled with lipids that are leached out by xylene in the tissue processing.

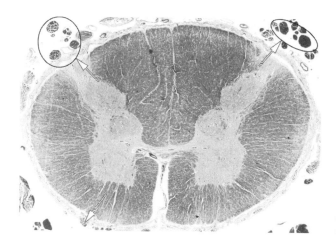

FIGURE 3.6. *Cross-sectional histology of upper lumbar spinal cord.*

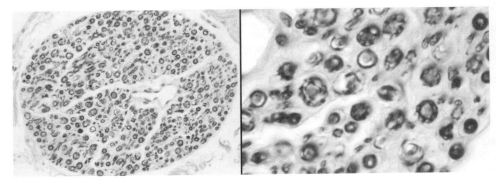

FIGURE 3.7. *Nerve root (H&E/ LFB stain). The left image is a low-power view, while the right is an enhanced high-power view.*

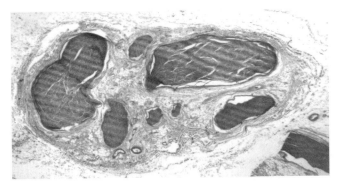

FIGURE 3.8. *Peripheral nerve cross section, stained with Masson trichrome stain.*

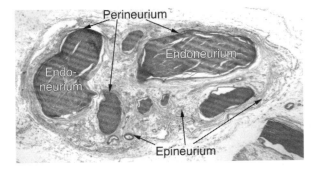

FIGURE 3.9. *Regional structures in a peripheral nerve.*

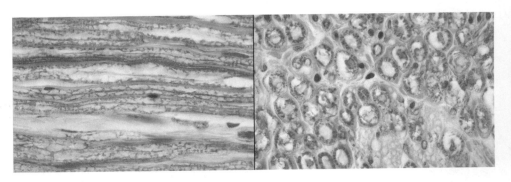

FIGURE 3.10. *High-power longitudinal (left) and cross-sectional views of peripheral nerve, stained with Masson trichrome stain. The axons have been accentuated on the left and the myelin sheaths accentuated on the right.*

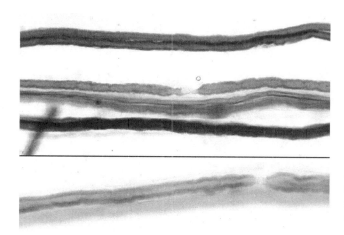

FIGURE 3.11. *Teased fiber preparation of peripheral nerve, stained with osmium to highlight myelin. The bottom photograph is at a slightly higher power than the upper.*

A3.7. Compared to the easily visualized large, myelinated axons, paraffin sections are nearly useless to look at the small unmyelinated fibers. The larger vessels are all contained in the epineurium; only capillaries, and the smallest arterioles are present in the endoneurial space. Collagen, which essentially holds the nerve together, is present in the endoneurium, perineurium, and epineurium. As in the LFB stain from the spinal cord, the myelin sheaths are like donuts around the axons.

Q3.8. Now examine the teased fiber microscopic slide preparation (Fig. 3.11) of a peripheral nerve. The slide has been painstakingly produced by separating out individual myelinated axons from a nerve bundle and then staining them with osmium. How long are individual Schwann cells, compared to their diameter? Does one axon have one Schwann cell, or many?

A3.8. Schwann cells are highly elongated cells that wrap the axon. While they may be 10 micrometers in diameter, they may extend up to a millimeter in length. Each Schwann cell wraps only one myelinated axon, while one axon is covered by many Schwann cells. In a demyelinating disease, loss of only one Schwann cell along the length of a single axon may lead to dramatic dysfunction of that axon. See Figure 3.12.

Q3.9. Figure 3.13 is a photomicrograph of the "thick section" of peripheral nerve. Describe the main components of a peripheral nerve.

A3.9. Several nerve fascicles are bound together with connective tissue and larger vessels to form the actual nerve. The big (black) blobs in the epineurium are droplets of fat. A larger vessel lies just off center in this figure. In addition to myelinated axons, nerve fascicles also contain capillaries and matrix material that glues all together. Each fascicle is composed of multiple myelinated fibers of various sizes, both large and small.

Q3.10. As a last look at nerve, examine the electron micrographs in Figure 3.14. Look first at the lower power figure and get a sense as to the types of fibers you can see. Would you say there are more large or small fibers? In the right panel compare the thickness of the myelin sheaths around larger and small axons. Explain how this feature would assist the axonal function. About how many fibers are unmyelinated versus myelinated? Which has the greatest total area in a peripheral nerve? Contrast the information conducted by myelinated and unmyelinated fibers.

A3.10. Assessing the number of small versus large fibers is nearly impossible at low power. To do this right at high power requires some sophisticated measuring techniques, since many small unmyelinated fibers are bundled together by single Schwann cells. What is clear is that the large, myelinated fibers occupy the largest area of the fascicle; it is these fibers that contribute the greatest extent to the nerve conduction studies (to be described in a subsequent chapter). The myelin thickness varies directly with the axon diameter. As larger diameter fibers conduct

Electron microscopy *When tissue is to be examined by electron microscopy, it is first fixed and then embedded in a plastic resin. This is stained and cut much thinner (one micrometer) than the usual paraffin block (four to eight micrometers or more), to choose the areas for further preparation. Finally, the tissue is cut extremely thin, laid on a fine copper grid, and coated lightly with a heavy metal. The metal grid acts as a conductor in the electron beam. The "one-micron" section is called a "thick section," in comparison to the ultra thin section examined under the electron microscope.*

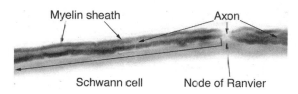

Myelin sheath   Axon

Schwann cell   Node of Ranvier

FIGURE 3.12. *Structures of individual myelinated axon in teased fiber preparation.*

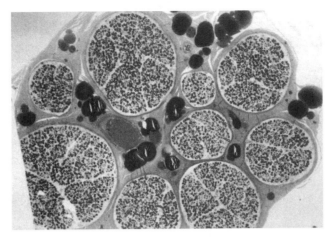

FIGURE 3.13. *Cross-section of peripheral nerve on a 1 micron-thick plastic section stained with Toluidine blue. (Modified from Biopsy Diagnosis of Peripheral Neuropathy by G. Midroni and J. M. Bilbao, © 1995, Butterworth-Heinemann, Boston, figure 2-2, page 15.)*

impulses faster, and thicker myelin also facilitates faster conduction, combining the two provides a maximal speed. Unmyelinated fibers, which conduct only slowly, represent about 50% of the axons in a peripheral nerve. These are the pain, temperature, and autonomic fibers, while the myelinated axons conduct motor and other sensory information.

SPINAL CORD

Q3.11. Examine again the microscopic section of spinal cord (see Figs. 3.15 and 3.16). Instead of focusing on the nerve roots, look at the cord itself. Look closely at the blue staining around the outside of the cord (see the squares in Fig. 3.15). What (hopefully) familiar tiny structures do you see in the myelinated areas? What do they look like? Can you guess the orientation of the structures (parallel or perpendicular)?

A3.11. *The spinal cord acts both as a major conduit of information going to and from the brain, as well as a local processing center for that information. The outer white matter ("blue matter" on the slide) is where the many long tracts lie. These by-and-large travel up and down the cord, and hence are oriented perpendicular to the slide. Just as in peripheral nerve, the white matter of the central nervous system is composed of myelinated axons, which also appear as blue donuts with pink centers on glass slides.*

Q3.12. Refocus your attention to the pinker areas within the center of the cord (see Fig. 3.17). Gray matter on an H&E stain appears pink, so this region is termed the

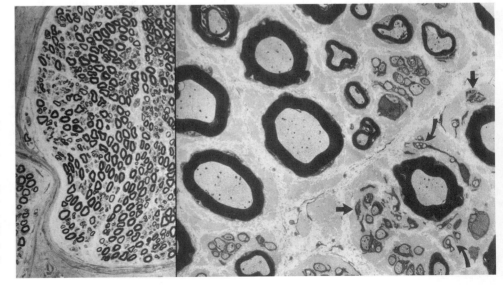

FIGURE 3.14. *Electron micrograph of a normal peripheral nerve, low power. (Left panel modified from Peripheral Nerve, by P. C. Johnson, in Textbook of Neuropathology, second edition, edited by R. L. Davis and D. M. Robertson, © 1991, Williams & Wilkins, Baltimore, figure 18.16, page 1015. Right panel modified from Biopsy Diagnosis of Peripheral Neuropathy by G. Midroni and J. M. Bilbao, © 1995, Butterworth-Heinemann, Boston, figure 2-8, page 21.)*

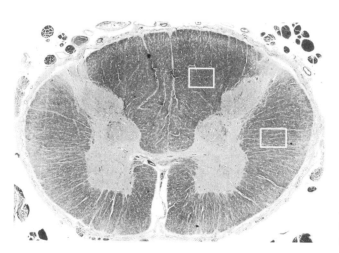

FIGURE 3.15. *Spinal cord histology, with squares on large white matter tracts.*

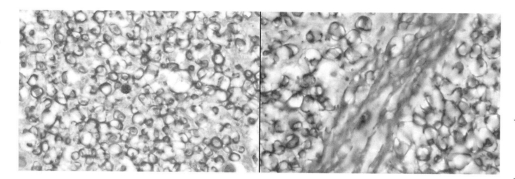

FIGURE 3.16. *Close-up histologic views of spinal white matter. The figure on the left has been slightly enhanced to show the axons within their myelin sheaths. On the right, a small bundle perpendicular to the main fibers lies in the middle of the image.*

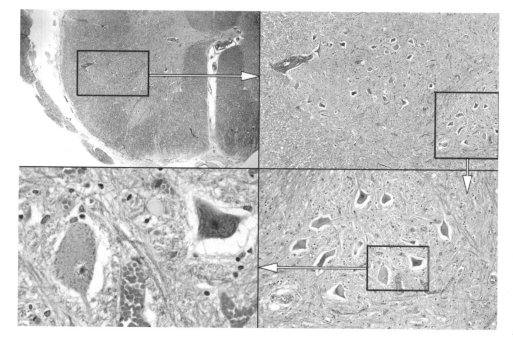

FIGURE 3.17. *Ventral horn of spinal cord, H&E/LFB stain. The images clockwise are at increasingly higher magnification, with boxes showing the approximate location of the next photograph.*

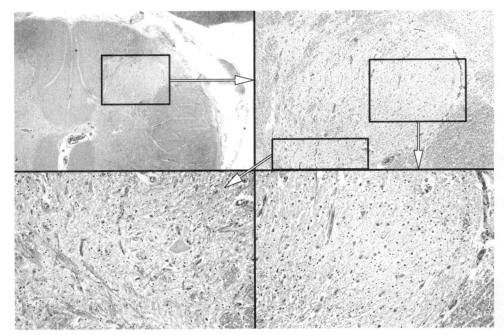

FIGURE 3.18. *Spinal cord dorsal horn, H&E/LFB stains, lower to higher powers clockwise. The dorsal horn contains multiple layers, each with different neuron types and projections.*

central gray (rather than the central pink, which sounds rather weak). On H&E stains, the synapses produced by unmyelinated axon terminals and dendrites, comprising the gray matter, stain as a fine pink and is termed neuropil. Some spinal sections will be larger (swellings) and represent either the cervical or lumbar enlargements. Look at the central gray in these, focusing on the larger ventral horn. How large are the largest neurons? The smallest? Specifically look at the myelin staining within and around the gray matter. How are the strands oriented now? What other cells are present in the gray matter?

A3.12. *The largest neurons are over 40 micrometers in diameter; they are big cells. You really can't be sure about the smallest neurons in the slide, since they can be close to the size of other small cells like oligodendroglia and endothelial cells. In the bottom-left photograph in Figure 3.17 these largest neurons are the lower motor neurons that innervate skeletal muscle.*

In contrast to the nearly universal perpendicular fibers in the outer tracts, the myelinated fibers in the gray matter have multiple orientations. They connect different regions of the spinal gray matter together. Specifically, they represent axonal connections from one neuron to another.

An important concept is that gray matter is not just a bunch of neurons, but that it contains dendrites and both myelinated and unmyelinated axons.

Q3.13. Examine the slide or Figure 3.18 to see how the cells in the gray matter change appearance from one portion to the next. Look at the smaller dorsal horn. Describe any cell groups you may see. How precise are they? What is the small cluster of cells in the center of the cord?

A3.13. *The spinal cord has several very distinct types of neurons. The huge cells with large nuclei and coarse cytoplasm on the ventral or anterior side are the* **motor neurons,** *while the smaller cells on the dorsal side are involved in processing sensory information. As you may have read in textbooks, the spinal cord is divided up into many* **lamina,** *which are really very long neuronal groups or nuclei (an unfortunate term, since "nucleus" may refer to both the chromosome-containing organelle of a cell as well as a collection of neurons).*

The concept of a "nucleus" will recur throughout this course. Individuals who study the brain tend to think of nuclei as little discrete boxes containing neurons and a bunch of wires. As you can see at first glance of the spinal cord gray matter, this black box concept is flawed. The boxes are not nice and neat, but rather blend with other adjacent parts, and themselves are composed of smaller sub-boxes. Nevertheless, the box concept has proved useful both clinically and scientifically.

Similarly the white matter is divided up into a series of tracts. But again, as you can see at a simple glance of the cord, the "tracts" blend imperceptibly into each other, and are by no

Neuropil *Gray matter. The term usually refers to the constituents outside immediate cell membranes, and includes synapses, dendrites, unmyelinated and myelinated axons, and the astroglial glue that holds it all together. At a light microscopic level it appears nearly uniform; only by electron microscopy can most of its components be distinguished.*

means discrete. While books and computer programs, including this manual, place nice circles over given tracts, you now know that this represents a gross human simplification of nature.

The small cluster of cells in the center of the cord is the ependymal remnant of the neural tube. No central canal remains, just broken lines of ependymal cells like stones from a fallen Roman temple.

NEURONS

Q3.14. As you have encountered in the spinal cord, the brain is made up of a plethora of different neuronal types. Examine a microscopic slide of the cerebellum. Focus only on the cortex (the convoluted outer portion; see Fig. 3.19). Describe the different types of cells present and where they are located. The brain is supposed to have axons connecting with dendrites. Where are these? Why can't you see these structures? Remember the color neuropil on H&E.

A3.14. *The cerebellar cortex has multiple neuron types, of varying sizes, shapes, and positions. See Figure 3.20. The smallest are the massive number of internal granular neurons, while the largest are the* **Purkinje cells,** *which lie only on the line dividing the granular layer from the outer "molecular" layer (a later chapter is devoted to the cerebellum).*

While all the different regions of the cerebellar cortex have their own types of connections, these are impossible to see in the slide. The slide has only been stained with agents that highlight either acidic or basic proteins. To see the connections, you would need a stain that is selective for the contents of neurons and their axons. To see the connections well, you would have to examine the tissue at a much greater power, using electron microscopy.

Q3.15. Compare the photomicrograph in Figure 3.21 of a Betz cell (the giant upper motor neurons in the cortex) with that of the cerebellar internal granular layer, taken at the same power. What is the size range of the neurons?

A3.15. *The puny internal granular neurons of the cerebellum may only be 6 to 7 micrometers across, while the gargantuan Betz cells range up to 100 micrometers. Thus the cell diameters differ over an order of magnitude and their volumes by well over three orders of magnitude.*

Q3.16. In Figure 3.22, contrast the dorsal root ganglion cell with the cerebellar Purkinje cell. What is the extension upward of material from the Purkinje cell?

A3.16. *The dorsal root ganglion cell has peripherally marginated (i.e., on the outer edge)* **Nissl substance** *and is huge. This cell body sustains axons that in some cases extend from the foot to the base of the brain. The Purkinje cell also sustains a long projection, but only within the*

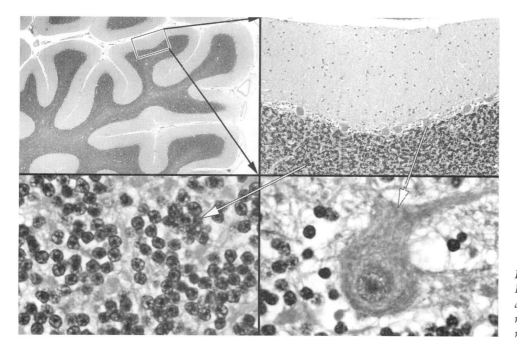

FIGURE 3.19. *Cerebellar cortex, H&E/LFB stains. The lower left image shows the internal granular neurons, while the right shows a Purkinje neuron.*

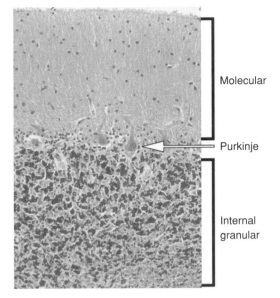

FIGURE 3.20. *Cerebellum cortical layers.*

cerebellum. *The long process extending from the Purkinje cell is its apical dendrite, which as you will see in a later laboratory, extends up into the cerebellar molecular layer. The small dark cells you see around the Purkinje cells are the same internal granular neurons you saw in the last question.*

Q3.17. Now examine the Golgi-stained preparation in Figure 3.23 of another Betz cell. (Even after a century, no one really knows how a Golgi stain works, so don't ask. Just know that a few of the neurons completely fill up with silver granules, out to their most distal processes, while others remain untouched.) Describe what you see. Can you identify the dendrites? Axon? How can you tell the difference (remember what makes them different)? How long is the axon? Does this fit into your preconceived notion of what a neuron looks like?

A3.17. *Golgi-stained sections of the brain have intrigued scientists for years, in large part for their beauty and detail. While it is easy to think of neurons as having dendrites at one end and an axon coming out the other, the Golgi stain reminds us just how simplistic this view is. The dendritic tree is truly*

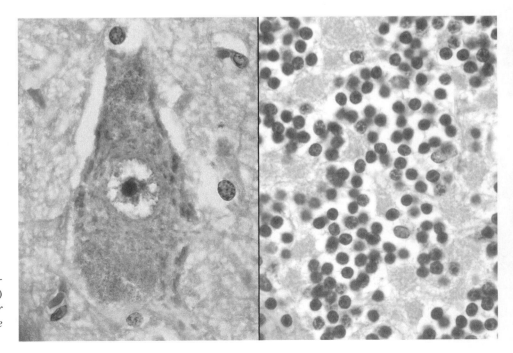

FIGURE 3.21. *Comparison between a cortical Betz neuron* (left) *with cerebellar internal granular neurons* (right), *taken at the same power. H&E stain.*

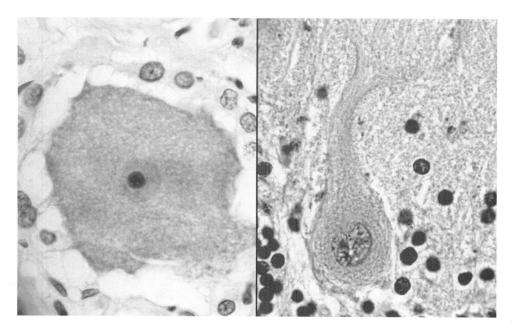

FIGURE 3.22. *Comparison between a dorsal root ganglion neuron* (left) *with a cerebellar Purkinje neuron* (right), *taken at the same power. H&E stain.*

a complex arborization of different units, located at different regions of the cell, and the axons may also branch. Dendrites may have many axons synapsing on them, and as in this Betz cell, may have knobs or spines at the sites of contact. In contrast, the lowly axon is devoid of spines. In this illustration the axon is the fiber coming out of the base of the cell body, just a bit to the left of center. Notice that it branches shortly after leaving the body. Axons can be extremely long. The one in the photograph extends well beyond the boundaries of the image and could extend down to the lower spinal cord.

OLIGODENDROGLIA

Q3.18. Oligodendrocytes are the central nervous system equivalent of Schwann cells. Re-examine the myelin-stained slide of the spinal cord and also examine a similar stain of cortical white matter (see Fig. 3.24). What do oligodendrocytes look like (they are

Oligodendrocytes *Myelinated axons in the central nervous system are ensheathed by oligodendrocyte membranes. Oligodendrocytes also provide support to axons and cluster around neuron cell bodies in gray matter.*

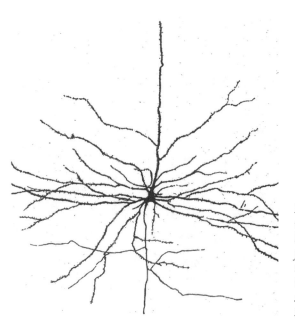

FIGURE 3.23. *Golgi-stained preparation of a Betz neuron, illustrated by Santiago Ramón y Cajal. (Modified from Histology of the Nervous System, volume II by Santiago Ramón y Cajal, reproduced by Oxford University Press, New York, © 1995, figure 370, page 468.)*

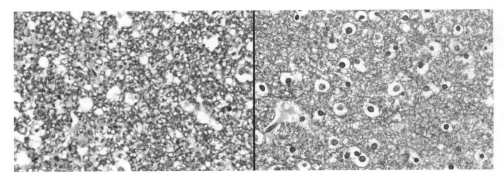

FIGURE 3.24. *White matter, H&E/ LFB. The left image is from the spinal cord, while the right is from below cortex. The enlargement of the subcortical nuclei on the right is probably due to the longer time it takes formalin to penetrate the thicker tissue and fix the tissue.*

Astrocytes *Interdigitating among all of the neurons and oligodendrocytes are the fingers of astrocytes. While neurons get most of the glory in the nervous system and the oligodendrocytes get best supporting actor, the astrocyte by contrast has until recently been relegated to a minor cast member, like a crowd that gathers around the king and queen. Our view of this cell is changing, as the astrocyte turns out to have many roles in brain function, including contributing to the blood-brain barrier and altering the extracellular matrix. Recently astrocytes have been shown to regulate neuronal synapses. More remains to be appreciated.*

the major cell in the white matter)? How does the spinal cord white matter differ from that in cortex?

A3.18. Oligodendrocyte morphology cannot really be appreciated on routine stains. In histological sections, they just appear as naked nuclei, small dark circles floating in a sea of blue. This primitive appearance belies their true complex form. In the spinal cord, oligodendroglial nuclei are few, the myelinated axons are large, and fibers in the columns are oriented together. In keeping with the (hopefully) more advanced functions of the cerebral cortex, myelinated axons in the subcortical white matter go in all directions.

Q3.19. To really appreciate the oligodendrocyte requires special techniques. Examine the immunofluorescence image in Figure 3.25 of oligodendrocytes in culture. The low-power left-hand image has been stained for O1, which stains a specific surface galactosyl-cerebroside of oligodendroglia, while the high-power right-hand image has been stained for myelin basic protein, a major constituent of myelin. How would you characterize the branches that extend from their cell body? Each branch represents the myelination of a different axon. Contrast this with a Schwann cell. Is the name "oligodendrocyte" appropriate?

A3.19. While oligodendrocytes got their name from having few processes [oligo — few + dendro — branch + cyte — cell], the older techniques used to examine them were insensitive to its true structure. Oligodendrocytes display a group of specific proteins; antibodies against these proteins clearly highlight the arborization of these cells. Today we know that a single oligodendrocyte wraps multiple axons within the central nervous system, in contrast to the single axon sheathed by a Schwann cell. On the routine myelin stains, all of the blue donuts around the pink axons are supplied by an oligodendrocyte somewhere.

ASTROCYTES

Q3.20. Examine again your spinal cord or cortex slide and look in the white matter for cell nuclei that have more "open" chromatin. These may be subtle and hard to find

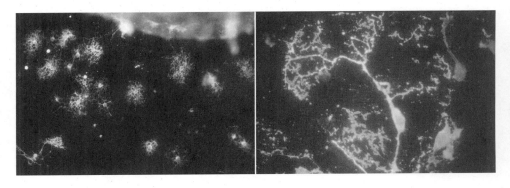

FIGURE 3.25. *Oligodendrocytes grown in culture. The left figure is a low-power image that has been stained for the antigen O1. The right is a higher power view that has been stained for myelin basic protein (MBP). (Images kindly provided by Dr. Timothy Vartanian.)*

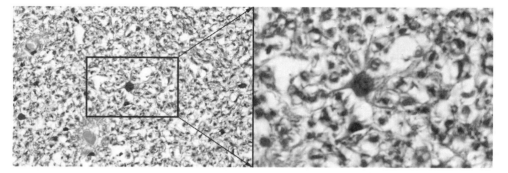

FIGURE 3.26. *Astrocytes in aged spinal cord. In order to obtain some contrast in these figures, the original photographs have been greatly enhanced to show the glial fibers around the nucleus.*

(see Fig. 3.26). Aside from the slightly larger nucleus and looser chromatin, how do these cells differ from oligodendrocytes? Any cytoplasm?

A3.20. *The astrocytes don't make myelin, but you can't really see myelin attached to oligodendrocytes on your slides. However, unlike oligodendrocytes, astrocytes may have fine wisps of pink-red cytoplasm around their nuclei. If your look really hard, and if your slide came from an aged brain, you may see that those pink fibers extend loosely over the background of the white matter, especially around vessels. These are glial fibers. They are similar to putting chicken wire in cement to make a stronger sidewalk.*

Q3.21. Examine the photomicrograph in Figure 3.27 taken from a region within an area of ischemia. Describe what you see. What are the features of the large cells in the center of the image?

A3.21. *The most easily visible cell is the astrocyte, the large cells with plump pink cytoplasm and pink processes. These cells have some extended processes, which will be better seen below. Other cells you may see are macrophages (discussed later).*

In addition to the ischemic damage in this case, astrocytes respond to many other types of injuries to neurons and axons, like Samurai protecting the Shogun.

Q3.22. The image in Figure 3.28 is another immunoperoxidase stain, this time using an antibody raised against the major intermediate filament in astrocytes, glial fibrillary acidic protein (GFAP). Why have these cells been given their name? Where is the GFAP staining, in addition to that around the cell bodies?

A3.22. *As you may have guessed, astrocytes derive their name from their similar appearance to stars. The GFAP stains emphasizes this dramatically. As astrocytes respond to various types of injury, they synthesize abundant GFAP and then distribute the intermediate filament out their long rays into the surrounding brain matrix, thus providing at least some additional support. While astrocytes support neurons and their processes, the glial scar that develops after a central nervous system injury also inhibits regrowth of axons.*

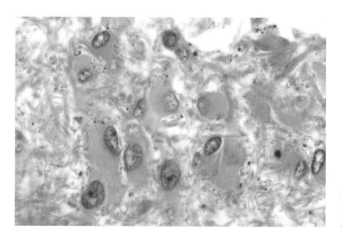

FIGURE 3.27. *Reactive astrocytes, enhanced H&E. These astrocytes were adjacent to a recent cerebral infarct.*

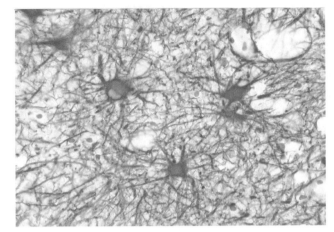

FIGURE 3.28. *Reactive astrocytes, glial fibrillary acidic protein immunostain.*

EPENDYMA

Ependyma *The epithelial ependymal cells line the ventricular wall and provide a loose barrier between the brain parenchyma and the CSF. These specialized glial cells allow a largely free exchange between the CSF and the brains extracellular matrix.*

Q3.23. In adults the ependyma lining of the ventricles may become denuded, either by wear and tear or artifactually from too much handling. Look at your glass slide of the caudate nucleus or hippocampus. Some ependyma should remain along the ventricular surfaces in both sections. How would you describe these cells? Squamous, cuboidal, columnar? Do you see any cilia? Now compare them with the image in Figure 3.29, taken from a 38-week-gestation infant. How do these ependymal cells differ from those in the adult?

A3.23. *The ependyma in an adult are usually a lining of cuboidal epithelial cells having cilia extending into the ventricle. These cells do not provide a significant barrier to the ventricular space, equivalent to the blood-brain barrier. Chemotherapeutic agents that don't cross the blood-brain barrier may be administered within the ventricle using catheters.*

In a fetus, the central canal remains open for a variable period, and then closes as the infant matures. Prior to closure the ependyma have a more columnar or pseudostratified morphology. In the adult, these cells remain in the central part of the spinal cord.

CHOROID PLEXUS

Choroid plexus *Cells of the choroid plexus use selective components of arterial blood to produce CSF.*

Q3.24. Examine the microscopic slide of hippocampus and Figure 3.30, which contains some choroid plexus. Depending on the age of the patient, you may see a variable amount of dark-staining junk. What is this stuff? Examine the structure of the plexus and the relationship between the lining epithelial cells and the blood vessels. How would you describe the cells lining the choroid plexus? Squamous, cuboidal, or what? Describe the layers from the surface to the vessels.

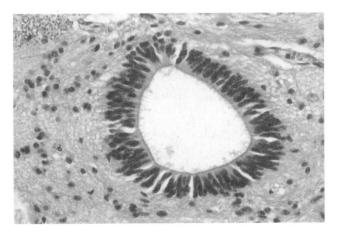

FIGURE 3.29. *Central canal taken from a 38-week-gestation infant spinal cord. The child died two weeks after birth from a profound muscle disorder.*

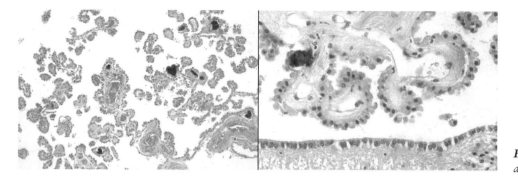

FIGURE 3.30. *Choroid plexus, low- and high-power views.*

A3.24. The choroid plexus is a tissue having a classic papillary structure: fingers containing a fibrovascular core and lined with epithelial cells. The plexus epithelium is cuboidal; pathologists would say "hob-nailed," although no one uses hob-nails anymore. These lie on a basement membrane. Between this membrane and the actual vessel is a variable amount of collagenous connective tissue.

As you age, several parts of your brain typically mineralize. These include the choroid plexus and the pineal gland. Something to look forward to during your long years of study. In the good old days before modern imaging, these crunchy spots were used to help localize brain lesions on X-rays.

VESSELS

Q3.25. Like other organs in the body, the brain requires energy, nutrients, and a method of waste disposal. All aspects of the nervous system have a full complement of vessels. Re-examine the spinal cord microscopic slide once again (see Fig. 3.31). Where are the largest vessels? How can you distinguish between an artery and a vein?

A3.25. In the spinal cord, the largest vessels are exterior to the parenchyma. The cord has a single ventral (anterior) artery and vein, which you can see just in front of the ventral horns containing the lower motor neurons. The artery has organized smooth muscle layers in its walls and a distinct internal elastic lamina. The wall of a vein is looser and lacks the prominent internal elastic lamina.

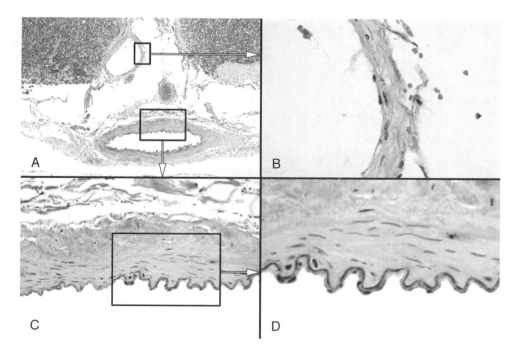

FIGURE 3.31. *Spinal vessels, H&E/LFB stain. A is a field view of the ventral spinal cord. B is the wall of a vein, while C and D are closer views of an arterial wall. B and D are at the same power. The dark wavy band in D is the internal elastic lamina.*

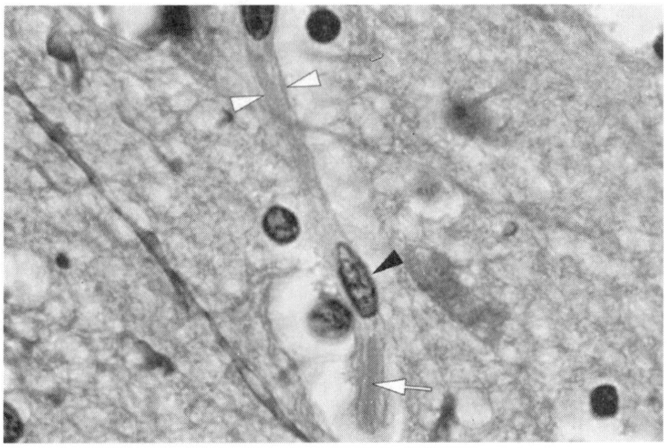

FIGURE 3.32. *Capillary, H&E/ LFB. An endothelial nucleus is marked with a black arrowhead and a red cell is marked with an arrow. The image has been enhanced to show the delicate capillary; a glass slide and a microscope are much better for viewing capillaries.*

Q3.26. Try to find some capillaries (see Fig. 3.32). Where do you find them? How are they distinguished from the larger vessels, aside from size?

A3.26. *Capillaries, which have no smooth muscle around them, are normally difficult to see. They may be clearly identified when they have a red blood cell within their lumen, as in Figure 3.32. Careful examination of any brain section will reveal many capillaries and small vessels distributed throughout the parenchyma.*

Microglia and Macrophages
Macrophages and their central nervous system resident equivalent, the microglia, are the trash collectors of the nervous system. They identify the garbage or damaged tissue, tell their bosses the lymphocytes about it, and then clean it up. These cells are one type of immune cell that may contribute substantially to inflammatory diseases such as infections or multiple sclerosis. Both of these cell types derive from bone marrow and both can phagocytose and digest dead brain tissue.

MICROGLIA AND MACROPHAGES

Q3.27. Examine the photomicrographs of a cerebral infarct in Figure 3.33 that has had time to partially organize. Notice the serpiginous border of the infarct in the low-power view. Describe the cells in the high-power view. Do they have distinct cytoplasmic border, or are they blurred? Some capillaries are also present in this view.

A3.27. *The infarct at this stage (about two weeks) is filled with macrophages. Most of the myelin has been digested by the macrophages; only a few have remaining dark-staining material. Macrophages classically have a distinct cell border, an eccentric nucleus, and foamy cytoplasm containing whatever they had phagocytosed. Capillaries have elongated and skinny nuclei in their endothelial cells. A close look at the artery in the bottom of the low-power figure will show thromboembolic material in its lumen.*

Q3.28. Now examine macrophages in Figure 3.34. The left figure is from the center of a three week old cerebral infarct, while the right is from a case of sarcoidosis. They are both taken at the same microscopic power. Describe what the macrophages look like. What organelle forms the bubbly material in the cytoplasm of the cells on the left? How does the cell on the right differ from those on the left?

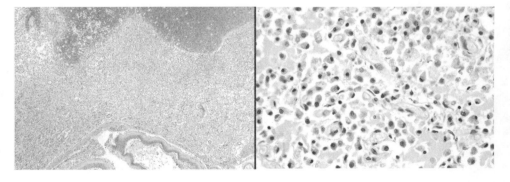

FIGURE 3.33. *Organizing embolic cerebral infarct, LFB/H&E stain. In the low-power view on the left, the remaining myelinated white matter is dark. The right panel is a high-power view of the same area.*

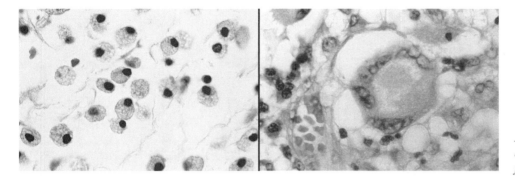

FIGURE 3.34. *Macrophages from a later organizing infarct* (left) *and from a case of sarcoidosis* (right).

A3.28. Activated macrophages in the left picture have a large, bubbly cytoplasm filled with lysosomes. The nucleus is round and slightly eccentric. At this stage, the lysosomes are filled with myelin debris, and hence may stain blue with the LFB stain. Later, the myelin breakdown products will loose their tinctorial properties and no longer stain. Some blood products may also be engulfed by the macrophages and end up as a relatively indigestible orange-yellow product, **hemosiderin.** *These cells do the major clean up of necrotic tissue in the central nervous stem. They are the sanitation engineers of the brain.*

The cell on the right is really a mass of macrophages that has fused to form a multinucleated giant cell. It differs from the usual macrophage in having multiple nuclei and being huge (hence the name). These are typically associated with "granulomatous diseases," such as sarcoidosis, tuberculosis, yeast infections, and foreign materials.

LYMPHOCYTES

Q3.29. Examine the photomicrograph in Figure 3.35, which is from a patient who died following Herpes encephalitis. Lymphocytes are somewhat disparagingly called "small round blue cells." Where are the lymphocytes in the photograph? Postulate why they accumulate at this site.

A3.29. In many types reactive brain diseases, lymphocytes cluster around blood vessels. Such perivascular lymphocytes accumulate at this site for several possible reasons. Lymphocytes in the brain originate from the blood and extravasate through the vessel walls. The Virchow-Robin space around the arteries, which is essentially topologically equivalent to the subarachnoid space, tracks down around vessels into the brain. Lymphocytes in this site, as in Figure 3.35, are nearly equivalent to having them in the subarachnoid space. Brain contacts with lymphocytes are first made in this region.

The brain normally contains few lymphocytes. However, in an inflammatory brain disease like Herpes encephalitis and multiple sclerosis, many of these lymphocytes leave the Virchow-Robin space and infiltrate brain. Since their nuclei are about the same size as oligodendroglial

Lymphocytes *These main effector cells of the immune system occasionally wander through normal brain.*

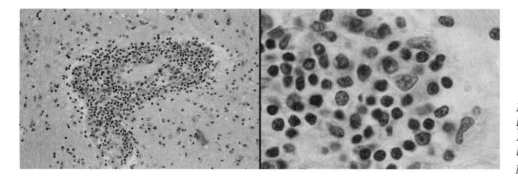

FIGURE 3.35. *Perivascular cuffs of lymphocytes in Herpes encephalitis, LFB/H&E stain. The left image is a low-power view, while the right is high power.*

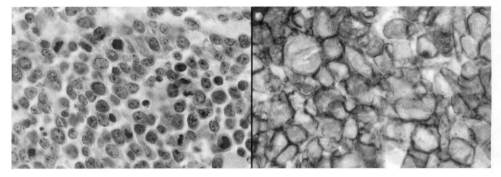

FIGURE 3.36. *High-power view of a primary central nervous system lymphoma. The left panel is a regular H&E stain, while the right is a slightly higher-power view immunostained for B-lymphocytes, using an antibody against the CD20 antigen.*

Virchow-Robin Space *The largest vessels supplying the brain remain primarily on the exterior surface. As these vessels branch and enter the parenchyma, they essentially retain their exterior topology and remain separated from the parenchyma by a pial barrier. This space between the vessel's adventia and the pia is named the Virchow-Robin space. It is an important site for specific inflammatory and neoplastic brain diseases.*

nuclei, an occasional, non-clustered lymphocyte may only be reliably recognized with special stains.

Q3.30. Examine Figure 3.36, which comes from a brain biopsy of a patient with a primary brain lymphoma. How do the cells in the left panel differ from those presented in Figure 3.35? Give several features. What does the right panel tell you?

A3.30. *These cells are larger than normal lymphocytes. They are also more "atypical," having coarser chromatin and irregular nuclear borders. Finally, frequent mitotic figures are scattered around the image. The right panel shows peripheral, nonnuclear staining for the B-cell marker CD20, which demonstrates that this tumor has a B-lymphocyte lineage. Essentially all primary central nervous system lymphomas derive from B-lymphocytes.*

POLYMORPHONUCLEAR LEUKOCYTES

Neutrophils *Otherwise called polymorphonuclear leukocytes or more affectionately "polys," are never a normal inhabitant of the brain parenchyma (although they pass through the vessels). Their presence always indicates disease, usually involving acute tissue destruction.*

Q3.31. The macroscopic photograph in Figure 3.37 (accurately called gross in this case) is from a case of acute bacterial meningitis. What has happened to the leptomeninges? Look especially at the close-up in the right panel. In what space is the purulent exudate (otherwise known as pus)?

A3.31. *The purulent exudate is in the subarachnoid space, which is best seen in the right coronal section. The pus surrounds the major arteries and pia mater over the surface of the brain, giving it a cloudy color. Release of inflammatory mediators by this inflammation can lead to vascular spasm and secondary brain ischemia.*

Q3.32. Now examine the photomicrograph in Figure 3.38. What is the predominant cell type? Where are they located?

A3.32. *In acute bacterial meningitis (or purulent meningitis), and other acute or necrotizing infections, polymorphonuclear leukocytes (also termed neutrophils or more affectionately "polys") are the predominant cell type. These cells ingest or phagocytize bacteria and also release a panoply of reactive radicals that destroy the invaders. The reactions may also seriously injure the underlying delicate brain. In an acute case, the polys are confined to the subarachnoid space. In*

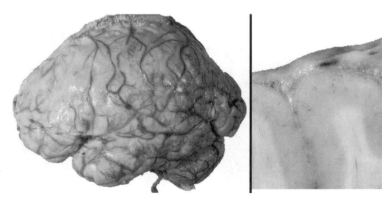

FIGURE 3.37. *Acute bacterial meningitis, lateral view and close-up of coronal section.*

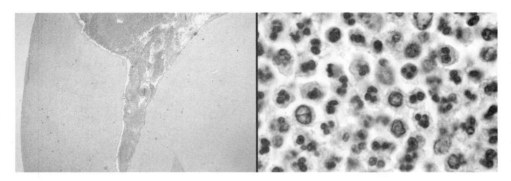

FIGURE 3.38. Low- and high-power photomicrographs of acute bacterial meningitis.

more necrotizing lesions, such as abscesses or fungal infections, the polys may also be within the brain.

CLINICAL CASE STUDY: PROGRESSIVE MULTIFOCAL LEUKOENCEPHALOPATHY (PML)

The patient was a 41-year-old man who contracted HIV seven years before his demise. His last CD4 count was 38 and the viral load was 130,000 per mL. In late September he presented with a clumsy and weak left hand. A lumbar puncture was normal, without cells. JC virus was identified by PCR in his cerebrospinal fluid. These features, combined with his MRI were considered diagnostic of progressive multifocal leukoencephalopathy (PML).

At the end of October, the patient was mildly inattentive, was unable to write his name, and had a prominent neglect of left hemispace; at one point he mistook the examiner's hand as his own. He had left upper motor neuron facial weakness. Motor examination showed a densely flaccid left hemiparesis. His reflexes were increased on the left side including a Babinski sign. By November, he was unable to visualize two fingers in his right hemifield. The patient expired at the end of November.

Q3.33. Examine the coronal view in Figure 3.39 showing a close-up view of his brain at autopsy. What do you see? What type of brain tissue is affected? What has happened to it?

A3.33. *The predominant injury is in his white matter. The gray matter is remarkably spared. Essentially, portions of this patient's white matter were nearly completely destroyed by the viral infection. Most of the cells in the white matter had undergone necrosis by the time of the autopsy. PML is white matter disease, hence the name "leukoencephalopathy."*

Q3.34. Now examine the giant section in Figure 3.40. This giant but very thin section of tissue has been stained for myelin with Luxol fast blue (dark) and with H&E (gray). Describe what you see. Is the injury bilateral? Symmetrical? Is some white

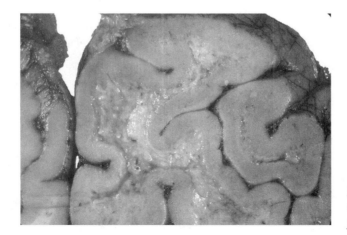

FIGURE 3.39. Close-up coronal view of progressive multifocal leukoencephalopathy.

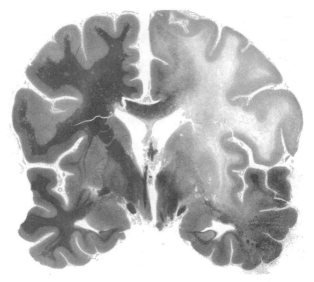

FIGURE 3.40. *Giant histologic coronal section of progressive multifocal leukoencephalopathy stained with Luxol fast blue for myelin (dark) and hematoxylin-eosin for cortex (gray). The right side of brain is on the right side of the figure.*

matter spared? Does the site of the lesion correspond to his dense flaccid left hemiparesis?

A3.34. *Where the myelin should be blue, it is pale. In this brain much of the white matter has no remaining myelin, and hence isn't white in the gross brain or blue in the myelin stain. As might be expected for an infectious process, the demyelination is not symmetrical and patches of myelin remain. You may be able to see some islands of demyelination in the opposite hemisphere, corresponding to new colonies of viruses. In some diseases, especially inherited diseases, the injury is symmetrical, but in most acquired diseases, especially infectious diseases, the damage is asymmetrical.*

The patient's dense left hemiparesis correlates with the massive involvement of the right hemisphere.

Q3.35. Look at the microscopic slide, or see Figure 3.41, which has also been stained with LFB and H&E. What do you see? What has happened to the myelin? How would you describe these lesions?

A3.35. *PML is a demyelinating disease, in which the viruses infect oligodendrocytes, reproduce in their nuclei, and kill the cell. The brain is basically like a culture dish, with viral colonies growing at different locations in the white matter, producing viral plaques. These plaques represent areas of oligodendrocyte death and demyelination.*

Q3.36. Now examine the microscopic slide at high power (see Fig. 3.42). What cells do you see in the center of large plaques (panel *B*)? What are the cells that contain round vacuoles filled with myelin (panel *D*)? Look at the uninvolved myelin. Examine the size of the oligodendrocyte nuclei. Compare them with the nuclear sizes at the periphery of a demyelinated plaque (panel *C*). What cell type is missing from this viral infection?

A3.36. *As the viruses replicate in the oligodendrocyte, its nucleus enlarges and become filled with viral particles (see panel* C; *the small nuclei are about the size of normal oligodendroglial nuclei).*

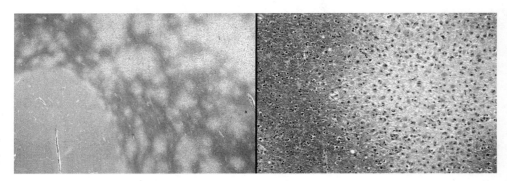

FIGURE 3.41. *PML field view. The left panel is a low-power view, while the right is at an intermediate power.*

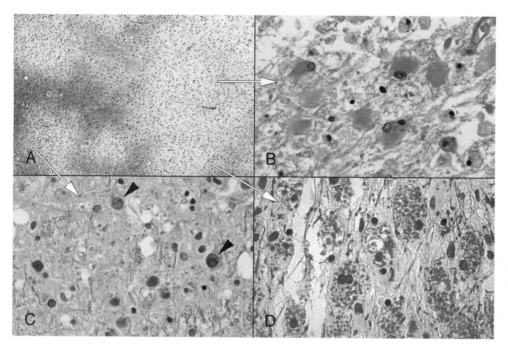

FIGURE 3.42. *Cell of progressive multifocal leukoencephalopathy. Panel A is a low-power view showing several plaques. Panel B is a high-power view from the center of a plaque. Panel C is from the white matter at the edge of a plaque (arrowheads on infected oligodendroglial nuclei). Panel D is at the edge just inside a plaque.*

When the oligodendrocytes die, their myelin sheaths degenerate and the various myelin proteins are engulfed and digested by macrophages (panel D). Although not readily apparent on this slide, the axons are initially spared by the disease, even though useful transmitted information is limited. Astrocytes and macrophages are the main cell types remaining in the plaque. Macrophages are greatest in areas of most active demyelination, while astrocytes are the survivors in the plaque centers. These latter cells may also be infected, but are not killed. The astrocytes take on a "reactive" appearance and lay down a matrix of GFAP, in a vain attempt to hold together a crumbling building.

The missing cell is the lymphocyte. Because AIDS and other immunocompromised patients have defective or missing T cells, they may essentially mount no immune response to the virus, which then replicates unchecked, eventually killing the patient. Other patients may be able to produce a variable lymphocytic and plasma cell response to this virus.

Q3.37. Examine Figure 3.43, which is a photomicrograph from the edge of one of the lesions. The tissue has been immunostained with an antibody against Papova viral epitopes. Arrowheads point to normal (noninfected) oligodendroglia. Where is the staining?

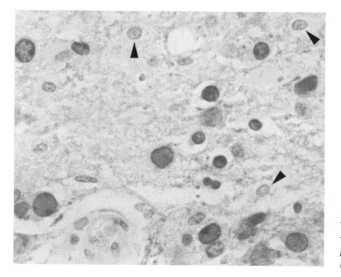

FIGURE 3.43. *Immunoperoxidase staining against Papova virus from a plaque edge in progressive multifocal leukoencephalopathy.*

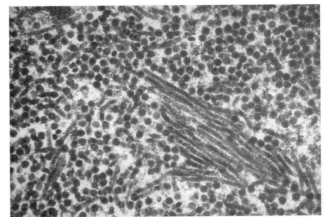

FIGURE 3.44. *Electron micrograph of an infected oligodendrocyte in progressive multifocal leukoencephalopathy.*

How do the stained cells compare with the uninfected cells? Where does the virus replicate?

A3.37. *The antibody was raised against the JC virus, which is the etiologic agent that produces PML. It shows nuclear staining, as might be expected, since this is where the virus replicates. Such immunostaining can confirm the diagnosis and helps define the type of viral infection.*

Q3.38. Finally, examine the electron micrograph in Figure 3.44 of an oligodendrocyte nucleus in a case of PML. What do you see? What shape are the viral particles? Is this what you might have expected from a viral infection?

A3.38. *Figure 3.44 contains densely packed virions. In PML, like all papova virus infections, the virions are found primarily in the nucleus, often in crystalline arrays. The particles are more or less spherical in shape. However, many elongated forms are also present. These represent "failed" particles, particles that failed to correctly incorporate their small ring of DNA into a compact protein shell. Nature is not always as neat and clean as it is supposed to be.*

REVIEW WORKSHEETS: CELLS OF THE NERVOUS SYSTEM

Cross section

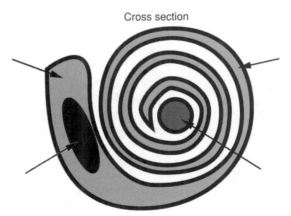

FIGURE 3.45. *Peripheral nerve cross section. Label indicated structures. How many axons does a single Schwann cell ensheathe?*

Longitudinal

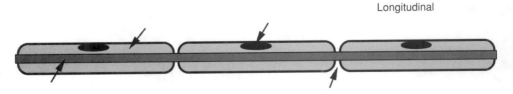

FIGURE 3.46. *Longitudinal peripheral nerve. Label.*

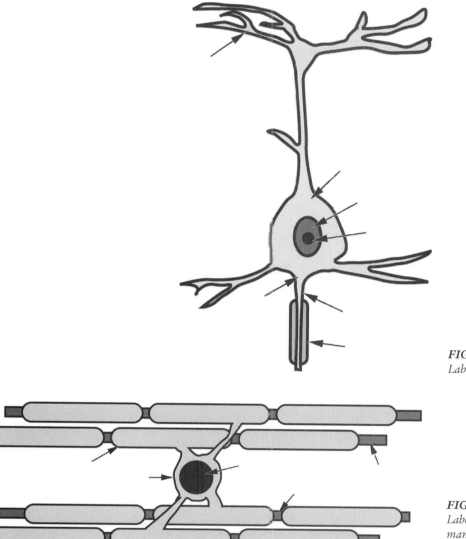

FIGURE 3.47. *Pyramidal neuron. Label indicated structures.*

FIGURE 3.48. *Oligodendrocyte. Label the indicated structures. How many axons does this oligodendrocyte ensheathe?*

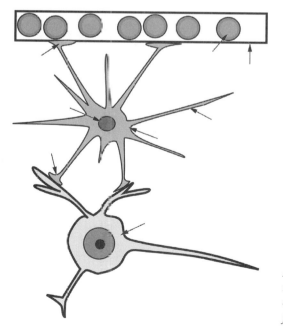

FIGURE 3.49. *Astrocyte. Label the indicated structures. Name three structures that receive the astrocyte endfeet.*

Chapter 4——NEUROIMAGING

While you have so far examined actual brains and pictures of brains, you hopefully won't be doing this too often on your future patients. However, at times you may wish that you could, to help you understand their diseases. Radiology is the next best thing (Although neuropathologists don't like to admit this, sometimes imaging is superior to real brain slices.)

In this laboratory you will examine several different types of imaging, each of which has its strengths and weaknesses. The laboratory only covers the basics of neuroimaging. In the remainder of the course you will be introduced to other more advanced techniques, most of which build on the fundamentals presented in this laboratory. Conventional angiography, which has been significantly supplanted by magnetic resonance angiography, receives excessive attention here because it illustrates so exquisitely the brain's vasculature.

Every generation of clinicians remembers the good old days when they had to make do with more primitive tools. The radiological tools presented in this laboratory will undoubtedly be considered primitive in your future. However, we live now and not later, and the brain will not change, at least for a while. Note: Much of the material in this laboratory was generously made available by Dr. Ellen Grant.

LEARNING OBJECTIVES

- Describe and contrast the basic principles underlying X-ray imaging (including CT scans and angiograms) and magnetic resonance imaging.
- Identify the main brain structures visualized in a CT scan.
- Identify the main brain structures visualized in an MRI scan. Contrast the different structures seen in T1 and T2 images.
- Identify the main cerebral vessels imaged in both angiograms and in MRA scans.
- Describe the technical and clinical advantages and limitations of CT scans, MRI scans, angiograms, and MRA imaging.
- Relate the neuroimaging to both the brain models as well as the brain itself, including the cerebral circulation.

INTRODUCTION

Our current structural imaging arsenal is based on a few physical principles. In this laboratory we will investigate two of these: penetration of X-rays in tissue and the precession of a proton in a

Functional Neuroanatomy: An Interactive Text and Manual, by Jeffrey T. Joseph and David L. Cardozo
ISBN 0-471-44437-5 Copyright © 2004 John Wiley & Sons, Inc.

magnetic field. Other techniques that we will not consider further, but that are clinically useful, include sound wave penetration of tissue (ultrasound) and release of different types of radiation by chemicals injected into the body (e.g., positron emission tomography or PET, single photon emission computed tomography or SPECT).

X-rays penetrate different tissue types to different degrees. Tissues containing heavier metals (e.g., calcium in bone, iron in blood) absorb more X-rays, lighter tissues absorb less, and air absorbs the least. It is the contrast in X-ray absorption between two media that we visualize by X rays.

The problem with the brain is that it is encased in bone. The intensity of radiation required to get through this bone limits our ability to distinguish the fine differences in absorption in the brain itself. In plain films of the skull, a staple in older medicine, very little of the brain was imaged well. Only sites that calcified or lesions that altered the skull were clearly seen. Pneumoencephalograms (ask an older neurologist about them), produced by injecting air into the ventricular system, were used to increase the contrast (remember, it is the difference between two media that you see).

CT (*computerized tomography*) circumvents many of the problems of plain films by using mathematical computations and more sensitive electronic sensors rather than film (chemical reactions). In a CT scanner, multiple angles of X rays penetrate the brain and are picked up by multiple sensors. Through a series of mathematical transformations, this information is reconstructed to produce an image. It is the difference in X-ray penetration of gray and white matter that allows them to be distinguished by CT scans. Since the two types of tissue don't differ greatly in radiation penetration, they still can only be moderately distinguished in the best CT scans. Because of the increased sensitivity and response of the electronic sensors, the computer can modify the projection to embellish specific features. The use of "bone windows" to look for fractures is an example. Bone still gets in the way; where it is thickest (e.g., posterior fossa, spine) the CT scan produces the poorest images.

The advantage of *magnetic resonance imaging (MRI)* is that chemical information, not radiation penetration, is used to differentiate tissues. If you remember back to your college chemistry, NMR was used to determine the chemistry of the proton. Slight differences in how the proton gives off radiation to the surrounding molecules allows the MRI to produce an image of the brain. Because we are really a big vat of Brownian motion, it is impossible to directly examine the radiation emitted by protons. To circumvent this problem, a very small percentage of the protons are lined up together in an immense magnet. They are then perturbed by pulses of radio waves. As they line back up, they emit more coherent radiation that can be detected. (Remembering back to college physics, changing magnetic fields produce an electric field and changing electric fields produce a magnetic field.)

Compared to NMR used in chemical analysis, much of the chemical information in MRI is ignored. Two main features are typically examined, the T1 and T2 "relaxation times." To use MRI scans, you don't really have to understand a bit about what these two terms mean. But once in your careers you should at least hear that T1 represents the time constant for the proton to realign itself with the magnetic field and T2 represents the time constant for the decay of the component perpendicular to the field. How they release this tiny bit of energy in part depends on the chemistry of the surrounding tissues, and it is these differences that allow you to see anything on a scan. An important point to remember is that although the energy differences produced by an individual proton are ridiculously small, we have and even more absurdly large number of protons in the small amount of tissue to make the signal detectable (remember Avogadro's number?). Even then, the detection in only in parts per million.

We can't go into how an MRI image is actually created, which would require advanced physics. Dr. William Copen has kindly provided a more detailed explanation in an appendix. Suffice it to say that the image is produced by a set of perpendicular radio wave gradients that are added onto the large magnetic field inside the magnet. So within the magnet's bore, various types of coils are placed around the patient's head to produce the radio frequency gradients and pick up the radio signals from the protons.

Various parlor tricks allow special types of tissue information to be acquired. *FLAIR* (*fluid-attenuated inversion recovery*) images use select sequences of radio frequency pulses to suppress the signal generated by fluids, notably cerebrospinal fluid. This technique accentuates the differences between normal and inflamed or edematous tissue. *Magnetic resonance angiography (MRA),* uses blood flow itself to produce an image of the vasculature. Normally moving objects don't image properly in MRIs since the protons have moved from where you labeled them to where they give off their energy. It is this information that is used and not wasted in MRA.

Last but not least, brain imaging uses a feature of most brain injuries to give greater delineation of the pathology. Normally contrast agents are of little use in the brain, since they can't cross the blood-brain barrier. However, in cases where tissue damage has occurred, say in a stroke, around a tumor, or in an active multiple sclerosis plaque, the blood-brain barrier breaks down. Contrast agents can now enter the tissue (at a low level) and can be imaged. X-rays, including CT scans, use contrast agents that are much more radio-opaque than normal tissue (e.g., iodine, barium). For MRI, agents are used that greatly shorten the T1 relaxation times of the protons, and so increase their signals. The typical agent for MRI is the rare earth (and expensive) element gadolinium.

INSTRUCTOR NOTES

This laboratory is the student's first formal introduction to neuroimaging. The main aim here remains neuroanatomy, not technique per se. But since students will much more likely view scans in their future, rather than slices of brain, it is key that they be able to recognize the anatomy on imaging.

Although the students have not yet formally covered horizontal brain sections, it will still be good to have them figure out the basic horizontal anatomy using their atlases. We're not asking for subthalamic nucleus on neuroimaging, just the basics.

Schedule (2.5 hours)
10   Plain film
30   CT
30   Angiogram
60   MRI
20   MRA

PLAIN FILM

Q4.1. Figure 4.1 is an almost historic view of the brain. The lateral view has an artifact on its left side. First try to discern the eye sockets and nasal passages. Explain how the sinuses are imaged so well. Can you see any brain? Can you identify the middle ear? Pituitary fossa? Spinal canal?

A4.1. *X-ray images reveal tissue contrasts in radio density. Sinus cavities, being filled with air, strongly contrast to bone, which is composed of a matrix of radio-opaque calcium salts. It is really difficult to say anything about the brain itself, except that its shell is intact. Within brain the X-ray absorption is much the same everywhere and similar to water. The pituitary fossa in the lateral view is the down-pointing dimple in the base of the middle cranial fossa, midway between the eyes and the ears. The middle ear, being filled with air, also shows well on these scans. Lastly, although you can't see the cord, you can see its vertebral protection and can visualize its path.*

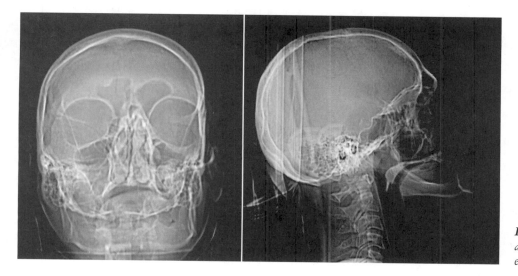

FIGURE 4.1. *Plain film of skull, anterior-posterior (AP) left and lateral right.*

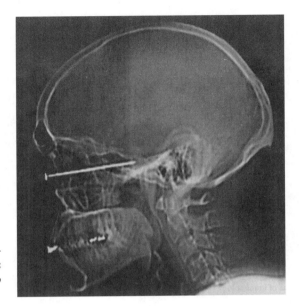

FIGURE 4.2. *Lateral plane skull X-ray. (Modified from W. X. Shandera & A. Hayman 2001. Nail injury to the skull. N Engl J Med 345: 339.)*

In the "old days" radiologists injected air into the CSF space to create an artificial contrast in the brain. As you can imagine, pneumoencephalograms were neither pleasant to administer nor to receive. In older patients the pineal and choroid plexus often are calcified and could act as landmarks in the plain film.

Q4.2. Examine the image in Figure 4.2. Suggest two possibilities about what you are seeing (real and possible artifact). What neuroanatomic structures could be close to the tip of this missile? If you had one more plain film to take, how could you answer this neuroanatomic question?

A4.2. *This carpenter had a nail driven into his face by someone else using a nail gun. From just this lateral view, you could be seeing this nail in the middle of his skull or you may be seeing it to one side or the other. You would need at least one more plain film to determine this. Just as in a CT scan (see below), the more angles you examine, the greater your anatomic resolution. The nail tip looks as though it is just millimeters from the pituitary fossa and a centimeter or so in front of the brainstem.*

The nail entered in the patient's left medial orbit and lodged in the sinuses and soft tissues below the skull base. It was removed and the patient suffered no sequelae.

CT SCAN

Normal CT Scans

INST Examine the normal CT scans in Figure 4.3. First try to determine the plane of the images on your own head and a model of the skull. Use landmarks you already know to guide you (e.g., eyes, ears).

Q4.3. On Figure 4.3 label the following structures:
- Cerebellum
- Fourth ventricle
- Medulla
- Pons
- Midbrain
- Aqueduct
- Pituitary
- Third ventricle
- Thalamus
- Lateral ventricle

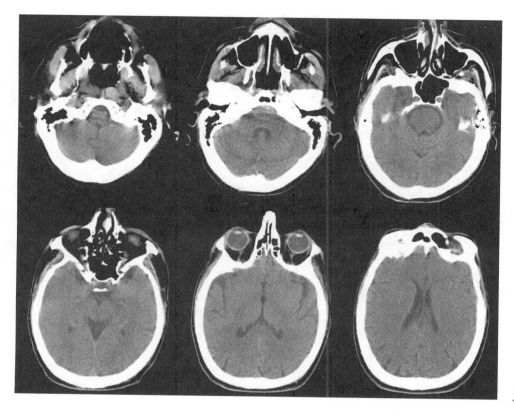

FIGURE 4.3. *CT scan.*

- Caudate nucleus
- Temporal lobe
- Occipital lobe
- Eye
- Ear

A4.3. See Figure 4.4.

Q4.4. What has happened to the medulla? What areas are imaged the best? In the upper right image, what is the radiodense material next to the pons, just at the base of the temporal lobes? How well can you distinguish brain structures on these images? What general type of information can you gain from these scans?

A4.4. The medulla is partially surrounded by the much more dense petrous bone and base of the skull. These structures produce significant artifacts on the CT scan and limit the resolution of CT scans in regions encased in thick bone (posterior fossa, spine). In contrast, when bone is less and brain is more, the images are good, especially in the upper cortex and deep gray structures. The radiodense material just at the base of the temporal lobes is a volume-averaging effect with the petrous ridge. Look at your human skull and think about where the temporal lobes lay.

Although these scans have limited information about the brain, you can discern several facts: The brain is symmetric, and so probably is devoid of large masses. It lacks hemorrhage. Major structures are intact; no large area has been destroyed by a pathologic process (e.g., infarct). The brain lacks significant atrophy. These are all useful data in specific clinical scenarios.

Volume averaging *Imaging modalities compress slabs of three-dimensional information onto a flat surface (film, monitor). All information in a line through the slab is averaged to produce a dot in the final image. On a slice of brain, you see only the surface, without averaging.*

CT Applications

In a CT the data are digital and have a much wider range of values than the eye can perceive on a video screen. The data are extracted so only portions are displayed. Bone windows display the range produced by the densest tissues (those showing the greatest absorption of X-rays), while soft tissue windows essentially overexpose the denser bones to best display the range of brain.

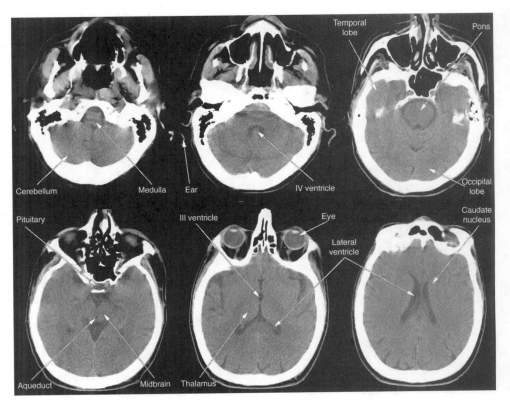

FIGURE 4.4. *Salient structures on CT scan.*

Q4.5. In Figure 4.5 the CT scan on the left has been optimized to enhance tissue contrast, while on the right only the densest tissues are imaged; you are looking at the "bone windows." Compare the two sides. Note on the left image the location of the lesion. What is the radiodense (white stuff) beneath the bone? What about the tissue above the bone? Remember the brain has two sides, so use its symmetry. Just by looking at the tissue windows, can you discern the underlying etiology of the tissue lesions? How do the "bone windows" help? What is the underlying pathology?

A4.5. *The more radio-opaque material beneath the bone is blood. X-rays don't penetrate blood (iron) as well as other soft tissues, and so blood is brighter on CT scans (this is not true in MRI scans). From the location of the blood and how it is layering, the CT shows it is an epidural*

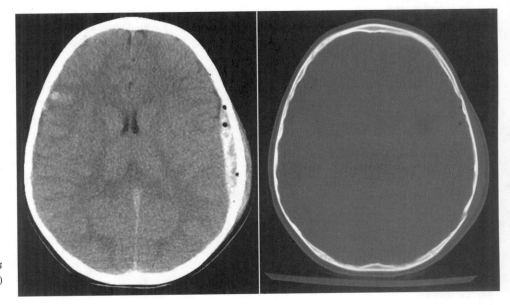

FIGURE 4.5. *Head CT scan after a fall. Tissue* (left) *versus bone* (right) *windows.*

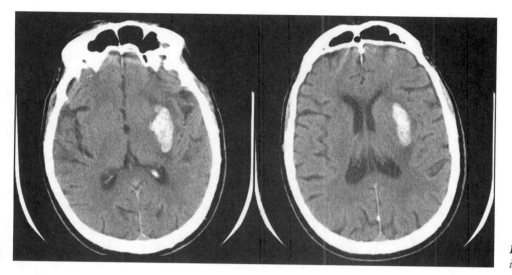

FIGURE 4.6. *Head CT scan showing intra-axial radiodense material.*

hematoma. *The soft tissue over the bone is also swollen and contains blood products, indicating that the patient struck his head on the left side. In the scans optimized for examining tissue, the bone is usually overbright. The bone windows allow you to discern the skull fracture that has produced the hemorrhages (it is the discontinuity in the bone on the left side of the brain).*

Q4.6. Referring to the images above, look at the skull thickness. Try to remember back to your anatomy course; does the skull look appropriately thick? How does the skull differ in thickness?

A4.6. *The skull varies in thickness, being thickest in the base around the ear ("rock" or petrous bone) and thinnest in the lateral temporal area ("temple"). In this case the skull is a bit thinner than that in most adults. The patient is a six year old who was injured in a fall.*

Astute students may also notice the radiodense lesion at the surface of the right frontal lobe in Figure 4.5. This is a contrecoup contusion on the opposite side of the brain, which has produced some tissue bruising and subarachnoid hemorrhage.

Q4.7. In the next CT scan (Fig. 4.6), where is the lesion? Be as specific as possible. Is the lesion more or less radio-opaque than bone? Justify your answer. What is the material? What effect has the lesion had on the surrounding brain? What arteries supply this site in the brain? Use your atlases to find the specific arteries. What major vessel feeds these arteries?

A4.7. *The radiodense mass lies within the left putamen and perhaps within part of the globus pallidus. It lies medial to the insula, just medial to the external capsule. Its volume has caused the left caudate nucleus to bulge into the lateral ventricle. In this CT the bone is completely opaque while the lesion has a mottled look, indicating it is less dense than bone. This material is blood, which is more dense than brain and less than bone. Blood, especially when it accumulates, is well imaged by CT scans. When it is spread out and lies next to the denser bone (e.g., a subdural hematoma), it is more difficult to visualize.*

This region of brain is supplied by the lenticulostriate (lentiform nucleus plus striatum) arteries, which arise at nearly right angles off the middle cerebral artery. This site, as well as thalamus, pons, and cerebellum are major sites for massive internal brain hemorrhages.

You may notice that this brain is somewhat atrophic. This suggests the scan is from an elderly patient.

Q4.8. The next patient had a gradual onset of clinical deficits, including some behavioral changes and a hemiparesis. Figure 4.7 shows the patient's contrast-enhanced CT scan. Where is the lesion? Name the anatomic structures that have been affected by this lesion. Would you say the lesion is a mass that pushes the brain away, or a lesion that infiltrates normal brain? Such distinctions help in identifying the pathology of the lesion. In the right image are two spikes in the patient's skull. What are they?

A4.8. *The patient had a glioblastoma multiforme, a cancer of the brain's astrocytes. It is located in the right caudate nucleus, internal capsule, corpus callosum, and probably putamen and thalamus.*

Lentiform nucleus *Includes the globus pallidus and the putamen. For those who's brain is governed by food, it has the shape of a lentil.*

Striatum *Includes the caudate nucleus and the putamen. The globus pallidus is sometimes included. It is the deep gray nuclei having prominent white matter striations coursing through them.*

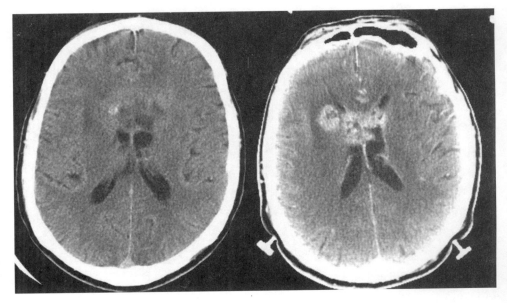

FIGURE 4.7. *Head CT scan of a patient with a glioblastoma multiforme. The right image is enhanced by contrast.*

It has crossed over the corpus callosum to the left side. In this case the lesion is BOTH a mass pushing away adjacent brain AND and infiltrative process, which is a characteristic signature of this tumor.

This CT was taken so that tissue could be sampled by a stereotactic biopsy. A frame is bolted onto the patient's skull (so it does not move) and the head and skull are imaged together. A coordinate system is then created and a needle is directed to the coordinates of the mass.

Q4.9. The brain is a highly vascular organ. Why does it not enhance everywhere? What do the sites of enhancement represent? In the middle of the enhancing areas in Figure 4.7 are some darker regions. What could these represent? Notice that surrounding the enhancing lesions the brain is actually less radiodense than the remainder of the brain. What does this represent?

A4.9. *Normal brain, except for a few regions we'll discuss later, has a barrier (blood-brain barrier) that blocks the contrast agent. Contrast enhancement on scans indicate that this barrier has been breached. In this case the disruption is due to malformed vessels. In other diseases it may be due to destruction of the endothelial cells that establish this barrier. Lack of enhancement in the center of the lesion usually indicates either degeneration or actual necrosis. The surrounding brain is less opaque than the remainder of the brain since it is edematous.*

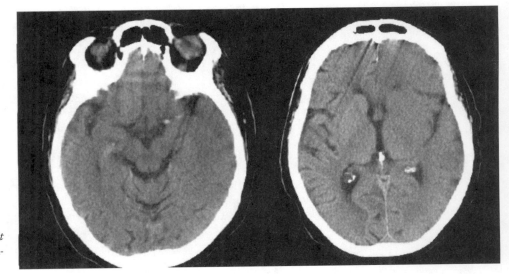

FIGURE 4.8. *CT scan of a patient with aphasia and right-sided weakness.*

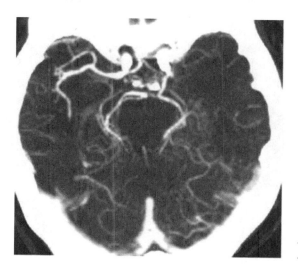

FIGURE 4.9. *CT angiogram from same patient.*

Q4.10. The patient imaged in Figure 4.8 was found on the ground, semiconscious and babbling. The emergency medical technicians noticed that he was not moving his right side. Where is the lesion in this picture? It is subtle. Look for asymmetries in the brain (which fortunately is normally bilaterally symmetric). Also look for sites where the normal cerebral convolutions become more obscured. What are the three bright spots, one in the center of the brain and the other two lateral to the central bright spot?

A4.10. *Compare the left and right sides, especially in the right-hand image. Notice how the gyri and sulci are not as clear on the patient's left (remember, it is the right side of the image) as on the right. Also notice how the left caudate nucleus bulges further into the lateral ventricles than on the right. This is due to edema, which has caused a mass effect and shift of left-sided structures to the right. You may also notice a small white dot in the left panel, just in front of the left medial temporal lobe. This is probably the origin of the left middle cerebral artery. It is dense on the CT scan since it is either occluded or affected by a large atherosclerotic plaque.*

Descartes thought that central bright spot was the "seat of your soul." It is the pineal gland. The more lateral and posterior bright spots are choroid plexus. These all become calcified as we age. Which may say something about our souls.

Q4.11. Now examine the CT angiogram from the same patient (Fig. 4.9). What is wrong? Where is the lesion? What region of brain would be affected by this lesion? Be as specific as possible. You may want to review your cerebral circulation again. Name the vessels arcing around the midbrain. What could have caused this pathology?

A4.11. *What is missing in Figure 4.9 is the left middle cerebral artery. You can identify the paired large bulbs just off of center at the top of the image. These are the internal carotid arteries coming up from the neck. On the left side of the image the right middle cerebral artery arises directly from the internal carotid. It is missing on the patient's left side.*

Obviously this type of proximal injury to a major artery would produce substantial clinical deficits. The left middle cerebral artery distributes blood to the lateral portions of the frontal, parietal, and temporal lobes. As you will learn later, for the majority of us, this lesion would produce a hemiparesis and a marked deficit in language.

The vessels around the midbrain would be the posterior cerebral arteries and the superior cerebellar arteries. At least on the left, the posterior cerebral artery circulation arises mostly from the left internal carotid artery, since the posterior communicating artery is well visualized.

The most likely etiology for such a blockage would be an embolus from a proximal source and less likely a thrombus developing at the vessel origin.

CT Artifacts

Q4.12. Describe what you see in Figure 4.10. Is the artifact created by something more or less radioopaque than bone? What type of material could this be? Guess what is causing the artifact. What produces the multiple lines radiating from the artifact?

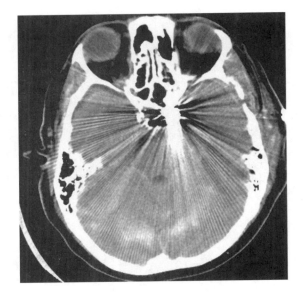

FIGURE 4.10. *CT artifact.*

A4.12. The bone of the skull is quite well imaged in this CT. The brain is nearly completely obscured by the artifact. Since bone does not produce this artifact, the material producing the radiating artifact must be more radio-opaque than bone, for example, metal.

While unwelcome foreign objects such as a bullet could potentially produce this image, the artifact arises in the region around the circle of Willis. Probably if a bullet reached this point, there would be no need to image the patient! This artifact is produced by an aneurysm clip.

A CT scan is constructed from data produced by X-ray sources arising at multiple angles. The lines thus represent each radiating beam normally used to produce the image.

ANGIOGRAM

While both CT and MR techniques can produce images of cerebral vessels, they lack the incredible resolution achievable using conventional angiograms. However, angiograms require an administration of a large amount of contrast agent through a catheter that has been threaded into an artery. In addition the patient receives a good dose of radiation. This technique is only used when the high level of resolution is required clinically, as in preparation for vascular surgery. For the novice, the images produced are also more difficult to interpret.

Part of the problem in understanding angiograms is that the patient is alive with a beating heart. The radio-opaque dye, instead of just filling the vessel of interest, flows through the artery into the capillary bed and then into the veins, all the while being diluted by additional blood. An angiogram is dynamic, requiring multiple snapshots over a short time to get a complete view of the vessels. An image taken early shows the main arteries, a bit later shows the end arteries and arterioles, later a capillary bed blush, and finally the veins.

Another problem in figuring out static images on a film is that they may have been taken in different planes. Remember that angiograms are a flat, two-dimensional compression of a three-dimensional structure. In modern angiography various subtractive techniques are used to obtain the final image (see the photographs below). They are also not a single, flat picture of the entire brain but select regions of "focus," somewhat like the depth of field in a photograph. Unlike CT and MRI, however, they are not a true "slice of brain."

Q4.13. Compare the unsubtracted angiogram on the left in Figure 4.11 with the image on the right. How do they differ?

A4.13. The unsubtracted image shows everything that absorbs X rays, including electrodes on the patient's skull (bright circles) and the dense petrous bone around the ear. After subtraction the anterior cerebral circulation becomes clear.

For the exercises below, use an atlas, available brains, texts, models, and your laboratory instructor to help you.

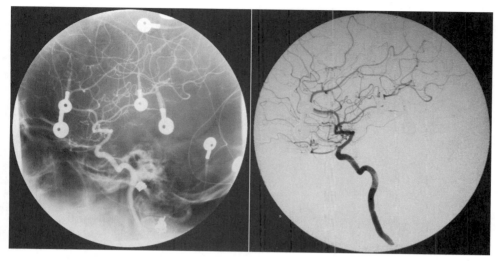

FIGURE 4.11. *Cerebral angiogram, unsubtracted* (left) *and subtracted* (right).

Q4.14. The angiograms in Figure 4.12 were taken in an anterior-posterior (AP) view. What vessels was injected? Remember, only the large, most proximal vessels are typically injected.

A4.14. *Carotid artery, one side.*

Q4.15. At 2.5 seconds, list the main vessels in the image. What arteries can you NOT see? Why are both anterior cerebral arteries visualized, but only one middle cerebral artery?

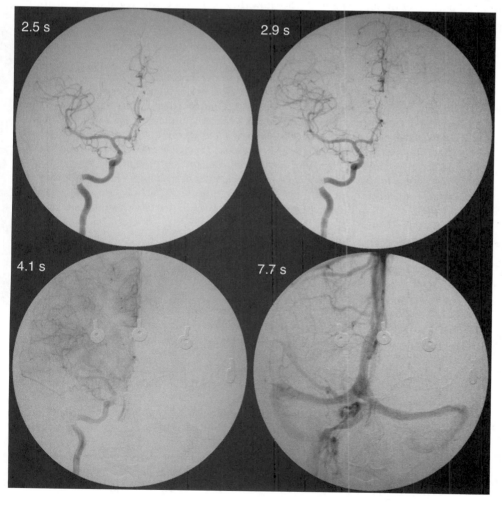

FIGURE 4.12. *Angiogram, AP view at select time points.*

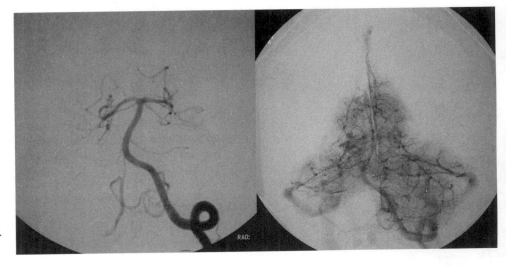

FIGURE 4.13. *Angiogram, AP view, early* (left) *and late* (right) *after injection.*

A4.15. *The images show the internal carotid artery feeding through the siphon (dark dot) and splitting into the anterior and middle cerebral arteries. The posterior circulation is not visualized (vertebral, basilar, posterior cerebral arteries). Some contrast has crossed the anterior communicating artery to fill both anterior cerebral arteries. The circle of Willis is really a "potential" anastomotic circle. As demonstrated here, the blood doesn't normally circulate to the opposite brain; hence only one middle cerebral artery is visualized.*

Q4.16. At 2.9 seconds, examine the distal branches of the middle cerebral artery (upper left portion of the angiogram). Notice how they curl back before reaching the brain surface. In what region of brain are these curled arteries? (Hint: Compare these images of the brain with the real thing.)

A4.16. *The middle cerebral artery branches feed into the deep insula and then curl back around its lips onto the outer surface of the brain.*

Q4.17. At 4.1 seconds, what does the diffuse gray in the image represent?

A4.17. *The capillary blush. These structures are too small to be resolved by angiogram.*

Q4.18. Finally, examine the image at 7.7 seconds. What are the main structures now visualized? Try to identify the components. Why has the unilateral dye become bilateral?

A4.18. *At this late time, the veins or cerebral sinuses contain the contrast agent. The central pillar of dye is the superior sagittal sinus (which overshadows the smaller inferior sinus). This large sinus drains in the back of the head into the two transverse sinuses. These in turn travel around the back of the skull, along the edge of the tentorium, to the sigmoid sinuses and jugular veins (not yet seen at this time).*

Q4.19. In the AP views in Figure 4.13 another major cerebral artery was injected with contrast. Which one?

A4.19. *Vertebral.*

Q4.20. On the left image trace this vessel up to where it joins its opposite. Name the main unpaired artery at this point. Notice the smaller curled vessel coming off the injected artery, before its major confluence. What is this artery. What structures does it supply? (Hint: Look at the right-hand image.)

A4.20. *The vertebral arteries join the basilar artery, which then ascends more or less straight upward (rostrally). Before the vertebral confluence, they give off the posterior inferior cerebellar artery, supplying the lateral medulla and inferior cerebellum, and the anterior spinal artery, feeding the anterior cord.*

You may wonder why the basilar artery has the same diameter as the vertebral. This is a frequent anatomic variation, in which one vertebral is dominant. In this case the injected vertebral artery was much larger than the noninjected one.

Q4.21. What structure does the basilar artery supply, as indicated in the right image of Figure 4.13? Notice the (nearly) paired arteries coming off both sides of the lower basilar. What is its name?

A4.21. *Arising from the basilar artery are a series of small penetrating and circumferential arteries that supply the pons and medial cerebellum. The main paired vessel is the anterior inferior cerebellar artery.*

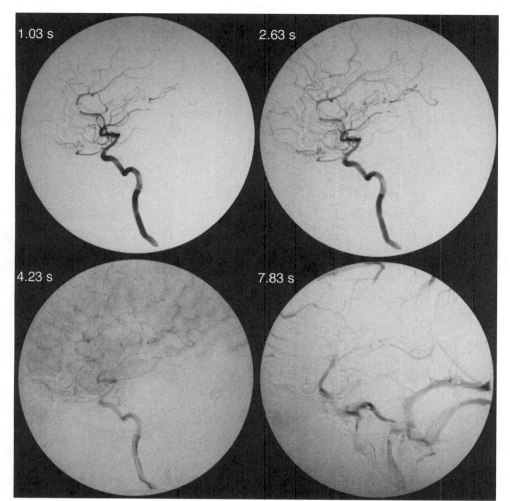

1.03 s

2.63 s

4.23 s

7.83 s

FIGURE 4.14. *Angiogram after carotid artery injection, lateral view.*

Q4.22. Describe what happens at the top of the main artery. Name the vessels it feeds and the structures the vessels supply.

A4.22. *At the midbrain, the basilar artery splits into the posterior cerebral arteries at the same point where the superior cerebellar arteries arise. The former vessels supply the inferior temporal and most of the occipital lobes, while the latter supply the superior cerebellum. Both give off small branches that supply the midbrain.*

The cerebral circulation varies from person to person, and never really follows "the book." About 15% to 20% of the time one posterior cerebral artery arises primarily from the carotid artery ("fetal circulation"). This may also be bilateral.

Q4.23. Figure 4.14 shows a lateral view after injection of the carotid artery. The circulation of the medial brain has been emphasized, while the lateral circulation is not as well seen. On which side of the image is the face? (Look at all of the pictures for help. You may want to compare these with a view of the sagittal brain from earlier labs.)

A4.23. *The face is on the left.*

Q4.24. At 1.03 seconds, trace the carotid upward through its tortuous path. Notice that at its top several arteries appear to branch off at right angles. Name the two main arteries at this point. Also at 1.03 seconds, notice the first artery coming off the internal carotid and going toward the face, before the carotid makes its sharp turn back to the left. What is this artery? (Hint: Look at what it supplies at 4.23 seconds, on the right.)

A4.24. *The anterior cerebral artery branches off the internal carotid shortly after it penetrates the dura. It is the vessel that forms a hook in the upper portions of the images. The middle cerebral artery is really a continuation of the internal carotid artery. It is not seen well in these images, although*

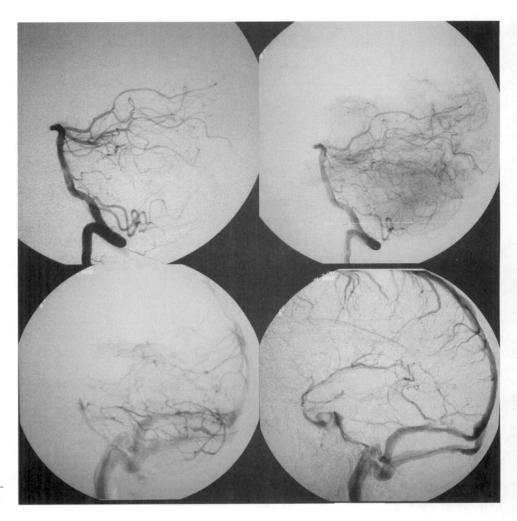

FIGURE 4.15. *Vertebral artery angiogram, lateral view.*

you can see some of the looping in the insula. Before the internal carotid reaches the dura, it gives off the important ophthalmic artery, which supplies the retina (left side at 4.23 seconds).

Q4.25. In the upper portion of the images, especially at 1.03 and 2.63 seconds, is the large, hooked-shaped artery that arose from the carotid. It travels forward, swings upward, then heads backward. What structure gives it this shape? At 4.23 seconds, notice how much of the medial brain it supplies.

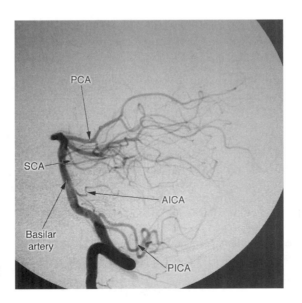

FIGURE 4.16. *Posterior cerebral circulation.*

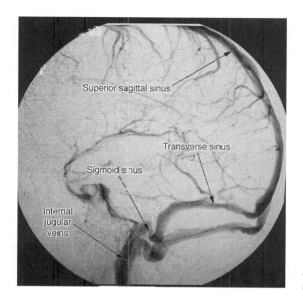

FIGURE 4.17. *Venous structures on angiogram.*

A4.25. The anterior cerebral artery supplies most of the medial brain. After arising from the internal carotid artery, it travels forward and then sweeps around the outside of the corpus callosum, which imparts a hook-shape on this lateral view.

Q4.26. Finally, examine Figure 4.15, which is a lateral-view angiogram produced after injection of a vertebral artery. Compare these with a sagittal brain slice. Try to identify the main vessels in the posterior circulation: posterior inferior cerebellar arteries (PICA), basilar artery, anterior inferior cerebellar arteries (AICA), superior cerebellar arteries, and the posterior cerebral arteries (PCA). Notice the capillary blush in the lower portion of the upper right image. What structures are usually supplied by the posterior circulation?

A4.26. The posterior circulation supplies the brainstem, cerebellum, and usually the occipital lobes and inferior temporal lobes. See Figure 4.16.

Q4.27. In the lower two images of Figure 4.15, the venous system contains contrast. Again, identify the superior sagittal sinus, transverse sinuses sigmoid sinuses, and now the internal jugular veins. Notice also the deep veins in the lower right image. Many of the same venous sinuses are imaged in these views as in the views above (compare with the venous phase of the first set of angiograms). What is this telling you?

*A4.27. See Figure 4.17. The veins in the brain differ from the arteries in several ways. One major difference is that veins form several different **anastomoses,** producing functional circuits or routes of drainage. This differs from say the circle of Willis, which in most people is not a functional circle. The venous structures, especially on the outer brain, also vary more from person to person. The posterior and anterior cerebral circulation injections both eventually fill some of the same venous channels because of their overlapping drainage. For example, posterior portions of thalamus are supplied by the posterior circulation, while the striatum receives blood from the middle circulation. These both drain into the thalamostriate veins and empty together into the vein of Galen, straight sinus, and eventually into the transverse sinuses.*

Angiogram Application

Q4.28. The MRI in Figure 4.18 (MRIs are proton density images; don't worry about the details) illustrates the anatomy of the patient's lesion. What anatomic structures are involved by the lesion (you will probably need to refer to your atlas, since horizontal sections have not yet been discussed in detail)? How would you describe the lesion (signal characteristics, morphology, etc.)? How well can you resolve the lesion? Guess what it might be.

A4.28. The scans show a mass in the left deep gray nuclei, including thalamus, globus pallidus, and putamen. The mass itself shows signal heterogeneity, including elongated structures devoid of

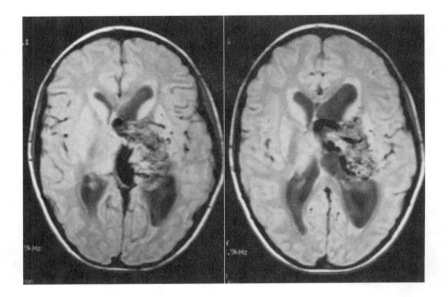

FIGURE 4.18. *Proton-weighted MRI showing intraaxial lesion.*

signal. The long structures are vessels, and this is a vascular malformation. More specifically, it is an arteriovenous malformation.

Q4.29. In the angiogram in Figure 4.19, taken of the same patient, the left internal carotid artery has been injected with contrast dye, and the patient has been imaged in an anterior-posterior view. The left figure is taken shortly after the injection (arterial phase), while that on the right is taken some time later (venous phase). Try to picture the flow of the blood up the left carotid and into the lesion. How would these images map onto the head. Are you looking at the front or the back of the patient's head? What does the blush of gray represent in the center of the lesion. Notice the size of the vessels in the two phases; how do the two phases differ? Contrast the resolution in these images with that in the MRI above.

A4.29. *Since you know the injection was in the left carotid, you must be looking at the face of the patient; the carotids arise more medially and then spread more laterally in the middle cerebral artery. The blush is the small vessel bed of the AVM that is fed by the carotid/middle cerebral artery. The veins imaged on the right are huge and tortuous. While the arteries on the left may also be too big, it is the veins that become greatly enlarged under the pressure of the arterial system (in an AVM, arterial blood is essentially being dumped into the venous system without undergoing the significant drop in pressure normally experienced across a capillary bed).*

The angiogram gives exquisite resolution of the vascular tree, and remains the study of choice in such lesions. It is greatly superior to other imaging modalities. Such studies remain useful in the day of the MR angiogram when the detailed vascular anatomy is needed, as in

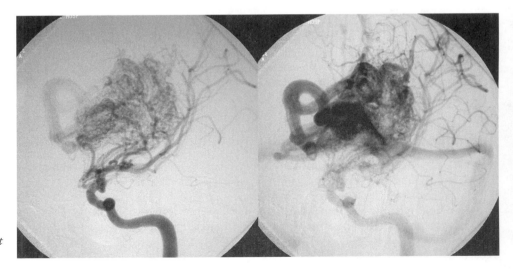

FIGURE 4.19. *Angiogram of patient shown in Figure 4.18.*

preparation for surgery. However, as you can see, no brain is imaged, which makes localizing the lesion more difficult.

Q4.30. Why are angiograms being replaced by MRA and CT angiography? Think about how angiograms work and think of some possible vascular malformations that may not be imaged well using this technique.

A4.30. *MRA scans don't require injection of large amounts of contrast and don't necessitate threading a catheter into the patient's vessels. In the more rapid CT angiograms the amount of contrast is much less than in conventional angiograms, and the dose of radiation is less.*

Angiograms require blood flow to work. Vascular malformations with no blood flow, for example, a clotted aneurysm, won't image well in an angiogram but can be imaged on a CT or MRI scan. Angiograms also require threading of a catheter into the arteries and injection of a large amount of contrast agent. These agents are not benign and can lead to problems such as renal failure.

MAGNETIC RESONANCE IMAGING

MRI Planes of Section

One of the great advantages of MRI is that you can view the brain in several orientations. To do this in a CT scanner you would need to make the bore hole as wide as the patient (although data from a CT can be used to reconstruct the other planes).

INST The three typical planes used in imaging are illustrated in Figure 4.20. For the middle and right scans, try to determine on your whole brain or brain model the slice used to obtain the images. See if you can match the middle image up with any of the coronal slices that you prepared in the second laboratory.

The MRI uses chemical data from protons to create images. In most clinically used instances, these involve receiving signals from protons as their spins relax in the magnetic field after being jolted by a pulse of radio waves. The most basic scans weight the data obtained from these relaxations, and are termed T1-weighted and T2-weighted (or just T1 and T2) scans.

In Figure 4.21, the left scan is T1-weighted and the right is T2-weighted, both taken at the same level.

Q4.31. What is the color of CSF in the T1 scan? In the T2 scan? In which scan can you more easily distinguish anatomic structures? What color is bone in the T1 and T2 images? What structures are better demonstrated on the T1 scan?

A4.31. *CSF is black in the T1 images and white in the T2 images. This rule may not apply to all of the radiologist's various scans, since with special sequences fluid signals can be either eliminated ("suppressed" or made black) or accentuated.*

Unlike CT scans, the MRI is picking up signals from PROTONS, not by how X-rays are blocked. Bone is black on both images, since it contains fewer protons (read: little water). Note, however, that bone marrow does produce signal, along with other soft tissues surrounding the bone.

In these images the T1 scan better demonstrates the choroid plexus in the atria of the lateral ventricles. It also shows some of the surrounding soft tissues better, like the temporalis muscle.

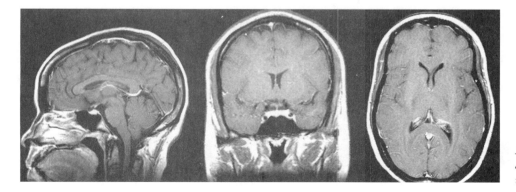

FIGURE 4.20. Sagittal, coronal, and horizontal T1 MRI scans. T1 versus T2

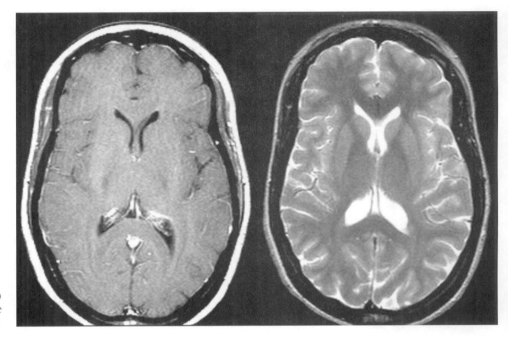

FIGURE 4.21. *Horizontal T1 (left) and T2 (right) MRI. A contrast agent has been administered in the T1 MRI.*

This scan was enhanced using a contrast agent, which is why these structures, with a loose blood-brain barrier, are bright.

Although, by just looking at these images, you may wonder why T1 scans are even done, these two forms of data are usually complementary. Also the T1 scan takes much less time than the T2, and so is used when examining contrast enhancement.

Q4.32. Now that you have had some experience looking at scans, look at the blown-up sagittal image in Figure 4.22. First, is it a T1 or T2 image? Compare this with the sagittal view of your half brain.

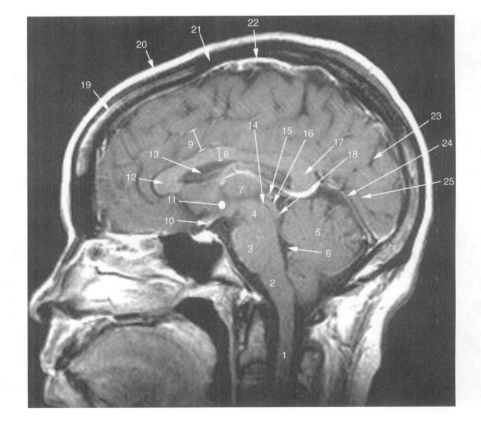

FIGURE 4.22. *Sagittal MRI.*

A4.32. The scan is an enhanced T1 image.

Q4.33. Using your resources (atlas, etc.), identify the structures indicated in Figure 4.22.

4.33.1 _____

4.33.2 _____

4.33.3 _____

4.33.4 _____

4.33.5 _____

4.33.6 _____

4.33.7 _____

4.33.8 _____

4.33.9 _____

4.33.10 _____

4.33.11 _____

4.33.12 _____

4.33.13 _____

4.33.14 _____

4.33.15 _____

4.33.16 _____

4.33.17 _____

4.33.18 _____

4.33.19 _____

4.33.20 _____

4.33.21 _____

4.33.22 _____

4.33.23 _____

4.33.24 _____

4.33.25 _____

A4.33 *4.33.1. Spinal cord*
   4.33.2. Medulla
   4.33.3. Base of pons
   4.33.4. Midbrain
   4.33.5. Cerebellar vermis
   4.33.6. Fourth ventricle
   4.33.7. Thalamus

4.33.8. *Corpus callosum*

4.33.9. *Cingulate gyrus*

4.33.10. *Optic chiasm*

4.33.11. *Third ventricle/hypothalamus*

4.33.12. *Genu of corpus callosum*

4.33.13. *Septum pellucidum/lateral ventricle*

4.33.14. *Aqueduct*

4.33.15. *Pineal*

4.33.16. *Superior colliculus*

4.33.17. *Splenium of corpus callosum*

4.33.18. *Inferior colliculus*

4.33.19. *Bone marrow*

4.33.20. *Scalp*

4.33.21. *Skull (frontal bone)*

4.33.22. *Dura*

4.33.23. *Parietooccipital sulcus*

4.33.24. *Tentorium*

4.33.25. *Calcarine fissure*

Q4.34. Figure 4.23 is a series of coronal T1 images. As above, identify the indicated structures.

4.34.1 _____

4.34.2 _____

4.34.3 _____

4.34.4 _____

4.34.5 _____

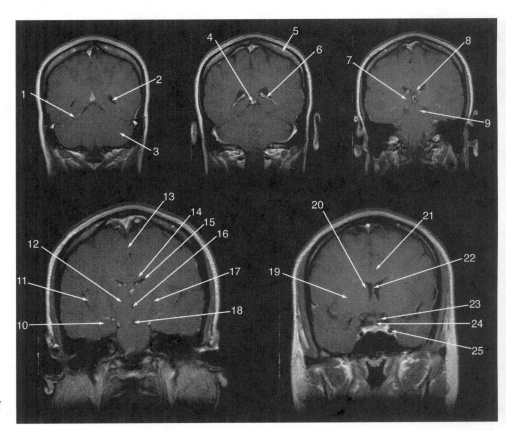

FIGURE 4.23. *Coronal T1 MRI scans; major landmarks indicated.*

4.34.6 _____

4.34.7 _____

4.34.8 _____

4.34.9 _____

4.34.10 _____

4.34.11 _____

4.34.12 _____

4.34.13 _____

4.34.14 _____

4.34.15 _____

4.34.16 _____

4.34.17 _____

4.34.18 _____

4.34.19 _____

4.34.20 _____

4.34.21 _____

4.34.22 _____

4.34.23 _____

4.34.24 _____

4.34.25 _____

A4.34. Structures in sagittal MRI.
   4.34.1. Tentorium vessel
   4.34.2. Occipital horn of third ventricle
   4.34.3. Cerebellum
   4.34.4. Pineal
   4.34.5. Bone marrow (NOT bone)
   4.34.6. Choroid plexus
   4.34.7. Posterior thalamus (pulvinar)
   4.34.8. Fornix
   4.34.9. Midbrain (tectum)
   4.34.10. Hippocampus
   4.34.11. Insula
   4.34.12. Thalamus
   4.34.13. Falx cerebri
   4.34.14. Corpus callosum
   4.34.15. Lateral ventricle
   4.34.16. Third ventricle
   4.34.17. Internal capsule
   4.34.18. Cerebral aqueduct

4.34.19. *Putamen/external capsule*
4.34.20. *Caudate nucleus*
4.34.21. *Cingulate gyrus*
4.34.22. *Septum pellucidum*
4.34.23. *Optic chiasm*
4.34.24. *Pituitary stalk*
4.34.25. *Internal carotid artery*

Q4.35. Compare the coronal images either here or at the end of the laboratory with those you sliced in the second laboratory. What is seen better on brain? What is seen better on MRI?

A4.35. *This is in part a matter of taste. You can certainly see more detail on the brain than in these scans. However, other types of scans, including the T2 MRI, will have more detail than in these coronal T1 images. Also MRIs can be made much finer in resolution, but at the expense of time. MRI scans have the advantage of showing the brain in the context of the body. Structures are NOT chopped off as they are at autopsy. They also demonstrate the full extent of the dura and show the cisterns that disappear when the brain coverings are removed. As you will encounter shortly, various MRI techniques (pulse sequences) have improved the identification of lesions. For example, subtle white matter changes may be difficult to visualize on sliced brain but are easy to see on a T2 MRI.*

MRI Applications

Q4.36. In Figure 4.24 is a set of four different types of images taken at the same level. First determine the plane of the cut and try to identify some landmarks (e.g., deep gray nuclei). Then try to figure out the types of the different scans. Contrast the upper right to the lower left image. How do they differ and how are they similar? Contrast the extent of the lesion in the lower right enhanced T1 image to that in the other images. Finally, briefly describe the pathology you see, and compare these images to the CT images above from a different patient with the same condition.

A4.36. *At this level of horizontal section, you can see the upper portion of the lateral ventricle and the body of the caudate nucleus along its outer edges. (Don't fret if you don't know your horizontal anatomy yet; you will get this in an upcoming laboratory.) The upper left image is T1-weighted, the right T2-weighted (CSF bright), the lower left is a FLAIR, and the lower right is enhanced.*

The CSF is bright on the T2 image and dark on the FLAIR. The FLAIR imaging sequences are designed to suppress fluid signals (the FLA stands for FLuid Attenuated), and so emphasize other tissue pathology. In this case the white matter pathology extensively involves both sides of the brain. You can better visualize the details of the mass in the FLAIR than in the overly bright T2 images.

The lower right enhanced image shows where the blood-brain barrier is disrupted, and also where no contrast agent penetrates. Notice how the area of enhancement is smaller than the total area of the lesion. Essentially none of the white matter infiltration on the left side of the brain, as revealed in the FLAIR scan, shows enhancement. Only around the central area of the tumor have the blood vessels become leaky; those in the white matter remain intact. Enhancement tells you something is bad, but the lack of enhancement does not mean it is good!

Like the CT scan above, this patient has a glioblastoma multiforme, a tumor of the brain's glia. Neoplastic glial cells migrate widely throughout the brain, as you can see especially well on the FLAIR sequence. The MRI is much superior to the CT scan for such imaging. Because of their better localizing properties, CT scans are used during stereotactic biopsies, as in the earlier image.

Q4.37. The patient shown in Figure 4.25 an acute onset of confusion and a right hemiparesis. Examine the images. Determine the type of scan and identify some major landmarks: midbrain, temporal lobes, occipital lobes, eyes. Where is the lesion? How extensive is it? How well demarcated is it from other brain tissues?

A4.37. *The scans are horizontal T2 images at the level of the midbrain and thalamus. Although subtle, the left side of the brain, in the lateral temporal lobe, has a greater T2 signal intensity than on the right side. Since so much of the brain shows a similar intensity of signal, it is difficult to discern the precise extent of this infarct.*

Q4.38. Figure 4.26 are the diffusion-weighted images on the same patient. Now where is the injury? How do you explain the hemiparesis? In what ways are these scans inferior

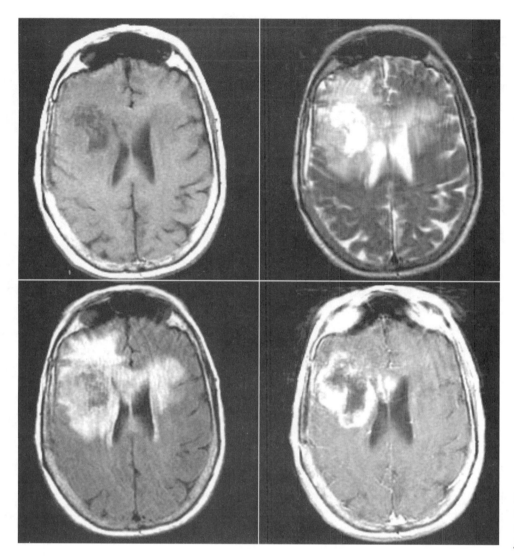

FIGURE 4.24. *MRI scans at the same level using different weighting and sequences, from a patient with a glioblastoma multiforme.*

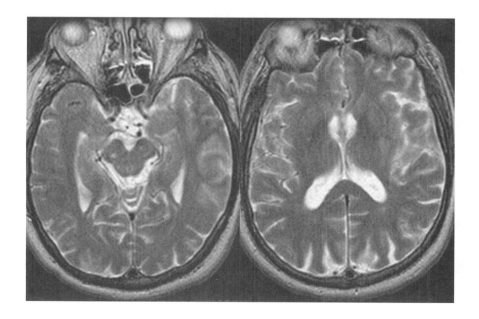

FIGURE 4.25. *MRI scans of a patient presenting with acute confusion and a right hemiparesis.*

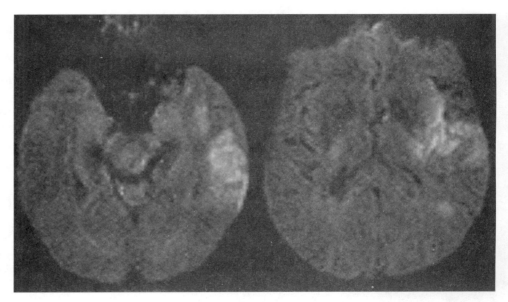

FIGURE 4.26. *Diffusion-weighted MRI scans from the patient presented in Figure 4.25.*

and superior to the regular T2 image? Anything in the image that might lead you astray?

A4.38. The **diffusion-weighted scans (dwi),** *in conjunction with some other images, highlight "diffusion abnormalities." Such abnormalities arise in the brain when cells are injured and diffusion is restricted. Through various sequences, those protons that don't move as far between the pulse and the data collection are bright. These scans are excellent for identifying and localizing acute infarcts. In this patient the area of limited diffusion is in the left inferior-lateral temporal lobe, but also extends into the deeper white matter and thalamus to near the ventricular surface. Beware of the bright signal in the front end of the brain. It is an artifact.*

Notice how grainy the images are. These scans have a much lower resolution than the T2 scans, and lack the beautiful anatomic detail of the latter. They do, however, better delineate the extent of the tissue damage. To examine these diffusion-weighted images properly, you need to go back and compare them with the T2, and sometimes with more primary (ADC or apparent diffusion coefficient) data.

As in all areas of medicine, to properly interpret this test, you need to put it into the context of the entire patient: clinical symptoms, patient's age, and risk factors. Scans can pick up lesions that really have nothing to do with the patient's current problem. The patient's hemiparesis is not readily explained in these images, since the diffusion abnormality does not directly affect the corticospinal tracts. However, the lesion would produce edema, which may secondarily impinge on the tract.

MRI Artifacts

Like other imaging modalities, MRI scans are susceptible to various artifacts. Unlike simpler techniques, however, MRI artifacts produce some very bizarre pictures.

Q4.39. Describe what you see in both images in Figure 4.27. Can you tell what type of MRI image they were supposed to be, T1 or T2? What produced this artifact? Can you "read through" the artifact on the left-hand image? How about on the right?

A4.39. *Both images shows a series of overlapping images, or rather the same image overlapped onto itself. Notice the complete degradation of the base of the left T1-enhanced image. You can still vaguely make out the multifocal ring-enhancing mass in this patient's frontal lobe, which is crossing the corpus callosum—a characteristic feature of glioblastoma. Any underlying pathology in the right-side T2 image (CSF is bright) is completely obliterated.*

This type of artifact is caused by patient motion. If you really needed the picture, then you would have had to sedate the patient or put them under general anesthesia. This would be routine in infants and young children. Such motion artifact, especially in an acute setting, perhaps with a patient seizing, is a major clinical limitation of MR scanning.

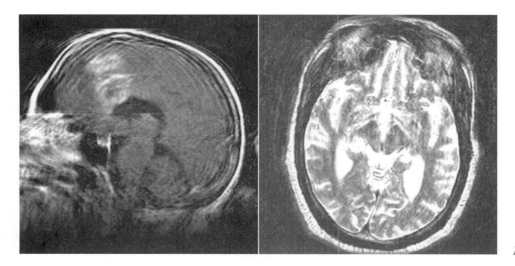

FIGURE 4.27. MRI artifacts.

Q4.40. Another interesting MRI artifact is pictured in Figure 4.28. First, describe what you see. How does this image differ from the motion artifact above? Can you still see anatomic detail, are these images still useful?

A4.40. *The false images pictured here are called "phase" artifacts. They result from how the MRI determines the position of a signal in space ("phase encoding"). The details of this are the province of magnetic resonance physicists and well beyond the scope of the text. The main point is to know that such artifacts exist. As you can see in these images, they really don't degrade the information substantially, although some minor pathology could be overlooked. They do make for occasional macabre humor.*

Q4.41. CT scans and MRI scans currently have distinct but overlapping uses. Compare and contrast both of these techniques. Specifically address:
- Resolution of images
- Speed of imaging
- Patient size
- Location of patient in scanner
- Relevance of ferromagnetic material
- Cost

A4.41. *This is an evolving topic. The outlay for an MRI unit is considerably greater than that of a CT scanner. The MRI requires an electrically isolated room, a large magnet, supercooled conductors, a fast computer, and several other pricey items, while a CT scan gets by on a much simpler apparatus. Hence a CT scanner is within reach of small community hospitals and even some large clinics, while MRI requires a wealthy entrepreneur or a larger hospital.*

An MRI also requires more time to acquire the image than a CT scan. These factors together make an MRI scan more costly than a CT scan.

In an acute setting, when speed is utmost, the MRI is a distant second to the CT. When a patient is medically unstable, say requiring a respirator and other mechanical equipment, then

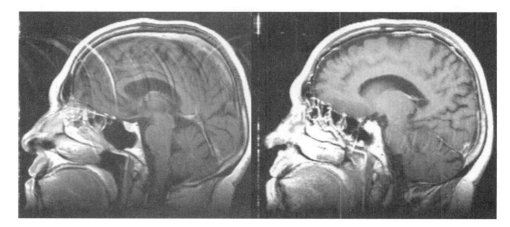

FIGURE 4.28. MRI artifacts.

CT is the only way to go. Also, if the patient has a ferromagnetic metallic object in their body, they cannot enter an MRI suite. Ferromagnetic metals and MRI scanners don't mix: in one case an oxygen tank inadvertently brought into the MRI suite whipped through the air and killed a child. Finally, the bore in the magnet is kept small, to increase its magnetic field strength; this also limits the diameter of the patient! Most magnets will not accommodate obese patients.

Some patients just cannot enter a magnet. Being inside the bore is much like being in a drainage pipe; not for the claustrophobic. Also patient movements degrade all imaging, but especially MRI, which generally requires a longer time to obtain data for the image. In children who can't stay still, general anesthesia, with all of its complications, is required to obtain useful images.

All this being said, the resolution and tissue differentiation offered by an MRI usually out-weighs any benefit provided by a CT scan, especially when the issue involves subtle differences in tissue characteristics provided by brain pathology.

MAGNETIC RESONANCE ANGIOGRAPHY

While a regular angiogram gives the highest resolution of the cerebral circulation, it does require threading a catheter up the arteries to the desired location, then injecting a good deal of contrast medium into the vessel, and finally zapping the patient with a significant dose of radiation. In contrast, with a few parlor tricks, the MRI can be adapted to illustrate vessels (MR angiogram or MRA) without the use of catheters or massive amounts of dye.

Q4.42. Figure 4.29 is one view produced by an MRA. Picture this image as if you are looking at just the vessels of a patient, viewed from the midline, either in front or behind. Although trying to interpret this picture is a bit like an inverted ink-blot test, try to map it onto your knowledge of the cerebral circulation. From where does the blood come? You know what vessels should be there. Find them! Label the indicated arteries.

4.42.1 _____

4.42.2 _____

4.42.3 _____

4.42.4 _____

4.42.5 _____

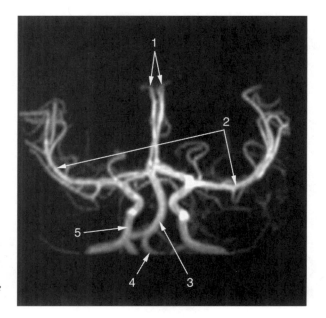

FIGURE 4.29. *Magnetic resonance angiogram, anterior-posterior view.*

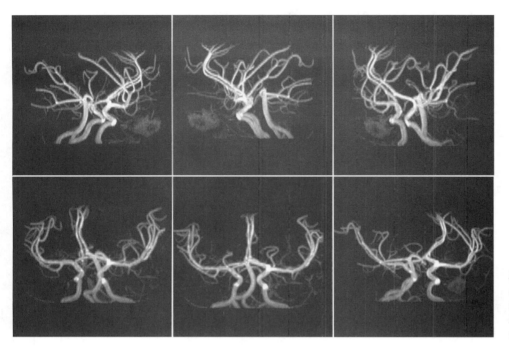

FIGURE 4.30. Magnetic resonance angiography in different views. The upper middle image is a lateral view. Beneath that is an anterior-posterior view.

A4.42. MRA vessels.
    4.42.1. Anterior cerebral arteries
    4.42.2. Middle cerebral arteries
    4.42.3. Basilar artery
    4.42.4. Vertebral artery
    4.42.5. Internal carotid artery
Q4.43. Where is the posterior cerebral artery? Anterior communicators? Posterior communicators? Vessels of the cerebellum?
A4.43. In this particular view these vessels are difficult to either distinguish from each other (e.g., posterior and anterior communicators) or visualize (e.g., posterior cerebral artery). This points to the need to examine these vessels in more than one projection.

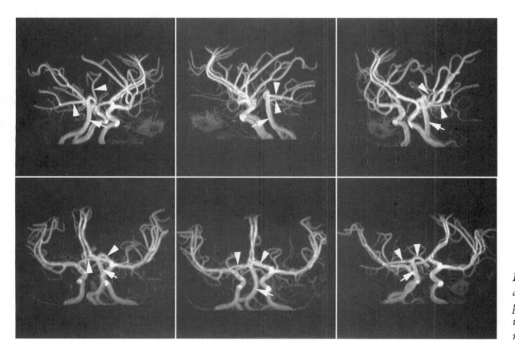

FIGURE 4.31. Magnetic resonance angiography (MRA). The white arrow points to the basilar artery, while the white arrowheads point to the posterior cerebral artery.

Q4.44. Figure 4.30 is a series of angiograms reconstructed at different projections, basically as if you were rotating the patient. The bottom middle image is what you examined in Figure 4.29. The top middle image is as if you a looking at the patient from the side, face to the left. In all of the images, first find the basilar artery. Knowing that the posterior cerebral arteries arise from the top of the basilar artery, find them in the upper middle panel. Now as the images rotates, try to follow the posterior cerebral arteries in the images and see if you can now see them in the original image above. Good luck!

A4.44. *This is not easy with static images! See Figure 4.31. While some of the vessels are easy to identify in some orientations, they can become obscured in other orientations by overlapping arteries. Portions of the posterior circulation nearly overlap the anterior circulation in the lower center panel. Radiologists can turn these images in real time, making identification much easier.*

Chapter 5—SOMATOSENSORY SYSTEM

The previous laboratories were introductory, appetizers for the main course. Beginning with this laboratory session we will systematically examine the nervous system's functional anatomy.

The central nervous system is an entire, integrated organ, so ideally we would want to learn about it all at once. However, since we can only receive information linearly over time, we will instead explore the brain by breaking it down into systems. You will examine the anatomy and function of several different systems, including sensory, visual, motor, and behavioral. Rather than only knowing the names of structures in the brain, you'll know what they do.

To explore the nervous system in more depth, you will need to know more of its overall architecture. Most of the remaining laboratories review specific neuroanatomy that is relevant to the selected systems. In this laboratory you will review in more detail transverse sections through the spinal cord and additionally get a first glimpse at brainstem. In the chapters to come, you will return to study these structures in more detail; this chapter is a first pass to embed the major landmarks in your mind.

Sensory systems have many modalities. This laboratory introduces and contrasts two: pain and touch sensations from the body. The next laboratory will put the head on the body.

LEARNING OBJECTIVES

- Conceptualize the three-dimensional anatomy of the vertebral column, spinal coverings, and spinal cord, including correlations on the MRI.
- Examine the spinal cord to understand its anatomy at several levels.
- Compare and contrast the receptors, fiber types, and entry into the spinal cord of the discriminative dorsal column/lemniscal pathway and the nociceptive spinothalamic or anterolateral system.
- Identify the major landmarks in the brainstem and trace both the lemniscal fibers and anterolateral system through the medulla, pons, and midbrain.

Functional Neuroanatomy: An Interactive Text and Manual, by Jeffrey T. Joseph and David L. Cardozo
ISBN 0-471-44437-5 Copyright © 2004 John Wiley & Sons, Inc.

INTRODUCTION

Various types of information must travel from your body to brain: Your right foot is on a stair. What is that thing in your hand? A hot stove burner is destroying your fingertip. These data ascend through the spinal cord, brainstem, and thalamus before reaching cortex. This chapter will explore touch/tactile sensations and pain associated with tissue destruction.

The Dorsal Column/Lemniscal System

When you reach into a backpack in search of a ballpoint pen, you find this object by its tactile qualities: round, smooth, a certain size, maybe a point. The information reaches your brain by a very specific system of receptors, pathways, and synapses. In the spinal cord the impulses travel in the dorsal columns and then dodge through the medulla, pons, and midbrain in the medial lemniscus, hence the name ***dorsal column/lemniscal*** system. This kind of sensory information has been called touch/tactile, or kinesthetic, or epicritic (the terms are pretty much interchangeable). We use this information to judge size and shape, weight, texture, or speed of movement. The information may or may not reach consciousness. Loss of this system leads to the following deficits: numbness or lack of feeling, inability to judge weight or size, and clumsy inaccurate movements. A person with a medial lemniscal deficit cannot button his shirt without looking at his fingers, and cannot walk around a room in the dark. Complete loss of dorsal column function will make a patient wheelchair bound, even though their strength may be normal.

Parts of the neurological examination directly test this system, including two-point discrimination (separation of two points lightly touching the skin), or stereognosis, which is the appreciation of the form of an object by touch (gnosis: knowledge; stereo: three dimensionality). This laboratory discusses some of these tests.

Some physiological features are characteristic of the dorsal column system. The nerve fibers are large, heavily myelinated, and conduct rapidly. Only a few synaptic relays intervene between the stimulus and its major central targets. Hence lemniscal information undergoes little processing in transit, but gets to its major target faster. At different levels the data undergo a degree of sharpening or enhancement of discrimination. This is carried out by a mechanism that is widespread in the central nervous system, known as lateral (surround) inhibition. Competing nearby stimuli are inhibited,

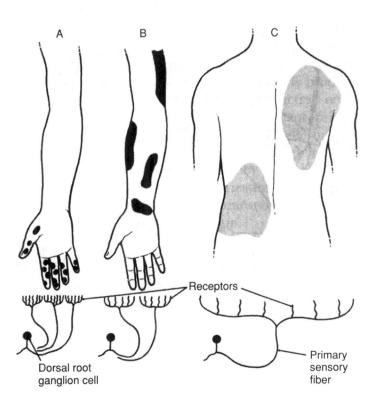

FIGURE 5.1. *Receptive fields. (Modified from Haines, D. E. Fundamental Neuroscience 2nd edition, © 2002, Churchill-Livingstone, New York, figure 17-3, page 258.)*

TABLE 5.1. Peripheral Touch and Tactile Sensory Receptors.

Cell Type	Sensation	Function/Signal
Meissner corpuscles	Tap or flutter	Texture, velocity
Hair follicle receptor	Movement, direction	Velocity
Pacinian corpuscle	Signal onset	Vibration, transients
Merkel cell	Light pressure	Edge detection
Ruffini complex	Unknown	Skin stretch or joint movement

thereby sharpening the perception. This accounts for our ability to accurately localize a sensation to a part of the body, and to judge its quality and intensity.

The first step in a dorsal column somatic sensation begins with a specialized receptor in the skin, muscle, or joint. The accuracy with which a stimulus can be detected and localized depends on the density of these receptors (see Fig. 5.1). They are particularly common in the lips and perioral region, the tips of the fingers, and the palms. You can judge this for yourself by seeing your own threshold for detecting two simultaneous point contacts as distinct. On the lips or tips of the fingers this distance is 1 or 2 mm, over the arm a centimeter, and over the back 10 cm, or so. Table 5.1 lists a few of the cutaneous receptive cell types and their functions. All of them are rapid conducting.

Receptive field   The distribution of sensation producing a response in a given neuron.

Other fibers and receptors derived from muscles and joints give information vital for balance, posture, and movement. These include the Golgi tendon receptors and the muscle spindle apparatus, which furnishes data on muscle tension. For the most part these receptor types do not supply signals that reach consciousness.

Information carried in the dorsal column/lemniscal system comes into the spinal cord on sensory nerve roots, travels through the spinal cord, makes a synapse in the low medulla, travels intact and unaltered through the pons and midbrain, and makes a second synapse in the sensory thalamus. Nerve roots that carry comparable kinds of information from the face and head travel in the trigeminal nerve, the fifth cranial nerve, and enter the brain at the level of the pons. We will trace this pathway in its entirety. You should gain an understanding of its specificity, power of resolution, and the losses of function observed when a lesion disrupts any point along this pathway.

Anterolateral–Spinothalamic System

The dorsal column–medial lemniscal system carries signals about the body's relationship to its environment. A separate form of information transmitted to the brain concerns potential or real tissue damage (see Fig. 5.2). Tap your finger with a pencil, and the information travels in the cuneate tract; release your finger and the sensation terminates. Hit your finger with a hammer, crush some cells and damage tissue, and your brain hears about things through a separate pathway, the ***spinothalamic*** or ***anterolateral system.*** After the damage has occurred, the signal continues (see Fig. 5.2). Nociception, temperature, and tissue stretching or squeezing sensations travel in this system.

The bite of a mosquito or sizzling flesh from a fire require a different response than, say, distinguishing a dime from a quarter. The brain therefore handles nociceptive and kinesthetic information quite differently. The core distinction between these two systems is that the nervous system processes pain information at multiple levels, starting from its entrance into the nervous system, while the dorsal column impulses travel relatively unexamined until reaching thalamus and cortex.

Nociception   The perception or sensation of pain, produced by tissue damage. Noci-derives from a Latin word meaning "to injur."

In the spinothalamic system, as the nerve fibers enter the spinal cord, they typically terminate near the point of entry, fanning out over several segments. Because of the wider distribution of its termini, these fibers lose some of their localizing specificity. Even in the dorsal horn the encoded data traverse several synapses before traveling on to the brain (see Fig. 5.3). (Note that the figure is informative but is not to be memorized!) Axons from second- or third-order projection neurons in the dorsal horn cross the midline of the cord just anterior to the ependymal remnants in the anterior white commissure and travel toward the thalamus in the ventrolateral half of the cord. The spinothalamic tract is poorly defined. You would have trouble picking out the ascending spinothalamic fibers from a myriad of other fiber-types in the same region of the cord.

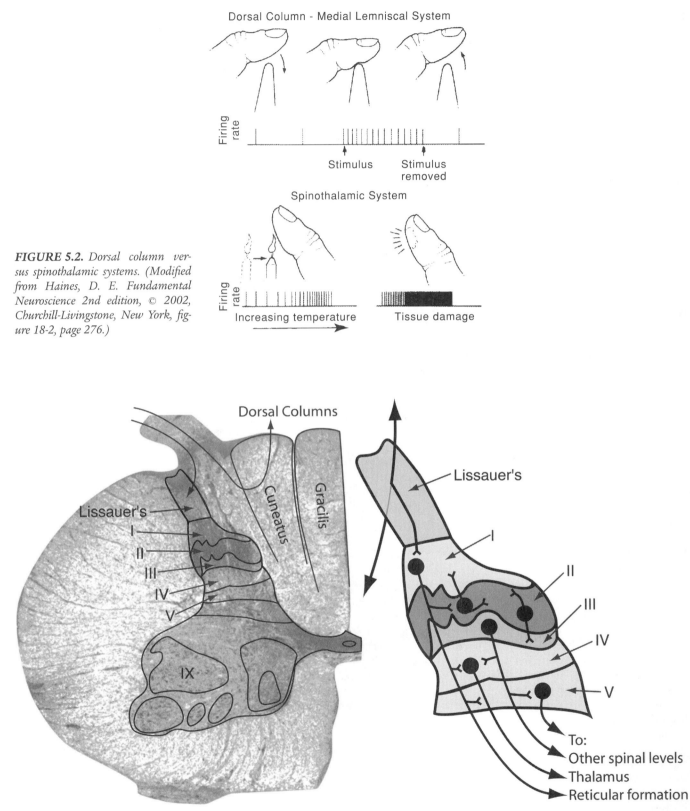

FIGURE 5.2. *Dorsal column versus spinothalamic systems. (Modified from Haines, D. E. Fundamental Neuroscience 2nd edition, © 2002, Churchill-Livingstone, New York, figure 18-2, page 276.)*

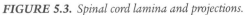

FIGURE 5.3. *Spinal cord lamina and projections.*

These two points must be emphasized:

- The spinothalamic fibers synapse near their level of entry and cross the midline prior to ascending.
- Dorsal column fibers travel ipsilaterally in the cord before synapsing and then crossing in the brainstem.

In marked contrast to the dorsal column system, the pain and temperature nerve endings do not have specialized cellular structures. They are found beneath the skin and in many other tissues as free nerve endings. How they come to detect different stimuli is an active area of investigation and is only now being worked out. Some neurons will detect nonnoxious temperature change of only a few degrees, some will detect potentially damaging heat, others potentially damaging tissue deformity (crushing). Recent work with cold-menthol temperature receptors and capsaicin-pain receptors is shedding new light on the mechanisms cells use to encode these modalities. A subset of these fibers conduct slowly in nonmyelinated fibers and are polymodal, responding to many kinds of stimuli.

Reticular formation An area in the medulla, pons, and midbrain where white matter fibers form a "net" around beds of neurons. Reticulum *is the Latin word for net. This area controls many visceral and diffuse functions.*

When you test pinprick sensation in a patient, using a small, well-localized stimulus, this information is carried on small, myelinated fibers (conduction velocity 5–30 m/s). These kinds of stimuli do not evoke much affective response; they are not "painful." The unmyelinated, slowly conducting fibers (speeds of 0.5–2 m/s) (C fibers) carry painful sensations. These are also the fibers that are easily blocked by local anesthetics like Lidocaine, producing analgesia (which is not quite the same as anesthesia).

The term spinothalamic is only approximately correct. Some fibers travel only a few segments in the cord, and then re-enter to participate in local reflexes. Others terminate in the reticular formation of the brainstem (spinoreticular fibers). A third group ends near the aqueduct in the midbrain, the spinotectal fibers. (The *tectum* is the most dorsal part of the midbrain.) For these reasons, the contemporary term for this tract is the "anterolateral system"; however, old timers (like the authors) use this term interchangeably with the spinothalamic tract. Specificity and fidelity of localization is reduced, compared to the lemniscal system.

To illustrate the anterolateral system, consider what happens when you touch a red hot object with your finger:

1. Your hand immediately pulls back. This is involuntary, and happens before you are aware that anything has gone wrong. Obviously this reflects local reflex actions within the spinal cord. They are *nociceptive reflexes,* which are not monosynaptic like the tendon reflex, but are very important, and phylogenetically ancient.
2. You are alerted, made wide awake. Some of this traffic goes to the ponto-mesencephalic reticular formation, and stimulates this activating system
3. About that time you feel two kinds of pain; an awareness of heat and burning and a second slower, sense of suffering.
4. You may be angry, frustrated, frightened, fearful, all reflecting the fact that the destination of the spinothalamic system, after the thalamus, is only partly to sensory cortex. It also is connected to the hypothalamus, the limbic system, and parts of the brain that express your emotional state. The experience has an emotional valance that you would not find arising from the DC/lemniscal system.

INSTRUCTOR NOTES

This laboratory has two interwoven themes. First is the presentation of more detailed anatomy, including the clinically important relationship between the spinal cord and its bony covering, as well as detailed spinal cord and introductory brainstem anatomy. Second is a comparison of the two main ascending sensory systems, the dorsal columns and pain.

The chapter covers a great deal of material; it is your job to see to it that the students don't get too bogged down in any one area. As they have seen spinal cord histology in the third chapter, this laboratory will discuss it in more detail. The students will also return to the spinal cord several more times in subsequent chapters. The brainstem introduction in this lab is just that, an introduction. As you may painfully be aware, this is a life-long pursuit. The goal of the lab is for the students to recognize (but not necessarily name) the major structures and to then follow the two main sensory pathways rostrally. The next laboratory will take these same pathways through thalamus to cortex and add on the trigeminal system. As in the spinal cord, the students will return to the brainstem in several later chapters, so don't swamp them now.

Make sure the students use any available laboratory materials, including the anatomic specimens, microscope slides, and skeleton models. In essence, it is these materials and you that make the lab more than just this manual. Add some of your clinical tidbits or research interests. Let these bring relevance to but not dominate the lab.

Schedule (2.5 hours)

20 Vertebral column
45 Spinal cord
10 Two point discrimination
60 Brainstem
15 Summary

VERTEBRAL COLUMN

Relationship of Vertebral Column to Spinal Cord and Roots

INST Examine a model of the human head and neck and compare it with the modified diagram in Figure 5.4. Note the location of the spinal cord in the vertebrae, where the nerves exit the bone, and the relationship of the nerves to the intervertebral discs. Be sure to distinguish front from back!

Q5.1. Where do the nerves exit the vertebral column? Where do the dorsal root ganglia lay? Where do the dorsal and ventral roots join to form the spinal nerves? List some of the important structures that immediately surround a spinal nerve.

A5.1. *The spinal nerves exit through the intervertebral foramen. The dorsal root ganglia lie within this space, just proximal to where the dorsal and ventral roots fuse. As the rootlets exit the spinal cord and join to form a nerve, they are first ensheathed by dura and more distally by the nerve sheath. They pass beneath one vertebral pedicle and above another, and lie along side the intervertebral disc.*

MRI Landmarks of the Vertebral Column and Spinal Cord

INST In these exercises it is also worth going to anatomic models or specimens to see the relationship among the spinal cord, its roots and nerves, and the bony structures that encase them.

Q5.2. Figure 5.5 is a diagram showing the spinal cord in the vertebral column. Make sure you know which side is ventral. Figure 5.6 compares a slice through a frozen human

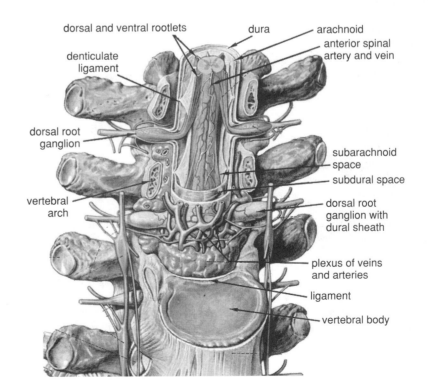

FIGURE 5.4. Spinal cord in vertebral column. (Figure adapted from C. D. Clemente, Anatomy A Regional Atlas of the Human Body, 3rd edition, © 1987, Urban & Schwarzenberg, Baltimore and Munich, figure 573.)

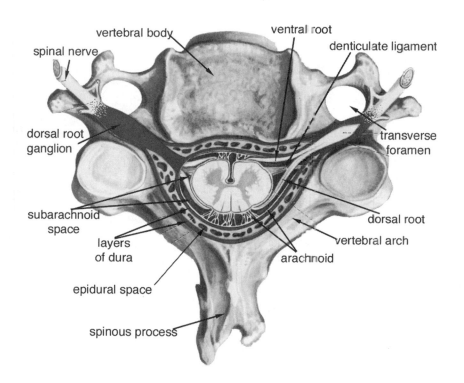

FIGURE 5.5. *Spinal cord in vertebral column (Figure adapted from C. D. Clemente, Anatomy A Regional Atlas of the Human Body, 3rd edition, © 1987, Urban & Schwarzenberg, Baltimore and Munich, figure 571.)*

with a routine cervical spine MRI. Use the diagram in Figure 5.5 to find the following structures in Figure 5.6:

- Vertebral body (body)
- Vertebral artery (VA)
- Dorsal root ganglion and spinal nerve (DRG)

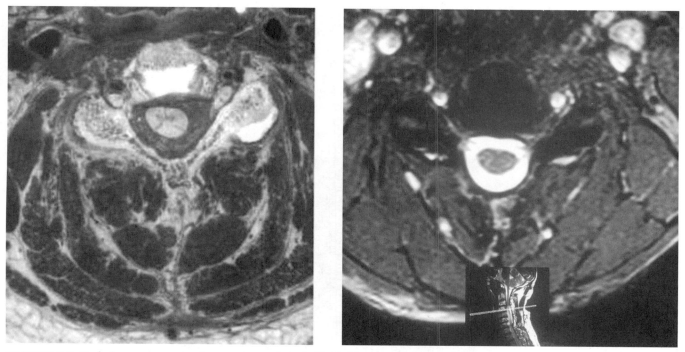

FIGURE 5.6. *Neck close-up comparison between images from the Visible Human Project on the left and a routine transverse MRI. (Left panel adapted from an image created by the Head Browser developed by the University of Michigan, Visible Human Project, National Library of Medicine.)*

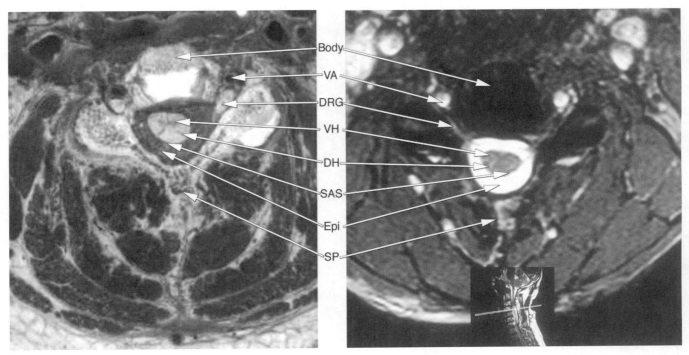

FIGURE 5.7. *Visible Human versus MRI salient structures.*

- Epidural space (Epi)
- Ventral horn (VH)
- Dorsal horn (DH)
- Spinous process (SP)

A5.2. *See Figure 5.7.*

Q5.3. Figure 5.8 compares the cervical level image above with one taken in the lumbar area. What are the little circular forms in the spinal canal in the right panel? Why are they in the lower half of the canal?

A5.3. *The circular forms in the right image are the spinal roots within the spinal canal. When a patient lies down, they settle to the back of the spinal canal.*

Spinal Epidural Space *Unlike the cranial dura, which has one side firmly adherent to bone, the spinal dural sheath remains separated from the vertebrae by a true, epidural space. This space lies between the dura and the periosteum lining the bone and contains loose connective tissue. It is the site where epidural anesthesia is administered.*

Back pain is pervasive in our bipedal species. Correcting an anatomic cause of the pain is a common surgical procedure. During a bilateral laminectomy for decompression, laminae on both sides are cut through and the spinous processes removed. This leaves a larger canal for the spinal cord.

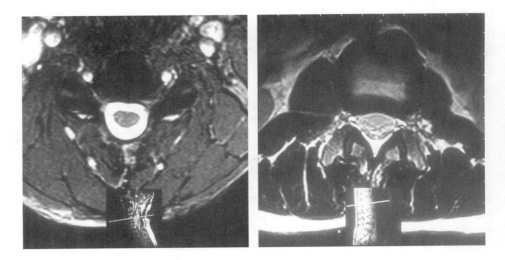

FIGURE 5.8. *Transverse spinal MRI. The left panel is from the cervical level and the right panel is from the lumbar level.*

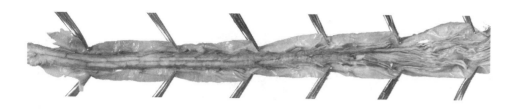

FIGURE 5.9. *Spinal cord gross diss-ection.*

SPINAL CORD

INST Examine again the spinal cord from the second laboratory (see Fig. 5.9). It should be cut along one surface.

- Identify the dura and the remaining portions of nerve roots still attached.
- Look for the cervical and lumbar enlargements. These may be truncated on some specimens.
- Compare the sizes of nerve roots from a lumbar and a thoracic level.
- Visualize the cauda equina.
- Look for blood vessels on the surface of the cord. Make sure you can distinguish anterior from posterior

Q5.4. As a review, which end is caudal? Which side is ventral?

A5.4. *The cauda equina (right in Fig. 5.9) is caudal (caudal is after all, toward the tail) and the side with the single central vessel is ventral or anterior.*

INST On the cut end of the cord, at its topmost level, look for the butterfly shape of the gray matter, surrounded by the ascending and descending tracts of white matter (see Fig. 5.10). No cortex here! White matter is on the outside, not the inside.

Spinal Sensory Roots

The primary cell bodies for the sensory system lie in ganglia outside the central nervous system. For the spinal cord these neurons lie in the ***dorsal root ganglia*** (DRG). Unfortunately for students (but fortunately for the rest of us), bony structures surround these ganglia (see Fig. 5.4), which means they often are left in the body at autopsy.

INST Find a couple of nerve roots from the upper region of the spinal cord on one side. Trace them to their cord level and observe where they enter the cord (dorsal or ventral). Now trace them back to where they have entered the dura. Flip the dura to the other side. This is where the ganglia should be (see Fig. 5.11). Does your specimen have a dorsal root ganglion? The ganglia are located at the

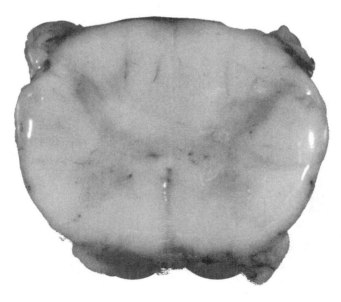

FIGURE 5.10. *Fresh transverse dissection of cervical spinal cord. The slightly darker, central "H" pattern is the gray matter, which is nearly completely surrounded by longitudinal white matter tracts. The gray-white distinction is greatest in unfixed tissue.*

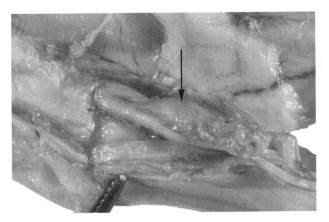

FIGURE 5.11. *Dorsal root ganglion. This photograph is a close-up from the exterior of the spinal dura. The arrow points to the ganglion.*

point where the ventral and dorsal roots penetrate the exit foramen between two vertebrae. Proximal to the ganglia the nerves have separate sensory and motor roots, while distal to the ganglia they form a mixed nerve. If you are able to find a dorsal root ganglion, show it to your lab partners!

Q5.5. Examine the histologic section of the dorsal root ganglion or Figure 5.12. What do you see? What type of cells are the largest?

A5.5. *You should see numerous large cells having a large nucleus, a prominent nucleolus, and peripheral Nissl substance. Around the large cells are many small cells. The largest cells are primary sensory ganglion neurons, and the smaller cells around them are supportive. These large neurons have processes going both to the periphery and centrally into the dorsal spinal cord.*

Anatomy of the Spinal Cord

Q5.6. Compare the spinal cord cross-sectional microscopic slides and the actual dissected cord (see Figs. 5.13 and 5.10). On both the gross specimen and in the slide, orient yourself to dorsal and ventral. Try to identify these structures on the tissue and in Figure 5.14:
- Exiting ventral roots
- Exiting dorsal roots
- Dorsal horn
- Ventral horn and its motor neurons
- Gracilis tract (medial posterior column)
- Cuneate tract (lateral posterior column)
- Corticospinal tract (good part of lateral column)
- Anterolateral (spinothalamic) tract
- Anterior spinal artery

Often you may need to examine a microscope slide at very low power. Try holding the section over a white piece of paper. You can also use a microscope ocular, reversed and held a few mm above

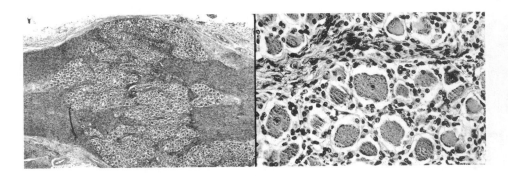

FIGURE 5.12. *Dorsal root ganglion histology, field view* (left) *and high-power* (right).

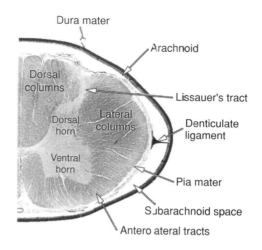

Dura mater
Arachnoid
Dorsal columns
Lissauer's tract
Dorsal horn
Lateral columns
Denticulate ligament
Ventral horn
Pia mater
Subarachnoid space
Anterolateral tracts

FIGURE 5.13. *Major divisions of the spinal cord.*

the slide; put the slide toward the sky. Or try to put the microscope slide directly on the light, below the stage. This latter trick gives you a distorted but low-power view.

> *A5.6. See Figure 5.15. We will return to the anterior horn motor neurons in the neuromuscular chapter; here we are emphasizing sensory pathways and functions.*

Cervical segments are the largest, contain the greatest amount of white matter, and tend to be oval. Thoracic segments are smaller, almost circular, contain the smallest amount of gray matter (in a clear "H" pattern), have a prominent dorsal horn, and two special features in the middle belt of gray matter (the pointed intermediolateral cell column laterally and Clarke's nucleus medially, containing large neurons). Lumbar segments have relatively more gray matter compared to cervical levels. At the lowest end of the cord, buried in the surrounding roots (cauda equina), are the much smaller sacral segments. We don't have tails anymore!

> Q5.7. Use the information above and your atlases to identify each spinal cord level on the microscopic slide and in Figure 5.16. As a help, label each section with the main structures indicated:
> - Dorsal columns
> - Corticospinal tract (CST)
> - Anterolateral tract
> - Ventral horn
> - Dorsal horn
> - Intermediolateral cell column (iml)
> - Clarke's nucleus
>
> *A5.7. The left section is from the lower lumbar level, the middle from the thoracic cord, and the right from the middle cervical level. See Figure 5.17.*
>
> Q5.8. Notice the different ratio of gray and white matter in the various levels of the cord. Explain why the cervical and lumbar cords contain more gray matter. Also explain

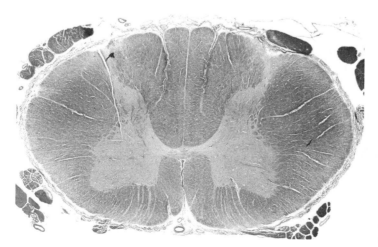

FIGURE 5.14. *Cervical spinal cord, H&E/LFB stain.*

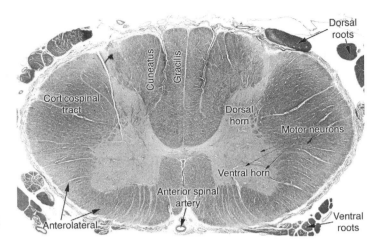

FIGURE 5.15. *Cervical spinal cord, transverse microscopic section.*

why the amount of white matter decreases in both ascending and descending tracts as you descend in the cord.

A5.8. *The prominence of the gray matter at any one level is determined by the number of neurons. The amount of white matter is determined by the number of fibers in the ascending and descending tracts at that level. You need more neurons to operate your feet and hands than you do to move your rib cage up and down, so the lumbar and cervical cords have more gray matter.*

As you travel down the cord descending tracts get off, and so decrease in size. Also, as you travel up the cord, the ascending fibers accumulate. This is similar to a subway; traveling either toward or away from the city, its cars will have few passengers at the end of the line but be full near town. Consequently both sets of tracts are thicker in the upper parts of the spinal cord.

If you feel queasy about your spinal cord anatomy, especially distinguishing levels, note these handy tips:

- Sometimes it IS difficult to distinguish cervical from lumbar. They both have large ventral horns and sometimes the gracilis tract in the lumbar cord looks divided (e.g., by a vessel). The key is the white matter: it is much more plentiful in the cervical cord than in the lumbar.

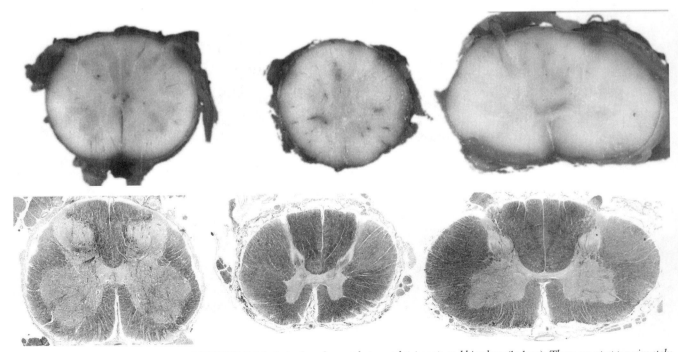

FIGURE 5.16. *Spinal cord gross photograph* (above) *and histology* (below). *These are at approximately the same level, but not from the same patient.*

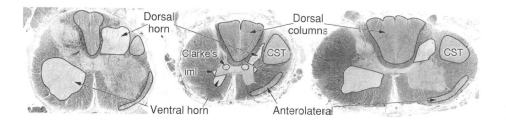

FIGURE 5.17. *Salient features at different spinal cord levels.*

- The intermediolateral and Clarke's columns SHOULD differentiate lumbar from cervical, but they don't travel very far down in the lumbar cord, and so their absence is generally uninformative.
- Thoracic cord is easy: it is small, has a miniscule ventral horn, and has both intermediolateral and Clarke's columns. While small, it still dwarfs the sacral segments.
- The uppermost cervical cord can be tricky to distinguish from thoracic cord, since it no longer has much in the way of ventral horns. But it is much larger than thoracic levels; hope that you have some levels to compare!

Root Entry Zone

INST Using the cross-sectional spinal cord slides, return to the root entry zone. Identify a lightly myelinated area between the top of the dorsal horn and the root entry zone. This is the dorsolateral fasciculus or ***Lissauer's tract*** (see Fig. 5.18, left). Nociceptive fibers travel in this tract for several segments before synapsing in the dorsal horn. Also find the ***substantia gelatinosa*** (see Fig. 5.18, right), a pink cap of gray matter in the dorsal horn that has only few myelinated fibers. This gray matter lamina processes nociceptive information.

The central gray matter is composed of layers of neurons, called zones. Rexed distinguished these zones and gave them numbers. Today, these are known as ***Rexed layers.*** Rexed layers I through VII make up the dorsal horn. While the substantia gelatinosa is easy to see, the others are less so. Several of these other dorsal horn lamina also receive and process nociceptive and temperature information and then send long fibers through the anterior white commissure to the contralateral anterolateral tracts (see Fig. 5.19). Details of Rexed lamination are beyond the use of all but die-hard neuroanatomists!

In contrast to pain and temperature information, kinesthetic impulses entering from dorsal roots that will join the dorsal column system bypass Lissauer's tract completely. They, instead, turn medially and directly enter the dorsal columns without synapsing. As you will encounter in many places in the nervous system, the dorsal column fibers have a somatotopic organization: those from the legs pile in first and so lie in the medial gracile column, while information from T6 up gets added on later and ascends in the more lateral cuneate fasciculus. (You are probably aware by now that medical terminology is designed to confuse; this gives us job security. Fasciculus, column, and tract are often used interchangeably).

The aim here is NOT details of Rexed lamination. The important points are:

- Dorsal column fibers enter the column somatotopically at their level.
- Dorsal column fibers travel ipsilaterally up the cord, and first synapse in the lower medulla prior to crossing.

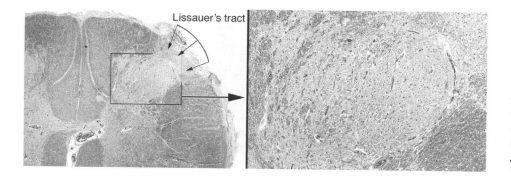

FIGURE 5.18. *Dorsal horn (left) and substantia gelatinosa (right). Lissauer's tract is the lightly myelinated tract exterior to the substantia gelatinosa and marginal zone (cap of the gelatinosa).*

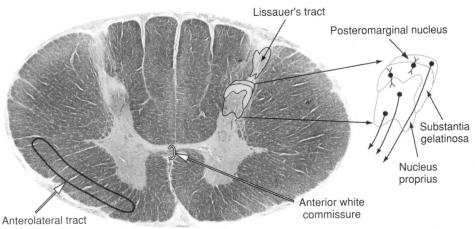

FIGURE 5.19. *Spinal cord dorsal horn and anterior white commissure.*

- Nociceptive and temperature fibers travel a few levels (in Lissauer's tract) and then synapse in the posterior horn.
- Nociceptive information is modified in the dorsal horn, for example, by descending impulses from the brainstem, prior to transmission onto thalamus.
- Nociceptive information crosses the cord near the level of entry and travels in the anterolateral portion of cord.

Q5.9. Compare the size of the dorsal columns in the cervical region with those in the lumbar (see Fig. 5.20). Which fibers are more medial, those from the leg or from the arm? How long is a single fiber of the gracile tract, derived from the big toe, until its termination at its other end? Why might the lengths of different fibers be significant for disease processes?

A5.9. *The dorsal columns in the cervical cord are much larger than in the lumbar, since they contain kinesthetic information from the body and arms, as well as the legs. The most medial fibers in the gracilis columns are added first and come from the lower limbs. Additional fibers are added from the dorsal root entry zone, and are more lateral; above the middle thoracic levels they become the cuneate tract.*
In a tall person a gracilis fiber could be up to 2 meters long, from toe to gracile nucleus in the medulla. Since many diseases act locally, for example, a focus of inflammation, long fibers are typically more frequently affected. This is also true of systemic diseases like diabetes. Toxins and ischemia have a greater probability of affecting a longer structure than a shorter one.

Q5.10. Contrast Lissauer's tract, sitting on top of the dorsal horn, with the posterior columns (see microscopic slide or Fig. 5.21). Then compare these with the substantia gelatinosa, and the remainder of the posterior horn. Specifically address the amount of myelin and gray matter in the latter structures.

A5.10. *The posterior columns are densely myelinated and are filled with "blue donuts." In contrast, Lissauer's tract is a sparsely myelinated (skimpy donuts). This latter tract carries "pain and temperature" fibers several spinal segments from the dorsal root ganglia before synapsing. The*

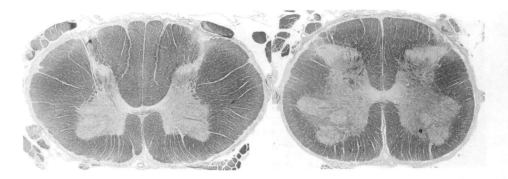

FIGURE 5.20. *Cervical and lumbar dorsal column comparison.*

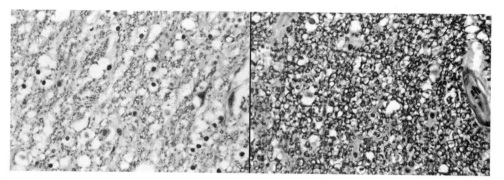

FIGURE 5.21. *Comparison of Lissauer's tract* (left) *with posterior column white matter* (right).

substantia gelatinosa is gray matter almost entirely devoid of myelinated axons (contains neurons, dendrites, and axon terminals—i.e., it's where processing occurs), while the gray matter in III and IV have some myelinated fibers. Notice the "cap" between the substantia gelatinosa and Lissauer's tract.

Q5.11. Neurons in the "cap" and in the deeper layers of the dorsal horn receive nociceptive information and then project this rostrally to the thalamus in the spinothalamic tract. Their axons cross the cord through the central commissure, and travel rostrally in the anterior-lateral portion of the cord. Contrast this with the posterior column lemniscal system. Specifically address the order of the neurons and the sites of decussation.

A5.11. *In the spinothalamic system (and as we will see in the next laboratory, its equivalent in the medulla) the second-order neurons are close to the entrance zone of the dorsal root ganglion neurons. In contrast, the second-order neurons of the posterior column system lie far away in the lower medulla. The primary nociceptive fibers travel a few segments before synapsing. The spinothalamic fibers cross the midline near their level of entry, while posterior column fibers cross in the lower medulla.*

Q5.12. On the left-hand image of Figure 5.22, draw the initial pathway of the left spinothalamic fibers. Draw ovals for the approximate ascending spinothalamic tracts. On the right-hand image, draw the dorsal column pathway. Starting with a right dorsal root ganglion neuron, distinguish fibers traveling from below from those entering at this level. Be sure to indicate where the cell bodies are for each pathway.

A5.12. *In Figure 5.23 the left image shows two projection neurons in the dorsal horn giving rise to the contralateral spinothalamic tract. The right image indicates a cuneatus fiber coming in from the arm. In gray is a fiber traveling up from the leg in the gracilis column.*

Q5.13. Review the anatomy above in slides and with atlases. Make sure you can locate these structures in Figure 5.24:
- Lissauer's tract
- Substantia gelatinosa
- Nucleus proprius (Rexed zones III and IV)
- Central or anterior white commissure
- Approximate location of spinothalamic tract
- Dorsal columns

A5.13. *See Figure 5.25.*

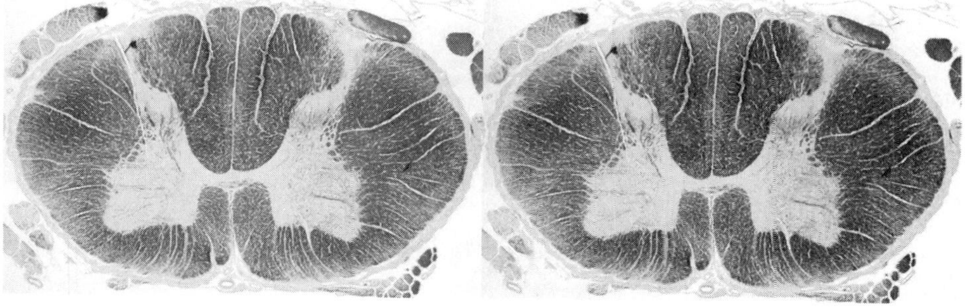

FIGURE 5.22. *Cervical spinal cord histologic sections, both at same level.*

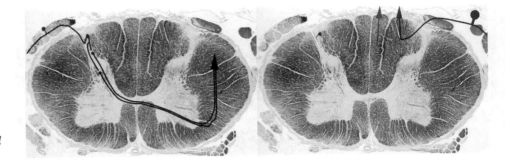

FIGURE 5.23. *Anterolateral and dorsal column systems.*

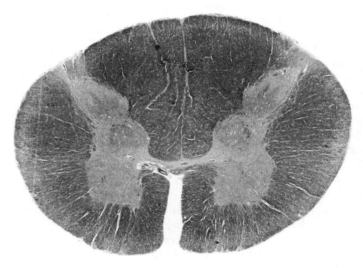

FIGURE 5.24. *Upper lumbar spinal cord histology.*

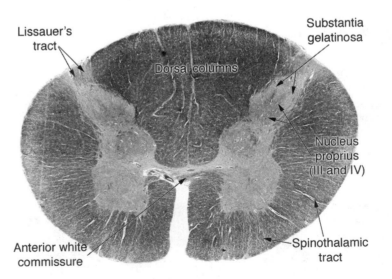

FIGURE 5.25. *Significant sensory sites in upper lumbar spinal cord (H&E/LFB stain).*

Two-Point Discrimination

INST Find a partner and pair up to give each other a two-point discrimination test. Use three or four zones of sensory perception: for example, the tip of the index finger, the lower lip, the dorsum of the forearm, and the middle of the back. (For the latter zone this can be done through light clothing.) Use two pencil points, or tips of two unfolded paper clips; the stimulus should be a small point but not sharp. Start with the two stimuli very close together, and see when the subject can detect that the two points are separate. For guidance, approximate thresholds are finger and lip 2 mm, forearm 1 to 2 cm, and back 10 to 15 cm.

Q5.14. What does this procedure test, the dorsal columns or anterolateral system?

A5.14. *Hopefully it tests the dorsal columns (although with excess force or sharp pins, it will also test pain)! This system provides fine discrimination; the test indicates the size of the receptive fields and excessively large fields suggests posterior column dysfunction.*

BRAINSTEM

You will now enter a bewildering area of the brain, the forest of nuclei and tracts that is the brainstem. Were you to be dropped here, you would surely get lost. However, in this chapter you will only fly over the region, following the two sensory tracts discussed in this laboratory.

While this laboratory discusses spinal cord anatomy in some detail, it only briefly introduces brainstem anatomy. The goal here is to follow the lemniscal and spinothalamic fibers through the brainstem. Word of caution: the brainstem is a life-study onto itself, so don't get bogged down on your first day! If you wonder about face sensation, that comes in the next laboratory. Two later chapters are devoted to the brainstem.

Cervicomedullary Transition

As you enter the lower medulla from the spinal cord, two major changes and a transition occur:

- The dorsal column fibers synapse on their second-order neurons.
- The pyramidal tract undergoes its decussation (as you have seen in the second lab and will return to later).
- The dorsal horn of the spinal cord becomes the spinal trigeminal nucleus (more on this nucleus in the next laboratory).

Q5.15. Using your atlas and texts, find the following structures in Figure 5.26, taken from the cervicomedullary junction:
- Decussation of the pyramids
- Gracilis nucleus
- Cuneatus nucleus
- Spinal trigeminal nucleus
- Location of the ascending spinothalamic fibers

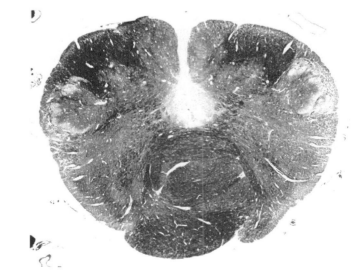

FIGURE 5.26. *Cervicomedullary junction.*

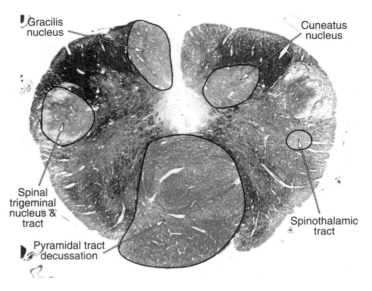

FIGURE 5.27. *Salient structures at the cervicomedullary junction.*

A5.15. *See Figure 5.27.*

Q5.16. Compare the structures in Figure 5.27 with those in the spinal cord (Figs. 5.15 and 5.19). Do the locations of the dorsal column nuclei (gracilis and cuneatus) "make sense"? What has happened to the spinothalamic tract? What is the medullary equivalent to the dorsal horn of the spinal cord?

A5.16. *The gracilis nucleus sits more or less directly on top of or rostral to its tract, while the cuneate nucleus lies a bit ventral and medial. The spinothalamic tract still sits anterior and lateral but is moving more posterior. This trend will continue as the tract ascends in the brainstem. For the head and neck, the gray matter equivalent to the spinal cord's dorsal horn is the spinal trigeminal nucleus. Analogously, Lissauer's tract corresponds to the spinal trigeminal tract. More on this in the next chapter.*

Medulla

To trace the two sensory systems higher in the brainstem, you will need some major landmarks to orient you in this foreign soil. These structures will serve as guideposts in your sojourns along tracts and around nuclei. When you return to the brainstem in later chapters, these guide posts will also help you. However, in this laboratory focus on the medial lemniscal and anterolateral system.

Q5.17. Examine the ventral medulla in either a model, the actual brainstem, or in Figure 5.29. Try to figure out where you would dissect Figure 5.29 to get the cross-sectional levels in Figure 5.28. (Hint: Look at the relationship between the pyramids and the inferior olivary nuclei.)

A5.17. *See Figure 5.30. The left histologic image in Figure 5.28 has just the beginning of the inferior olivary nucleus, and so is in the lower third of the medulla. The right photo has a full-blown olive. As always, these figures are approximate; use them to get a sense of where you are in the brainstem rather than as gospel.*

Q5.18. Use your atlases and diagrams to label the main features of the medulla in Figure 5.28:
- Pyramids (e.g., pyramidal or corticospinal tract) on the ventral surface of medulla.
- Inferior olivary nucleus (ION), just dorsolateral to the pyramids.
- Fourth ventricle (iv), beginning about a third of the way up the medulla and enlarging as one moves rostrally.
- Hypoglossal (XII) nucleus.
- Solitary tract and nucleus, easy to identify, important for taste sensation and for various cardiovascular reflexes.
- Spinotrigeminal nucleus (V n.) and tract (V tr.).
- Medial lemniscus (ml).

As in the spinal cord, the spinothalamic fibers are not as tightly organized as the posterior column fibers.

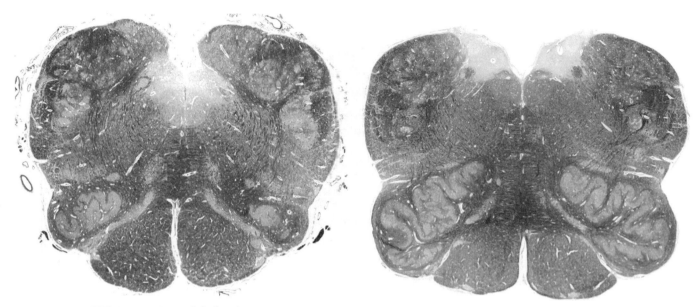

FIGURE 5.28. *Medulla histologic sections, caudal third and middle.*

A5.18. See Figure 5.31.

Q5.19. Locate in the left panel of Figure 5.31 the gracile and cuneate nuclei. This is the termination point for the dorsal column fibers. They form synapses here with second-order sensory neurons that continue on upward to thalamus. The strict somatotopic organization of the fibers is preserved through this synapse. Synaptic connections from modulatory neurons nearby and from other systems modulate the signals.

Streaming ventrally from the cuneate and gracile nuclei toward the ventral midline are thin arcs of myelinated fibers (see Fig. 5.31). What is the name of these fibers? These fibers decussate or cross the midline at this point, just as they enter the medial lemniscus.

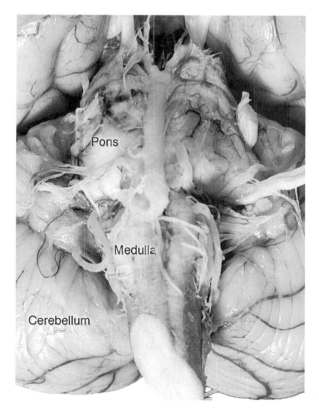

FIGURE 5.29. *Ventral view of medulla and pons.*

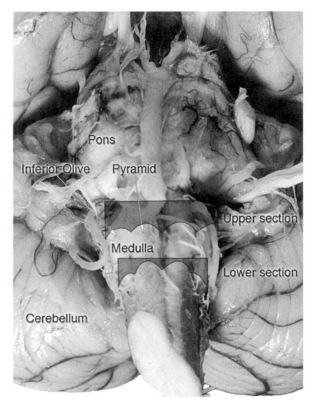

FIGURE 5.30. *Slices in Figure 5.28 through lower third and middle of medulla.*

With the help of your atlas and texts, also locate the ascending pain and temperature fibers (spinothalamic fibers) in Figure 5.31 as they travel upward in the medulla.

A5.19. *The fibers arcing off the posterior column nuclei are the internal arcuate fibers. They cross the midline in small bundles and immediately form the medial lemniscus. They are the axons from the second-order neurons of the lemniscal system. Remember, this is the site where posterior column sensory information crosses to the contralateral side. See Figure 5.32.*

The gracilis and cuneate nuclei basically sit on top of their respective columns. The gracilis neurons lie slightly caudal to those of the cuneate; as such they contribute their fibers earlier to the medial lemniscus. The gracilis, and hence leg fibers, lie more ventral to the those of the cuneate. Arm fibers are added on top, making the well-known body without a head. The head kinesthetic fibers are added in the pons. More of this in the next laboratory.

Pain and temperature fibers remain in the lateral aspects of the medulla.

Q5.20. What large nucleus lies dorsal to the spinothalamic tract? Which one lies ventromedial to it? Axons in this tract make extensive connections in the reticular formation. Locate this area in the figure. What is the anatomic relationship between the lemniscal and anterolateral fibers?

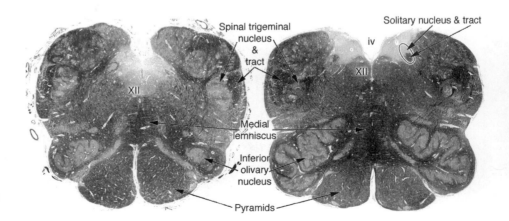

FIGURE 5.31. *Salient structures in the medulla.*

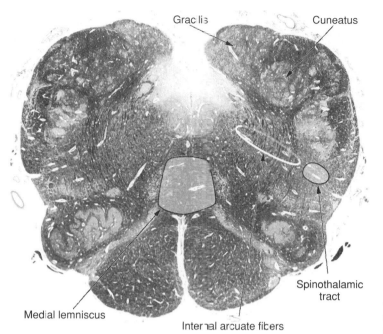

Gracilis   Cuneatus

Spinothalamic
tract

Medial lemniscus   Internal arcuate fibers

FIGURE 5.32. *Somatosensory nuclei and tracts in medulla. Arrows on decussation of medial lemniscal fibers.*

A5.20. *Dorsal to the spinothalamic or anterolateral fibers are the spinal trigeminal nucleus and tract, and dorsal to that the vestibular nuclei. Ventromedial to it is the magnificent inferior olivary nucleus. The spinothalamic fibers travel in the lateral aspect of the reticular formation, synapsing on nearby neurons as it ascends rostrally.*

In the medulla the two ascending sensory systems remain separated in its medial and lateral aspects. They become juxtaposed more rostrally, but the information remains separate. In the medulla the spinothalamic fibers are located lateral to the nucleus ambiguus, in a separate vascular territory compared to the lemniscal fibers. Hence this is one part of the CNS where a lesion may produce a dissociated sensory loss affecting one system and not the other, as can happen after small a stroke. A lateral medullary stroke (in the territory of the posterior inferior cerebellar artery or PICA) is one of the common ways to get this kind of sensory loss. As the lemniscal fibers rotate in the pons, they move laterally and then abut the already lateral anterolateral fibers. As the spinothalamic system reaches the midbrain, many of its fibers split off and project to the reticular formation and periaqueductal gray matter. Pain and temperature fibers from the face add to the anterolateral tract throughout the medulla (more in the next laboratory).

Dissociated sensory loss *Loss of different sensory modalities (especially dorsal column—medial lemniscal and nociception, and temperature) on opposite sides of the body or face. This most often indicates pathology in either the spinal cord or lower brainstem, where the two major systems remain separate.*

Q5.21. The medial lemniscus maintains a somatotopic organization as it ascends to thalamus. In the medulla the medial lemniscus contains a body without a head, with the feet pointing ventrally. Draw a headless body in Figure 5.33

A5.21. *See Figure 5.34.*

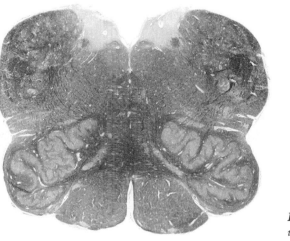

FIGURE 5.33. *Medulla, about midway up.*

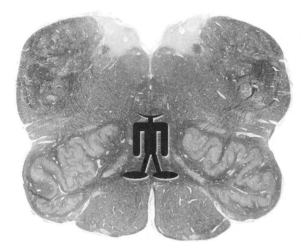

FIGURE 5.34. *Somatotopic organization of medial lemniscus in medulla. Note that this representation is only approximate, to emphasize that the medial lemniscus in the medulla is a body standing up, but without a head.*

Pons

Q5.22. In order to trace the medial lemniscus through the pons, first label its main landmarks in Figure 5.35:
- Fourth ventricle (iv). Its walls are the cerebellar peduncles.
- Basis pontis. This is the large bulge in the ventral pons. The bulge is formed from various motor tracts and fibers, many of them related to the cerebellum. (We will return to them in later chapters.) Many small and large neurons are embedded in the basis pontis.
- Trigeminal complex (V). Located in the lateral part of the midpons. It is a complex nucleus, containing motor fibers for the muscles of mastication, and sensory fibers for deep and superficial structures of the face and head.
- Abducens nucleus (VI). Controls one extraocular muscle.
- Facial nucleus (VII). Furnishes motor innervation for the muscles of the face.

A5.22. *See Figure 5.36.*

Q5.23. Using your atlases and texts, locate the lemniscal pathway in Figure 5.37. How has its orientation changed since the medulla? Knowing that the headless person in the medulla has laid down with his or her feet pointed laterally and gotten a head, draw this person on the figure.

A5.23. *The medial lemniscus stands up in the medulla (and looks like a headless person, with arm fibers dorsally and leg fibers ventrally) and lays down in the pons. The crossed head fibers, added medially, give this laying person a head. The feet are lateral, the head medial. See Figure 5.38.*

Unlike the spinothalamic fibers, which synapse extensively in the brainstem, lemniscal fibers travel without further connection on to thalamus. However, in the pons the body gets a head: fibers from the contralateral face and head (homologous to the dorsal column fibers) join onto the medial edge

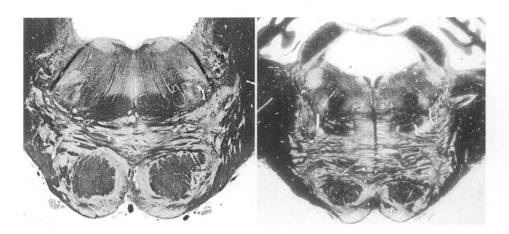

FIGURE 5.35. *Pons transverse histology. The left figure is from the lower end of the pons, showing cranial nerve nuclei VI and VII, while the right is at the level of cranial nerve V.*

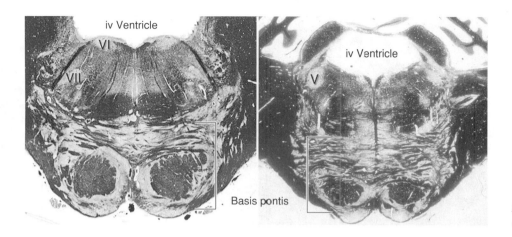

FIGURE 5.36. *Salient pontine structures.*

of the lemniscus. By the middle of the pons, the medial lemniscus contains kinesthetic information from the entire opposite side of the body and face.

Q5.24. What happened to the spinothalamic fibers? Try to locate them in Figure 5.37.

A5.24. *These fibers have now joined to the lateral end of the medial lemniscal fibers. In essence, the medial lemniscus has moved lateral and met up with the already lateral anterolateral fibers (see Fig. 5.39).*

Midbrain

Q5.25. Again, label these main landmarks in Figure 5.40.
- Cerebral aqueduct. The fourth ventricle narrowed down to a small tube.
- Oculomotor nucleus (III). Large cells innervating the muscles of eye movement.
- Cerebral peduncle. Large descending motor fibers, some of which are destined to go all the way down to the spinal cord, some of which will terminate in the pons and make connections with the cerebellum. (More on this in later chapters.)
- Red nucleus (RN). A rounded or oval structure with motor system functions.
- Substantia nigra (SN). Between the peduncle and the red nucleus, containing pigmented cells hence its color, and also concerned with motor tone and movement.

A5.25. See Figure 5.41.

Q5.26. Using your references, position the lemniscal system in the midbrain in Figure 5.40. What structures lie medial to this great tract? Ventral? All of the fibers are unchanged in function. Where are the anterolateral fibers now? Using the previous somatotopic diagram above, identify the leg, thorax, and arm (and head) regions.

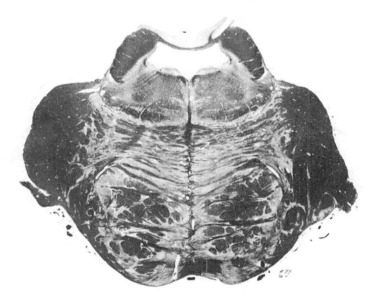

FIGURE 5.37. *Pons, middle-rostral level.*

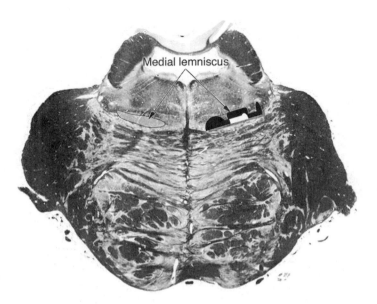

FIGURE 5.38. *Medial lemniscus in rostral pons. The somatotopic map is only approximate.*

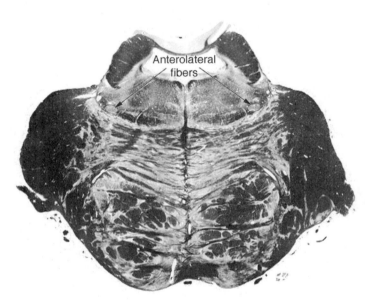

FIGURE 5.39. *Approximate location of anterolateral fibers, including the spinothalamic tracts.*

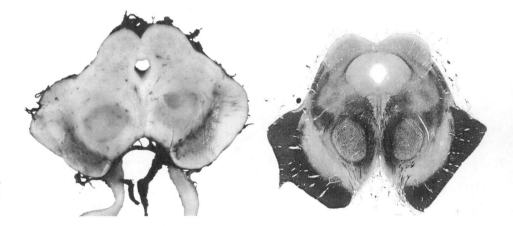

FIGURE 5.40. *Midbrain. The left image is a gross picture and the right is a histology section stained for myelin.*

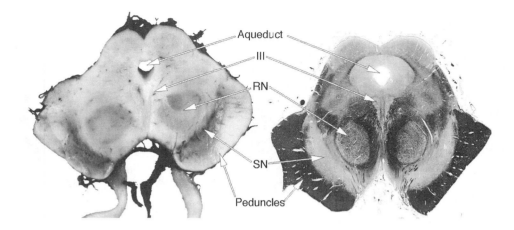

FIGURE 5.41. *Salient midbrain structures.*

A5.26. See Figure 5.42. Medial to the lemniscus pathway (which, to make your life difficult, is now lateral in the midbrain) lie the red nucleus, the oculomotor nucleus, and the aqueduct. Ventral to these fibers are the substantia nigra and the cerebral peduncle. The anterolateral fibers are juxtaposed with the lemniscal fibers, on its dorsolateral edge.

Q5.27. The next synaptic relay is found immediately above the midbrain, in the sensory nuclei of the thalamus. The thalamus is the gateway for the cortex. All non-olfactory sensory information passes through the thalamus. Our next laboratory will discuss this and hemispheric primary sensory structures.

Note that the thalamus lies immediately above the midbrain. Predict the relative location of the leg and head neurons in thalamus.

A5.27. The leg neurons are in the lateral aspect of thalamus (VPL), just above the leg fibers in the midbrain. Similarly facial information is more medial (VPM) in both structures.

ANTEROLATERAL VERSUS MEDIAL LEMNISCAL PATHWAYS IN BRAINSTEM

Q5.28. As a summary, trace the spinothalamic fibers through the brainstem, using the panel on the left in Figure 5.43. Then trace the medial lemniscal fibers from the gracilis nucleus through the midbrain on the panel to the right. Feel free to use your atlas and other references.

A5.28. See Figure 5.44.

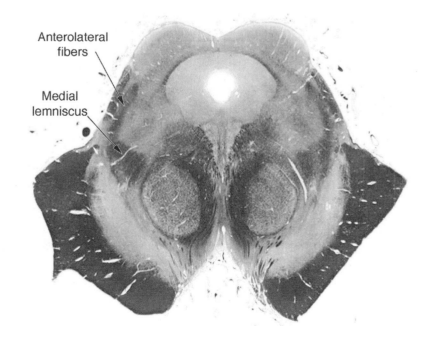

FIGURE 5.42. *Approximate positions of the medial lemniscal and anterolateral fibers. While atlases and textbooks show these fibers systems as segregated in the midbrain, they both head for adjacent regions of thalamus and so must be blending before reaching their targets.*

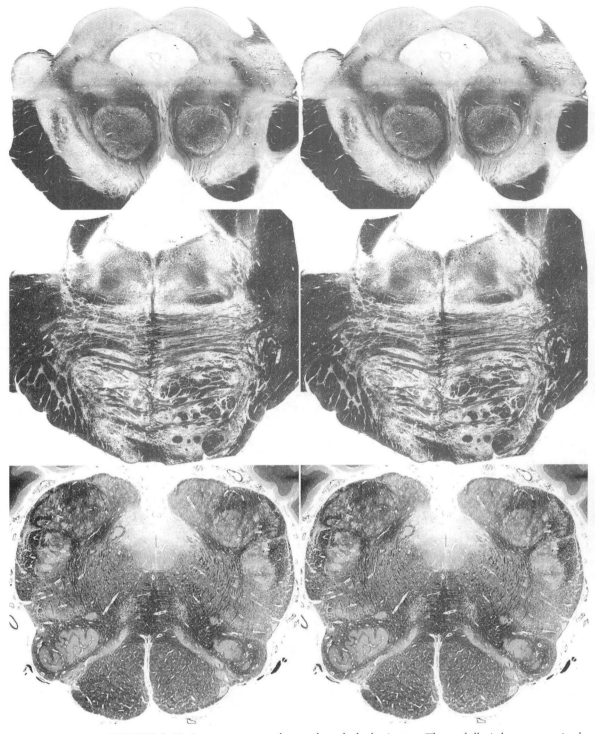

FIGURE 5.43. *Somatosensory pathways through the brainstem. The medulla is lowest, pons in the middle, and midbrain at the top.*

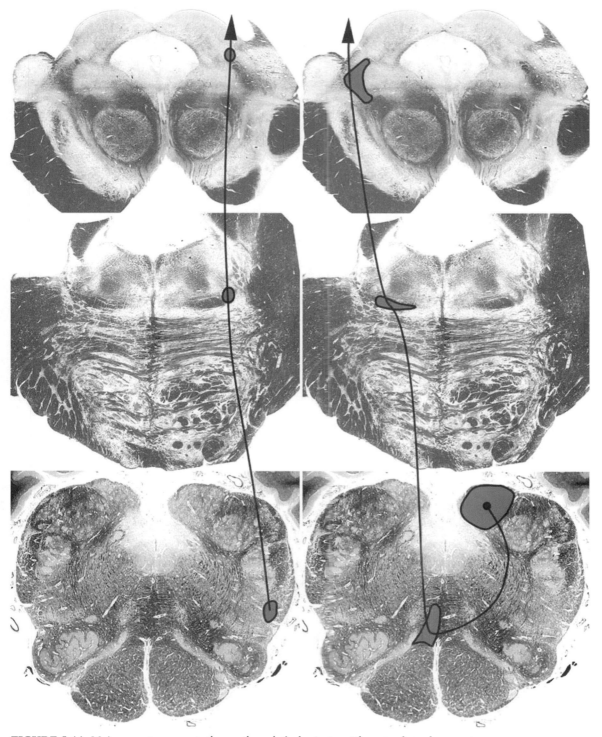

FIGURE 5.44. *Major somatosensory pathways through the brainstem. The anterolateral system is on the left, while the medial lemniscal system is on the right.*

Chapter 6—CRANIOSENSORY SYSTEMS

Y ou have delivered sensory information to the top of the midbrain. However, you are missing the head, and you still need to get all of this data to the cortex. In this chapter you continue to follow the two main sensory tracts through the thalamus to cortex, and you'll add the head to the body by adding on the trigeminal system.

Our head is what truly distinguishes vertebrates from invertebrates. It is what allowed our distant ancestors to better eat their neighbor than to be eaten by them. It possesses several special sensory modalities, including hearing, vision, and taste. You will visit these in later chapters. This chapter will focus on the pathways shared with the body: pain, temperature, and kinesthetic sensations.

To better appreciate the brain's three-dimensional structure, you'll examine horizontal slabs of brain. Look at the brain carefully; you may not get to see it in such detail again. Use all resources you have available to reinforce the spatial anatomy of the brain.

LEARNING OBJECTIVES

- Obtain a working knowledge of the gross anatomy of the cerebral hemispheres, by examining eight horizontal sections through the brain.
- Continue to track the dorsal column–medial lemniscal and anterolateral systems through the thalamus to their termination in the postcentral gyrus.
- Understand the two main sensory components of the trigeminal system, one traveling in parallel with the lemniscal fibers, carrying sensory impulses from head and face, and the other carrying nociceptive and temperature information in the anterolateral system.
- Compare and contrast the anterolateral and the lemniscal systems.

Functional Neuroanatomy: An Interactive Text and Manual, by Jeffrey T. Joseph and David L. Cardozo
ISBN 0-471-44437-5 Copyright © 2004 John Wiley & Sons, Inc.

INTRODUCTION

Thalamus

Sensory traffic undergoes considerable modification and modulation in the thalamus. While relay neurons preserve the precise somatotopic sensory organization ascending from below, small interneurons in the ventrobasal complex serve to enhance or inhibit their transmission. Some of the fibers are also sorted out anatomically. For example, fibers dealing with position sensations arrive at columns of cells a distance away from those dealing with touch, although still organized by receptive field.

The thalamus is like a compact cortex. Its nuclei have connections with specific regions of cortex, and correspondingly, most areas of cortex, including all of the neocortex, have close connections with their own thalamic nuclei. These thalamocortical circuits are especially prominent in the frontal and parietal lobes. The thalamocortical circuit that has been studied in greatest detail interconnects the thalamic lateral geniculate nucleus and the visual cortex (next chapter).

Those sensory fibers from the last laboratory, involving sensations from the body, project to the ventral posterior-lateral (VPL) nucleus of thalamus. (The thalamus, like all other areas of neuroanatomy, is a collection of confusingly named substructures that are often hard to identify. For example, the VPL is neither particularly ventral nor particularly posterior and is not easily distinguished from its neighbors.) Third-order neurons in the VPL project on to cortex.

Cortex and Homunculus

Fibers from the VPL travel through the internal capsule, into the centrum semiovale. Many somatosensory fibers terminate in the postcentral gyrus of the anterior parietal lobe. In this gyrus the somatotopic fidelity is preserved. Recordings from cells in the cortex will show sharp localization to regions of the body. Body regions with small receptive fields, and hence having a greater density of representative lemniscal fibers, will project to a disproportionately larger region of sensory cortex. Watching an infant bring new objects to their lips emphasizes their tactile sensitivity; lips, face, fingers and thumb are all over-represented in sensory cortex (see the "sensory homunculus" diagram in Fig. 6.1). Within the sensory cortex, organized columns of neurons respond to particular kinds of stimuli. Some respond to edges, others to various textures. At each level of the three neuron chain, somatotopic fidelity, although modulated, is preserved.

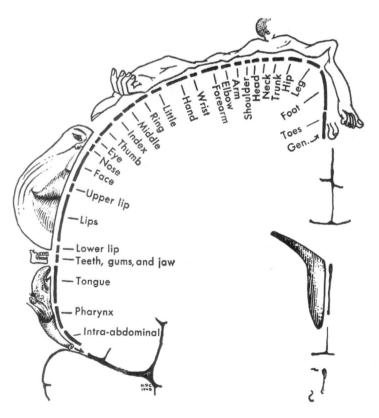

FIGURE 6.1. *Sensory homunculus (Figure modified from Penfield and Rasmussen, The Cerebral Cortex of Man, Macmillan Company, New York, 1952, figure 17, page 44.). These neurosurgeons empirically determined this mapping during craniotomies by directly stimulating the cortex and asking the awake patient what they sensed.*

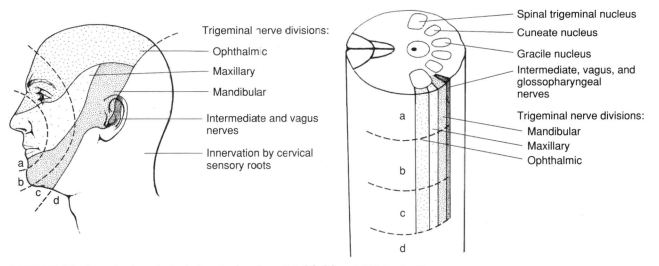

FIGURE 6.2. *Organization of spinal trigeminal nucleus. (Modified from J. H. Martin, Neuroanatomy: Text and Atlas, second edition, © 1996, Appleton & Lange, Stamford, CT, figure 12-7, page 369.)*

Lemniscal System; Adding Trigeminal Input

The trigeminal system is responsible for relaying sensory information from the face, oral and nasal cavities, and the cornea. These sensations arise from receptors similar to those elsewhere in the body. For example, some receptors in the periodontal tissue are extremely sensitive to tooth displacement and bite force, allowing us to use teeth to assess size, hardness, and other qualities.

The trigeminal assemblage is a complex system, with a motor component, nociceptive and temperature sensory fibers that track downward through the medulla to the spinal trigeminal nucleus, and a chief sensory nucleus. This latter nucleus is the homologue of the cuneate and gracile nuclei in the medulla. The homologue of the dorsal root ganglion, situated on the fifth nerve in front of the pons, is the trigeminal or Gasserian ganglion. This structure is often neglected, since it lies in the middle cranial fossa underneath the dura. (Remember it from the sheep brain!)

Like the medial lemniscal system, second-order neurons from the chief sensory nucleus project to the contralateral thalamus. Fibers from the chief sensory nucleus cross to the opposite side, and follow along with the lemniscal fibers to the thalamus. They enter into the ventrobasal complex traveling in company with the medial lemniscus. The body will now get a head. Their destination is the ventral posteromedial (VPM) nucleus, medial to ventral posterolateral nucleus (VPL). However, the trigeminal system reflects the head's complicated phylogenetic past (the cranial nerves have a relationship to the gill slits). Second-order sensory neurons form two bundles, determined by their origin; those derived from the face and from the oral cavity travel by different routes. The fibers from face travel ventrally, while those from the oral cavity lie in the trigeminal mesencephalic tract, nearer the aqueduct. They both eventually arrive at the VPM nucleus.

Trigeminal Input into Anterolateral System

Fiber systems homologous to the spinothalamic system come from the face and head. These fibers enter the pons, but in contrast to the lemniscal system, they turn caudally, and descend in the medulla down into the first cervical segment. Along this descending spinal trigeminal tract they make second-order connections with neurons in its associated nucleus. This nociceptive system then includes a long descending tract and a long spinal trigeminal nucleus. Like the trigeminal contribution to the lemniscal system, the spinal trigeminal nucleus and tract are also somatotopically organized. However, the anatomic relationships are complex, as demonstrated in Figure 6.2.

INSTRUCTOR'S NOTES

This laboratory is a continuation from chapter 5. The same two sensory pathways are emphasized. The first part of the chapter is really a digression into gross neuroanatomy, using horizontal slices of brain. The remainder of the activities in part build on the horizontal sections to illustrate the sensory thalamus and its relationship to the sensory cortices.

As always, make sure students look at the brain in some detail. They will want to look at pictures and diagrams, but the real thing will stick with them much longer. You may wish to play "dump the brain," in which you take their carefully cut and laid out slices of brain, mix them up, and have the students put them back together. Excellent training to learn what is where and who is next to whom.

Schedule (2.5 hours)
45 Horizontal slabs
30 Thalamus
30 Trigeminal pain and kinesthetic system
15 Sensory cortex
30 Clinical aspects

HORIZONTAL SLABS

We will cut slabs from the brain in order to get an idea of the 3D anatomy of the main structures in unstained tissue. Correlate what you see with atlases, and sections of brain cut in other planes, sagittal and coronal. You may also want to refer back to the neuroradiology images from the fourth lab. Using the ventricular system as a landmark is very helpful, and you should also review models of the CSF containing spaces of the brain as you go along.

INST   Review the external anatomy of the hemisphere before you start. Pre-mark the precentral gyrus with India ink, as you did in the second laboratory. Remove the posterior fossa structures from the cerebrum by cutting transversely across the upper midbrain, making an even slice from the superior colliculus dorsally through the peduncles anteriorly, just behind the mammillary bodies. See Figure 6.3. SAVE the brainstem and cerebellum in a bag for a later lab! A dehydrated cerebellum is not a pleasant sight.

INST   Section the hemisphere along the planes outlined in Figure 6.4. Carefully lay out the slices so that you know their order, front from back, and right from left.

Q6.1. Examine the highest slice (Fig. 6.5). Note the large amount of white matter present. It is composed of three kinds of fiber tracts, which you cannot easily distinguish by gross inspection. Some travel across the corpus callosum and connect homologous parts of cortex on the two sides of the brain (callosal fibers). Some are ascending or descending fiber tracts, carrying motor or sensory information to and from lower levels. Some run anterior-posterior, making corticocortical connections, often between

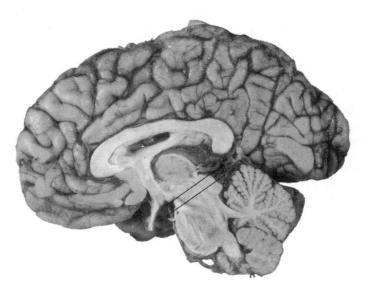

FIGURE 6.3. Location of cuts to remove the brainstem from the hemispheres.

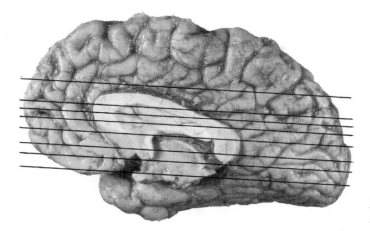

FIGURE 6.4. *Approximate slice positions for horizontal dissection.*

association cortices (association fibers). Altogether this large area of white matter is called the ***centrum semiovale,*** a term which applies to hemispheric white matter located dorsal and lateral to the lateral ventricle. Use your atlases of the brain to locate these structures on your slices and in Figure 6.5:

- Central (Rolandic) sulcus. This divides frontal and parietal lobes.
- Precentral gyrus (remember the India ink)
- Postcentral gyrus
- Centrum semiovale
- Cingulate gyrus

A6.1. *See Figure 6.13.*

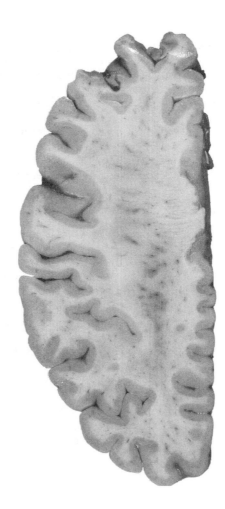

FIGURE 6.5. *Slice 1, above the ventricles. This cut passes through the cingulate gyrus.*

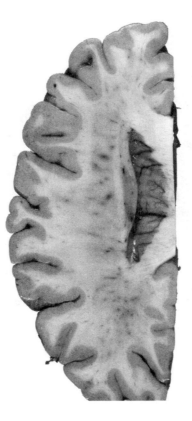

FIGURE 6.6. *Slice 2, through the upper portion of the lateral ventricle, into corpus callosum and superior caudate nucleus.*

Q6.2. In the next slice (see Fig. 6.6), look down into the lateral ventricle and see the smooth ependymal surface with some overlying vessels. Use atlases and texts to find these structures on your brain and in Figure 6.6:
   • Central sulcus (again)
   • Genu of the corpus callosum, connecting white matter of the frontal lobes
   • Centrum semiovale
   • Body of the corpus callosum (variably present, depending on the cut)

A6.2. *See Figure 6.13.*

Q6.3. Uses atlases to find the following structures on your slices and in Figure 6.7:
   • Caudate nucleus, head and body
   • Corpus callosum
   • Centrum semiovale
   • Genu of the corpus callosum

A6.3. *See Figure 6.13.*

Q6.4. On your slices and in Figure 6.8, identify the following:
   • Head of the caudate nucleus.
   • Buried portions of the cortex of the Sylvian fissure. Use atlases to understand the infolded cortex forming the insula (island) underneath the frontal and tip of temporal lobes; note that you are below the ventral end of the central sulcus.
   • Thalamus (egg-shaped structure). You are just reaching the dorsal and superior portion of the egg.
   • Fornix, within the cavity of the lateral ventricle.

A6.4. *See Figure 6.13.*

Q6.5. In this next slice the cortex of the Sylvian fissure reaches almost to the basal ganglia; you are below the level of the centrum semiovale. Identify the following in the slices and in Figure 6.9:
   • Head of the caudate
   • Tail of the caudate
   • Putamen
   • Anterior and posterior limbs of the internal capsule

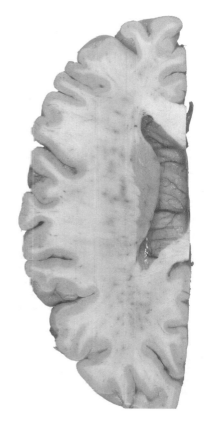

FIGURE 6.7. *Slice 3, through the lateral ventricle and below the body of the corpus callosum.*

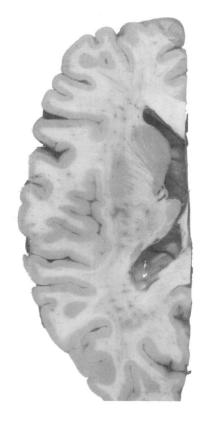

FIGURE 6.8. *Slice 4, through the dorsal part of the thalamus, and almost below the corpus callosum.*

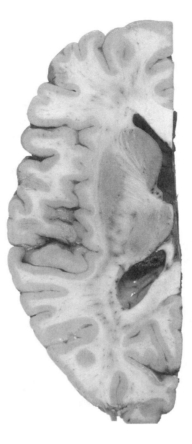

FIGURE 6.9. *Slice 5, through the main gray matter nuclei of the hemisphere, specifically the basal ganglia and the thalamus.*

- Lateral nuclei of thalamus
- Anterior nuclei of thalamus
- Fornix
- Occipital cortex (calcarine cortex)
- Choroid plexus of the lateral ventricle

A6.5. *See Figure 6.13.*

Q6.6. The body and temporal horn of the ventricle still remain. The basal ganglia and thalamus are reaching their full glory. Identify in Figure 6.10 and in your brain slice:
- Head of the caudate nucleus
- Putamen
- Claustrum
- External and extreme capsules
- Anterior and posterior limbs of the internal capsule
- Thalamus "ventral tier" nuclei (now approximately the midportion)
- Pulvinar (back bulge of thalamus)
- Fornix
- Anterior commissure, running between the two temporal lobes (visibility depends on cut)
- Splenium of corpus callosum

A6.6. *See Figure 6.13.*

Q6.7. Use a lateral view of the brain surface to make sure you understand cortical structures in this next slice, including the tip of the temporal lobe, the buried Sylvian (insular) cortex, and the medial portion of the occipital lobe. Identify in Figure 6.11 and on the gross brain slice:
- Nucleus accumbens (limbic part of basal ganglia)
- Putamen
- Globus pallidus
- Tail of the caudate (not easy to find)

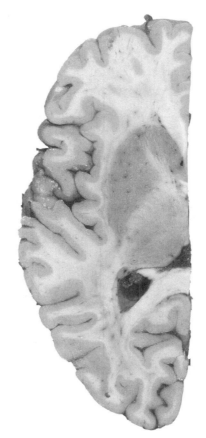

FIGURE 6.10. *Slice 6, below the lateral ventricle in the frontal horn.*

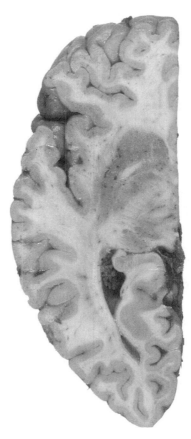

FIGURE 6.11. *Slice 7, at the level of the anterior and posterior commissures.*

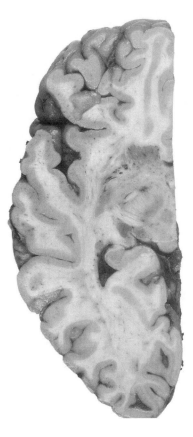

FIGURE 6.12. *Slice 8, through the upper midbrain and lowest reaches of the thalamus and basal ganglia.*

- Hippocampus
- Thalamus (only the basolateral part remains)
- Choroid plexus of the lateral ventricle
- Insula

A6.7. *See Figure 6.13.*

Q6.8. Notice in Figure 6.12 that although slice extends into the midbrain (the red nucleus is visible), it also contains the back end of the thalamus. Both geniculate nuclei dangle laterally off the back end of thalamus. Identify on your slice and in Figure 6.12:
- Medial and lateral geniculate nuclei (these are both part of the thalamus, at its posterior and inferior margin)
- Cerebral peduncles (in the rostral midbrain)
- Red nucleus (in midbrain)
- Temporal horn of the ventricle
- Tail of caudate nucleus
- Hippocampus

A6.8. *See Figure 6.13.*

TRIGEMINAL SYSTEM

You have been following two main sensory tracts up the nervous system and are poised to reach the cortex. But we still have a body without a head. For a sound mind and a sound body, we best add the head before terminating in cortex.

Sensory information from the face enters the brain via the trigeminal nerve. As in the spinal cord, the information dissociates: pain and temperature impulses project into the medulla while kinesthetic signals project to the pons.

Q6.9. On the right in Figure 6.14 showing the medulla, locate the spinal trigeminal nucleus. Compare this with the spinal cord section of the left. What region of spinal cord

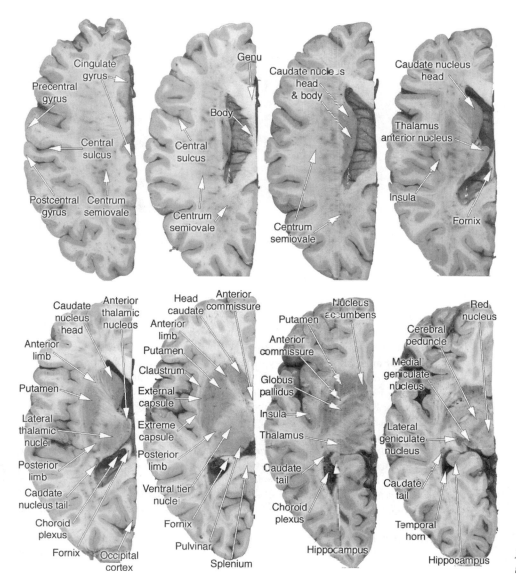

FIGURE 6.13. *Some salient structures on horizontal sections.*

corresponds to the this nucleus (ignore the posterior column nuclei, which have no analogue in the spinal cord)? Knowing that Lissauer's tract carries nociceptive inputs in the spinal cord, locate its analogous spinal trigeminal tract in the medulla on the right. Remembering where trigeminal fibers enter the brainstem, would you expect this tract to increase or decrease in size as you travel down in the medulla?

Also locate the anterolateral fibers in these two figures. From which side of the body does its information arise? Compare that to the adjacent spinal trigeminal nucleus. Describe the change in pain perception if a patient had a small lesion involving just these two structures, say midway up the medulla.

A6.9. *The spinal trigeminal nucleus corresponds to the dorsal horn of the spinal cord. Its fibers enter the pons and then travel down in the spinal trigeminal tract (equivalent to Lissauer's tract). As they synapse in the nucleus, the tract decreases in size and so gets smaller caudally. See Figure 6.15.*

Information in the anterolateral (spinothalamic) fibers is from the contralateral body, while that in the trigeminal nucleus and tract is from the ipsilateral face and oral cavity. A focal lesion involving these two structures would produce ipsilateral facial and contralateral body anesthesia. However, fibers leaving the spinal nucleus of V cross the medulla and join the contralateral spinothalamic fibers. So higher up in the medulla, the same lesion would produce increasing contralateral facial anesthesia. These decussating fibers spread over much of the medulla and do not form a nice tight bundle like the anterior white commissure in the spinal cord. By the middle pons you have a complete representation of pain and temperature sensation for the

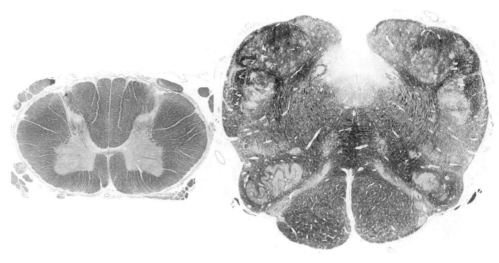

FIGURE 6.14. *Comparison of cervical spinal cord and caudal medulla.*

entire opposite side, face and body, in the combined tracts consisting of anterolateral and medial lemniscal fibers.

Q6.10. Using your atlas, now locate in the histologic image of the middle pons in Figure 6.16 (pontine tegmentum) the large trigeminal nuclear complex. Separately identify the motor and principal sensory divisions. Which is lateral? Where is the dorsal root ganglion for this sensory nucleus? What order neurons are in the principal sensory nucleus of V? This nucleus lies in the pons about midway between the medulla and midbrain. Knowing that these fibers add the head to the lemniscal "body," indicate also where these kinesthetic trigeminal fibers travel in relation to the medial lemniscus. Again note that the fibers cross before entering the lemniscus.

A6.10. *Throughout the brainstem, sensory functions are more lateral than their corresponding motor functions. See Figure 6.17. As indicated in the introduction, the dorsal root ganglion equivalent of the trigeminal nerve is the trigeminal, semilunar, or Gasserian ganglion (called different names to confuse students), which lies on the floor of the middle cranial fossa, outside the dura but inside the skull. Its first-order neurons send axons to synapses on the second-order neurons in the principle sensory nucleus of V.*

In this single exception some "dorsal root ganglion" neurons are actually in the central nervous system, within the trigeminal mesencephalic nucleus. The fibers of this nucleus participate in the jaw jerk, which is equivalent to the patellar reflex, or knee jerk, and perhaps evolved to more finely control mastication.

Q6.11. As a last step before entering thalamus, reexamine the midbrain in Figure 6.18. Always orient yourself; which side of the picture points toward the face? Again locate

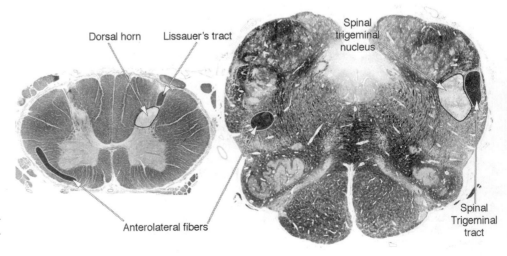

FIGURE 6.15. *Comparison of spinal and medullary nociceptive systems.*

Dorsal horn

Lissauer's tract

Spinal trigeminal nucleus

Anterolateral fibers

Spinal Trigeminal tract

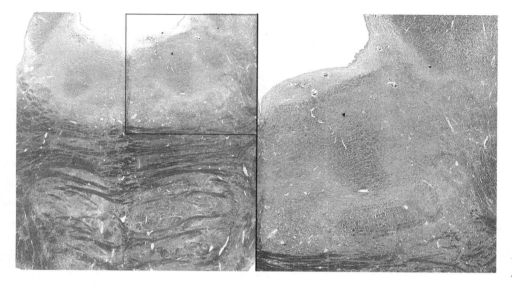

FIGURE 6.16. *Trigeminal nuclei in pontine tegmentum.*

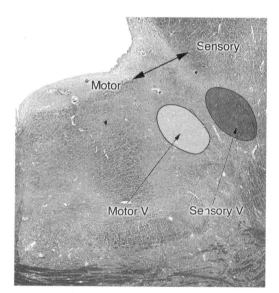

FIGURE 6.17. *Trigeminal complex in the pontine tegmentum.*

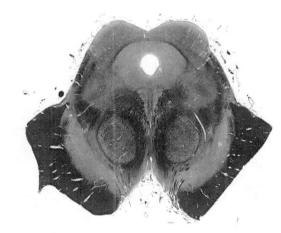

FIGURE 6.18. *Midbrain at the red nucleus level.*

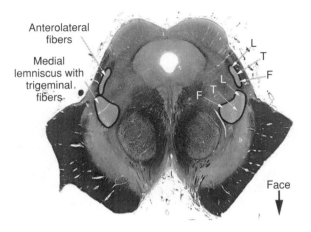

Anterolateral
fibers

Medial
lemniscus with
trigeminal
fibers

Face

FIGURE 6.19. *Sensory fibers in midbrain. Note: While it is relatively easy to mark these tracts on a picture, determining them is much more difficult! Their exact positions and somatotopy are really only known imprecisely, especially in humans.*

the medial lemniscal fibers in Figure 6.18 (you may want to refer to the previous chapter). Where are the head, arm, and leg fibers? Locate the anterolateral fibers. Knowing that these also have a head on the body, guess about the somatotopic organization of facial pain and temperature fibers.

A6.11. *The bottom of the image is ventral and so is in the direction of the face. This is opposite from the orientation you see in typical horizontal brain sections or routine neuroimaging. See Figure 6.19*

In both the medial lemniscus and in the spinothalamic tract, the head fibers are medial while the arm, trunk, and leg fibers are more lateral.

As when you learn anything the first time, much of the information presented here and in other parts of the text has been simplified. While the basic information is correct, it is woefully incomplete. For example, both the kinesthetic and pain systems have some bilateral projections to thalamus, and several other thalamic nuclei also receive this information. However, in a "first pass" through this material and for most clinical uses, this level of detail is adequate.

INTRODUCTION TO THALAMUS

Q6.12. If you get a good idea of where the thalamus is in the brain, your life will be much easier. What is above the thalamus? What region of brain lies below it? Can you identify any structures, using your prior dissections? What major white and gray structures lie lateral to the thalamus? What lies medial? Finally, what is in front of and behind the thalamus? Use the previous figures and the MRI in Figure 6.20 to assist you.

A6.12. *Above the thalamus is the lateral ventricle. The thalamus is part of the diencephalon. Below the thalamus are several major structures, including the hypothalamus and midbrain (mesencephalon). You may be able to see the upper portions of the substantia nigra and red nucleus.*

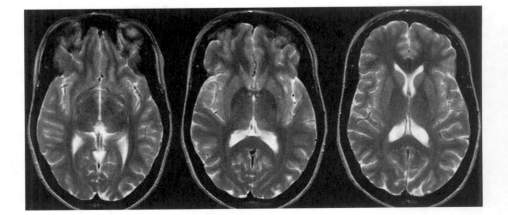

FIGURE 6.20. *Horizontal MRI scans of thalamic region.*

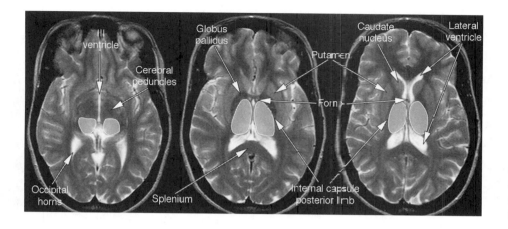

FIGURE 6.21. Thalamic regional structures on MRI scan. The approximate location of the thalamus is indicated by the lightened areas.

Look back on your coronal sections for guidance. With sharp eyes and a well-placed cut you may also find the subthalamic nucleus, which you will revisit in one of the motor laboratories.

Immediately lateral to the thalamus is the internal capsule, which will carry thalamic sensory fibers to the cortex. Lateral to the internal capsule lie both the globus pallidus and putamen. The medial surface of the thalamus bounds the third ventricle. At the front end of the thalamus is more of the lateral ventricle and the caudate nucleus, while the back end is near the occipital horns of the lateral ventricles, the splenium of the corpus callosum, and the vast reaches of the occipital cortex. See Figure 6.21

Q6.13. Keeping the horizontal and coronal slices separate, select those slices that contain thalamus, and lay them on separate trays. Use your atlas and the histologic sections in Figure 6.22 to again identify the major anatomic divisions of thalamus:
- Anterior nucleus (more on this in the limbic laboratory)
- Ventral tier nuclei
- Medial nuclei (especially the medial dorsal nucleus—more on this in the cortical laboratories)
- Posterior nuclei (pulvinar)
- Geniculate nuclei (medial and lateral—more on these in the next laboratory)

A6.13. See Figure 6.23.

Q6.14. Try to identify the main ascending sensory pathways in the midbrain in the left side of Figure 6.22. Then try to identify them on the higher resolution images in Figure 6.24. Observe how it enters the thalamus from the midbrain. What are the thalamic nuclei directly above these fibers?

A6.14. See Figure 6.25. As you might have guessed, these sensory fibers project upward into the ventral posterior-lateral and medial nuclei. Again, while the lines in this figure are precise, our knowledge

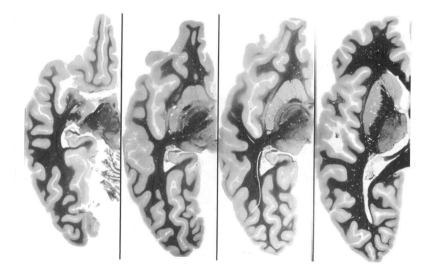

FIGURE 6.22. Horizontal histologic sections of brain, stained for myelin.

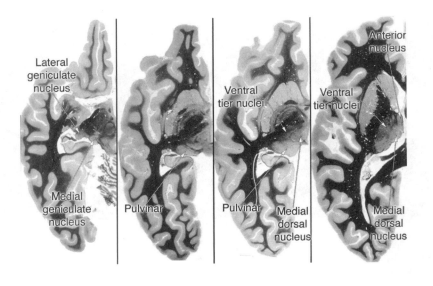

FIGURE 6.23. *Salient thalamic structures.*

is not. These locations should be considered only approximate. The exercise emphasizes that ascending sensory fibers travel through the dorsolateral midbrain and lead directly into their target nuclei in thalamus.

Although you may not realize it, the goal here is not to learn detailed thalamic anatomy. What has been presented is mostly to get your bearings. Few students would retain any detailed thalamic anatomy longer than microseconds after learning it. The goal is to know how the thalamus is placed in the brain, that it has subdivisions, that each division serves a distinct system, and that the thalamus is the gateway to most of the cortex. Make sure you understand these principles.

Q6.15. The organization of the sensory relay nuclei in thalamus mimic those of their input fibers from the midbrain. Sensory neurons serving the body lie in the ventral posterior-lateral (VPL) nucleus, while sensations from the face and part of the head project to the ventral posterior-medial (VPM) nucleus. What is the order of the kinesthetic neurons in thalamus (e.g., how many neuronal synapses have we encountered)? Remembering that the VPL/VPM complex lies directly above the ascending sensory

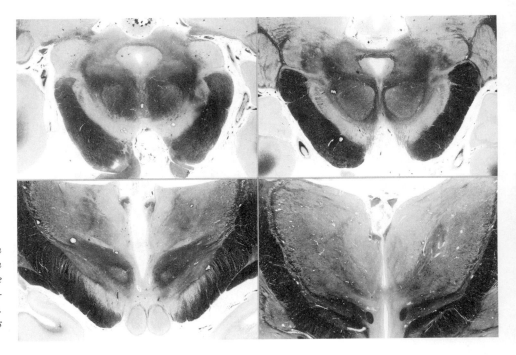

FIGURE 6.24. *Transition between the midbrain and thalamus, myelin stain. The four images are transverse sections, taken approximately perpendicular to the axis of the brainstem. Because of the sectioning, the thalamus images are not precisely horizontal.*

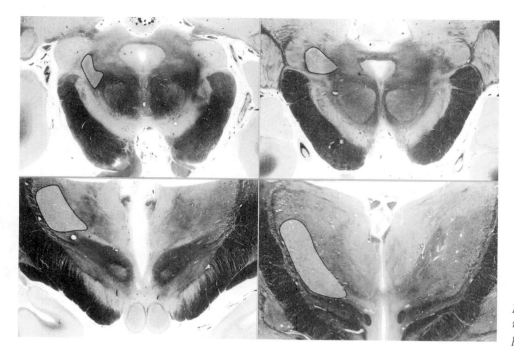

FIGURE 6.25. *Sensory fibers and nuclei in the mesencephalic-diencephalic transition.*

fibers and that the VPM is medial, in the coronal histologic section in Figure 6.26, identify:
- VPM
- VPL
- Caudate nucleus (CN)
- Red nucleus (RN)

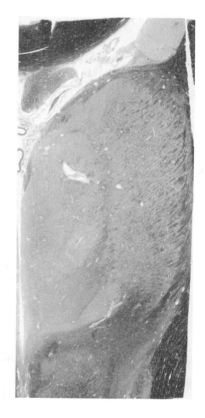

FIGURE 6.26. *Coronal thalamus histology.*

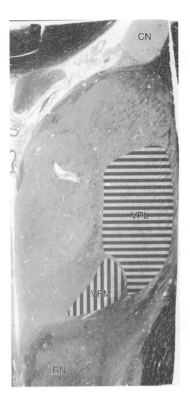

FIGURE 6.27. *VPL and VPM in coronal section of thalamus.*

A6.15. *The kinesthetic neurons and many nociceptive neurons are third order. See Figure 6.27*
Note that although kinesthetic and nociceptive fibers project to the same general areas in thalamus, their neurons remain distinct and their cortical projections differ. These indeed are two different systems.

SENSORY CORTEX

Q6.16. Review the cut horizontal slabs of brain and locate the postcentral gyrus (in back of the ink) in the slices, on the uncut brain, and in Figure 6.28. Histology shows that the primary sensory cortex differs significantly from adjacent association cortices and from the anterior motor cortex. You can't see this grossly, but it is a very

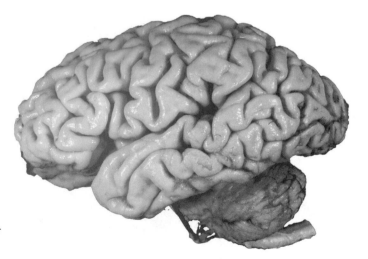

FIGURE 6.28. *Lateral view of brain.*

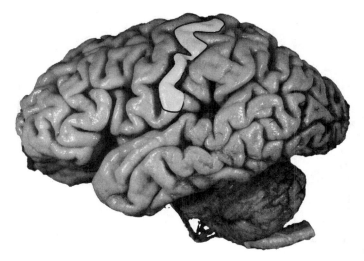

FIGURE 6.29. *Postcentral gyrus.*

obvious difference under the microscope, which you will see in a later chapter. If you get a good section, compare the thicknesses of the gray matter in the precentral and postcentral gyri.

A6.16. Not surprisingly, the **postcentral gyrus** *is just behind the* **precentral gyrus** *(see Fig. 6.29). The central sulcus is one of the deepest in the brain, and is flanked by the thickest cortical area, the precentral gyrus, and one of the thinnest areas, the postcentral cortex. Its great depth in high horizontal brain sections (above the corpus callosum) discloses its location and hence reveals the pre- and postcentral gyri.*

Q6.17. On the sensory homunculus of the primary sensory cortex in Figure 6.30, indicate the region receiving information from the dorsal columns and separately indicate the region receiving trigeminal information.

A6.17. See Figure 6.31.

Q6.18. What is the relative proportion of primary sensory cortex used to represent the face compared to the body? How does the cortical area correlate with the sensory receptive fields?

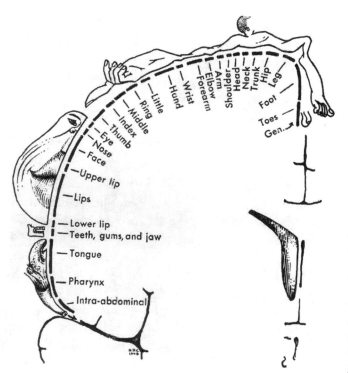

FIGURE 6.30. *Sensory homunculus (Figure modified from Penfield and Rasmussen, The Cerebral Cortex of Man, Macmillan Company, New York, 1952, figure 17, page 44.). These neurosurgeons empirically determined this mapping during craniotomies by directly stimulating the cortex and asking the awake patient what they sensed.*

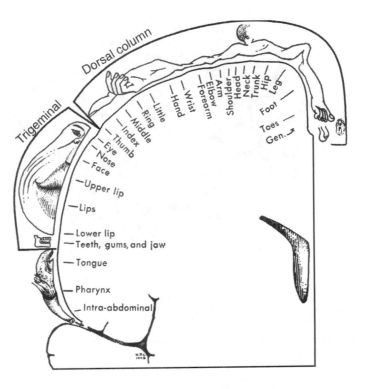

FIGURE 6.31. Sensory homunculus (Figure modified from Penfield and Rasmussen, The Cerebral Cortex of Man, Macmillan Company, New York, 1952, figure 17, page 44.). These neurosurgeons empirically determined this mapping during craniotomies by directly stimulating the cortex and asking the awake patient what they sensed.

A6.18. The face takes up about a third of the primary sensory cortex, even though it occupies only a small proportion of the body's surface area. However, the receptive fields for the face are the greatest in the entire body. You have only to watch an infant put every new object to their lips to realize this. The cortical area devoted to a particular region of the body roughly correlates with the size of the receptive field for that region.

Q6.19. In Figure 6.32 a functional MRI (fMRI) was used to study the segregation of cortical activation by somatosensory information. An fMRI can detect increased brain activity

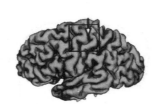

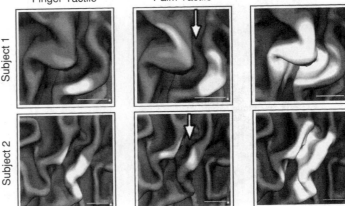

FIGURE 6.32. Segregation of somatosensory cortical activation. The arrow marks the depth of the central sulcus (CS) overlying Brodmann area 3a. PreCG is the precentral gyrus, while PoCG is the postcentral gyrus. (Adapted from Moore, C. I., et al. (2000). Segregation of somatosensory activation in the human Rolandic cortex using fMRI. J. Neurophysiol 84: 558–596.)

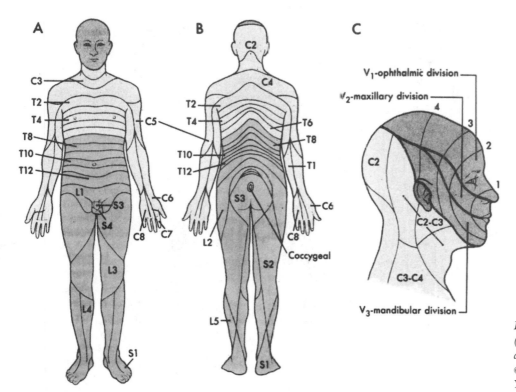

FIGURE 6.33. *Dermatome map. (Modified from Haines, D. E., Fundamental Neuroscience, 2nd edition, © 2002, Churchill-Livingstone, New York, figure 18-4, page 278.)*

by sensing subtle changes in the blood flow. In this modified version, more active regions are white and control regions are gray. The subjects had fMRI imaging done while they had their finger or palm brushed with a fine brush, or while they flexed their fingers. What area is most active during pure sensory stimulation (finger and palm tactile)? What other area is also active? Compare these areas with those activated by hand flexion. Any surprises? Do these make sense?

A6.19. *As was discussed above, the postcentral gyrus or primary somatosensory cortex showed the greatest activation when the subjects received a pure sensory stimulation. Hopefully you won't ever forget this. However, the precentral gyrus, otherwise known as the motor strip or primary motor cortex, was also activated, even though the subjects were not moving. Similarly the precentral gyrus showed the greatest activation during movement, at least in the first subject. However, the postcentral gyrus was also activated by movement. While at first pass, this may be a surprise, it makes sense; to move your fingers you need to know where they are!*

Note that the depth of the central sulcus was not activated by tactile sensation, even though it still represents sensory cortex. This part of somatosensory cortex (area 3a) responds to deep receptor and proprioceptive inputs, rather than tactile sensations. Although the details are beyond this first course in neuroscience, the experiment does illustrate the fine divisions and integration of all types of information in the brain.

CLINICAL ASPECTS

Dermatomes

Q6.20. Imagine that two nerve roots have been cut on one side, just distal to the dorsal root ganglia of C6 and C7. What would be the clinical deficit? Would it be motor plus sensory? Look below at a map of the **dermatomes** (the skin territory innervated by the different nerve roots). Identify the distribution of C6 and C7.

A6.20. *The dermatome maps were constructed by outlining sensory deficits in patients with monoradicular syndromes (see definition), often from herniated discs, or nerve root tumors, or cases of herpes zoster.*

Radicular *Referring to a spinal root, between its exit from the spinal cord and when it joins its mate to become a mixed nerve. A monoradicular syndrome means a deficit that localizes to just one spinal root.*

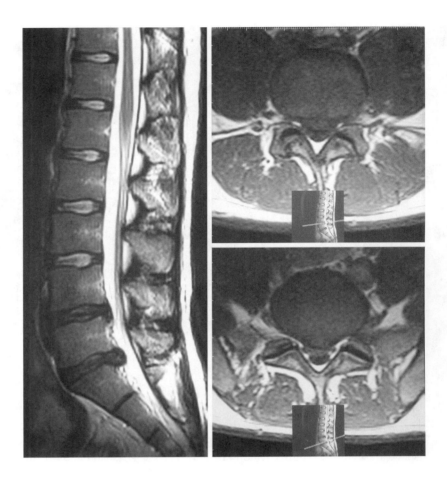

FIGURE 6.34. MRI of herniated disc. The herniation is central and nearly symmetrical.

Since the cut is just distal to the dorsal root ganglion, it would cut the closely apposed motor and sensory nerves. (This is also true if the cut were immediately proximal to the ganglion, before the fibers diverge to opposite sides of the cord.) As such, it would produce both motor and sensory deficits. Since all sensory modalities enter via the posterior root, they would all be affected by the cut. However, the target regions on the skin for a given nerve overlap, so the clinical deficit would be smaller than the precise distribution on the dermatome maps.

Herniated or "Slipped" Disc

Q6.21. Examine the MRI images in Figure 6.34, which illustrate a herniation (protrusion) of a portion of the intervertebral disc. This material is rubbery, firmer than a nerve root, and will compress the root if it herniates into the intervertebral foramen. The patient will have radicular (root) pain in the territory of that root, and may lose motor and sensory function in the muscles and sensory territory innervated by that root. Is the herniated disc extradural or intradural? Why would there be both motor and sensory deficits? Identify the level of the herniated disc. Referring to your dermatome map, where would be the clinical deficit?

A6.21. *The herniated disc is extradural, between L4 and L5 and another between L5 and S1; the dura is pushed inward by its presence. Both anterior and posterior roots are involved, and so would produce both sensory and motor function loss.*

The deficit would involve the fibers exiting at these levels, the L4 and L5 roots; these would innervate the medial and lateral sides of the lower leg and foot.

Lateral Medullary Infarct

A lateral medullary stroke, resulting from an occlusion of the posterior inferior cerebellar artery (PICA) can produce a mixture of sensory findings. Such an infarct is illustrated in Figure 6.35.

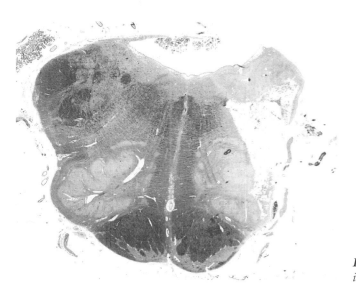

FIGURE 6.35. *Lateral medullary infarct.*

Q6.22. Describe which sensory structures are injured and which are spared in Figure 6.35. Let right be the right side.

A6.22. *At this level the medial lemniscus is spared, while the right ascending fibers from the spinothalamic fibers in the lateral medulla are destroyed. The right spinal trigeminal nucleus and tract have also been eliminated.*

Q6.23. See if you can figure out why these odd patterns sometimes occur:
 • Impairment of sensation of pinprick and cold, but not for light touch.
 • Impairment of sensation of pinprick and cold on the opposite side of the body but not over the face and head.

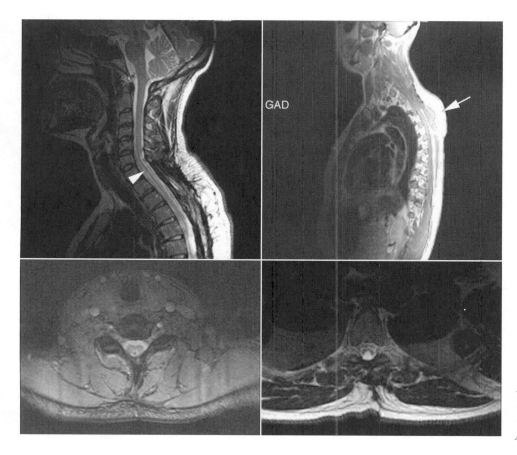

FIGURE 6.36. *Neuroradiology. The top panel has sagittal MRI scans, while the bottom has axial scans taken at different levels.*

- Impairment of sensation of pinprick and cold over the opposite side of the body *and* the face.
- Impairment of sensation of pinprick and cold over the opposite side of the body and *both* sides of the face

A6.23. *In this lateral medullary infarct, the necrotic area involves the anterolateral fibers and the spinal trigeminal nucleus just above these fibers in the lateral medulla. The lesion touches the inferior olivary nucleus but spares both sides of the medial lemniscus, as well as the hypoglossal nucleus.*

    Since the injury does not affect the medial lemniscus, but only the spinothalamic fibers, only pain and temperature are affected. As the spinothalamic fibers cross in the cord, the deficit would be on the opposite side of the lesion.

    The clinical variations discussed in the question are produced by different extents of infarction after occlusion of the PICA. If the lesion is higher, at a level where many of the trigeminal fibers have joined the anterolateral tract, then pinprick and temperature sensation will be impaired on the contralateral side of the body. Since the trigeminal fibers are crossing over to the contralateral anterolateral tract as they exit from the nucleus, large lesions will impair the trigeminal fibers along with the anterolateral fibers, giving sensory impairment on both sides of the face and on only the contralateral side of the body.

    Note that lateral medullary infarcts typically injure other structures, which we have yet to examine. Some of them we'll visit in later chapters.

Posterior Column Deficit

The patient is a 35-year-old woman who had undergone multiple neurosurgical procedures. She was previously diagnosed with a Chiari I malformation and had cervical and thoracic syrinxes. Also she had several accidents and other events that aggravated her problems, including a fall on the ice, two motor vehicle accidents, and a spinal abscess. To alleviate her symptoms, she had undergone multiple surgical procedures, including shunt placements and revisions. She came into the hospital with a new complaint of pressure in her back and lack of coordination of her legs.

    She had been able to swim about a mile, several times a week. About a month before admission she felt a pressure sensation in the center of her back, slightly above her scapulae. A week prior to admission she arose from a seated position and suddenly felt that her legs lacked all coordination. She could not stand. She developed excruciating pain in her back that would come in waves.

    Examination showed a normal mental status and cranial nerves. She had normal bulk and tone, with at most 4+ out of 5 weakness in her left wrist and right toe flexion. Sensory examination showed intact light touch, pinprick, cold, vibration, and proprioception in her upper extremities, except for a decrease in all modalities in the left arm in a C8/T1 distribution. In contrast, her legs bilaterally showed a marked decreased-to-absent sensation to light touch, vibration, and proprioception. Cold sensation was intact, and she had hyperesthesia to pin in an L3–L5 distribution. Her reflexes were increased in her biceps, quadriceps (patellar), Achilles tendon, and her toes were upgoing (Babinski sign). Rapid, alternating movements were slow in the left hand and both legs showed "very sloppy" heel-to-shin testing. She could not walk without assistance. When she did walk, her gait was wide-based and slow. She had a right foot drop and could not lift her left foot fully off the floor. She had a dramatic Romberg sign.

    Her neuroradiology is presented in Figure 6.36.

Q6.24. This is a complex case, with distinct aspects. Examine her MRI in Figure 6.36 and try to correlate the anatomic findings with her signs. What may be causing her left arm and wrist sensory loss and weakness? Look closely at panels 1 and 4.

A6.24. *She has a syrinx (basically, a hole) in her cervical spinal cord at the arrowhead in the first panel of Figure 6.36 and better seen in the fourth panel. The syrinx involves the posterior columns in this view. How this actually has injured the cord is uncertain from these scans alone. The loss of left sensory and motor modalities at the C8-T1 level suggests a root lesion at this level.*

Q6.25. She seemed to have full strength in her legs, yet she was unable to walk without assistance. In addition, she performed poorly on classic "cerebellar" testing. What is going on? Use the MRI scans to help you answer. Especially look at panels 1 and 5 in Figure 6.36.

A6.25. *The multiple surgeries and shunts for her prior syrinx (see panel 2) created a second pathology in her dorsal columns. Panel 5 in Figure 6.36 shows a massive, enhancing lesion that has pretty much destroyed her posterior columns below that level. Posterior column information is also important for regular cerebellar testing. You can't run your heel on your shin if you aren't quite sure where either one is. Although she has essentially full strength in her leg muscles, she has lost sensory knowledge of their location and state of contraction. Her excruciating pain and limited hyperesthesia to pinprick are probably related to root damage from her dorsal spinal cord disease. From the scans, most of her spinothalamic tract remains unaffected by the lesion.*

This patient illustrates the importance of the posterior column information. She is strong but can't walk. When first evaluated in the emergency room, physicians thought she was malingering. However, major posterior column pathology can be nearly as debilitating as corticospinal tract injury. In this patient the etiology of the enhancing lesion was not determined. No organisms grew in cultures of the tissue.

COMPARISON OF LEMNISCAL AND ANTEROLATERAL SYSTEMS

Q6.26. Compare these two sensory system by completing Table 6.1:
A6.26. See Table 6.2.
Q6.27. On Figure 6.37, diagram the entire anterolateral pathway on the left and the posterior column pathway on the right, from cord to cortex, starting at the right dorsal root ganglion. Shade the appropriate structures on each "slice," label it, and connect these sites with lines between the levels. Especially note the site of decussation, where synapses are found, and the "order" of the neuron at these synapses.
A6.27. See Figure 6.38.

TABLE 6.1. Comparison of Lemniscal and Anterolateral Systems: Worksheet

	Lemniscal System	Anterolateral System
Receptors		
First-order neurons		
Path of first-order axons		
Second-order neurons		
Site of decussation		
Path of second-order axons		
Third-order neuron		
Cortical target		

TABLE 6.2. Comparison of Lemniscal and Anterolateral Systems

	Lemniscal System	Anterolateral System
Receptors	Specialized, cutaneous and subcutaneous corpuscles	Free, naked axonal nerve endings
First-order neurons	Peripheral process of cell in dorsal root or trigeminal ganglion	Peripheral process of cell in dorsal root or trigeminal ganglion
Path of first-order axons	Enters and ascends in posterior column or projects to chief sensory trigeminal nucleus	Travels for short distance in Lissauer's or spinal trigeminal tract
Second-order neurons	Gracilis, cuneatus, or chief sensory trigeminal nucleus	Arise in spinal cord posterior horn or spinal trigeminal nucleus
Site of decussation	Axons cross in lower medulla (arcuate fibers) or in pontine tegmentum	Axons cross in anterior white commissure or medulla near spinal trigeminal system
Path of second-order axons	Ascend in medial lemniscus	Ascend in anterolateral cord and medulla
Third-order neuron	VPL/VPM of thalamus	VPL/VPM of thalamus (neurons distinct from lemniscal neurons); also reticular and intralaminar nuclei
Cortical target	Projects to primary sensory cortex	Projects to primary sensory cortex and other areas of cortex, including lip of insula; fibers may be third order or beyond

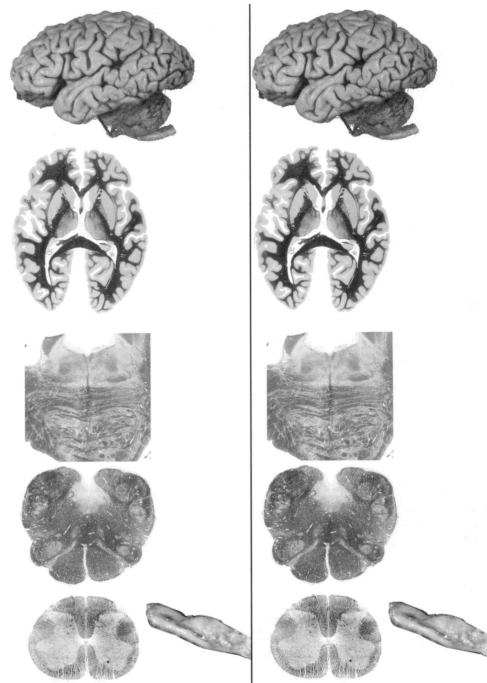

FIGURE 6.37. *Comparison of anterolateral* (left) *and posterior column/ lemniscal system* (right) *worksheet.*

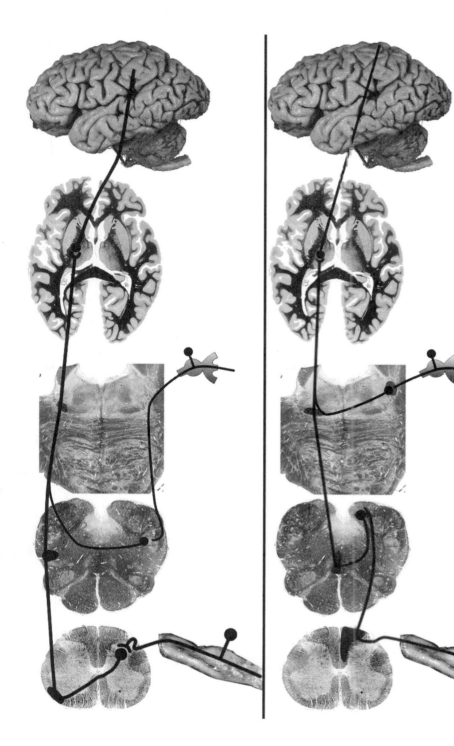

FIGURE 6.38. *Comparison of anterolateral* (left) *and posterior column/lemniscal system* (right).

Chapter 7——VISION AND HEARING

You heard the cry from the far-off trees at the edge of the forest: a fellow chimpanzee had seen a leopard and screamed an alert. These cats can climb trees, so you had to scatter to the outer branches. Swinging through the foliage requires you to judge three-dimensional distances, assess limb strength, and target your limbs appropriately.

As humans, having evolved from tree-swinging apes, we have a keen sense of vision and hearing. While dogs have our nose beat a hundredfold, we are the masters of vision and intricate sounds. Unlike most mammals, we and our great ape relatives can also see in color.

The visual pathways sweep widely through the diencephalon, midbrain, and cerebrum (more than a third of the fibers in the forebrain carry some sort of visual information), so that CNS lesions, whatever their nature, have a relatively high probability of impinging on the visual system. Analysis of visual function at the bedside or in the physician's office offers an excellent opportunity for localization of many different types of disease through clinical-anatomical correlation. Unlike the highly segregated visual system, the auditory system has a largely bilateral representation within the brain. This makes hearing relatively poor for neurologically localizing central lesions. However, it is still useful to investigate peripheral diseases and is an important sense for talkative humans.

LEARNING OBJECTIVES

Vision

- Learn the anatomy of the visual system from the retina to primary visual cortex (area 17).
- Identify and understand the logic of visual field deficits resulting from typical lesions along the visual pathway.
- Understand the basic receptive field properties of neurons in the visual system.

Audition

- Learn the anatomy of the auditory system from the cochlea to primary auditory cortex.
- Understand the effects of unilateral lesions in the auditory system.

Functional Neuroanatomy: An Interactive Text and Manual, by Jeffrey T. Joseph and David L. Cardozo
ISBN 0-471-44437-5 Copyright © 2004 John Wiley & Sons, Inc.

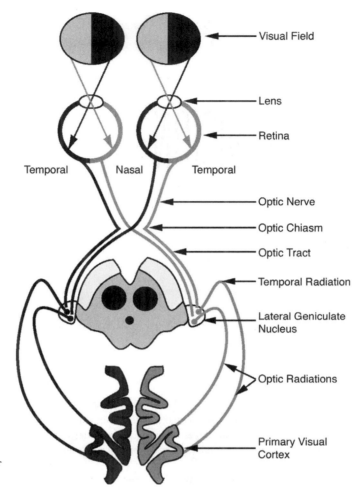

Visual Field

Lens

Retina

Temporal   Nasal   Temporal

Optic Nerve

Optic Chiasm

Optic Tract

Temporal Radiation

Lateral Geniculate Nucleus

Optic Radiations

Primary Visual Cortex

FIGURE 7.1. *Schematic diagram of visual pathway.*

Integrative

- Learn the relationships between the CN II and VIII and the skull.
- Compare the overall organization of the two systems.
- Compare the consequences of unilateral lesions in these systems.

INTRODUCTION

Transformation of visual signals into simple and more complex perceptions takes place in the cell layers of the retina, in the cell populations and distinctive layers of the lateral geniculate body, and in a hierarchy of cortical layers and regions. The most salient features of the visual system are shown in Figure 7.1.

The Optic Nerve and Its Projections

The *optic nerve* is actually not a nerve at all, but an externalized, myelinated central nervous system fiber pathway that passes from one area of central nervous system (the retina) to other parts (hypothalamus, thalamus, midbrain, and cerebral cortex). Virtually the entire visual pathway maintains a topographically organized representation of the retinal surface, which, in turn, reflects the visual field. Several areas of visual cortex sustain this retinotopic organization. The very orderliness of this organization often enables a physician to locate the site of a lesion as it encroaches upon the visual pathway by analysis of the visual field defects from each eye. Because of the visual pathway's long trajectory through the brain, visual field tests are often employed to aid in diagnosing a variety of neurological abnormalities. Figure 7.2 diagrams the topographic organization and orientation of the

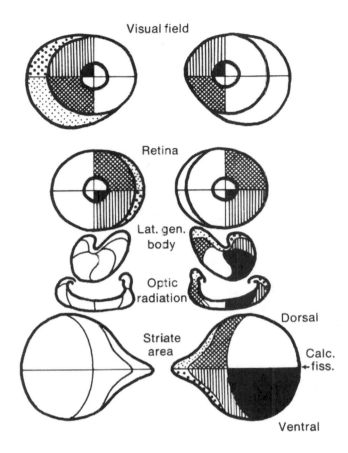

Visual field

Retina

Lat. gen.
body

Optic
radiation

Striate
area

Dorsal

Calc.
←fiss.

Ventral

FIGURE 7.2. The Topography of the
visual system. The different patterns
are used to indicate different parts
of the visual field in order to trace
their neural representations at various
stages along the visual pathway. (Modified from A. Brodal, Neurological
Anatomy, 3rd Edition, Oxford University Press, 1981. figure 8-3, p. 583.)

visual pathway from the retina to the visual cortex. (It is interesting to note from Fig. 7.2 that the
projection from the retina to the lateral geniculate nucleus undergoes a 90° counterclockwise rotation,
which accounts for the topography in the nucleus.)

Examination of the visual field is performed separately for each eye; the patient covers one eye
and fixes the uncovered eye on a distant object. The examiner moves a small object slowly into and
across the visual field of the patient. The patient keeps his eye fixed, and reports in set intervals
whether he can see the object. These responses are recorded on a perimeter chart. Discrete "blind
spots" or scotomas can occur within the visual field, either temporarily, as during migraine attacks,
or permanently, resulting from glaucoma, vascular, or metabolic/toxic damage to the retina or from
lesions of the optic nerve or higher visual centers. Such lesions, if present in only one eye or optic
nerve, result in monocular field defects. A unilateral lesion beyond the optic chiasm results in a
binocular contralateral field defect noted when each eye is tested separately, as explained below.

Compression by tumors expanding upward from the pituitary gland often impinge on the middle
of the optic chiasm. The crossing fibers of the optic nerves are injured and visual functions from the
nasal halves of each retina are lost. The result is a scotoma in the temporal field of each eye, called
bitemporal heteronomous hemianopsia.

A lesion in the visual pathways behind the chiasm (e.g., destruction of an optic tract) severs
fibers from the same half of each retina. If the right tract is damaged, visual information from the right
halves of both retinas is blocked. In this situation the patient is blind in the left half of each visual
field, a condition known as left homonymous hemianopsia.

A defect restricted to one quadrant in the field of vision may result from a lesion in the optic
radiation or primary visual cortex. A loss in the lower quadrant indicates involvement of the upper bank
of the calcarine sulcus or the optic radiations that innervate it. These radiations traverse a relatively
direct path from the lateral geniculate body back through the parietal lobe. Loss in the upper quadrant
of the visual field indicates involvement of the lower bank of the calcarine sulcus or fibers of the
radiation that reach it by passing through the temporal lobe and more laterally around the temporal
horn of the lateral ventricle. In principle, similar defects could arise from small lesions of the optic
tract or the lateral geniculate nucleus, but such small lesions are rare.

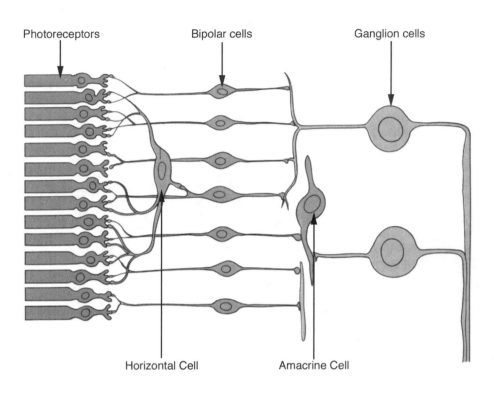

Photoreceptors   Bipolar cells   Ganglion cells

Horizontal Cell   Amacrine Cell

FIGURE 7.3. Organization of the retina. (Adapted from D. H. Hubel, Eye, Brain, and Vision, © 1988. W. H. Freeman, New York, page 52.)

The Retina

The organization of the retina is diagrammed in Figure 7.3. The first level of sensory information processing is the retina. It transforms electromagnetic signals representing the spectrum of visible light into a neural code. Approximately 100 million photoreceptors convert energy from light into an electrical potential, which modulates the release of neurotransmitter. The signal is passed on to bipolar cells and then to the retinal ganglion cells, which are the output neurons for the retina. The horizontal and amacrine cells modulate the signal being passed from photoreceptors to the *ganglion cells.* The optic nerve consists solely of ganglion cell axons (there are about a million of them), so that what we "see" results from retinal ganglion cell activity.

Central Auditory Pathways

The auditory system maintains a tonotopic organization from the level of the primary receptors on the curving sheet of the cochlear basilar membrane in the inner ear, buried within the temporal bone, to the auditory cortex on the superior bank of the temporal lobe (superior temporal gyrus). The central auditory system is organized with exquisite precision and complexity, which is accomplished by a wide range of neuronal shapes, clustering patterns of neurons into nuclei, and synaptic arrangements. These features allow localization of sound sources, based both on the different times when impulses arrive at a given neuron in the brainstem and on the different intensities of impulses arriving in each ear. We are able to recognize an extraordinary variety of auditory patterns and to select and attend to an auditory stimulus of personal interest even when it is mingled among other simultaneous auditory stimuli.

The key stations in the central auditory pathway are diagrammed in Figure 7.4. The *organ of Corti* in the cochlea transduces sound wave vibrations into nerve impulses in primary sensory neurons, whose cell bodies are in the spiral ganglion within the inner ear. Axons from the ganglion enter the brain at the cerebello-pontine angle, at the confluence of the cerebellum, pons, and medulla, to synapse on target neurons in the dorsal and the two ventral cochlear nuclei. These nuclei drape over the external surface of the inferior cerebellar peduncle as the peduncle ascends into the cerebellum. Without getting bogged down in a wealth of detail, you should recognize the processing stations further upstream: the superior olivary complex, the inferior colliculus, and the medial geniculate nucleus.

The main tracts in the brainstem, as diagrammed, are the lateral lemniscus and the brachium of the inferior colliculus. Some axons of ventral cochlear nucleus neurons ascend in the lateral lemniscus on

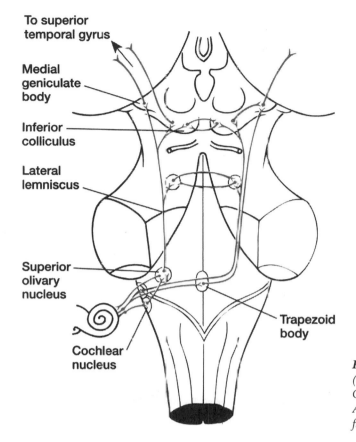

To superior
temporal gyrus

Medial
geniculate
body

Inferior
colliculus

Lateral
lemniscus

Superior
olivary
nucleus

Cochlear
nucleus

Trapezoid
body

FIGURE 7.4. Auditory Pathways. (Adapted from Stephen G Waxman, Correlative Neuroanatomy, 23rd, Appleton & Lange, Stamford, 1996, figure 16-6, p. 233.)

the ipsilateral side to the inferior colliculus, both directly and indirectly after making an intermediate synapse in the superior olivary complex. The majority of axons of neurons in the cochlear nuclei cross to the opposite side through the prominent trapezoid body and in less visible, more dorsal positions. The trapezoid body is a topographic name for the second-order auditory fibers from the cochlear nuclei that cross and may synapse in the ventral part of the caudal pontine tegmentum. At this level the trapezoid body intersects with the medial lemniscus. As they course up the brainstem and perhaps synapse at several way stations, almost all ascending fibers make synaptic connections in the inferior colliculus, especially its central nucleus. These in turn project to the medial geniculate via the brachium of the inferior colliculus. From there they project via the auditory radiations to primary auditory cortex, which is located in a buried portion of the superior temporal gyrus known as Hechl's gyrus.

INSTRUCTOR'S GUIDE

This chapter has several key points that students should retain. Most important clinically is the field cut diagram. Memorizing a list of eponymous syndromes is essentially useless and will be quickly forgotten. The idea of the pathways of visual information, including the reversal of all data by the lens and the splitting and segregation of the information at the chiasm, can be retained and will be useful. Given that the visual system travels through much of the brain and that many brain lesions can impact on it, the students should also know the visual system's major regional anatomy.

Visual Cortex Histology

To locate the visual cortex on histological material, first look at the slide on a white piece of paper. In myelin-stained sections, notice the line in the center of the gray matter along the longest sulcus. This is the **line of Gennari** or layer IV of the primary visual cortex. It is blue on this myelin-stained slide since it contains abundant myelinated fibers arriving from the lateral geniculate nucleus. It is also filled with small blue cells, mostly small neurons, and is itself divided into sublayers. While this site gets a lot of press, the cortex is actually quite thin; you can compare it with the surrounding area 18 association cortex, which has a smaller layer IV and a better developed layer V. Since the myelin in area 17 is thick, you can see it on the gross brain specimens. Note, however, that if you look closely at many other areas of cortex, they also have a white line; it is just smaller in other sites.

Auditory System

Since central auditory pathways bilateralize so extensively, they have little clinical utility. It is extremely rare for an auditory lesion to be localizing. Nevertheless, since so much of our socialization occurs through language, the auditory system should not be neglected. Most clinicians, including neurologists, know little of this system, aside from the names of several key structures. Try to impart more than just these anatomic names, and emphasize some of the information processing that goes on at the different sites.

Schedule (2.5 hours)

10	Dissection of eye
20	Macroscopic visual anatomy
10	Retina
10	Blind spot
30	Visual pathways
10	Visual cortex
20	Visual field cuts
10	Auditory system
30	Cases

VISUAL SYSTEM

Dissection of the Eye

Q7.1. First examine the external eye from a cow (see Fig. 7.5). Identify the optic nerve and the extraocular muscles that form a ring around the posterior aspect of the eye. Next cut on the cow's eye sagittally in the plane of the optic nerve (middle panel). Identify the following structures:
  • Optic nerve
  • Extra ocular muscles
  • Cornea
  • Lens
  • Pigment epithelium
  • Retina
  • Optic disk

A7.1. *See Figure 7.6.*

Q7.2. What is the optic disk?

A7.2. *It is the point of convergence of the axons from the retinal ganglion cells which form the optic nerve. It is devoid of photoreceptors, and hence is the eye's "blind spot."*

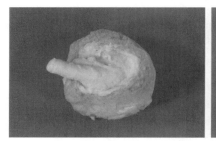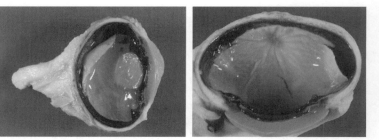

FIGURE 7.5. *Dissection of the cow eye.*

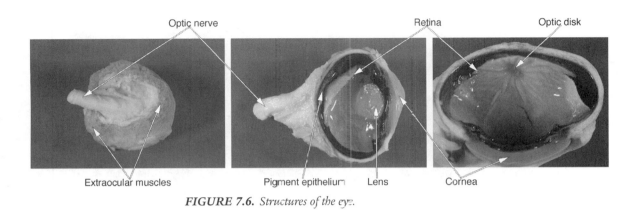

Optic nerve   Retina   Optic disk

Extraocular muscles   Pigment epithelium   Lens   Cornea

FIGURE 7.6. *Structures of the eye.*

Relationship to Skull

Let's begin by tracing the path that visual information follows into and through the brain.

Q7.3. Using the skull or Figure 7.7, locate the entrance site for the optic nerve and note its relationship to the sellae turcica and the pituitary fossa. What other structure passes through this foramen?

A7.3. *Optic canal. The ophthalmic artery also passes through the optic canal. See Figure 7.8.*

Retina

Q7.4. Examine the histological section from the center of the retina in Figure 7.9. Referring back to the diagram in Figure 7.3, identify the location of optic pit, the layers containing ganglion cells, amacrines and bipolars, and the photoreceptors. What is the significance of the optic pit?

A7.4. *The principal cell types are indicated in Figure 7.10. Note that the retina has an "inside-out" organization in so much as light passes through the other cell layers to reach the photoreceptors. The optic pit is the location of the fovea in the center of the retina. It has the highest packing of photoreceptor cells and is consequently the area of highest visual acuity.*

Retinal Ganglion Cell Physiology

Q7.5. On the left side in Figure 7.11, the outer circle indicates what is termed the cell's ***receptive field.*** It represents the area of the retina for which the presence of light stimulus can affect the cell's activity. Light falling anywhere outside the circle has no influence on the cell's firing. The inner circle indicates

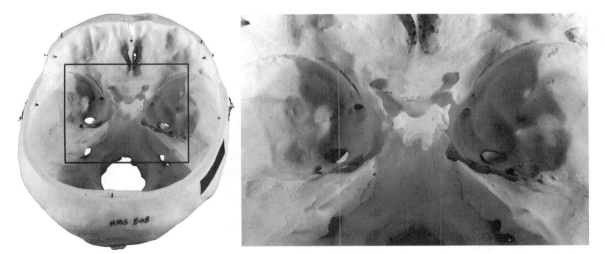

FIGURE 7.7. *Skull worksheet.*

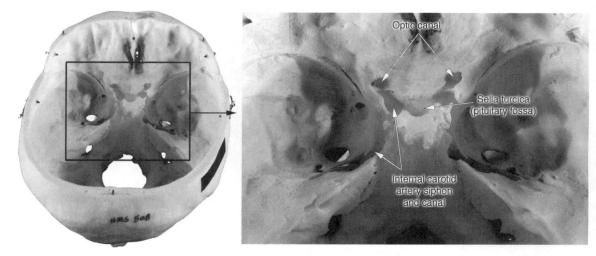

FIGURE 7.8. *Optic canal.*

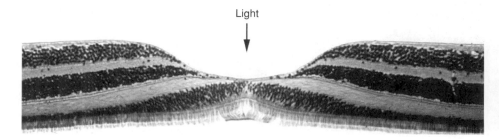

FIGURE 7.9. Histology of the retina. (Courtesy of Dr. Elio Raviola.)

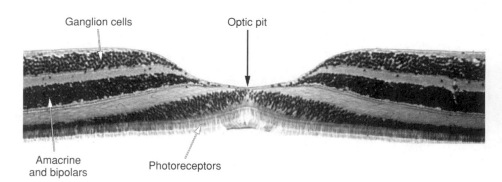

FIGURE 7.10. Salient histologic structures of the retina.

FIGURE 7.11. *Receptive fields of retinal ganglion cells. In this experiment, a spot of light was shone on the retina, while the activity of a single retinal ganglion cell was recorded with a microelectrode. The left hand panel indicates where the spot of light was presented, and the right hand panel shows the neuron's response to the stimulus. In the right panel, each vertical line represents an action potential, and the horizontal lines indicate the period of stimulus presentation. Three trials (A-C) are shown.(Modified from figure 2, S. W. Kuffler, The single-cell approach in the visual system and the study of receptive field. Investigative Ophthalmology 12:794–813, 1973.)*

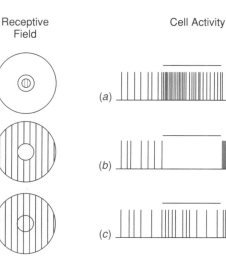

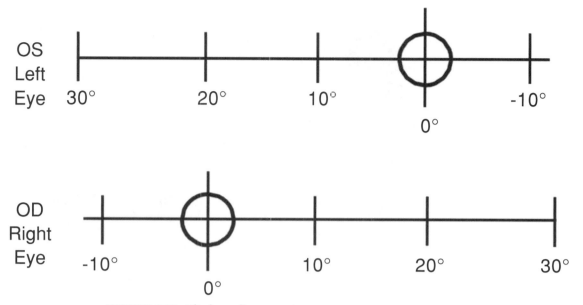

FIGURE 7.12. *Blind spot diagram.*

the central area of the receptive field. The vertical hatch marks indicate where in the receptive field the stimulus was presented. In *A*, the light was shone in the field's center, in *B*, in the "surround" part of the field, and in *C*, the entire receptive field was illuminated.

Describe which areas of the receptive field excite the cell and which inhibit it. What happens when the entire receptive field is illuminated?

A7.5. *Stimulation of the center of the receptive field excites the cell, while an annulus of light presented in the surround inhibits the cell. Simultaneously stimulating the whole receptive field has no effect on cell firing.*

This is a classical center-surround receptive field organization. It is termed an "on-center" cell because of the excitatory effect of light falling in the receptive field's center.

Q7.6. Would diffuse light be a good stimulus for this cell?

A7.6. *Completely filling the cell's receptive field with light results in no significant change in cell activity, so diffuse light would not stimulate the cell well. The cell signals a difference in the level of light in its receptive field center versus its surround. It is a contrast detector.*

> **Receptive field** *The entire extent of a stimulus that can influence a cell's firing. The stimulus may inhibit or stimulate the cell. Cells subserving each sensory modality (e.g., vision, hearing, touch) have their own types of receptive fields.*

Blind Spot

Q7.7. Use the visual field plot in Figure 7.12. Close one eye. With the open eye, fixate directly over the 0° target, keeping your eye about six inches (one pen length) from the page. Now take your pen, place its tip at 0°, then slowly move it outward. Keeping your eye fixed at 0°, at what angle does the tip disappear? This is your blind spot. If you have difficulty finding it, slowly sweep the pen back and forth in the horizontal plane. You'll start to notice its disappearance and reappearance. Does this correlate with the location of the optic disk?

A7.7. *The optic nerve exits the eye ball at about 12° off-axis. Your blind spot should also be about 10° to 15° eccentric in the horizontal plane.*

Visual Pathways

Q7.8. Examine the base of the brain using a specimen or Figure 7.13. Identify the following visual structures and landmarks:
- Optic nerve
- Optic chiasm
- Optic tract
- Lateral geniculate nucleus

A7.8. *See Figure 7.14.*

Q7.9. Locate the most medial fibers in the left optic nerve. Information from what part of the visual field is carried by these fibers?

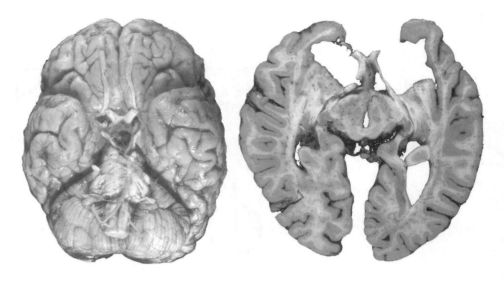

FIGURE 7.13. *Anatomy of the visual system, worksheet.*

A7.9. *Light from the left visual field will fall on the nasal or medial half of the left retina. This information then will travel in the medial side of the left optic nerve. These medial fibers will decussate, carrying the information from the left visual field to the right hemisphere.*

Q7.10. Now locate the most medial fibers in the left optic tract. What information are they carrying?

A7.10. *The light is from the right visual field falling on the nasal half of the right retina. These fibers crossed at the optic chiasm.*

Q7.11. Figure 7.15 a close-up photograph of a coronal section through a fixed brain. The contrast has been enhanced slightly. What do the layers in structure 1 represent? Name the indicated structures:

7.11.1 _____

7.11.2 _____

7.11.3 _____

7.11.4 _____

A7.11. *The layers in the lateral geniculate nucleus, six in all, represent the segregated inputs from each eye; three ipsilateral and three contralateral. The layers are in topographic register, so that cells directly above and below in adjacent layers are dedicated to the same point in the visual field.*
7.11.1. Lateral geniculate nucleus
7.11.2. Hippocampus

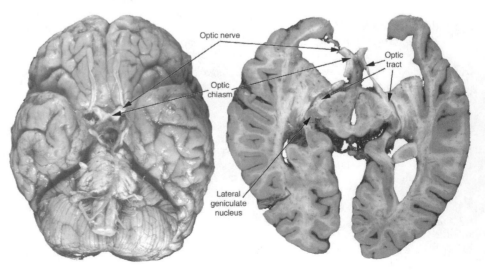

Optic nerve

Optic tract

Optic chiasm

Lateral geniculate nucleus

FIGURE 7.14. *Anterior visual pathway.*

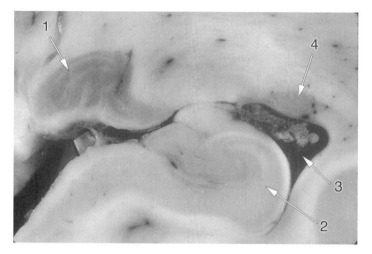

FIGURE 7.15. *Coronal section of brain, close-up.*

7.11.3. Temporal horn of the lateral ventricle
7.11.4. Tail of the caudate nucleus
Q7.12. Identify the labeled structures in Figure 7.16:

7.12.1 _____

7.12.2 _____

7.12.3 _____

7.12.4 _____

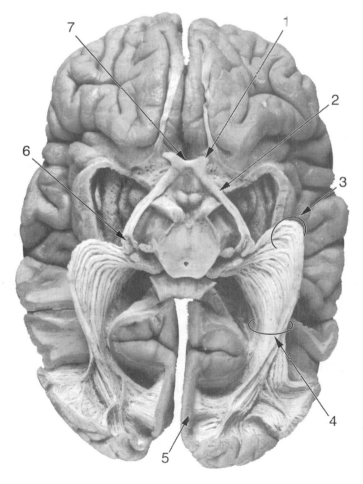

FIGURE 7.16. *Optic pathways. This beautiful specimen was made by freezing and thawing the brain several times, then carefully dissecting out the white matter tracts. (Modified from Gluhbegovic and Williams, The Human Brain, a Photographic Guide. © 1980, Harper & Row, figure 5-24, page 147.)*

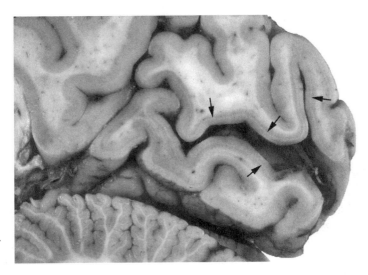

FIGURE 7.17. *Sagittal close-up of the primary visual cortex.*

7.12.5 _____

7.12.6 _____

7.12.7 _____

A7.12. *7.12.1. Optic nerve*
7.12.2. Optic tract
7.12.3. Meyer's loop (lower optic radiation in temporal lobe)
7.12.4. Optic radiation
7.12.5. Primary visual cortex
7.12.6. Lateral geniculate nucleus
7.12.7. Optic chiasm

Q7.13. What is the significance of Meyer's loop?

A7.13. Meyer's loop consists of the optic radiations that loop anteriorly around the posterior horn of the lateral ventricle coursing through the temporal lobe before sweeping posteriorly to the calcarine cortex. Damage to the temporal lobe can destroy these fibers while sparing the remainder of the optic radiations thus producing a superior quadrantanopia.

Q7.14. In Figure 7.17 or on your gross specimens, identify the labeled structure. What is its significance? Why is it white?

A7.14. The stripe of Gennari contains a large density of myelinated axons projecting to cortex. Many of these originate in the lateral geniculate nucleus. It demarcates primary visual cortex. Because of the high density of myelinated fibers, it appears as a white line on a slice of brain.

Q7.15. Using the sagittal brain anatomic specimen or Figure 7.17, find the calcarine fissure. What is its significance?

A7.15. The calcarine fissure represents primary visual cortex, which is the first level of cortical processing of visual information. It separates the upper and lower occipital lobes on the medial brain.

Q7.16. What kinds of stimuli activate cells here?

A7.16. The cells in layer IV, which receive the input from the lateral geniculate nucleus via the optic radiations, have center-surround receptive fields similar to those of cells in the retina and the lateral geniculate nucleus. Cells in other layers have more complex receptive fields, responding to bars, lines, and so on.

Visual Cortex

Q7.17. Examine the microscopic slide of primary visual cortex that has been stained for cell bodies and for myelin (see Fig. 7.18). Note again the ***stripe of Gennari.*** This defines the extent of primary visual cortex. Locate layer IV, which receives the projection fibers from the geniculate. What type of neurons do you find? Notice the layer's thickness. Contrast the thickness with layer IV here with its thickness in adjacent areas of brain.

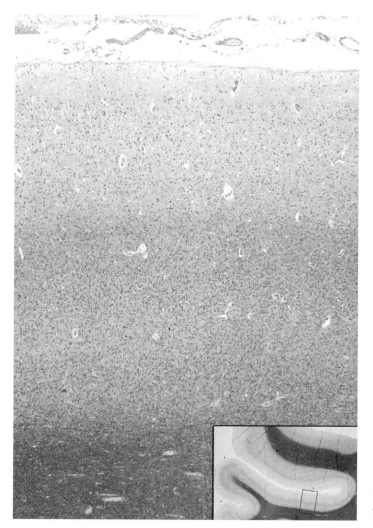

FIGURE 7.18. *Histology of the primary visual cortex (LFB/H&E stain).*

Why do you think it's different? Compare the appearance of neurons in layer IV with that of neurons in the layers above and below.

A7.17. Layer IV (**granular cortex**) *is remarkably thick and is packed with small, round neurons. These are the cells with the center-surround receptive fields mentioned above. This layer is much thicker in visual cortex than in adjacent cortex due to the massive sensory input from thalamus.*

Cortical Representation of the Visual Field

A most remarkable aspect of the visual system is the manner in which the topography of visual space projected onto the retina is preserved in the geniculate and in the cortex. This topography can be experimentally established in many ways. Two are shown in Figure 7.19 and Figure 7.20. In both cases brain activity is measured while a specific part of the visual field is stimulated. This allows a correspondence to be established between an area of visual space and a brain region. The first example identifies active neurons in a monkey by visualizing uptake of a radioactive tracer in response to a visual stimulus. The second study uses fMRI on human subjects.

Figure 7.19 is a flattened preparation of a monkey's left primary visual cortex that has been photographed using the 2-deoxy glucose method. The arrows point to corresponding points on the target and the cortical surface. In this way the topographic representation of the visual field is demonstrated.

Q7.18. Compare the data in Figures 7.19 and 7.20 with the cartoon of the visual fields in Figure 7.2. Do they agree?

A7.18. Figure 7.20 shows that the lower right visual field maps onto the upper bank of the left calcarine cortex, as diagrammed in Figure 7.2. Figure 7.19 demonstrates that intersecting lines in the visual field faithfully map onto the retina.

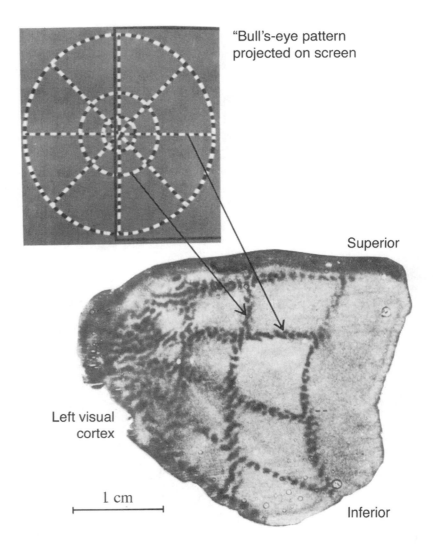

"Bull's-eye pattern projected on screen

Superior

Left visual cortex

1 cm

Inferior

FIGURE 7.19. *Topography of the retina. A monkey was injected with radioactive 2-deoxyglucose while it's eyes were focused on a bull's-eye pattern. The 2-deoxyglucose was taken up by the brain cells that were most active at the time (2-deoxyglucose is not metabolized, and hence remains within the neurons). After sectioning, the tissue was place against X-ray film to detect areas that had taken up the tracer. Since this is the left visual cortex, it responds to the right half of the stimulus figure. (Contributed by Roger Tootell)*

Q7.19. What is the blood supply to primary visual cortex?
A7.19. *The blood supply to the visual cortex is carried by the posterior cerebral artery.*
Q7.20. What is macular sparing?
A7.20. *Macular sparing is the preservation of a portion of the center of the visual field following massive damage to one or both visual cortices. While it is not entirely understood, it is believed to be due to the relatively large portion of cortex dedicated to the center of gaze, making it a difficult target to wipe out entirely.*

Visual field stimulation

Activity in left visual cortex

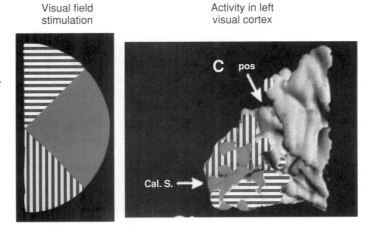

FIGURE 7.20. *Functional MRI of visual cortex topography. The image was made by recording blood flow changes in the cortex (representative of neuronal activity) while a subject watched a visual display. The location of the cortical visual field representation was mapped onto the brain. (Adapted from figure 2, DeYoe et al. 1996. Proc Nat Acad Sci 93: 2386.)*

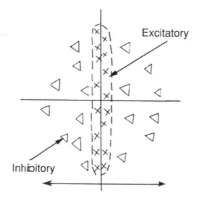

FIGURE 7.21. *The receptive field properties of a "simple cell" in cat primary visual cortex. The figure shows the results of a single cell recording made in response to a visual stimulus in a manner similar to the experiment described for the retinal ganglion cell in Figure 7.11. The X's indicate the part of the receptive field excited by light, and the triangles indicate the portion inhibited by light. (Provided by David Hubel)*

Cell Physiology in the Primary Visual Cortex

We saw how retinal ganglion cells had circular, center-surround receptive fields. Those in the lateral geniculate nucleus and in layer IV are similar. When physiologists studied the other layers of visual cortex, they found more complicated receptive field properties. An example is shown in Figure 7.21.

Q7.21. What would be the optimal stimulus for this cell?

A7.21. A vertically oriented bar of light that just filled the central region of the receptive field would optimally stimulate the neuron.

Q7.22. Examine Figure 7.22, in which the cell was stimulated with bars of varying orientations. What do these results tell you about the receptive field of this particular neuron?

A7.22. This neuron, like that in Figure 7.21, responds best to a vertical bar.

Visual cortex contains an orderly arrangement of cells, like the one shown, that respond to lines of each possible orientation. It is hypothesized that such cells function as edge detectors that serve to analyze image contours.

Q7.23. Hypothesize how the type of receptive field illustrated in Figure 7.21 could be built up from contributions from neurons having the center-surround receptive field properties shown in Figure 7.11?

A7.23. Figure 7.23 shows how a cell responsive to a bar could be created by summing inputs from an oriented grouping of neurons with center-surround properties. This scheme was first proposed Hubel and Weisel, and experimental evidence in support of the idea has recently been provided by Clay Reid.

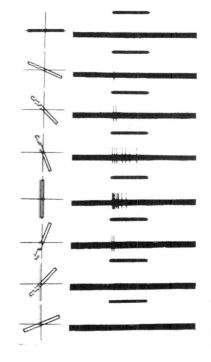

FIGURE 7.22. *Response of a visual cortical neuron to oriented lines. The left-hand panel indicates the orientation of the line. The right-hand panel indicates the cell's response. Vertical lines indicate action potentials, and the horizontal bars indicate the period of stimulus presentation. (Provided by David Hubel.)*

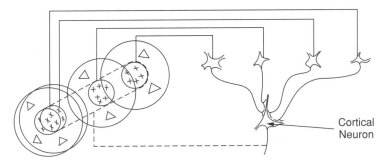

FIGURE 7.23. *Creating an oriented receptive field by grouping inputs from cells with center-surround response properties. The cortical neuron cartooned at right receives inputs from four cells having receptive field properties indicated at left. The cortical neuron's receptive field is built up from a summation of these inputs. The center of its receptive field is indicated by the dotted cylinder encompassing the centers of the inputs' receptive fields. The optimal stimulus for the cortical neuron would be a bar of light that was oriented in such a manner as to simultaneously excite its inputs. (Contributed by David Hubel)*

FIGURE 7.24. *Recording from a cell responsive to faces. The study was done in a macaque monkey. The area in which neurons were tuned to faces is indicated by the shading in A. In B, an example of a recording is shown from a cell that fired in response to the presentations of images of faces. The vertical bars represent the neuronal activity averaged over many trials. The horizontal bars indicate the period of stimulus presentation. The right hand panel shows the neuron's response to a scrambled version of the face presented at left. (Adapted from figures 1 & 6, 1984. Desimone et al. J. Neurosci 4: 2051–2062.)*

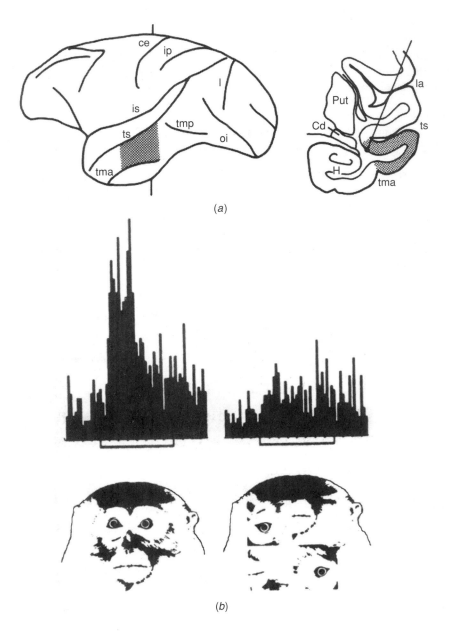

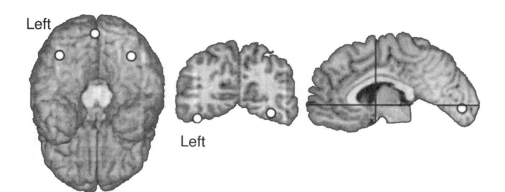

FIGURE 7.25. *Region of neuronal activation response to the presentation of faces. Subjects were shown a variety of images, including color and black-and-white faces, animal faces and bodies, and diagrams of faces. The white dots represent the average location of greatest neuronal activity when ten subjects viewed photographs of human faces, compared to animal faces, bodies, and diagrams. Activity was detected by changes in the local magnetic field. The data are superimposed upon one of the subject's MRI. The responses were independent of the color of the photograph and of the emotional valence of the person imaged. (Modified from Figure 6, Halgren et al., 2000. Cerebral Cortex 10:69–81.)*

Higher Visual Cortical Areas

Vision processing doesn't stop at primary visual cortex. Research has identified at least 25 visual areas beyond the calcarine gyri. These higher areas are often conceptually organized as dorsal ("where" pathway) and ventral ("what" pathway) streams. The dorsal stream of visual information moves into parietal cortex, where much of the processing concerns the location and trajectory of visual stimuli. The ventral stream moves into temporal cortex, where much of the analysis has to do with the identification of objects. Two examples of studies of visual areas that are responsive to faces are given in Figure 7.24 and Figure 7.25. In the first study electrophysiological recordings were made in the temporal lobe of the macaque monkey, where neurons were specifically activated in response to images of faces.

Q7.24. A human example of the "what" pathway is shown in Figure 7.25. It demonstrates neuronal activity recorded specifically in response to human faces. The spots indicate areas of maximal activity in response to faces. What brain area has been activated in response to faces?

A7.24. *The basal cortices of the occipital and temporal lobes show the greatest response to human faces. More specifically, the occipitotemporal or fusiform gyrus contains the sites of greatest activation.*

Q7.25. Suppose that a patient has a lesion in this area of brain. Predict the patient's clinical deficit.

A7.25. *You would expect the patient to be unable to recognize human faces. In practice, these patients can recognize that a face is human but cannot further identify the specific face, be it of a friend, a famous person, or even their own. The neurologic term for this deficit is prosopagnosia.*

Visual Field Deficits

Q7.26. Figure 7.26 is a diagram of the visual system with specific lesions indicated at different sites along the visual pathways. Imagine this brain slice is viewed from above, so the left visual field is on the left and the right is on the right. First identify the principal structures indicated using the blanks on the left. Then, for each "lesion," map out the patient's resulting visual field deficit in each eye. Shade in the visual field deficits using the charts to the right. Each oval represents what the corresponding eye would see. Make sure you understand the logic of each deficit.

A7.26. *See Figure 7.27.*

AUDITORY SYSTEM

Anatomy

Q7.27. Examine the skull or Figure 7.28. Locate and label the orifices important for hearing. What travels in the internal auditory meatus? External auditory meatus?

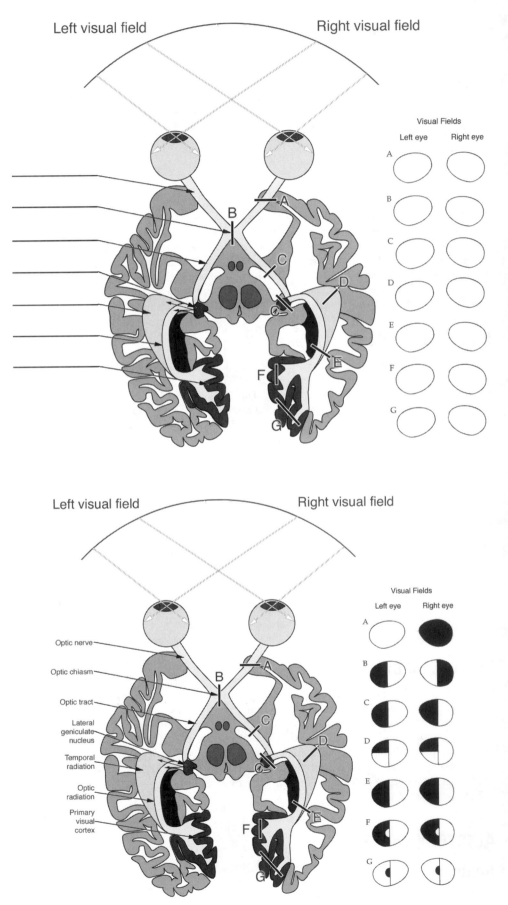

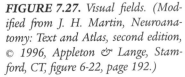

FIGURE 7.26. Visual field worksheet. (Adapted from J. H. Martin, Neuroanatomy: Text and Atlas, second edition, © 1996, Appleton & Lange, Stamford, CT, figure 6-22, page 192.)

FIGURE 7.27. Visual fields. (Modified from J. H. Martin, Neuroanatomy: Text and Atlas, second edition, © 1996, Appleton & Lange, Stamford, CT, figure 6-22, page 192.)

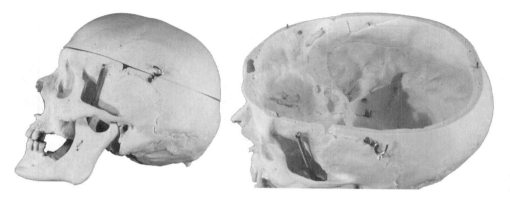

FIGURE 7.28. *Skull auditory worksheet.*

A7.27. *See Figure 7.29. The auditory, vestibular, and facial nerves all enter or exit through the internal auditory meatus. Sound waves travel into the external auditory meatus.*

Q7.28. Identify the auditory structures in Figure 7.30.
      7.28.1
      7.28.2
      7.28.3

A7.28. *7.28.1. Inferior colliculus*
      7.28.2. Medial geniculate nucleus
      7.28.3. Heschl's gyrus

Q7.29. Figure 7.31 diagrams several major brainstem auditory nuclei. Label these. Then wire the brainstem's auditory pathways, starting at the left cochlear nucleus.

A7.29. *See Figure 7.32. As mentioned previously, the system has extensive bilateral connections, only some of which are diagramed here. Because of these crossings, past the cochlear nucleus the auditory system is poor for localizing neurologic deficits.*

Q7.30 Look at Figure 7.33 below showing averaged fMRIs taken from musicians and nonmusicians while they were listening to musical tones. What differences do you see? What other type of input shows such a significant asymmetry?

A7.30. *In the upper panel the strongest activation is in the left primary auditory cortex. This cortex is located in the transverse temporal gyrus (of Heschl) on the superior surface of the temporal lobe and is mostly buried in the lateral sulcus. In the middle panel, the right **Heschl's gyrus** is most strongly activated. In the case of the nonmusician, most of the processing is also on the right. Although you may not know it yet, language for most people is "located" on the left: destroy parts of the left brain and the person becomes aphasic. This study shows that perfect-pitch musicians seem to process tones more like language, while others process it like regular sound. This is an example of hemispheric asymmetry in which corresponding areas of each hemisphere have differing roles or emphasis. In this case the left gyrus of Heschl may be involved with the symbolic interpretation of musical notes while the corresponding right gyrus of Heschl is processing music as a "real time" sensory experience. We will discuss more examples of hemispheric asymmetries later in the text when we study the cortex.*

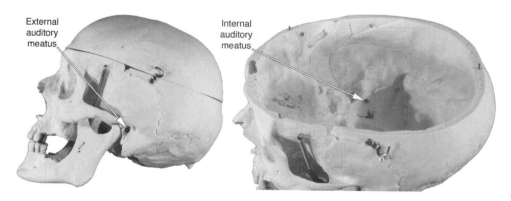

External auditory meatus

Internal auditory meatus

FIGURE 7.29. *Skull auditory orifices.*

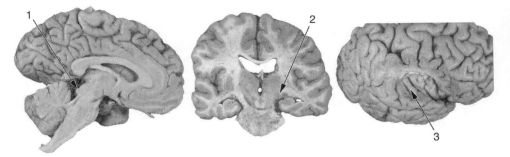

FIGURE 7.30. Brain auditory structures.

Receptive Fields in Auditory Cortex

The receptive field properties of neurons in the auditory system have been studied in a manner similar to that for cells of the visual system. As for the visual system, different classes of cells have different receptive field properties, analyzing such features as timing, intensity, location, and frequency of an auditory stimulus. Examples of receptive fields for two cells in the auditory cortex of the owl monkey are shown in Figure 7.34. The receptive fields were mapped out by correlating a neuron's firing with the stimulus that preceded the onset of activity.

Q7.31. Describe the receptive field properties of neuron *A*.

A7.31. *Neuron A's optimal stimulus is a sequence of two tones. The first tone is a bit above 4 Hz and of 50 ms duration. It is followed by a second tone just below 4 Hz and of 25 ms duration.*

Q7.32. Describe the receptive field properties of neuron *B*.

A7.32. *Neuron B best responds to a tone steadily increasing in frequency from about 2 to 4 Hz, over a period of approximately 50 ms. Combining signals from such chirp-responsive cells to produce language will occupy neuroscientists for decades!*

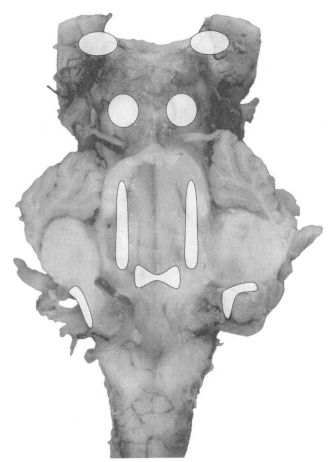

FIGURE 7.31. Brainstem auditory pathway worksheet.

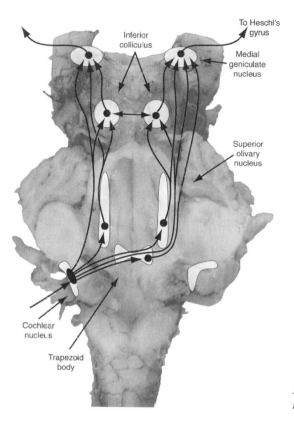

FIGURE 7.32. *Auditory pathways in the brainstem.*

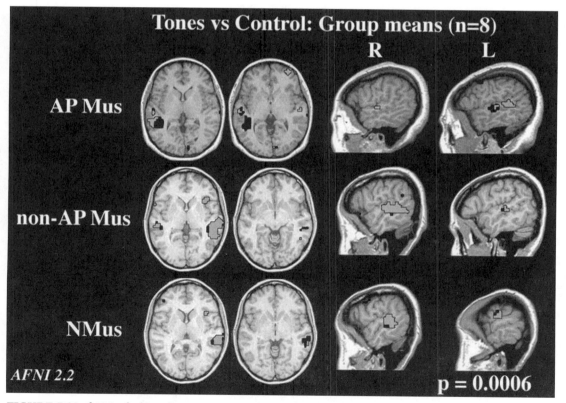

FIGURE 7.33. *fMRIs of subjects listening to tones. Black and gray indicate the areas of highest activity. The upper panel shows the data for musicians with perfect pitch, the middle panel for musicians lacking perfect pitch, and the lower panel for nonmusicians. On the horizontal images, the left is on the left. (Contributed by Gottfried Schlaug)*

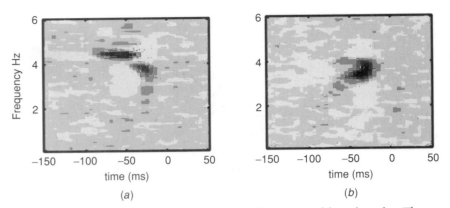

(a)   (b)

FIGURE 7.34. *Receptive field plots for 2 neurons in auditory cortex of the owl monkey. The properties of the sound stimulus activating each neuron are plotted with respect to frequency and time. The stimulus frequency is plotted on the Y axis and time on the X axis. Time "0" indicates when the cell first responds, negative time indicates the period preceding the cell's response. Black areas indicate the stimulus properties that excited the cell. (Adapted from figure 2, deCharms et al., Science 280: 1439–1443, 1998.)*

CLINICAL CASES

Visual Case 1

A 14-year-old boy complained of headaches. Initial examination of the cranial nerves showed only a partial loss of vision in the upper quadrants of the temporal fields bilaterally. The visual deficit increased over time until it included the entire temporal fields bilaterally.

Q7.33. Make a rough plot of his initial visual fields using Figure 7.35. Remember that the visual fields map space right-to-left and top-to-bottom on the retina, and segregate at the chiasm. Where is the lesion in this patient?

A7.33. *See Figure 7.36. The lesion is at the optic chiasm.*

Q7.34. Why does a lesion within the chiasm affect only the temporal visual fields bilaterally?

A7.34. *A compressive lesion at the optic chiasm can produce this type of field defect which is a bitemporal (heteronymous) hemianopsia. Fibers from both nasal retinal fields cross at the chiasm. Each nasal retina subserves the temporal field of its eye, so a lesion affecting the nasal fields of both eyes would be expected to produce a temporal field cut (deficit) in each eye. This is called a* **heteronymous** *deficit because the field cut is on the right in one eye and on the left in the other eye, in contrast to a* **homonymous hemianopsia,** *in which the deficit is in the same position in the visual field of each eye (due to a postchiasmatic lesion of the optic tract, lateral geniculate, optic radiations, or visual cortex).*

Q7.35. What structure lies just below the optic chiasm?

A7.35. *The pituitary.*

Q7.36. Now look at the MRI for this case shown in Figure 7.37. First, determine the plane of each image and the type of scan. Describe what you see. Indicate important surrounding anatomic structures. Suggest a diagnosis.

A7.36. *The upper four images are horizontal T2 scans and the lower images are sagittal and parasagittal enhanced scans.*

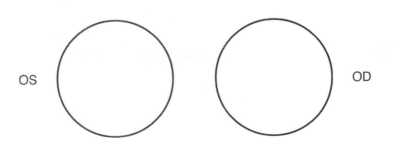

OS   OD

FIGURE 7.35. *Case 1 worksheet.*

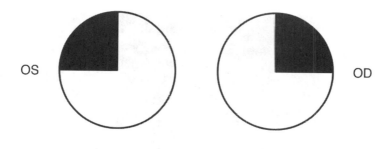

OS   OD

FIGURE 7.36. *Case 1 visual field deficit.*

    Sitting between the two carotid and middle cerebral arteries, just in front of the midbrain and mammillary bodies, is a strongly and uniformly enhancing mass. This mass has essentially obliterated the sella turcica.
    The lesion is a pituitary adenoma with suprasellar extension, compressing the optic chiasm.

Q7.37. Why were the upper quadrants of the temporal fields affected before the lower quadrants?

A7.37. *The upper quadrants were first affected because the lower most fibers in the chiasm, derived from the lower regions of both nasal halves of the retinas, were the earliest damaged by the compression from below.*

Auditory Case 1

Q7.38. A 73-year-old woman noticed that she couldn't hear her callers when she put the telephone receiver to her right ear. She had no history of dizziness or vertigo. Upon examination, she exhibited unilateral hearing loss. An image from her MRI is shown in Figure 7.38. Describe what you see. Where is the lesion? Name the adjacent brain structures in this image. How could this lesion get so large without producing more neurologic deficits? Suggest the diagnosis?

A7.38. *On this coronal, enhanced MRI is a brightly but not completely uniformly enhancing mass arises next to the pons and just below the hippocampus. Notice how the mass impinges on the pons. Had this mass arisen quickly, the patient would either be dead or comatose (as you will learn*

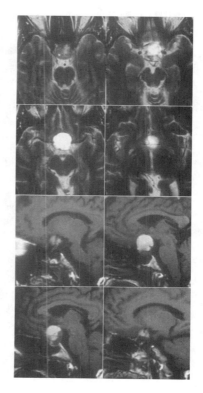

FIGURE 7.37. *MRI scans on visual case 1.*

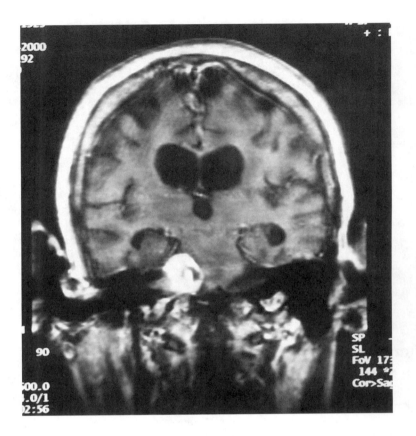

FIGURE 7.38. MRI scan on auditory case 1.

later, the reticular activating system lives in the pons and midbrain). That she only has a hearing deficit indicates the tumor has grown very slowly and been there a long time.

She had a right vestibular nerve Schwannoma. The main differential diagnosis would be a meningioma, and then a laundry list of more unusual tumors.

Visual Case 2

A 70-year-old right-handed woman complained that she was having trouble walking, and having trouble seeing out of her left eye. She seemed to walk into objects on her left side and in one instance, bruised her left hand by accidently swinging it into a table edge. The problem came on rather suddenly and no other neurological symptoms were present.

Q7.39. How might you distinguish whether the patient's attribution of impaired vision in the left eye actually corresponded to a deficit limited to the left eye or whether the deficit related to the left side of space?

A7.39. *To get accurate information you must conduct visual field testing separate for each eye. In this case testing the right eye will distinguish left eye blindness or a left hemianopsia.*

Q7.40. The results of the patient's visual field testing are given in Figure 7.39. How would you describe her deficit?

A7.40. *She has a bilateral left homonymous hemianopia, or in language that anyone can understand: a deficit in the left visual field for both eyes.*

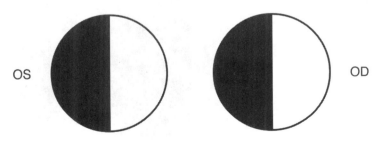

FIGURE 7.39. Visual case 2 field plot.

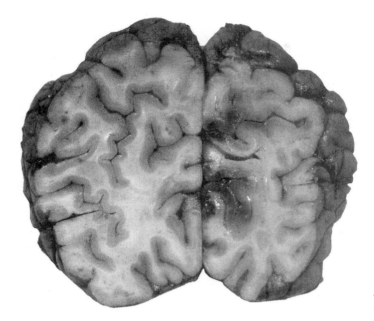

FIGURE 7.40. *Pathology on visual case 2. Coronal section.*

Q7.41. Where would you localize the lesion responsible for this patient's deficit?

A7.41. *Since the lesion affects the same area of visual space for both eyes, it has to be behind the optic chiasm, where the information from the two eyes comes together. In theory, the lesion could be anywhere along the path from chiasm to visual cortex. In your mind you should march like Sherman to the sea, through the connections including optic tract, lateral geniculate nucleus, optic radiations, to visual cortex. In a case where the deficit is purely visual, one tends to suspect a cortical lesion. The lateral geniculate nucleus is a very small target, and it is unlikely to be affected exclusively. Similarly, if the deficit is in either the optic tract or the radiations, you would expect some of the grey matter through which the fibers course to be affected, and this would produce additional symptoms.*

Q7.42. Look at Figure 7.40, which illustrates the lesion. Describe the location and nature of the lesion. Does this make sense?

A7.42. *This is a right PCA hemorrhagic infarct, which includes the primary visual cortex. More or less where you would predict.*

Chapter 8—
NEUROMUSCULAR SYSTEM

You have seen and smelled what you want. To taste it requires action. Time to move.

Having mastered the two main somatic sensory systems we will now turn attention to the motor systems, and will begin with the peripheral aspects first. We will examine the structure of muscle, its innervation, types and locations of motor nerves, and the motor neuron.

LEARNING OBJECTIVES

- Discuss the concept of motor unit, including its role as the final common pathway in the motor system, the sequence of firing of motor units and their main subtypes.
- Understand muscle fiber structure, different types of fibers and how these are detected by histo-chemistry. Review some diseases of muscle, especially muscular dystrophies and some of their molecular abnormalities.
- Become familiar with the basic concepts of electromyogram (EMG) and nerve conduction, including compound muscle action potential, fibrillation, and fasciculation.
- Identify the location of anterior horn cells and their function.
- Review diseases affecting motor nerves: axon degeneration, demyelination, transection, or in-farction. Discuss their consequences to muscle. Indicate what happens with chronic denerva-tion/reinnervation, including fiber type grouping.

INTRODUCTION

Virtually every neurological examination includes a good whack on the knee cap. In doing this, the doctor is examining the stretch reflex, which provides a window into the integrity of the nervous system's local control over the muscle. The circuit underlying this response is shown in Figure 8.1. The tap with the hammer distends the patellar tendon, which activates stretch receptors embedded in the tendon. The receptors are located in the terminal processes of **_dorsal root ganglion_** (DRG) neurons causing them to fire. The DRG cells synapse on the lower motor neurons controlling the

Functional Neuroanatomy: An Interactive Text and Manual, by Jeffrey T. Joseph and David L. Cardozo
ISBN 0-471-44437-5 Copyright © 2004 John Wiley & Sons, Inc.

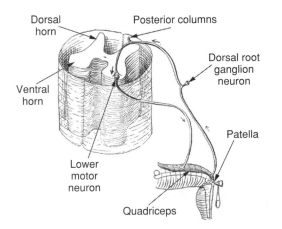

FIGURE 8.1. *Circuit underlying the patellar stretch reflex. (Adapted from Krieg, Functional Neuroanatomy, Blakiston Co., Philadelphia, 1942, figure 19, pg. 41.)*

quadriceps muscle, causing it to contract and thereby opposing the stretch. All somatic muscles with the exception of the extra-ocular muscles, have this circuit. It's believed to be involved in adjusting and maintaining muscle tension. In order for the reflex to be normal, all the components, including the muscle, the sensory neuron and its processes, the motor neuron, and its axon have to be functioning normally. The efferent arm of this reflex consists of the lower motor neurons, their axons and their nerve terminals synapsing on muscle fibers at the neuromuscular junction.

In approaching the neuromuscular system, we need to be familiar with its principal components, including the lower motor neurons situated in the ventral horn of the spinal cord, the nerves going to and from muscle, the muscle tissue, and the sensory innervation of the muscle. The neuromuscular system and its pathologies can be considered using several approaches, including localization of lesions based on anatomical considerations, histological examination of tissue, and electrophysiological testing of nerve and muscle function.

The Motor Unit

Examine Figure 8.2. Fundamental to understanding the neuromuscular system is grasping the concept of the motor unit. A given unit consists of a lower motor neuron, its axon, and all of the myofibers it innervates. Implicit in this definition is the concept that a single myofiber is innervated by only one motor neuron, while a single motor neuron may innervate many muscle fibers. Motor units vary in size from the smallest units containing only a few muscle fibers to units in the largest muscles, with more than a thousand fibers. In the healthy state, every time a lower motor neuron fires, the muscles fibers comprising its motor unit contract. (Muscle fiber has no counterbalancing inhibitory inputs.) Since their activity dictates the state of the muscles, the lower motor neurons are the final common pathway.

Whether or not a muscle contracts depends only on whether or not its anterior horn cells fires. Every movement we make, with a few unimportant exceptions like cramps and fasciculations, is the result of the orderly firing of motor units. Whether or not the anterior horn cell fires is the product of two things: its background tone (actually its resting potential) and the sum of all the excitatory and inhibitory inputs to it. Some of these inputs are local reflexes, some come from descending tracts, some from nearby, and others from far away in the motor cortex.

Structure and Function of Skeletal Muscle

From previous work in Chapter 3, you are familiar with the basic structure of muscle. The organization of muscle is shown in Figure 8.3.

Periodic thick Z-bands divide a longitudinal muscle into small subunits. Between the bands lie bundles of the contractile proteins actin and myosin. During each contraction, these filaments slide next to each other, in a process requiring calcium ions. As you have seen in the histology laboratory, muscle nuclei are usually near the periphery of their fiber. Since a muscle may be many centimeters long, it may contain thousands of nuclei and millions of mitochondria. The proteins making up the thousands of myofibrils in a single myofiber are slowly replaced over several weeks by protein synthesis. When a muscle enlarges, due to training or usage, the number of fibrils increases; while with atrophy or disuse their number falls.

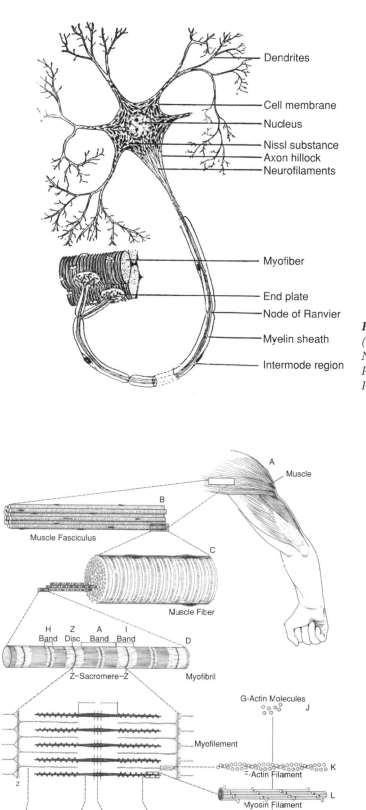

Dendrites

Cell membrane

Nucleus

Nissl substance

Axon hillock

Neurofilaments

Myofiber

End plate

Node of Ranvier

Myelin sheath

Intermode region

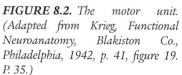

FIGURE 8.2. *The motor unit. (Adapted from Krieg, Functional Neuroanatomy, Blakiston Co., Philadelphia, 1942, p. 41, figure 19. P. 35.)*

A Muscle

B

Muscle Fasciculus

C

Muscle Fiber

H   Z   A   I
Band Disc Band Band   D

Z–Sacromere–Z   Myofibril

Myofilement

G-Actin Molecules   J

F-Actin Filament   K

Myosin Filament   L

Myosin Molecule

Z

F   G   H

Light   Heavy
Meromyosin   Meromyosin

M

N

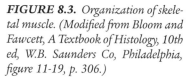

FIGURE 8.3. *Organization of skeletal muscle. (Modified from Bloom and Fawcett, A Textbook of Histology, 10th ed, W.B. Saunders Co, Philadelphia, figure 11-19, p. 306.)*

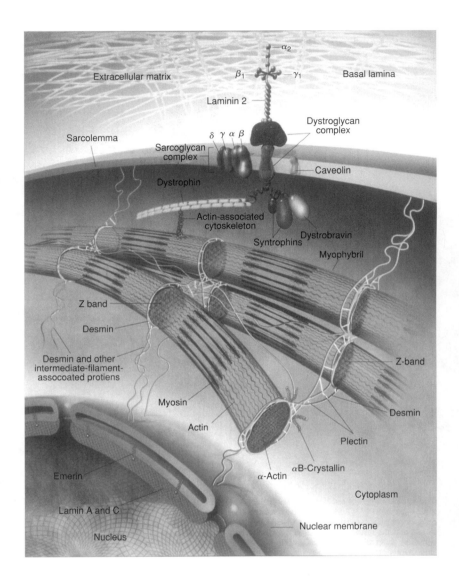

FIGURE 8.4. *Muscle proteins associated with inherited muscular dystrophies. (Modified from figure 5, Dalakas, M. C., et al. Desmin myopathy, a skeletal myopathy with cardiomyopathy caused by mutations in the desmin gene. 2000. N Engl J Med 342: 770–780.)*

The contractile proteins would do nothing, were they not tethered to the muscle membrane and extracellular matrix. A large group of structural proteins provide the necessary anchoring. It is these proteins that are associated with many genetic disorders of muscle, collectively named the muscular dystrophies. Some of the different components of the sarcolemmal membrane are shown in Figure 8.4.

X-linked dystrophies involve the muscle protein dystrophin, a very large protein located inside the muscle membrane, and presumably responsible for its structural integrity. Depending on how abnormal the dystrophin molecule is, boys with this disease have mild (Becker type) or severe (Duchenne type) dystrophy. Spanning the muscle membrane, and attaching dystrophin to the extracellular matrix, are several other glycoproteins, particularly the sarcoglycans. Mutations in the mostly autosomal genes for these proteins also cause dystrophies, although with a different clinical picture. The habit of naming the different types of dystrophy for their original describers is slowly fading, and the relevant protein is now more often the source of the name, for example, dystrophinopathy.

Muscle Innervation and Denervation

The integrity of skeletal muscle fibers depends on its innervation. Deprived of any nerve supply, a myofiber will slowly atrophy. Eventually it will degenerate into a small bag of neurons enclosed in a membrane. Such knots of nuclei can persist for a long time.

After denervation of a muscle fiber, it can receive innervation from an adjacent motor unit by means of axon sprouting at the nerve terminal. *Poliomyelitis* was a disease that was epidemic in the United States in decades gone by, and still exists in pockets on other continents. It is caused by an

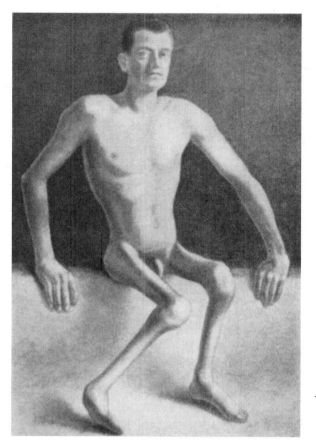

FIGURE 8.5. *Drawing of a patient with polio. Note the atrophy in the muscles of the lower limb. (Modified from Bing and Haymaker, Regional Diagnosis of the Brain and Spinal Cord, 11th ed, © 1940, Mosby Co., St. Louis, figure 12, page 48.)*

acute loss of motor units due to viral infection of the anterior horn cell. Adjacent surviving motor neurons, if any, would send out sprouts and take over the lost territory. Some of the largest motor units ever observed are seen in prior polio victims. They may have units containing many thousands of muscle fibers, firing somewhat asynchronously.

The same process occurs in ***amyotrophic lateral sclerosis*** (*ALS,* a degenerative motor neuron disease). Unlike polio, this disease is progressive and ultimately, all of the anterior horn cells are lost and sprouting will fail. In both of these diseases, reduced innervation leads to a characteristic atrophy of the affected muscle.

Damage to the motor unit at any point produces denervation. Polio and ALS damage the anterior horn cell. A herniated disc will damage a nerve root. Peripheral neuropathy damages the motor axons as they course through the peripheral nerve. Wherever the unit is damaged, its distal parts will degenerate. This process is analogous to the degeneration of central axons we saw in the Chapter 2, and is also termed ***Wallerian degeneration***.

Figure 8.6 shows several general processes that may follow injury to a peripheral nerve. An injury may crush or transect the nerve, thereby producing distal Wallerian degeneration and compensatory changes to the neuron cell body. Toxins and degenerative diseases may inflict damage specifically to the axon or its neuron. Inflammatory diseases and certain inherited diseases may damage the myelin sheath around axons. These processes are equally important for sensory and motor axons. Destruction of the myelin sheath may occur as a result of a direct attack upon myelin or secondarily following axon loss.

Axonal neuropathies account for about 90% of the neuropathies that are clinically recognized. They all share these features: symmetrical, distal muscles most affected, atrophy of muscle visible, features of denervation by electromyogram (EMG), no evidence of slowing of conduction velocity, both motor and sensory fibers affected.

Demyelinating neuropathies are important for two reasons: they can be very severe to the point of being life threatening, and they are treatable. The majority of demyelinating diseases are autoimmune. They are treated with some combination of high dose steroids, plasma exchange, and immunosuppressive drugs. Most cases also show axonal damage, so some of the features of axonal neuropathy

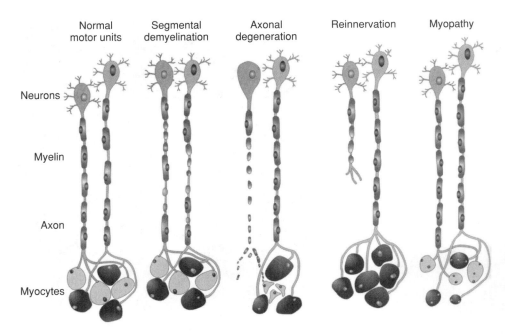

are present, but you can also find these features: paralysis without atrophy, proximal or asymmetric weakness, and evidence of conduction slowing or conduction block.

To localize the level of a spinal nerve injury, you need to know its sites of distribution. Nerve myotome tables and dermatome maps, like the ones shown in Figure 8.7, while not identical for every individual, are most useful to localize the site of the lesion. For each muscle the myotome table indicates both the level of spinal cord containing the associated lower motor neurons, and the peripheral nerve through which their axons travel. The dermatome chart does the same for the somatosensory distribution. The reasoning is quite simple. After determining the pattern of muscle weakness and sensory deficit, a skilled neurologist (who carries this chart in his head) deduces whether the deficit is best explained by peripheral nerve damage, central lesion(s) or some combination of both.

Clinical Electrophysiology

Electrophysiological testing is a useful tool for studying the integrity of the neuromuscular system. There are three basic types of testing, as well as several other more specialized and sophisticated tests. The basic tests consist of (1) nerve conduction studies, (2) measurement of the compound muscle action potential following nerve stimulation, and (3) electromyography.

Nerve Conduction Studies

Figure 8.8 is an illustration of the setup for recording nerve conduction. Recordings are made using surface electrodes placed over the nerve of interest. In this case the ulnar nerve is being examined. A stimulating electrode is placed at one point over the nerve, and a recording electrode is moved to different positions along its course. The stimulation electrode depolarizes all of the axons in the nerve, causing them to simultaneously fire action potentials. The signal obtained at the recording electrode represents a summation of the action potentials of the individual nerve fibers. It is examined for velocity, amplitude, and shape of the waveform. The conduction velocity is calculated by dividing the distance between the stimulating and recording electrodes by the time of travel (latency) of the action potential. This value can be compared to age-matched standards or in the case of unilateral lesions, to the performance of the contralateral unaffected nerve. Decreased conduction velocity suggests a problem with axonal myelination. The amplitude of the signal is indicative of the number of axons firing, and consequently a decrease in amplitude indicates axonal loss or complete conduction block for some of the fibers. Finally the shape of the recorded signal yields information concerning the synchrony of fiber activity. Since all of the axons in the nerve are depolarized by the stimulating electrode at the same time, to the extent that they are in perfect synchrony, the signal will resemble a giant single action potential. The ideal situation doesn't exist because there is normal variation in the conduction velocities recorded, due to the differing diameters of myelinated fibers contributing to the

Muscle	Nerve root level	Action
Rhomboids	Dorsal scapular N C4-C5	Adduction – scapula
Supraspinatus	Suprascapular N C4-C5	Abduction – arm
Infraspinatus	Suprascapular N C4-C6	Lateral rotation – arm
Serratus anterior	Long thoracic N C5-C7	Draws scapula forward during pushing
Subscapularis	Subscapular N C5-C6	Medial rotation – arm
Latissimus dorsi	Thoracodorsal N C6-C8	Adduction, medial rotation – arm
Teres major	Lateral subscapular N C5-C7	Adduction, extension, medial rotation – arm
Deltoid	Axillary N C5-C6	Abduction – arm
Biceps brachii	Musculocutaneous N C5-C6	Flexion – forearm; Supination – hand
Triceps	Radial N C6-C8	Extension – forearm
Brachioradialis	Radial N C5-C6	Flexion – forearm
Extensor carpi radialis	Radial N C5-C7	Extension, abduction – hand
Supinator	Radial N C5-C7	Supination - hand
Extensor digitorum	Radial N C6-C8	Extension – wrist, phalanges
Extensor carpi ulnaris	Radial N C6-C8	Extension adduction – hand
Abductor pollicis longus	Radial N C6-C8	Abduction - thumb
Extensor pollicis longus	Radial N C6-C8	Extension - second phalanx (thumb)
Extensor pollicis brevis	Radial N C7-T1	Extension - first phalanx (thumb)
Pronator teres	Median N C6-C7	Pronation - hand
Flexor carpi radialis	Median N C6-C7	Flexion, abduction – hand
Flexor digitorum sublimis	Median N C7-T1	Flexion - second phalanx (fingers)
Flexor digitorum profundus	Median N C7-T1	Flexion - terminal phalanx (fingers)
Flexor pollicis longus	Median N C6-C8	Flexion - second phalanx (thumb)
Abductor pollicis brevis	Median N C7-T1	Abduction - thumb
Opponens pollicis	Median N C7-T1	Abduction, flexion - thumb
Flexor pollicis brevis	Median N C7-T1	Adduction, flexion - thumb
Flexor carpi ulnaris	Ulnar N C7-T1	Flexion, adduction - hand
Abductor digiti quinti brevis	Ulnar N C8-T1	Abduction – little finger
Flexor digiti quinti brevis	Ulnar N C8-T1	Flexion – little finger
Opponens digiti quinti	Ulnar N C8-T1	Abduction, flexion – little finger
Adductor pollicis	Ulnar N C8-T1	Adduction - thumb
Interossei	Ulnar N C8-T1	Dorsal – abduction fingers from middle finger
Lumbricals	1,2 – Median N / 3,4 – Ulnar N C8-T1	Palmar – adduction fingers toward middle finger
Neck flexors	C1-C6	Flexion – neck
Neck extensors	C1-T1	Extension – neck
Diaphragm	Phrenic N C3-C5	Diaphragmatic breathing
Abdominal muscles		
Upper	T5-T9	
Lower	T10-L3	
Iliopsoas	Femoral N L2-L4	Flexion – thigh at hip
Adductor magnus, longus, brevis	Obturator N L2-L4	Adduction – thigh
Gluteus medius & minimus	Superior gluteal N L4-S1	Abduction, medial rotation - thigh
Gluteus maximus	Inferior gluteal N L4-S2	Extension, lateral rotation – thigh
Quadriceps femoris	Femoral N L4-S1	Extension – leg at knee
Hamstrings	Sciatic N L4-S1	Flexion – leg at knee
Tibialis anterior	Deep peroneal N L4-L5	Dorsiflexion, inversion – foot
Extensor hallucis longus	Deep peroneal N L4-S1	Extension – great toe; Dorsiflexion – foot
Extensor digitorum longus	Deep peroneal N L4-S1	Extension – lateral four toes; Dorsiflexion - foot
Extensor digitorum brevis	Deep peroneal N L4-S1	Extension – all toes except little toe
Peroneus longus brevis	Superficial peroneal N L5-S1	Eversion – foot
Gastrocnemius & soleus	Tibial N L5-S2	Plantar flexion – foot
Tibialis posterior	Posterior tibial N L5-S1	Inversion - foot
Flexor digitorum longus	Posterior tibial N L5-S2	Plantar flexion – toes
Flexor hallucis longus	Posterior tibial N L5-S2	Plantar flexion –great toe
Foot intrinsics	Posterior tibial L5-S2	

FIGURE 8.7. *Nerve myotome table and peripheral sensory nerve figure. (Left table adapted from J. Gilroy, Basic Neurology, third edition, © 2000. McGraw Hill, New York, table 1-9, page 45–46. Right figure adapted from Brock, Basis of Clinical Neurology, Williams & Wilkins, Baltimore, 1938, figure 1, page 18.)*

signal. In normal nerves, though, the waveform has a reasonably sharp appearance, while in diseased nerve, the shape of the wave can be significantly altered as a result of the contributions of fibers in varying states of demyelination.

Compound Muscle Action Potential (CMAP)

A second electrophysiological approach is measurement of the compound muscle action potential (CMAP). In this form of recording, the nerve is stimulated in the same manner as discussed above, but the recording electrode is placed over the muscle innervated by the nerve (see Fig. 8.9). The resulting signal represents the depolarization of the muscle fibers below the electrode. Since the recorded signal originates from muscle fibers alone, only these fibers and the motor axons providing their innervation are being tested. Although in a mixed nerve the sensory fibers are also depolarized by the stimulating electrode, their activity does not contribute directly or indirectly to the CMAP. In order for the signal to be normal, the peripheral motor axons, the neuromuscular junction, and the muscle fibers, all have to be in working order.

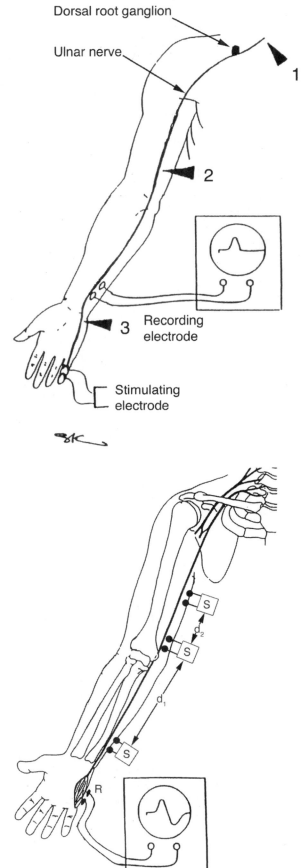

Dorsal root ganglion

Ulnar nerve

1

2

3 Recording
electrode

Stimulating
electrode

FIGURE 8.8. *Recording the sensory action potential in the ulnar nerve. The numbered arrowheads indicate three different recording sites along the nerve. (Contributed by Dr. Shahram Khoshbin.)*

S

d₂

S

d₁

S

R

FIGURE 8.9. *Recording the compound muscle action potential. (Drawing by Shahram Khoshbin.)*

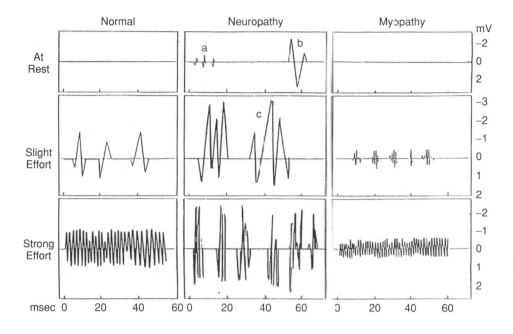

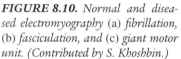

FIGURE 8.10. *Normal and diseased electromyography* (a) *fibrillation,* (b) *fasciculation, and* (c) *giant motor unit. (Contributed by S. Khoshbin.)*

Electromyography (EMG)

A third major approach in clinical electrophysiology is electromyography. In EMG studies a recording electrode is placed directly in the muscle and recordings are made of the depolarization of the muscle fibers following voluntary contraction. Typically the recordings are made under three conditions: (1) muscle at rest, (2) the patient exerting minimal effort, and (3) the patient exerting maximal effort.

Typical results for an EMG study are illustrated in Figure 8.10. The EMGs shown are for a normal subject, a patient with a neuropathy, and a patient with a myopathy. In the normal state, the EMG is completely flat at rest, as there are no motor neurons that are active. This is shown in the uppermost left-hand panel. With slight effort EMG can detect the depolarization of the first motor unit activated. This is pictured in the second panel on the left, in which three spikes can be observed, representing three firings of the same motor unit. The recording during maximal effort is shown in the third panel. Its complexity is due to fact that a very large number (perhaps nearly all) of the muscle fibers are activated so that no single motor unit can be resolved, causing what is termed an "*interference pattern.*"

The middle panel shows the results one might find in a case where there is pathology at the level of the motor neuron or its fiber. At rest, the trace is not flat. Two types of spontaneous depolarizations are present. The smaller of the two is termed a *fibrillation* and the larger depolarization which is the same size as a single motor unit, is termed a *fasciculation.*

As myofibers become denervated, their membrane is much less stable and they may fire spontaneously to produce fibrillations. These effects are not be visible externally. Fasciculations represent the spontaneous firing of a motor unit, which are often visible to eye. They are caused by the unregulated activity of a motor neuron. Although they can be benign (everyone has them once in a while), they are also present in motor neuron pathology.

The middle panel shows the recording following slight effort from a patient with a chronic neuropathy. As was the case for normal muscle, single motor units can be resolved with minimal effort. In this case, however, the single unit is much larger and is termed a "giant motor unit." This results from denervation followed by reinnervation as shown in Figure 8.6. The surviving neurons will have much larger motor units as they have taken over the abandoned muscle fibers. Finally, there is much less complexity with full contraction because the loss of motor neurons has resulted in fewer motor units.

The right panels show the case for myopathy. At rest, fasciculations will not be seen because the motor nerves are healthy. Fibrillations may or may not be seen depending on the pathology. With minimal contraction, the motor unit amplitude will be smaller due to the loss of muscle fibers. With maximal effort, there will be a full interference pattern since the normal number of motor units is present. The amplitude of the signal will nevertheless be diminished because there are fewer fibers contributing to it.

Schedule (2.5 hours)

15 Muscle
30 Myopathy
45 Innervation of muscle
10 Spinal cord
20 Clinical electrophysiology
30 Clinical cases

MUSCLE

INST Review the cross-sectional slides of muscle stained with H&E, which you saw in Chapter 3. See Figure 8.11. Review the monotonous pattern of fibers, which have pretty much the same size and same shape, with nuclei near the periphery.

Q8.1. Knowing that the myofibrillary filaments are long and in register, how are you viewing them on the slide or in Figure 8.11? Where are most of the proteins located that are pictured in Figure 8.4? Focus up and down on the slide; you'll get an idea of the myofibrils within each fiber.

A8.1. *Snap-frozen muscles are usually cut in cross section (right, Fig. 8.11), while paraffin-embedded muscle may be embedded in any direction. If you see striations, you are looking at a longitudinal view (left, Fig. 8.11). If the myofiber contains an array of dots, with some larger blobs, the myofilaments most likely point directly out of the slide (right, Fig. 8.11). In cross-sectional view you may see some areas having more thin filaments (predominantly actin) and some having more thick filaments (predominantly myosin) because they are end-on, you can no longer see the sarcomere structure (A-bands, I-bands, Z-disc). In longitudinal sections the sarcomeric structure comes out in its full glory (left, Fig. 8.11).*

The membrane-associated proteins pictured in the muscular dystrophy figure are on only the surface of the myofiber (the dystrophin-related proteins). The nuclear proteins, of course, reside only in the peripherally marginated nuclei. Most of the muscle is composed of contractile proteins.

In a muscle sample its fibers all seem pretty much the same, except for some slight variation in their size. Yet they are quite different in their physiological characteristics. Recall from Chapter 3 that type I fibers (one slow red ox) are nonfatigable, since they predominantly utilize oxidative phosphorylation and contain larger amounts of enzymes of the oxidative pathways. Because of the cytochrome content of mitochondria, these fibers are red. So type I fibers are SLOW twitch, RED, and OXidative. At the other end of the spectrum are the type II fibers, which are high threshold and contract rarely, are high in glycolysis, and are easily fatigued. Muscles that contract rarely but do so with high force have a lot of these fibers.

Q8.2. Review the ATPase histochemical stain of a cross section of muscle in Figure 8.12. Do you see the two main fiber types? You may recognize some intermediate types too. All the muscle fibers that are innervated by one ventral horn motor neuron share the same physiological and histochemical characteristics. The properties of the motor neuron determine the fiber type of all myofibers in its motor unit. In animals such as the rat, where muscles are more separated by type (i.e. reddish muscles which are slow twitch, and white muscles which are fast twitch type) you can switch the innervation

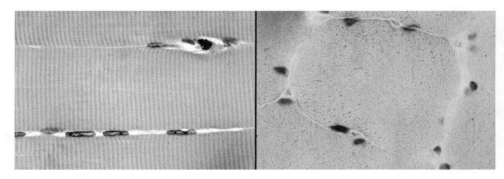

FIGURE 8.11. *Normal muscle histology, H&E. Both views were taken at the same microscopic power.*

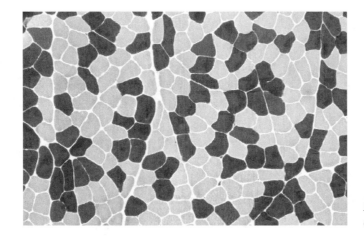

FIGURE 8.12. ATPase histochemical stain.

surgically, and after some time the muscle will switch from "red" to "white" or vice versa.

MYOPATHY

Case 1: Duchenne's Muscular Dystrophy

A 5-year-old boy appeared to be normal at birth, but his muscular movements were soon noticed to be somewhat weaker than would be expected. He began to crawl at three months, but not vigorously. He was slow in walking and his gait was seen to be clumsy and waddling. He could not run well and had difficulty in arising from a lying position. Two male cousins on his mother's side died in childhood with a similar history.

On examination, he displayed moderate weakness of all the muscles of the trunk and limbs, but less prominent weakness in the small muscles of the hands and feet. The calves were relatively bulky, appearing hypertrophied; the large muscles were abnormally firm to palpation. Muscle stretch reflexes were obtainable but were sluggish. Plantar responses ("Babinski test") were normal (flexor). He had no fasciculations or sensory changes. Laboratory studies showed a ***creatine kinase*** (CK, CPK) of 17,000 (normal less than 200).

Q8.3. Would you say his weakness more significantly involved his proximal or distal muscles? What information suggests that his nerves were fine?

A8.3. As is typical of a myopathy, his weakness primarily involved his large, more proximal postural muscles rather than the muscles of his hands and feet. He still had stretch reflexes and had no fasciculations or sensory changes, indicating his peripheral nerves were all right.

Q8.4. Briefly review the introductory figure of the muscle membrane and then examine a microscopic slide from another boy with this disease (see Fig. 8.13). How does this muscle differ from the normal (Fig. 8.11)? Muscle sizes? Fiber shape? Connective tissue between fibers (panel *B*)? Do you see any fiber death (panel *C*)? Notice the occasional large-diameter reddish fibers. These large fibers are useful artifacts: when the muscle is removed, some of its fibers become hypercontracted. Knowing the function of dystrophin, suggest how this may happen? What is happening in panel *D* (the fibers are bluish on the slide)?

A8.4. The muscle has significant variation in fiber size, and includes some degenerating fibers that are being eaten by macrophages (clusters of cells around a dying fiber; see panel C). Rather than the usual polygonal fibers, the myofibers are rounded and embedded in a great deal of secondary connective tissue (see the gray fluff between the myofibers in panel B). The large diameter, hypercontracted fibers form when the muscle's filamentous proteins contract without being anchored to the cell surface (prominent myofibers in panel A).

Dystrophin tightly tethers the myosin-actin contractile network to the surface glycoproteins (e.g., sarcoglycans). Other surface proteins, in turn, link the sarcolemma to the extracellular matrix. These networks of proteins normally prevent hypercontraction of the myosin-actin filaments by anchoring them. Any failure of these network proteins leads to filament hypercontraction resulting in the large red cells you see in the slide.

Creatine kinase When skeletal or heart muscles are damaged they release their enzymes into the blood. Creatine kinase is mostly found in striated muscle, so it is a good, easily measured marker for muscle pathology.

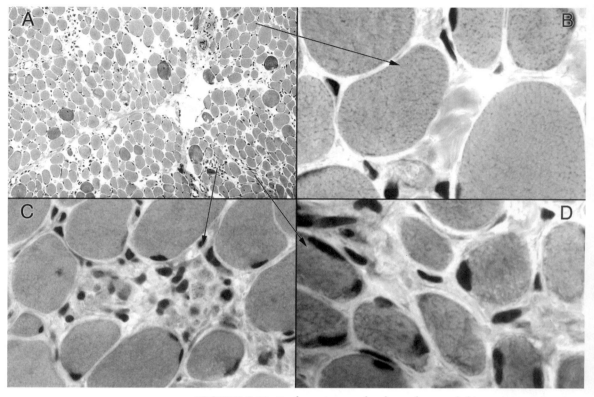

FIGURE 8.13. *Duchenne's muscular dystrophy, muscle biopsy.*

Panel D shows smaller, bluish (under the microscope) or basophilic fibers with enlarged nuclei. These are satellite fibers attempting to regenerate. The basophilia is due to increased amounts of mRNA and ribosomes in the sarcoplasm. Basophilic regenerative fibers are a common feature to many myopathies.

Elucidation of the Duchenne's gene was one of the first big success stories of modern molecular genetics. Its protein product, dystrophin, bridges the muscle's contractile proteins with the myofiber plasma membrane (sarcolemma).

Case 2: Polymyositis

A 37-year-old woman began having transient joint pain in the knees and shoulders five months before hospital admission. Three months later, weakness of the limbs developed. She became unable to climb stairs, arise from a chair, raise her arms for dressing, or to fix her hair. She had no muscle pain.

The abnormal findings on physical examination consisted of severe weakness of the muscles of the trunk and limbs, more severe at the shoulders and hips, than in the hands and feet. She showed no sensory deficits. Muscle-stretch reflexes were present. Laboratory studies showed a creatine kinase of 300 (normal less than 200).

Q8.5. Would you say her weakness more significantly involved her proximal or distal muscles? What information indicates that her disease involved her muscles but not her nerves?

A8.5. *Polymyositis patients present with proximal weakness, with or without a skin rash. As is typical of a myopathy, her weakness was of her larger, postural muscles. In addition her laboratory tests indicated the presence of muscle fiber damage. Her sensory examination was normal, and stretch reflexes were present, suggesting her nerves were uninvolved.*

Q8.6. Examine a microscopic slide of a biopsy from a patient with polymyositis (see Fig. 8.14). Do you see additional nonmuscle cells in the tissue? Where are they located (panel *B*)? Do all the muscle fibers look healthy (panel *C*)? Panel *D* is an immunoperoxidase stain prepared with antibodies against the T-lymphocyte antigen CD-8. What does this tell you?

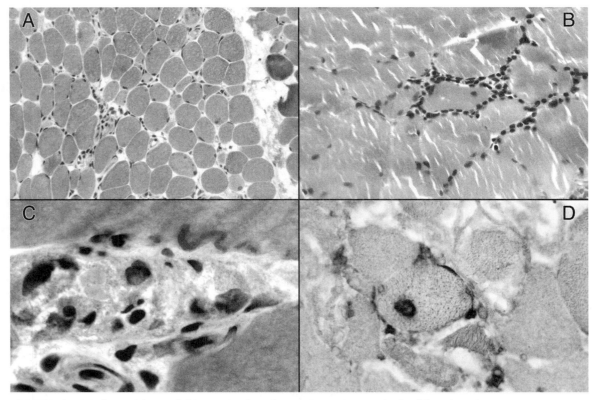

FIGURE 8.14. *Polymyositis muscle biopsy. Panels A through C are H&E stained, while D is an immunoperoxidase stain against the T-lymphocyte antigen CD-8.*

A8.6. *Polymyositis has lymphocytes predominantly, but not exclusively, within the muscle itself rather than mostly around vessels (panel B). Individual muscle fibers may show evidence of necrosis (pink-red), individual small round fibers, and sometimes regeneration (small and bluish). In sites of necrosis, the fibers are often undergoing phagocytosis (panel C). Although it may not look as though the muscle has much destruction, don't forget that even a small area of through and through necrosis of a muscle fiber will put the whole fiber out of commission, making it unable to contract.*

The CD-8 stain in panel D shows a T-lymphocyte that has invaded into a muscle fiber, which has not yet been destroyed. This pattern of lymphocyte activity suggests that the immune response is directed at muscle fibers themselves, rather than another component of the muscle.

Inflammatory diseases of muscle include polymyositis and dermatomyositis. Current understanding of these diseases is that in polymyositis the primary immune response is directed against the muscle, while in dermatomyositis, the response is mounted against small vessels, including capillaries.

INNERVATION OF MUSCLE

Localization of a Lesion

A 43-year-old female suffered a fall from a ladder resulting in a fractured femur. The bone was set in a cast. Following removal of the cast, she had wasting of the quadriceps muscle, weakness of knee extension, loss of the knee jerk reflex, and impaired sensation for vibration and pinprick, on the anterior portion of the thigh.

Q8.7. Using the nerve myotome table and sensory nerve diagram in Figure 8.7, locate the lesion.

A8.7. *The main motor deficits are due to weakness in the quadriceps. The lesion is in the femoral nerve. It arises from the lumbar plexus, passes under the inguinal ligament, then innervates the iliacus proximally, and more distally, the sartorius, and quadriceps muscles. The sensory loss localizes to the anterior cutaneous branches of the nerve. See Figure 8.15.*

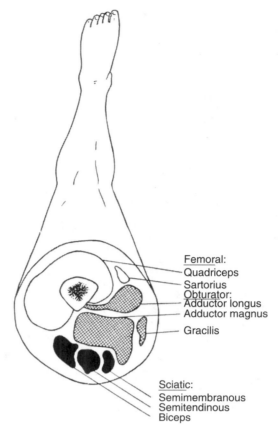

FIGURE 8.15. *Innervation of muscles of the thigh. (Adapted from Bing and Haymaker, Regional Diagnosis in lesions of the Brain and Spinal Cord, 11th ed, Mosby Co, St. Louis, 1940, figure 24, pg. 79)*

Nerve Histology

Q8.8. Examine Figure 8.16, which shows a drawing of a low power cross section through an entire human ulnar nerve. What are the large, round dark structures and what do they contain?

A8.8. *Fascicles containing bundles of axons.*

Q8.9. Identify the structures labeled 1 through 5. Refer back to Chapter 3 on histology if necessary.

8.9.1

8.9.2

8.9.3

8.9.4

8.9.5

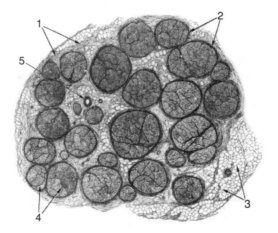

FIGURE 8.16. *Cross section of human ulnar nerve. (Adapted from Bloom and Fawcett, A Textbook of Histology, 10th ed, W.B. Saunders Co, Philadelphia, figure 12-24, p. 359.)*

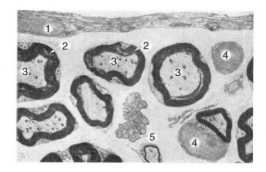

FIGURE 8.17. *Cross section of mouse sciatic nerve. Magnification 9,000X. (Adapted from Rhodin, An Atlas of Ultrastructure, © 1963, W.B. Saunders Co., Philadelphia, page 43.)*

A8.9.   8.9.1. *Epineurium*
        8.9.2. *Perineurium*
        8.9.3. *Adipose tissue*
        8.9.4. *Endoneurium*
        8.9.5. *Blood vessel*

Q8.10. Figure 8.17 shows a high-power electron micrograph of a cross section of mouse sciatic nerve. Identify the indicated structures.
        8.10.1
        8.10.2
        8.10.3
        8.10.4
        8.10.5

A8.10. 8.10.1. *Perineurium*
        8.10.2. *Myelin sheath*
        8.10.3. *Myelinated axon*
        8.10.4. *Schwann cell*
        8.10.5. *Unmyelinated axon*

Q8.11. Besides the presence of myelin, what other differences do you notice between the myelinated and unmyelinated axons?

A8.11. *The myelinated axons are much larger, being about 5 to 8 times greater in diameter than the unmyelinated axons. Also the more compact, unmyelinated axons tend to cluster in small bundles.*

Q8.12. Examine Figure 8.18, which shows an isolated, myelinated axon. What structures do the arrows indicate and what is their significance?

A8.12. *The arrows indicate the nodes of Ranvier. These are the points where the axon is not invested with its myelin sheath. The node of Ranvier is densely packed with the ion channels that provide the currents necessary for maintaining the action potential.*

Q8.13. Using a ruler, compare the length of a node and an internode. What is approximate ratio?

A8.13. *About 200 : 1. Myelin is such a good insulator that very little of the electrical charge propagating the action potential down the axon is expended. Consequently the nodal regions necessary for recharging are few and far between. Myelin reduces the metabolic load on the axon and it dramatically speeds the conduction velocity of the action potential.*

Figure 8.19 shows the compound action potential recorded by Gasser and Grundfest following stimulation of the entire saphenous nerve. These authors were able to relate the complex waveform to the sum of individual action potentials of different velocities, with the fastest action potentials having velocities of around 80 m/s contributing to the early, left-hand portion of the waveform.

Q8.14. Looking at Figure 8.17, which axon type is most likely to contribute to α peak, and which type to the δ peak?

A8.14. *The large, myelinated axons (now termed A fibers) are the fastest conducting and are the ones whose sum shapes the α peak. The δ peak is formed by the contributions from the unmyelinated,*

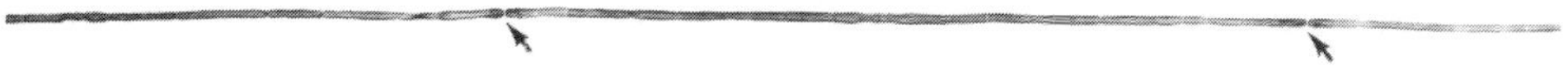

FIGURE 8.18. *Longitudinal view of a section of myelinated axon. (Modified from Schaumburg et al., Disorder of Peripheral Nerves, F. A. Davis Co., Philadelphia, 1983, Figure 4, pg 4.)*

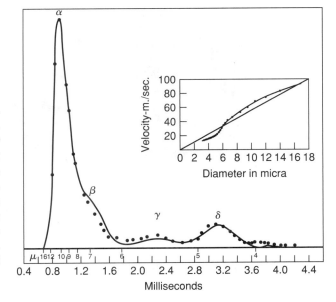

FIGURE 8.19. *Compound action potential recorded from saphenous nerve. Four peaks of the wave are indicated by the letters above. The Y axis represents voltage and the X axis represents time in ms. The inset displays the conduction velocity measured for individual nerve fibers as a function of fiber diameter. Just above the X axis in the main figure, is a scale relating fiber diameter to contribution to the complex wave form. (Adapted from figure 9, Gasser and Grundfest, 1939. Am J Physiol 127:393.)*

slowly conducting axons, now termed C fibers, with conduction velocities of less than 5 m/s. All of the a motor neurons controlling motor units are fast-conducting A type fibers. Recall from the sensory chapters that the A class fibers also carry information about touch, vibration, and position sense. The slowest conducting C fibers carry sensory information concerning pain and temperature.

The Motor Unit

As discussed in the introduction, the motor unit consists of the lower motor neuron and the muscle fibers that it innervates. Early in the last century, anatomists and physiologists conducted experiments to estimate the size of the motor units innervating different muscles. The approach that they took was quite simple, but very detailed and time-consuming. With great care they counted the number of muscle fibers in a given muscle and the number of motor axons innervating that muscle. Some of the results for human muscles are shown in Table 8.1.

Q8.15. Complete the fifth row of Table 8.1 to determine the innervation ratio for each of the muscles.

A8.15. *Dividing the number of muscle fibers by the number of axons yields the following innervation ratios:*
   8.15.1. Platysma: 25
   8.15.2. Biceps brachii: 750
   8.15.3. Gastrocnemius medius: 1720
   8.15.4. Brachioradialis: 390

TABLE 8.1. Nerve and Muscle Fiber Counts for Some Human Muscles

Muscle	Nerve Supply	Motor Axons	Muscle Fibers	Innervation Ratio
Platysma	Facial nerve, cervical branch	1096	27,100	
Biceps brachii	Musculocutaneous	774	580,000	
Gastrocnemius medius	Tibial	580	1,000,000	
Brachioradialis	Radial	330	130,000	

Source: Data from Buchthal and Schmalbruch, *Physiolog. Rev.,* 60 (1): 91–142, 1980; and Feinstein et al., *Acta Anat.* 23: 127–142, 1955.

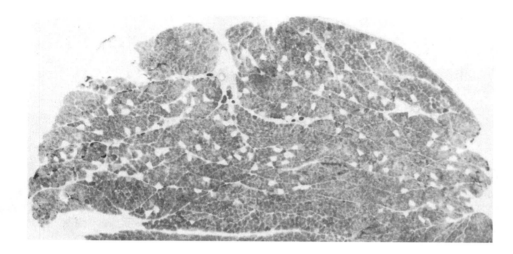

FIGURE 8.20. *Single motor neuron stimulation of cat soleus muscle, followed by glycogen staining. Fibers innervated by the single motor neuron were depleted of their glycogen by the repeated stimulation, and thus did not stain in this preparation. (Modified from figure 4, page 9, S. Chamberlain and D. Lewis. 1989. Contractile Characteristics and Innervation Ratio of Rat Soleus Motor Units. Journal of Physiology 412: 1–21.)*

Q8.16. The preceding method produces an average size of motor units for each muscle, but it doesn't provide insight into the variation in motor unit size within a given muscle. In order to determine the sizes of individual motor units and their topographic relationships to the muscle, they have to be examined one at a time. Look at Figure 8.20, which is a section of cat soleus muscle stained for glycogen. Prior to removal and fixation of the muscle tissue, a single motor neuron innervating the soleus was stimulated for a prolonged period of time, basically causing glycogen depletion of all the muscle fibers that it innervated. In this manner, the composition of that neuron's motor unit could be determined. Look at the distribution of fibers lacking glycogen. They appear as white trapezoids in the figure. Estimate the number of fibers in this motor unit. Discuss the distribution of the fibers within the entire muscle. What are some advantages of this partitioning?

A8.16. *In this case the motor unit has about 150 fibers. The size of the motor units varies widely within a given muscle and additionally the composition of motor units is different for different muscles. The smallest motor units found are from 7 to 10 fibers, and the largest contain several thousand fibers. While it may at first seem logical that all of the fibers of a given motor neuron would be grouped together, in life they are distributed over a wider range. This distributes the generated force over more of the muscle.*

Q8.17. What do you imagine are the differing roles for motor units of different size?

A8.17. *The smallest motor units exert the finest control and tend to be the first activated, while the larger motor units tend to be recruited later in a movement, and generate the greatest amount of force.*

Q8.18. Consider just an extraocular muscle and a back muscle. Which would have the large motor units, and which would have small units?

A8.18. *The extraocular eye muscles may have as few as 7 to 10 fibers in a unit, while the postural back muscles have much larger units, some with over a thousand fibers. This is consistent with the differing requirements of the muscle groups. The extraocular muscles are called upon to make exquisitely precise movements but are not required to generate a significant amount of force. The opposite is true of the back muscles.*

Q8.19. Examine Figure 8.21, which shows a muscle biopsy stained for ATPase from a patient who has amyotrophic lateral sclerosis (ALS). In this disease the motor neurons slowly degenerate. How is the pattern different from the normal staining? Still a checkerboard? Discuss the fiber size. How has the distribution changed?

A8.19. *The muscle differs from the normal checkerboard pattern of ATPase staining in two ways: (1) the muscle has groups of fibers all of the same type and (2) many fibers in the groups are diminutive.*
This is a classic example of neurogenic muscular atrophy. However, understanding how this pattern of staining evolves takes some time.

Q8.20. Consider what happens in ALS: as individual motor neurons in the spinal cord die, others not yet dead reinnervate the orphan muscle fibers. Using the information from the cat muscle above, what would the muscle look like a short time after you had destroyed the motor neuron (rather than stimulate it)? Consider only the early appearance. Now imagine that the remaining motor neurons have had time to reinnervate

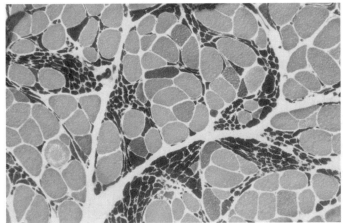

FIGURE 8.21. *Muscle biopsy of ALS patient, basic ATPase histochemistry. Dark-staining fibers are type II.*

the muscle fibers. What would it look like? How could you get the experimental muscle to match that of a patient with motor neuron disease?

A8.20. *Immediately after denervating a muscle, you would see no change; morphologic changes require protein loss and take time. After losing a motor neuron, the associated myofibers will atrophy. In the cat muscle, those fibers previously depleted of glycogen and distributed over the muscle would now be shrunken and atrophic. After reinnervation, those fibers would take on the characteristic of the motor neuron that had taken them over. On regular stains (e.g., H&E) the muscle would appear normal. Since such sprouting comes from a close axonal twig, several fibers of the same class may become grouped together. The muscle would begin to lose its checkerboard appearance and show grouping of the same types of fibers. This is nearly impossible to detect after loss of only one motor neuron but becomes quite obvious after many have died. The massive large group changes in ALS come from the continued loss of motor units, followed by reinnervation from the few remaining neurons. This loss, followed by reinnervation, followed by more loss, sequence eventually leaves only a few giant units remaining.*

SPINAL CORD

Q8.21. Review your histologic slides of cross sections of spinal cord. This is a good time to review the ascending and descending tracts again. Find these pathways on your slide or in Figure 8.22:
- Corticospinal tracts (descending)
- Dorsal columns, gracilis and cuneatus
- Spinothalamic tracts
- Location of lower motor neurons

A8.21. *See Figure 8.23.*

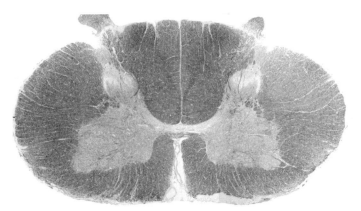

FIGURE 8.22. *Histologic section of normal cervical spinal cord.*

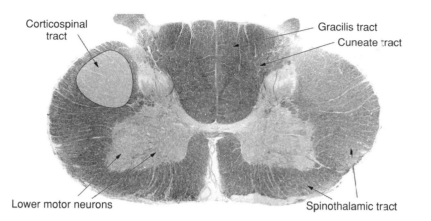

Corticospinal tract

Gracilis tract

Cuneate tract

Lower motor neurons

Spinothalamic tract

FIGURE 8.23. *Major structures of spinal cord.*

Q8.22. Review the location, size, and configuration of the ventral horn and the alpha motor neurons (see Fig. 8.24). Especially in the cervical region, where there are many nerve cells giving rise to motor fibers to the hands and arms, you will be able to see two main groups, medial and lateral. The medial group is present at most spinal levels, while the lateral is only in the lumbar and especially the cervical region. Suggest which categories of muscle are innervated by the medial versus the lateral groups.

A8.22. *The lateral group runs to the most distal muscles, including the small muscles of the hands. The medial group innervates the large proximal muscles. The medial group is more concerned with posture and general body tone. Those cells are more continuously discharging and are better connected to reflexes that have to do with body position, such as vestibulospinal input. The lateral group are more likely to have a direct corticospinal input and to be involved in conscious, volitional movement.*

Several distinct diseases primarily or significantly affect the ventral motor neurons. These include the viral infectious disease poliomyelitis, the degenerative disease amyotrophic lateral sclerosis, and the childhood genetic disease spinal muscular atrophy (SMA).

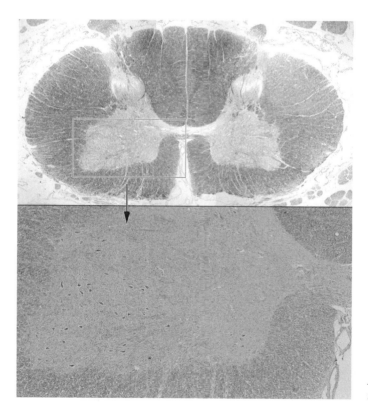

FIGURE 8.24. *Histology of the ventral horn.*

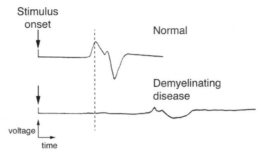

FIGURE 8.25. *Normal compared with pathological nerve conduction results.*

CLINICAL ELECTROPHYSIOLOGY

Q8.23. Examine the traces in Figure 8.25 showing nerve conduction recordings performed on a normal nerve and for a nerve undergoing demyelination. What differences are present? How can you explain them?

A8.23. *The compound action potential for the damaged nerve is slower, of smaller amplitude, and the waveform is less sharp. The slowing of the signal is caused by demyelination. The diminished amplitude is due to complete conduction failure in a number of fibers. The wave is more spread out because it's summing action potentials that are arriving over a wider range of time. This is due to fibers being in various stages of the demyelinating process.*

Q8.24. The trace shown in Figure 8.26 at right is from an EMG of a patient who had polio as a child. This trace resulted while the muscle was at rest. The amplitude of the wave is the same as for a single motor unit. Describe the trace and explain what caused it.

A8.24. *This is a fasciculation. It is caused by the spontaneous firing of a anterior horn cell, and is indicative of pathology in the lower motor neuron or its axon.*

Q8.25. Finally, examine Figure 8.27, which shows the spinal cord pathology of an older adult patient who had polio as a child. Compare panels *C* and *D*. What is the pathology in the ventral horn?

A8.25. *Panel C shows a near-complete loss of lower motor neurons. Many of the smaller cells are reactive astrocytes. Had this been an acute rather than chronic case of poliomyelitis, the spinal cord would have shown the features of any encephalitis, including infiltrates of lymphocytes, microglia, and macrophages.*

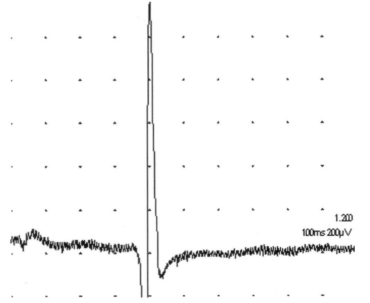

FIGURE 8.26. *EMG trace while muscle was at rest, from a polio case. The dots are spaced at 200 mV and 100 ms. (Contributed by Dr. Hannah Briemberg)*

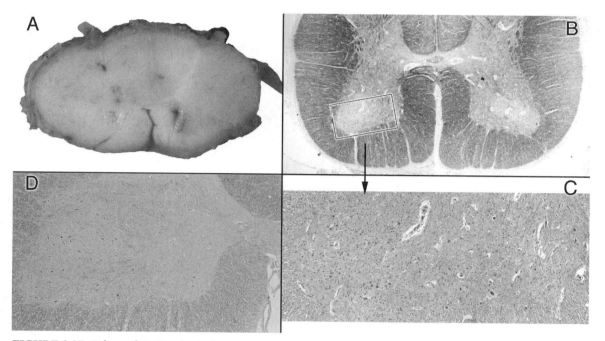

FIGURE 8.27. *Poliomyelitis. Panel* A *is the macroscopic spinal cord, while* B *and* C *are higher power views of the histology. Panel* D *is a normal cervical spinal cord.*

CLINICAL CASES

Case 1. Weakness in Hand without Sensory Deficits

A 62-year-old man notes painless weakness and atrophy of his right hand, developing over months. He has trouble snapping his fingers, turning a key in a car ignition, or pinching. Neurological exam is normal in all other respects. He had a series of blood tests showing no abnormalities. MRI study of his cervical spine showed no important abnormalities. He was referred for clinical electrophysiology.

Results

1. Nerve conduction velocity (NCV) for radial, median, and ulnar nerves is normal through forearm and hand.
2. Amplitude of the CMAP of the abductor pollicis brevis (a median nerve muscle) is less than 50% of normal.
3. Amplitude of the CMAP of the first dorsal interosseous (an ulnar muscle between the thumb and index finger) is 20% of normal.
4. EMG of intrinsic muscles of hand shows profuse fibrillations.
5. EMG of the proximal muscles of that arm, of the paraspinal muscle, and the left forearm shows both fasciculations and fibrillations.
6. EMG of the tongue also shows fasciculations and fibrillations.

Q8.26. What do the NCV results suggest?
A8.26. *Normal velocities indicate that this is not a demyelinating disease.*
Q8.27. What do the diminished CMAP's indicate?
A8.27. *There is problem in the peripheral motor pathway somewhere from the lower motor neuron to the muscle fiber.*
Q8.28. How do the presence of fibrillations and fasciculations narrow down localization of the lesion?
A8.28. *They point to an ongoing process of loss of innervation to the muscle. The diffuse nature of the deficits (including the upper extremity and tongue), combined with the finding of normal nerve conduction velocities, suggests anterior horn cell disease.*

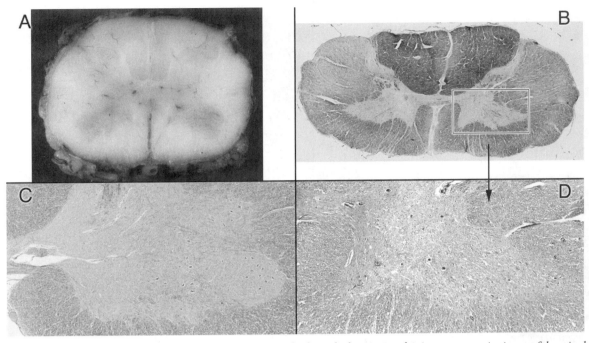

FIGURE 8.28. *Pathology of amyotrophic lateral sclerosis. Panel A is a macroscopic picture of the spinal cord, while B and D show the histology. Panel C is a normal spinal cord ventral horn.*

Q8.29. Now examine the pathology in Figure 8.28 from the spinal cord of a similar patient. What white matter tract is primarily affected? Where are the cell bodies for this tract? How do you explain this finding? Compare panels *C* (normal) and *D* (ALS). Describe what you see.

A8.29. *In ALS the descending pyramidal tract is often gliotic, which grossly looks sclerotic. Hence the name lateral sclerosis. The primary cell bodies for these axons arise in the primary motor cortex and the premotor cortex. In addition to the upper motor neurons, lower motor neurons are lost. In panel D few if any remain. Some of the dark dots are actually vessels, rather than neurons. Also the anterior horn is shrunken, again indicating loss of neurons and neuropil produced by this disease.*

Case 2: Acute Onset of Distal Numbness and Weakness

A 25-year-old fourth-year medical student was in San Francisco to interview for residency positions. He visited a street fair on Market Street and bought a stick of grilled meat from a street vendor. He noticed that through the strong spicy taste there was an odd aroma. Late that night he had profuse diarrhea and vomiting, which lasted for 12 hours. Four days later, back at home, he found that his feet felt numb. This was followed by a rapidly increasing weakness of arms, legs, and the right side of his face.

He arrived at the hospital emergency ward 18 hours after the first symptoms of numbness were perceived. Examination by the ward physician showed:

He was alert and frightened. Ocular movements and vision were preserved. The right side of his face was weak, especially for eye closure. He had very marked proximal weakness of all four limbs. For example, he could not lift either leg off the examining stretcher. Distal strength was 4/5. He had a vague, generalized muscle pain. Sensory function was normal other than loss of vibration sense up to the knees. All tendon reflexes were absent. Plantar response (Babinski sign) was not present. A lumbar puncture showed 5 lymphocytes/ml in the CSF. The total protein was 110 mg%.

He underwent electrophysiological testing:

1. Nerve conduction testing indicated a reduced velocity and reduced amplitude in several of the peripheral nerves.
2. When the ulnar CMAP was elicited by stimulation at the wrist, it was 8.5 mV (normal). When the ulnar CMAP was elicited by stimulation in the upper arm, it is 1.2 mV (very low) and the waveform was prolonged and polyphasic.

Q8.30. What do the combination of slowing and reduced amplitude indicate?

A8.30. *A demyelinating process in which a significant number of the fibers are sufficiently demyelinated to cause complete conduction block.*

Q8.31. Explain why the ulnar CMAP was normal when the nerve was stimulated at a site near the muscle but very reduced in amplitude and prolonged when the stimulation site was in the upper arm.

A8.31. *Between the two stimulation sites is a conduction block. Stimulation near the recording site yielded a full size potential, while proximal stimulation elicited a CMAP greatly reduced in amplitude. This indicates that along the forearm 75% of the ulnar fibers are blocked from conducting. This, along with the reduced conduction velocity in nerve, is the characteristic finding in demyelinating disease. The prolonged waveform is due to fibers with different conduction velocities because of varying states of demyelination.*

Q8.32. What is the diagnosis?

A8.32. *The clinical pattern is that of Guillain-Barré syndrome, an acute demyelinating inflammatory polyneuropathy. The differential diagnosis would include various kinds of neuromuscular block such as myasthenia and botulism, but the electrophysiology settles it. The spinal fluid was also abnormal and indicates a process within the spinal subarachnoid space (i.e., the nerve roots). The patient was treated aggressively with plasma exchange and made a good recovery. He was able to return to his classes three months later. The 10 day stay in the ICU was a period he would vividly recall forever.*

Chapter 9—BASAL GANGLIA

Were we living in a simple world, we might be able to get by with a sensory cell, a sensory neuron, a motor neuron, and a muscle. You have worked with the pyramidal motor system, connecting the motor cortex with its target neurons in the spinal cord. But as you have seen in the sensory laboratories, our nervous system displays a complex degree of information processing. In these next two laboratories you will be introduced to mechanisms that fine-tune the control of movement. Our motor activity and other behaviors are so elaborate, they require planning and refinement for their execution. In a simplistic view, the basal ganglia plan our behaviors while the cerebellum refines them. The thalamus acts as a sophisticated routing center for these activities. This laboratory will focus on the basal ganglia, while the subsequent lab will explore the cerebellum.

For future physicians, you will encounter patients with diseases of the basal ganglia. Parkinson's disease is a common degenerative disorder characterized by bradykinesia and tremor. As a contrast, Huntington's disease patients suffer from excessive movements, chorea, and athetosis. Understanding the basal ganglia helps in comprehending these manifestations; its study has and will continue to produce better therapeutic interventions.

LEARNING OBJECTIVES

- Identify the regional anatomy around the basal ganglia.
- Understand the three-dimensional structure of the basal ganglia, especially with reference to the ventricles.
- Define the components of the basal ganglia, including their inputs, projections, and principal transmitters.
- Describe the basic circuits connecting the cortex, basal ganglia, and thalamus, and their relationship to extrapyramidal disease.
- Discuss Huntington's disease, including its presentation, pathology, neuroanatomic basis, and genetics.

INTRODUCTION

Structures of the Basal Ganglia

The term *basal ganglia* refers to the gray matter structures deep in the cerebrum. Thalamus, having a different type of function, is excluded from the usual definition basal ganglia, although, as you will

Functional Neuroanatomy: An Interactive Text and Manual, by Jeffrey T. Joseph and David L. Cardozo
ISBN 0-471-44437-5 Copyright © 2004 John Wiley & Sons, Inc.

see, it is intimately connected with parts of these structures. You have seen the major components of the basal ganglia in previous laboratories: caudate nucleus, putamen, nucleus accumbens, and globus pallidus. In addition the two parts of the substantia nigra (reticular part and compact part), as well as the slightly more obscure ventral tegmental area and subthalamic nucleus, all belong to the basal ganglia system.

One of the more difficult concepts for the novice to understand about the basal ganglia is its three-dimensional architecture. During early development the basal ganglia structures lie in the ventral portion of the neural tube, with the caudate nucleus directly abutting the ventricular wall. In our eternal competition with other organisms, our brain has tremendously increased in complexity, outpacing its enclosure. In this process the cerebrum has folded back on itself to form a "C." As you have seen in prior laboratories, the ventricular system follows this C-shape. The caudate nucleus, being along the ventricular wall, also follows this shape. It lies ventrolateral to the ventricular system in the middle of the brain, but as the temporal lobes curved underneath, the body and tail of the caudate nucleus have taken up topologically equivalent positions in front of and then dorsal to the lateral ventricle. The hippocampus, to be encountered in detail in later laboratories, has suffered an analogous fate.

The other difficulty in initially facing the basal ganglia is the confusing, overlapping terms used to describe these nuclei. Because the putamen and globus pallidus together reminded early investigators of lentils, they lumped these together as the "lentiform nucleus"; it remains a convenient descriptive term, but lumps and splits neuroanatomically different nuclei. The *striatum,* by definition, refers to the gray matter with obvious striations or thick white matter bundles coursing through them. Technically, the *neostriatum* refers to the caudate nucleus and putamen, while the *paleostriatum* would indicate the globus pallidus. However, in working practice, most people refer to the former just as the "striatum" and the latter as the "pallidum." Once in your lives, you may hear the term "Luys' nucleus," usually in the context of the very rare triple repeat disease dentatorubropallidoluysian atrophy (DRPLA); you can impress your associates by indicating that this refers to the subthalamic nucleus.

Basal Ganglia Connections

While a panoply of wiring diagrams exist to explain select aspects of the basal ganglia, several general principles apply. Different areas of cerebral cortex map excitatory input onto specific regions of the striatum. These regions then project inhibitory impulses onto specific regions of the pallidum. From here, two major pathways arise, a direct and an indirect. The direct pathway maps inhibitory signals directly onto thalamus, while the indirect pathway has an inhibitory and then an excitatory interlude before giving off its final inhibition to thalamus. Dopamine selectively modulates both the direct and indirect circuits. The circuits end by projecting excitatory information back to cortex.

Major functional regions of the cortex (e.g., motor, association, visual processing, limbic) map onto specific regions of the basal ganglia and form their own circuits. The motor cortex projects to the lateral putamen, while the frontal association cortices send axons to the head of the caudate nucleus. The caudate and putamen then connect either to the internal segment of the globus pallidus via the direct pathway or to the external segment, and onto the subthalamic nucleus via the indirect paths. Limbic areas follow slightly different pathways through the nucleus accumbens and then onto the ventral striatum (that part of the globus pallidus lying underneath the anterior commissure).

However, reducing the basal ganglia to wiring diagrams grossly simplifies their actions. As an example, the caudate nucleus contains a population of interneurons (aspiny neurons) that modulate the information. The substantia nigra produces dopamine and projects to striatum but acts in an opposite manner on the direct and indirect pathways: dopamine augments the direct pathway via D1 receptors and inhibits the indirect pathway using D2 receptors.

Concept of the Extrapyramidal System

In you sojourn in clinical medicine, you will hear the expression "extrapyramidal disease." The term is used loosely to mean any disease of the motor system that does not directly relate to the pyramidal tract or upper-to-lower motor neuron connections. If you have an infarction of your pyramidal tract, you will initially have weakness. In contrast, diseases of the "extrapyramidal" system lead to rigidity or uncontrolled movements. Since the "extrapyramidal" system really means anything not pyramidal, it encompasses several distinct and sometimes disparate diseases. It is a clinical term, rooted in the past, when our understanding of brain function was less sophisticated. You will hear it, you will probably even use it. Just know that a patient with "extrapyramidal dysfunction" could have a disease in one of several different systems. It is not simply "extrapyramidal."

Experimental Anatomic Techniques

The information in these laboratories has taken well over a century to accumulate. By the time the knowledge has been distilled down to a tonic presentable to students, it often has lost all of its fire. To rectify this problem, as least to a small degree, some laboratory exercises will introduce a few of the techniques used to study neuroanatomic connections.

Probably the most easily conceived method of studying connections between neurons is to inject the cell body at one site and look for the tracer in another. Different types of tracers may either be transported *anterograde* or *retrograde* from the site of injection to the target or the source of the projection. *Lectins* are a frequently used anterograde tracer, while *horse radish peroxidase* is retrogradely transported.

Knowing who is connected to whom is just the first step in analyzing the pathways. You generally also want to know if the connections are excitatory, inhibitory, or modulatory. Knowing which transmitter is used by a given neuron assists in teasing these apart. Certain transmitters, notably the catecholamines, may be directly stained, using their chemical properties. Antibodies that bind to serotonin may also directly identify this transmitter when applied to a tissue section. Enzymes that synthesize transmitters are also useful. You will see an example of immunostaining for *tyrosine hydroxylase,* an enzyme in the pathway to catecholamine synthesis.

Further refinement in understanding the neuroanatomic connections involves dissecting out the types of receptors used by a given transmitter. Antibodies raised against specific receptors may be used to stain for the protein itself, thus telling you where the protein is present. To determine in which neurons the receptor is synthesized, you can localize its mRNA using in situ hybridization. To the person initially trying to understand neuroanatomy, the entire field of receptor subtypes can seem like an activity suited to monks or insect taxonomists. But such study has born fruit. For example, the specific subtypes of the dopamine receptor are now thought to each play their own roles in movement disorders, thought disorders, and attentional deficits. Much of this refinement and the techniques used to tease the data apart is beyond the scope of this text; its introduction here is to give you a flavor for how we have come to know what we think we know.

Schedule (2.5 hours)
50   Coronal dissection
20   Model structures of basal ganglia around ventricles
20   Basal ganglia components
30   Basal ganglia circuits
30   Case: Huntington's disease

CORONAL DISSECTION

In the second laboratory, when you didn't know anything, you made several cuts through the basal ganglia. Today you will refine those cuts, so you can see more detail in these slices.

INST   Your first task will be to orient the slices you have already cut. Put them in order, from anterior to posterior, making certain you know medial from lateral in each piece. Select the pieces extending from where you first find caudate nucleus anteriorly to the splenium of the corpus callosum posteriorly. Lay these thick slabs flat on the cutting board and slice them to between 0.5 and 1 centimeter. This is a tricky business; you don't want to see fingers with brain. Give yourself plenty of room. Carefully cut through the slice, parallel to the board. Keeping you knife wet will help a lot.

Q9.1.   Now lay the slices all out in order on your brain tray (or table if you need space). See Figure 9.1 for photographs of coronal slices. You should first make sure you can identify these structures in each slice where they occur (as well as in Fig. 9.1):
- Caudate nucleus (CN)
- Putamen (Put)
- Nucleus accumbens (Acc)
- Globus pallidus (both segments, GPi and GPe)
- Thalamus (Th)
- Subthalamic nucleus (STN)
- Top end of substantia nigra (SN)
- Internal capsule (ic)

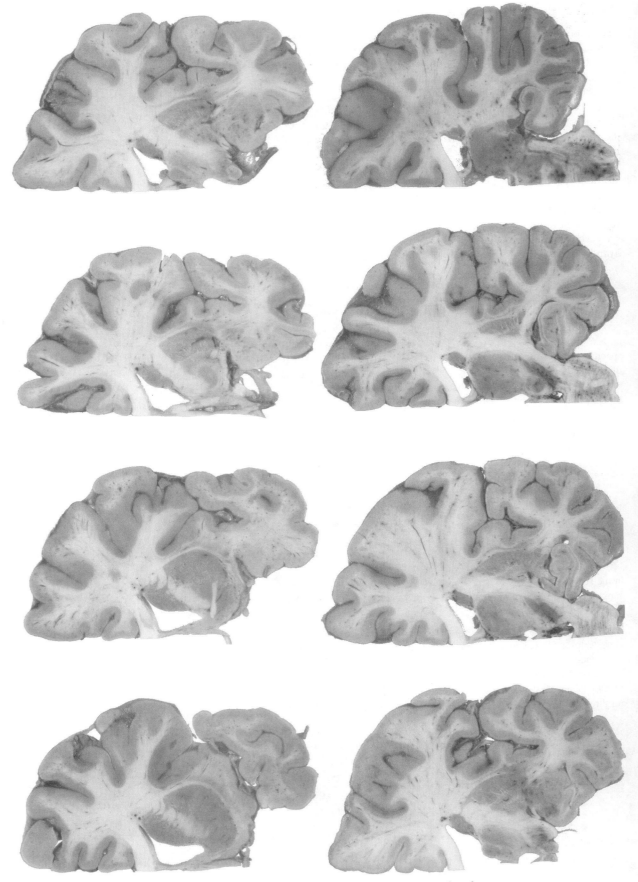

FIGURE 9.1. *Coronal dissection of cerebrum.*

Also identify these regional structures and white matter tracts:

- Corpus callosum (cc)
- Cingulate gyrus (Cing)
- Insular cortex (Ins)
- External capsule (ec)
- Optic chiasm and tract (oc and ot)
- Fornix (fx)
- Anterior commissure (ac)
- Amygdala (Amyg)
- Lateral geniculate nucleus (LGN)
- Medial geniculate nucleus (MGN)
- Hippocampal formation (Hip)
- Centrum semiovale (centrum)

A9.1. See Figure 9.2.

Q9.2. Now go back to your carefully laid out slices and trace the entire caudate nucleus. Along which parts of its course does it lie next to the ventricle? How does its size change from anterior to posterior? Where does the head end and the body begin? How far back can you trace its course? What major structure is located near its tail end? What white matter tract passes by its head and body?

A9.2. The caudate nucleus always lies next to the ventricle, which provides a sure landmark for lost souls. Its greatest mass is at its most anterior portion, the head. Unlike mammals, the head, body, and tail merge imperceptibly into each other, all the while continually decreasing in diameter. The internal capsule separates the caudate from the putamen. The tail ends in the roof of the temporal horn of the lateral ventricle, across the CSF from the hippocampus. It is lateral to the lateral geniculate nucleus in this region. The corpus callosum lies dorsal to the caudate, while the internal capsule is ventrolateral.

Q9.3. How does the putamen differ in gross structure from the caudate nucleus? Where does it contact the ventricular system? Where does it merge with the caudate nucleus? Notice the white matter bundles coursing through the putamen (striatum). To where do they go? What white matter tract lies lateral to the putamen? What structures are lateral to the white matter tract?

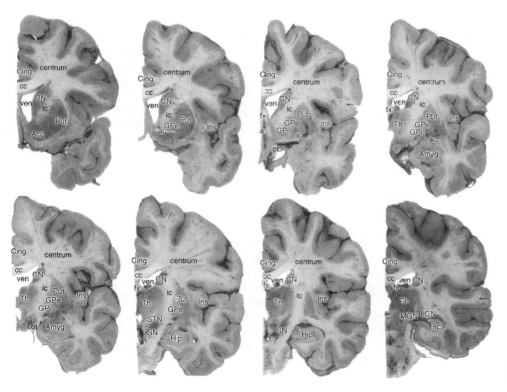

FIGURE 9.2. *Salient structures on coronal dissection.*

A9.3. *The putamen never contacts the ventricular system. The internal capsule separates the putamen from the caudate nucleus. However, these two structures appear to merge in their most medial and ventral parts. This confluence is the accumbens nucleus. The specific boundaries separating these striatal structures are somewhat arbitrary. The white matter bundles coursing through the putamen give it its name "striatum" and are the pencillary fibers of Wilson (of Wilson's disease fame) that project to the globus pallidus. Lateral to the putamen, in order, are the external capsule, claustrum, extreme capsule, and insular cortex. You will encounter some of these sites again in later laboratories.*

Q9.4. Identify the globus pallidus in the different coronal slices. Distinguish between the external and internal segments. Do both segments extend forward and backward to the same degree? What great white matter bundle lies along the side? What gray matter structures lie medial to the globus pallidus? Identify the white matter bundle crossing underneath the globus pallidus. What other white matter bundle lies on the surface of the brain inferior to the globus pallidus?

A9.4. *The external and internal segments are separated by a thin lamina. The external segment three-dimensionally wraps around the internal segment, so when only one segment is present, it is the external. The internal capsule rides down (and up) along the medial side of the globus pallidus. Medial to the globus pallidus is the thalamus, but also the subthalamic nucleus, seemingly buried in the internal capsule. Directly beneath the globus pallidus is the* **anterior commissure,** *which connects the anterior temporal poles and olfactory tracts. Traveling on the surface of the brain beneath this region is the optic tract coursing back to the lateral geniculate nucleus.*

Q9.5. The *subthalamic nucleus* is sometimes difficult to find, depending on your cut. Find it anyway; it is shown on one of the photographs. Make any extra cuts you may need to see it. How would you describe the shape of this nucleus? What round gray matter structure lies beneath and to the back of the subthalamic nucleus? What other pigmented structure lies lateral and caudal to it? What gray matter nucleus lies dorsal and medial to the subthalamic nucleus?

A9.5. *The subthalamic nucleus is shaped like a lens, and so no matter how you cut it, it still more or less looks like a lens. It lies in a small region containing important structures controlling motion. These include the red nucleus and substantia nigra below (remember, the midbrain lies directly beneath the diencephalon), the thalamus dorsomedially, and the "lentiform" nucleus (globus pallidus and putamen) laterally.*

Q9.6. The motor thalamus lies in the anterior and lateral part of the thalamus. Use your atlas to try to find the *ventral anterior* and *ventral lateral* thalamic nuclei. Which thalamic nucleus lies medial to these? Which lies superior and medial, separated from the other parts by white matter? You may be sick of it by now, but what great white matter structure separates the lentiform nuclei from motor thalamus?

A9.6. *In this course we will not delve too deeply into the multitude of different thalamic nuclei. However, it is useful for you to appreciate the major divisions of this cortical gatekeeper. Medial to the motor thalamus lives the* **medial dorsal nucleus,** *which has cognitive association functions. The* **anterior nucleus,** *part of the limbic thalamus, sits on the top of the other nuclei and is surrounded by white matter. And of course, the internal capsule lies just lateral to the thalamus and separates it from the lentiform nuclei.*

Q9.7. You should dig out your brainstem dissection from the second laboratory to find the substantia nigra. Find the several slices of midbrain containing this pigmented structure. Notice where you see pigment. How is the pigment distributed, in an oval, a line? What is the major white matter bundle lying ventrolateral to the substantia nigra? As you move rostrally, what structure appears between the pigmented area and this white matter bundle? What round gray matter structure lives dorsomedial to the nigra?

A9.7. *The substantia nigra, as you have read, has two distinct divisions: the pigmented part (or pars compacta) and the non-pigmented reticulated part (pars reticulata). The pigmented neurons lie in two somewhat broken lines, and the pars reticulata is between the pars compacta and the cerebral peduncle. The pigmented part has its greatest extent caudally, and becomes smaller rostrally, while the opposite is true for the reticulated part. The reticulated part is neuroanatomically equivalent to the internal segment of the globus pallidus. Medial to the nigra is the decussation of the superior cerebellar peduncles and above that the red nucleus. The most rostral end of the substantia nigra may also be visible on the coronal slices containing the subthalamic nucleus.*

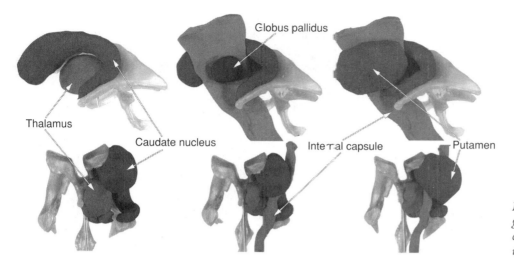

FIGURE 9.3. *Clay model of basal ganglia, molded onto a ventricular cast. The upper images are lateral, while the lower are from the anterior.*

MODEL STRUCTURES OF BASAL GANGLIA AROUND VENTRICLES

To gain a better working knowledge of basal ganglia anatomy, you will reconstruct its principal structures onto the ventricles. Use your atlas and the coronal sections from the first part of the laboratory to build the caudate nucleus, putamen, internal capsule, and thalamus onto the models of the ventricular system. You will need several colors of clay.

INST Refer to Figure 9.3 as a model. Build these deep nuclei from medial to lateral. First fit the thalamus onto the model, using blue clay. Remember it lies next to the surface of the third ventricle. Along the medial surface of the lateral ventricle is the caudate nucleus. Add this using green clay. Separating the thalamus and caudate nucleus from the putamen and globus pallidus is the internal capsule. Add the internal capsule using yellow clay. Remember it runs from beneath these nuclei on up to cortex, so let a little extra stick out of both ends. Try to figure out where the globus pallidus fits, and add this in red. Use the green clay again to add the putamen. (Why the same color as caudate? What is the region called where they merge?) You can double check your masterpiece by removing it from the ventricular model and performing a coronal dissection; how close were you to the actual brain?

BASAL GANGLIA COMPONENTS

Q9.8. To further reinforce the basic anatomy of the basal ganglia, examine the giant section from the Yakovlev collection in Figure 9.4. These thinly sliced brain sections were

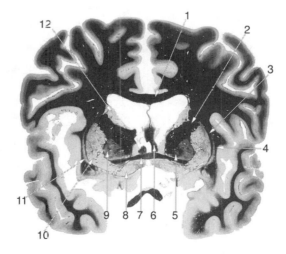

FIGURE 9.4. *Coronal section at the level of the globus pallidus internus.*

stained for myelin, so the dark areas represent myelinated white matter, and the light areas are gray matter (i.e., white is black and gray is white). Label the indicated structures:

9.8.1 _____

9.8.2 _____

9.8.3 _____

9.8.4 _____

9.8.5 _____

9.8.6 _____

9.8.7 _____

9.8.8 _____

9.8.9 _____

9.8.10 _____

9.8.11 _____

9.8.12 _____

A9.8. *See Figure 9.5.*

Q9.9. Now examine the histologic section of the basal ganglia. Make sure you can identify the following in the slides and in Figure 9.6:
- Caudate nucleus (CN)
- Putamen (Put)
- Nucleus accumbens (Acc). Connects the caudate and putamen ventromedially.
- Globus pallidus (GP). Has external and internal segments.
- Internal capsule (ic).
- Lateral ventricle.

A9.9. *See Figure 9.7. For your edification some other nearby structures have been added.*

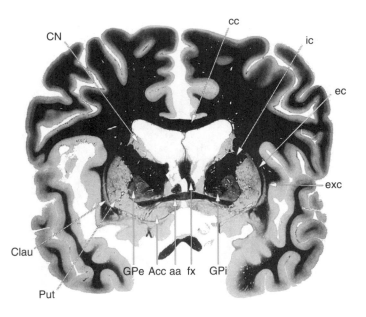

FIGURE 9.5. *Salient parts of the basal ganglia and regional structures. Coronal section at the level of the globus pallidus internus.*

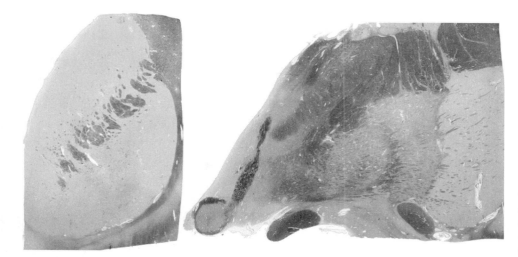

FIGURE 9.6. *Basal ganglia low-power histology. The left section shows the confluence of the caudate, accumbens, and putamen nuclei, while the right shows the lentiform nuclei.*

Q9.10. Using your histologic slide or Figure 9.8, describe the histology of the caudate nucleus and putamen. What does the gray matter look like? How many different types of neurons can you distinguish in the caudate nucleus and putamen? Notice the bits of branching gray matter spanning the internal capsule. What are these?

A9.10. *Both the caudate nucleus and putamen have small, tight white matter bundles originating in them and projecting to the globus pallidus. These* **pencillary fibers of Wilson** *are more sparse toward the edges of the striatum and increase in size as they approach the globus pallidus. Little myelin is present between the bundles.*

Within the caudate and putamen are two distinguishable neuron types using this stain: smaller, much more numerous neurons and a few (1 in 200–400) larger neurons (see arrowhead in the lower left panel in Fig. 9.8). The larger neurons may be difficult to find; look for them on your slide. You cannot distinguish the patchwork of striasomes on these stains. The bits of gray matter spanning the internal capsule are reminders that the caudate and putamen are really one structure, split in two later in evolution by the internal capsule fibers subserving the burgeoning frontal lobes. These are most developed in humans. In rodents the two nuclei are much closer together.

Q9.11. How do the caudate and putamen compare with the globus pallidus? White matter? Neurons? See Figure 9.9.

A9.11. *Except for the small bundles of white matter in the caudate/putamen, the striatal neuropil contains few myelinated axons. In contrast, the globus pallidus contains many myelinated fibers, fewer neurons, and less fine neuropil (the pink-staining mesh of axons and dendrites). Because of the increased amount of myelin, the globus is paler on gross examination, hence its name "pale body."*

Spiny versus aspiny neurons.
Golgi stains distinguish these two classes of striatal neurons. Long axons projecting beyond the striatum arise from medium size spiny neurons. These have numerous dendritic spines and use GABA and either substance P on enkephalin as transmitters. A subpopulation of large, aspiny neurons lack spines and produce acetylcholine for local connections.

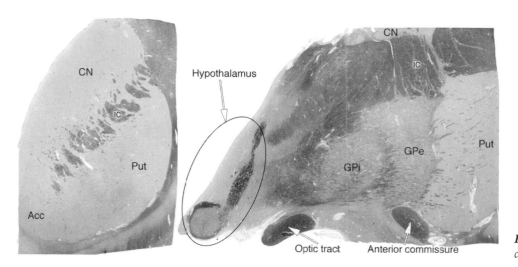

FIGURE 9.7. *Salient histologic structures.*

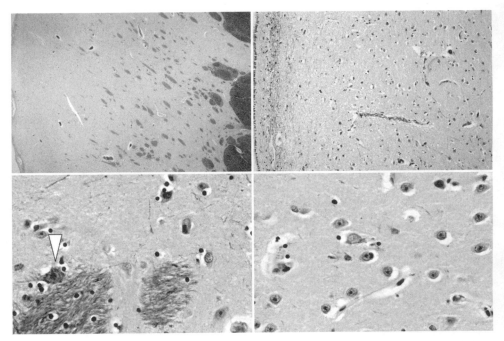

FIGURE 9.8. *Histology of the caudate nucleus. The two upper figures are at low and midrange power, while the lower figures are at high power.*

BASAL GANGLIA CONNECTIONS

Dopamine System

INST Orient yourself by revisiting the transverse slices from your prior dissection of the midbrain. Identify: substantia nigra, red nucleus, superior cerebellar peduncle, cerebral peduncles, and inferior and superior colliculi.

Q9.12. Examine the microscopic section of the midbrain, focusing specifically on the pigmented neurons (see Fig. 9.10). Where are these neurons? Some fall outside the substantia nigra; where? Distinguish between the pars compacta, where the pigmented neurons live, and the pars reticulata, which is similar to the internal segment of the globus pallidus and contains GABAergic neurons.

A9.12. *Neurons in the substantia nigra lie just dorsal and slightly medial to the peduncles. They generally lie in two tiers, although sometimes these are not clearly distinguished. However, some pigmented neurons spread medially away from the substantia nigra proper into the medial portion of the midbrain. This site is termed the* **ventral tegmental area** *(VTA).*

Q9.13. Next inspect the photograph of the human striatum stained with an antibody to tyrosine hydroxylase. Although TH highlights both dopamine and norepinepherine projections, in this region the majority of TH staining is from dopaminergic fibers.

Ventral Tegmental Area *The medial tier of the substantia nigra pars compacta has pigmented neurons flowing into the ventromedial aspects of the midbrain. These dopaminergic neurons belong to the ventral tegmental area. They mainly project to the cortex of the frontal lobe and are considered important in the dopaminergic dysfunction associated with schizophrenia.*

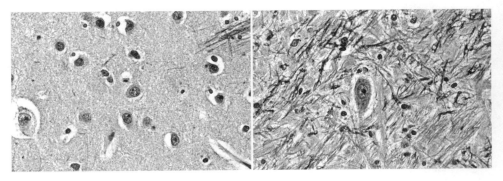

FIGURE 9.9. *Caudate/putamen* (left) *and globus pallidus* (right), *LFB/H&E stain.*

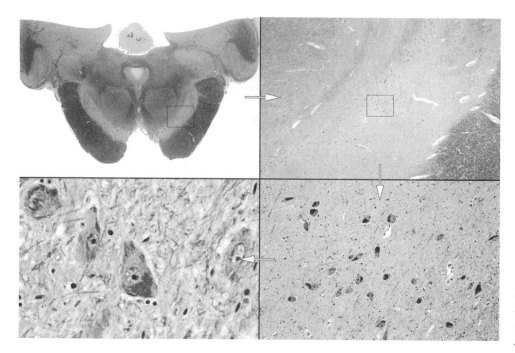

FIGURE 9.10. *Histology of the substantia nigra. H&E/LFB stain. The lower panels are close-up views of the pars compacta.*

Label the specific structures. Where is the staining most intense? What portion of the basal ganglia has the least staining?

9.13.1 _____

9.13.2 _____

9.13.3 _____

9.13.4 _____

9.13.5 _____

A9.13. 9.13.1. *Caudate nucleus*
9.13.2. *Putamen*
9.13.3. *Globus pallidus*
9.13.4. *Accumbens*
9.13.5. *Internal capsule*

The majority of the dopamine projection from the substantia nigra is to the striatum. In Figure 9.11 the greatest staining is in the caudate nucleus, followed by the accumbens and then the putamen. The globus pallidus has no significant staining; it receives no input from the ascending nigral dopaminergic system.

Cocaine blocks the re-uptake system of several agents, including dopamine, norepinepherine, and serotonin. While cocaine interacts with the three amine systems, major antidepressants like desipramine only block re-uptake of the latter two. Another antidepressant, bupropion, only blocks dopamine.

Q9.14. Examine Figure 9.12, which illustrates cocaine binding to the brain. Name the principal sites of binding. Compare the image of cocaine binding with that of dopamine. Postulate why cocaine may have addictive effects, while desipramine does not.

A9.14. *As in the tyrosine hydroxylase immunostaining, the sites of binding include the caudate nucleus, putamen, and accumbens nucleus (in addition to the olfactory tubercle). The image is nearly identical with the tyrosine hydroxylase-stained figure.*

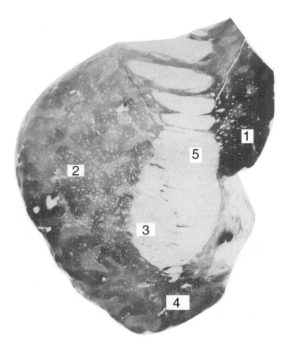

FIGURE 9.11. Striatum immunostained with antibody to tyrosine hydroxylase (TH) (Adapted from J. Pearson, G. Halliday, N. Sakamoto, and J.-P. Michel, Catecholaminergic Neurons, in The Human Nervous System, ed. G. Paxinos, © 1990, Academic Press, San Diego, figure 31.10, page 1038).

Cocaine's addictive effects are currently thought to correlate with its ability to block the re-uptake of dopamine, especially in the limbic portion of the striatum, the accumbens nucleus. Data in animals suggest that amphetamine operates in a similar manner. The addictive actions of nicotine are thought to be mediated by presynaptic cholinergic enhancement of dopamine transmission.

Connections with Cortex

Q9.15. The different divisions of the striatum have relationships with distinct areas of cortex. Complete the table below.

Striatal Structure	Associated Cortex	Associated Function
Caudate nucleus		
Putamen		
Accumbens		

A9.15. *Corticostriatal associations:*

Striatal Structure	Associated Cortex	Associated Function
Caudate Nucleus	Frontal Cortex	Organization of behavior and personality
Putamen	Cortical motor areas	Motor
Accumbens	Cingulate gyrus	Affect and motivation

Each division of the basal ganglia contributes to a separate cortical–striatal–pallidal–thalamic circuit. A portion of caudate associates with the ventral anterior and medial dorsal thalamus, which in turn projects to the lateral orbitofrontal cortex. The accumbens nucleus has more limbic functions, receiving projections from the anterior cingulate gyrus and projects to the ventral pallidum. The putamen is considered the motor striatum. It receives fibers from the supplementary motor cortex and projects to the globus pallidus and onto the ventral lateral thalamus. Posterior parts of caudate form similar circuits with occipital cortex.

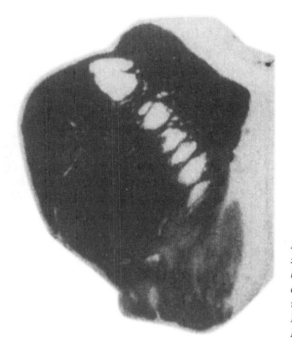

FIGURE 9.12. *Cocaine binding to striatum. This image was prepared by binding a tritiated analog of cocaine, [3H]CFT, to whole slices of monkey brain (Adapted from figure 3, Kaufman, M. J., Spealman, R. D. and Madras, B. K., 1991. Synapse 9: 183.)*

Basal Ganglia Intrinsic Connections

As you will recall from the introduction, the basal ganglia connectivity has been determined largely by retrograde and anterograde studies. Two examples are shown in Figure 9.13 and Figure 9.14. In Figure 9.13, horse radish peroxidase (a protein) was injected into the caudate nucleus and retrogradely labeled neurons in the cerebral cortex, thereby demonstrating the corticostriate projections (results tabulated in Table 9.1). Similarly, in Figure 9.14, an anterograde tracer injected into globus pallidus labeled axons terminating in the subthalamic nucleus, thus establishing the pallidal-subthalamic connections (results also indicated in Table 9.1). These structures are outlined in Figure 9.14 so make sure you can identify them.

Q9.16. To further refine our understanding of these connections, the projection studies above can be combined with histological studies to determine the transmitters used by the neurons involved. For instance, tracing studies demonstrate that the striatal neurons project strongly to the globus pallidus. The projection neurons are inhibitory. All use GABA as their primary transmitter but differ in their peptide cotransmitter. These subtypes may be distinguished using substance P (direct pathway) and met-enkephalin (indirect pathway) staining. Examine Figure 9.15 of the basal ganglia, stained on the left for substance P and on the right for met-enkephalin. Identify the anatomic structures labeled with substance P and those with met-enkephalin.

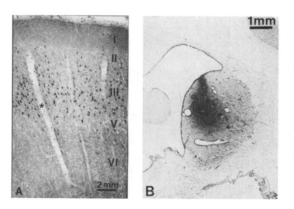

FIGURE 9.13. *Retrograde labeling of corticostriatal project. Horseradish peroxidase (a protein) was injected into the caudate nucleus (shown in the left image) and retrogradely labeled neurons in the cerebral cortex (right). (Modified from figures 1 & 4, Royce, G. J., Laminar origin of cortical neurons which project upon the caudate nucleus: a horseradish peroxidase investigation in the cat. 1982. J. Comp. Neurol. 205: 8–29.)*

FIGURE 9.14. *Anterograde labeling of pallidoluysian projection. An anterograde tracer that was injected into globus pallidus (left figure) labeled axons terminating in the subthalamic nucleus (right figure). (Adapted from Carpenter, M. B., et. al. Interconnections and organization of pallidal and subthalamic nucleus in the monkey. 1981. J Comp Neurol 197; 579–603.)*

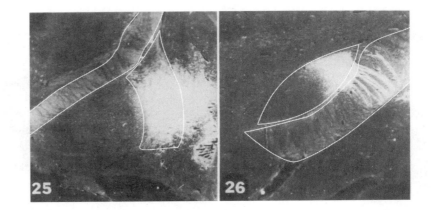

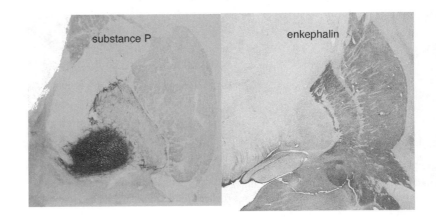

FIGURE 9.15. *Basal ganglia stained for substance P (left) and enkephalin (right). (Raw data generously donated by Dr. Clifford Saper)*

TABLE 9.1. Tracer Study Results

Structure	Transmitter Synthesized	Anterograde Tracing Results	Retrograde Tracing Results
Cerebral cortex	Glutamate	Caudate + putamen	Motor thalamus (VA/VL)
Caudate + putamen	GABA + met-enkephalin	External segment globus pallidus	Cerebral cortex, substantia nigra compacta
Caudate + putamen	GABA + substance P	Internal segment globus pallidus	Cerebral cortex, substantia nigra compacta
External segment globus pallidus	GABA	Subthalamic nucleus	Caudate + putamen
Internal segment globus pallidus/ reticular part of substantia nigra	GABA	Motor thalamus (VA/VL)	Caudate + putamen and subthalamic nucleus
Subthalamic nucleus	Glutamate	Internal segment globus pallidus / reticular part of substantia nigra	External segment globus pallidus
Substantia nigra (pigmented compact part)	Dopamine	Caudate + putamen	Many
Motor thalamus (VA/VL)	Glutamate	Cortex	Internal segment globus pallidus, reticular part of substantia nigra

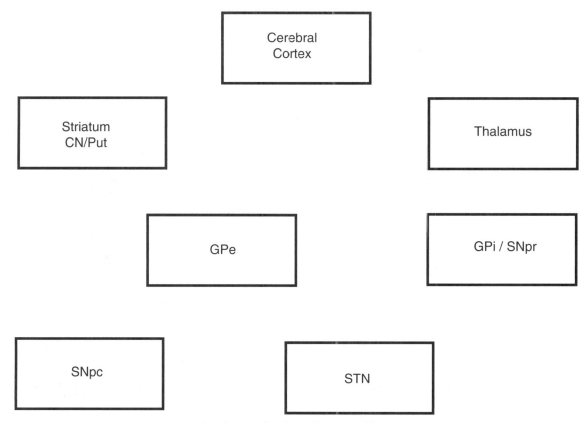

FIGURE 9.16. *Template for basic basal ganglia wiring diagram.*

A9.16. *Substance P highlights the internal segment of the globus pallidus (along with the reticular part of the substantia nigra, not seen in this section). Met-enkephalin stains the external segment of the globus pallidus (and also shows staining of the putamen.) In other preparations they both would stain the ventral pallidum, demonstrating that this "limbic" portion of the pallidum lacks the anatomic distinction between the direct and indirect pathways that is present in the motor and association regions. These results are also summarized in Table 9.1.*

Q9.17. Use the results in Table 9.1 from axonal tracing studies to create your own wiring diagram for the basal ganglia motor system in the box diagram in Figure 9.16. Indicate the transmitter used and whether the signal is excitatory or inhibitory.

A9.17. *See Figure 9.17.*

Q9.18. Similarly to how you filled in the box diagram above, on the anatomic diagram in Figure 9.18, draw arrows to indicate the direction of signal transmission and indicate whether the synapses are excitatory or inhibitory. Relevant nuclei have been enhanced on the right side of the figure.

A9.18. *See Figure 9.19. You now know why these diagrams are usually presented as boxes.*

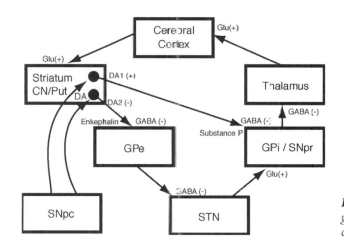

FIGURE 9.17. *Simple wiring diagram of basal ganglia interconnections.*

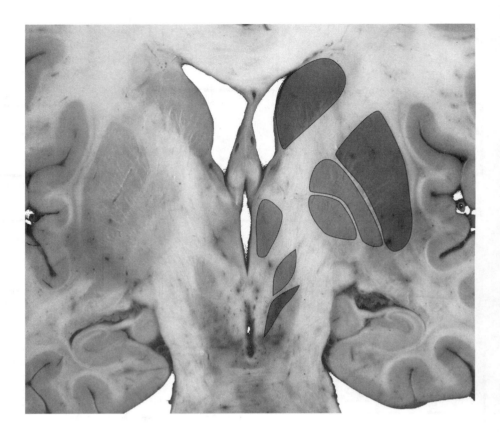

FIGURE 9.18. *Anatomic template for basal ganglia interconnections.*

INST Your wiring diagram will have included both the "direct" and the "indirect" pathways. The standard model (Penne and Young) claims that striatal neurons in the direct pathway are activated by dopamine (via D1 receptors), while neurons in the indirect pathway are inhibited by dopamine (via D2 receptors). Add this feature to your wiring diagram.

Q9.19. On the block diagram in Figure 9.16, identify the site of injury in Parkinson's disease. Knowing that this abnormality must eventually affect the primary motor cortex for its clinical manifestations, try to explain these patient's bradykinesia based on the wiring diagram and the distribution of D1 and D2 receptors in the striatum.

A9.19. *See Figure 9.20. The end result of the nigral cell loss is diminished excitatory glutamate transmission to the cortex. This is thought to underlie the bradykinesia.*

Q9.20. How do you explain tremor with this model?

A9.20. *The model fails to explain the tremor of Parkinson's disease. Some other diseases that also affect the substantia nigra do not have an associated tremor, which suggests that this aspect of Parkinson's is not yet well understood.*

BASAL GANGLIA PHYSIOLOGY

Lesions in the basal ganglia circuitry suggest that it is involved in the initiation of movement. Figure 9.21 shows some results from a classic electrophysiological study by Schultz and Romo (1988) in the monkey, in which the activity of two striatal neurons (*A* and *B*) was recorded prior to, and following the initiation of movement. These movements were spontaneous; no external signal was given for the monkey to move. The locations for all of the recordings in the study (of which only two are shown) are indicated by the dots and dashes in panel *C*.

Q9.21. First, be sure you can identify the caudate nucleus, the putamen, the internal capsule, and the lateral ventricles in panel *C*. When do these neurons generally fire, in relationship to the onset of movement? Compare the activity profiles of the two neurons shown in *A* and *B*; how do they differ? (Remember, the lower traces are EMGs to show muscle movement.)

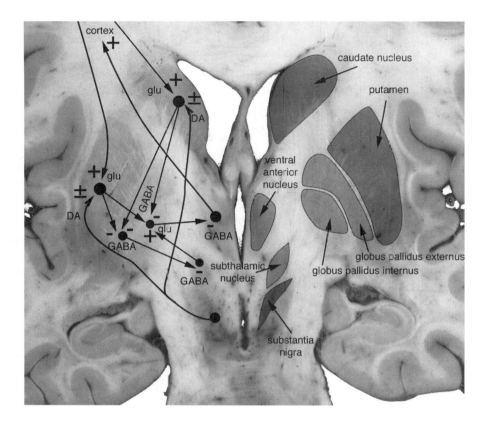

FIGURE 9.19. *Simplified basal ganglia wiring diagram.*

A9.21. For the structures in panel C, see Figure 9.11. Both neurons commence firing more than 1 second before the start of muscle contraction. The striatal neuron shown in A ceases firing at the onset of movement, while the neuron in B continues to fire during muscle contraction.

Q9.22. What do the activity records indicate about the relationship between basal ganglia activity and movement?

A9.22. The two striatal neurons are active well in advance of the initiation of movement as indicated by the EMG activity, which is consistent with the hypothesis that the basal ganglia are involved in the initiation of movement.

Q9.23. The next experiment, shown in Figure 9.22, is a functional MRI study of the striatum. Subjects were asked to repeatedly move their toes, move their fingers, move their lips, or move their eyes. During these tasks they were imaged. The figure shows those areas of the basal ganglia in which blood flow increased during these tasks. Make sure you can orient yourself; map these onto your clay model. Describe the "homunculus" of the basal ganglia. What regions are activated by these tasks? How might you change this study to determine other representations of the basal ganglia?

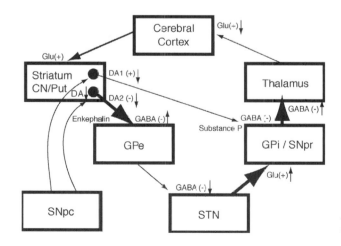

FIGURE 9.20. *Parkinson's disease wiring diagram.*

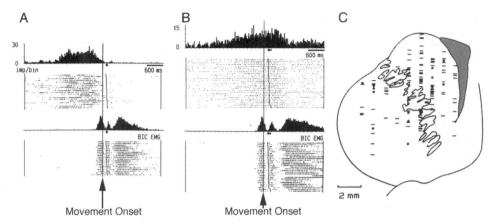

A   B   C

Movement Onset   Movement Onset   2 mm

FIGURE 9.21. *Electrophysiology data from electrodes placed in the basal ganglia. Panel C shows the location of the electrodes (the lateral ventricle is shaded gray). In these experiments, a monkey was spontaneously reaching for a food reward. Each trial consisted of one reaching movement by the monkey, during which both striatal neuron firing and muscle activity (EMG) were recorded simultaneously. Two representative trials are shown in A and B. In each case, the upper panel shows the neuronal firing activity and the lower panel shows the electromyography from a prime mover muscle, in this case, the biceps brachii (BIC). The arrow indicates the onset of movement, which was recorded optically. The histograms above the firing data represent the cumulative results from multiple trials, with the individual trials displayed below the histograms. Each horizontal line represents one trial, and each tick represents an action potential during that trial. (Adapted from figures 2 & 3, Schultz, W. and Romo, R. Neuronal activity in the monkey striatum during the initiation of movements. 1988. Exp Brain Res 71: 431–436.)*

A9.23.   *The toes are represented more dorsolaterally, while the lips more ventromedially. The body of the caudate nucleus has more visual functions connected to eye movement, which reflects its interconnections with the occipital lobes. These repetitive movements activate primarily the central region of the basal ganglia. While not part of the study, you may predict that more complex movements (e.g., playing a piano piece or manipulating a jeweler's screwdriver) would activate more anterior parts of the caudate nucleus, which has greater interconnections with the frontal lobes and planning.*

CLINICAL CASE: HUNTINGTON'S DISEASE

This case is derived in part from L. Sudarsky, R. Myers, and T. M. Walshe *J. Med. Genet.*, 20: 408–411, 1983).

The patient had a twin brother. Their biologic father developed Huntington's disease in his early thirties and died at age 42.

The patient had been raised with six other siblings in the home of his biological parents. He had a history of alcoholism from the age of 20. His family declined to press charges for repeated episodes of assault involving his mother and siblings. He was admitted to a psychiatric hospital at the age of 42 for drunkenness. He had choreic movements present on admission. Six months after being discharged, he assaulted his mother with a kitchen knife, and was admitted to a chronic care facility at the age of 42. He had active psychotic delusions. He was disoriented and had severe dysarthria.

FIGURE 9.22. *Representation of body areas in the basal ganglia. (Adapted from Gerardin, E, Lehericy, S. Pochon, J.-B., du Montcel, S. T., Mangin, J.-F., Poupon, F., Agid, Y., Le Bihan, D., and Marsault, C. 2003. Foot, hand, face and eye representation in the human striatum. Cerebral Cortex 13; 162–169.)*

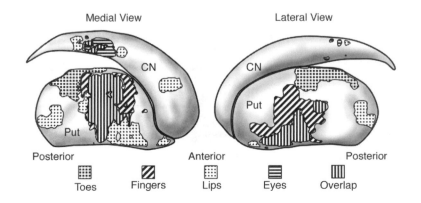

Medial View   Lateral View

CN   CN

Put   Put

Posterior   Anterior   Posterior

Toes   Fingers   Lips   Eyes   Overlap

Walking required assistance and he had marked chorea. His reflexes were brisk and his toes upgoing. Later in his course, he had minimal volitional lateral gaze but retained doll's eyes movements. He had perioral choreic movements, which included his lips, tongue. and face. The patient continued to decline and died at the age of 68. He had spent his last 26 years cf life in a hospital.

The patient's twin brother was raised as an only child by a paternal uncle and his wife. At age 39, during a routine physical examination, he had chorea. Prior to this, he had a 10 year history of "aggressive outbursts and moodiness" and had experienced movements of his hands for four years. He was admitted to a psychiatric hospital at the age of 42 following two episodes of violent behavior associated with alcohol. Finally, at the age of 44 he was admitted to the same chronic care facility as his brother. On examination, he was inattentive and had an inappropriate lack of concern. His speech was dysarthric, but his comprehension, repetition, and object naming were good. He had diffuse chorea and bilateral ankle clonus. Early during his course, he had repeated falls and had assaulted a nurse. Later he could make only vocal utterances, lost volitional lateral gaze, but retained doll's eyes movements. He had marked oral-buccal-lingual chorea.

Q9.24. How similar or different would you characterize these twin brothers' presentation?

A9.24. *Both brothers presented with psychiatric problems. Remembering that the frontal cortex more or less gives you your personality and that the frontal cortex projects to the caudate nucleus, this at least superficially makes sense. Often it is their psychiatric manifestations that bring Huntington's disease patients to the medical system. The incidence of suicide is high in these patients.*

Q9.25. The patient's family tree is indicated in Figure 9.23. Although you probably already know the inheritance pattern of Huntington's disease, try to convince yourself of it using the figure. Does anything about this family tree strike you as unusual?

A9.25. *The pattern of inheritance is classic for a dominant disease. In this tree well over 50% of the offspring are affected (16 out of a total number of 22). Also the progeny are mostly males (17 out of 22). It is not possible to make further conclusions from these data alone.*

Q9.26. The patient's brain is illustrated in Figure 9.24. What do you find most striking? Lists the sites where you think the brain is atrophic, as well as those sites in which it is normal. Identify: caudate nucleus, putamen, globus pallidus, thalamus, frontal cortex, and temporal cortex.

A9.26. *The brain (which you hopefully guessed is on the right side) is amazing for how little remains. Rather than the nice convex bulge of the caudate nucleus into the lateral ventricle in the normal specimen, these structures form a concave depression in the same region. If you think you can successfully identify any components of the basal ganglia in this patient, you are probably having visual hallucinations. However, if you look only at the basal ganglia you will miss this patient's generalized atrophy. You can see the incredibly thin frontal cortex and the highly atrophic temporal cortex. You may also be able to make out a bit of the optic tract and hypothalamus. Note the withered corpus callosum.*

Q9.27. Now examine Figure 9.25 from a patient with less severe disease. Compare it with the adjacent "normal" brain. What structure show the most marked degeneration?

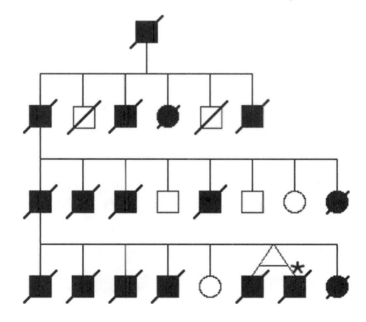

FIGURE 9.23. Family tree, showing affected family members.

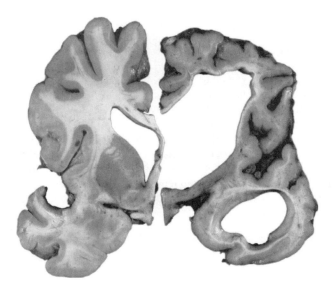

FIGURE 9.24. *Coronal half-section of a relatively normal brain* (left) *and the patient* (right).

Which others have degenerated? Remembering what areas of cortex map onto the basal ganglia, suggest an explanation for some of the clinical manifestations in the patient presented above.

A9.27. *In this image the caudate nucleus is most severely atrophic, followed closely by the putamen. However, the cerebral cortex is also atrophic; witness the differences in thickness between the corpus callosum in the two brains. Remember, through this structure, cortex talks to cortex.*

Huntington's disease doesn't only affect the caudate nucleus, it just affects it early. Damage to the putamen soon follows the caudate degeneration, as shown in both Figure 9.24 and Figure 9.25. The deprogramming of movements that follows degeneration of the motor striatum presumably leads to the choreoathetosis so typical of Huntington's disease. However, this disease affects other regions as well, and many areas of the brain will degenerate, given enough time. The patient presented here spent most of the last years of his life in a fetal position.

Q9.28. As the brain is so atrophic, interpretation of the gross specimen is nearly impossible. Figure 9.26 shows a histologic section of this patient's entire hemisphere and Figure 9.27 shows a close up of the deep nuclei. Now try to label the structures indicated by the numbers in Figure 9.27.

9.28.1 _____

9.28.2 _____

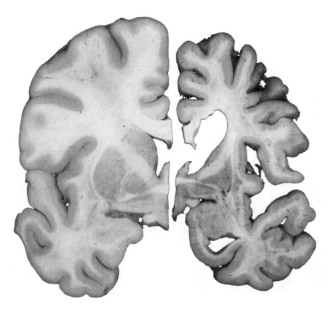

FIGURE 9.25. *Huntington's disease brain* (right) *compared to a normal brain* (left). *(The photograph was kindly supplied by Dr. Jean Paul Vonsattel)*

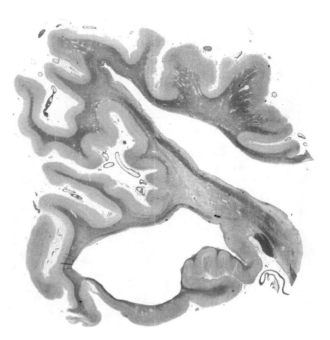

FIGURE 9.26. *Histologic whole-mount coronal section from the patient, at the level of the amygdala, H&E/LFB stain.*

9.28.3 _____

9.28.4 _____

9.28.5 _____

9.28.6 _____

9.28.7 _____

A9.28. *The histology is not much easier!*
    9.28.1. *Insular cortex*
    9.28.2. *Claustrum*
    9.28.3. *Internal capsule*
    9.28.4. *Putamen*
    9.28.5. *Caudate nucleus*
    9.28.6. *Globus pallidus, external and internal segments*
    9.28.7. *Temporal horn, lateral ventricle*

Q9.29. Compare the microscopy from a mild case of Huntington's disease with that of the normal basal ganglia (see Fig. 9.28). If available, compare the two slides on a white piece of paper. How do the caudate nuclei differ? Now look at the slide. Are there more or less cells in the caudate nucleus? More or less neurons? What has happened to the neuropil?

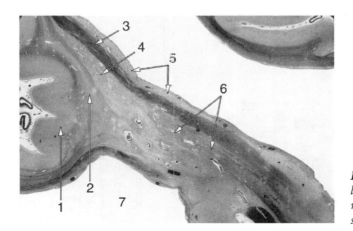

FIGURE 9.27. *Close-up from histologic giant section, showing what remains of the basal ganglia. H&E/LFB stain.*

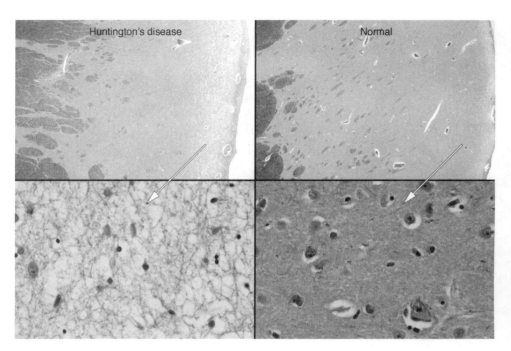

FIGURE 9.28. *Histology of Huntington's disease* (left) *versus normal caudate nucleus* (right).

A9.29. Compared to the normal basal ganglia, the caudate is not as thick. In more advanced cases it is often relatively concave. Microscopically it may at first appear to have more cells than the normal caudate nucleus. However, the number and density of neurons is decreased; much of the extra cellularity are reactive astrocytes and other residual glia left after the neurons have died. To study this accurately, you would have to determine the density of neurons and then account for the loss in total volume of the nucleus. With the loss of neurons is a concomitant loss of their connections. Hence the neuropil is paler and more vacuolated than in the normal.

Q9.30. In the next figure are the results of genetic testing for Huntington's disease on a series of patients. The test determines the number of triple repeats in the huntingtin gene, specifically of the CAG repeats that encode the polyglutamine tract within the protein. The arrow indicates a repeat length of 18 (18 triple repeats). Determine the number of repeats in each of the patients listed. Remember that we all have two chromosomes, so there should be two major bands for each individual. The test is considered positive when the number of repeats is greater than 38 and negative when it is less than 32. Does this particular patient (patient *J*) have Huntington's disease? How would you council this patient?

A9.30. The official reading for all of these patients is as follows:
A: 22/17, B: 22/18, C: 23/18, D: 45/15, E: 24/17, F: 44/19, G: 18/16, H: 18/15, I: 40/20, J: 42/28, K: 42/28, L: 22/18, M: 28/17, N: 18/17, O: 17/12, P: 28/17, Q: 40/23, R: 41/17
Our patient has 42 repeats and has Huntington's disease.

FIGURE 9.29. *DNA triple repeat analysis. Radio-labeled primers from the flanking regions of the repeat region were used in polymerase chain reactions to amplify the repeats. These reaction products were then run out on a gel. Each letter represents the reaction product for a given patient. The largest fragments run the slowest in the gel, and so are nearer the top. Each band represents many reaction products of a given length. The highest two major dark bands give the length of the region on each chromosome. (Data kindly supplied by Dr. Jean Paul Vonsattel.)*

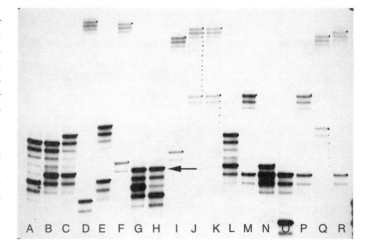

Chapter 10—CEREBELLUM

The car had traveled from side to side down the road, often crossing into the oncoming traffic lane. The police officer smelled a strong odor of whisky after he had stopped the car and came to the window. Asked to stand by his car, the driver reeled slightly and leaned a bit on the fender. He fumbled to get his driver's license from his back pocket. When the officer asked the man to walk a straight line, he staggered back and fourth, barely catching himself on the side of the car. The driver could not accurately follow the officer's finger with his eyes.

The cerebellum, which literally means "little cerebrum," takes up about 10% of the volume of the human brain but accounts for about 50% of the neurons. So dense a population of cells coordinates our actions. A cerebellar hemisphere controls movement on the same side of the body. The graded contraction of extensor muscles in the arm as one reaches for an object in space and the reciprocally graded relaxation of flexors in the arm happen without much apparent ado, but a great deal of information gets shared by discrete and various cortical and subcortical structures for such actions to take place without wild lack of control. The sensory system plays a part, supplying data on both the external and internal world: where the object is in space and where the arm is in relationship to the object, from one moment to the next. As attested to by the drunken driver, the cerebellum also maintains posture; this also requires extensive sensory information about the environment and our relationship with gravity. Yet another job of the cerebellum is producing accurate eye movements. Without this little brain, you would not be able to track the baseball with moving eyes in a turning head on a mobile body. Current research also points to major participation of the cerebellum in cognitive functions, including in visuospatial tasks, abstract reasoning, and personality.

This chapter reviews cerebellar anatomy, including its functional divisions and connections.

LEARNING OBJECTIVES

- Identify major features of cerebellar anatomy, including its major divisions, vascular supply, and relationship with regional structures.
- Describe the inputs, outputs, and circuitry of the cerebellum, including important relay nuclei.
- Describe general clinical aspects of cerebellar diseases, including nystagmus, control of movement, and ataxia.

Functional Neuroanatomy: An Interactive Text and Manual, by Jeffrey T. Joseph and David L. Cardozo
ISBN 0-471-44437-5 Copyright © 2004 John Wiley & Sons, Inc.

INTRODUCTION

Function of the Cerebellum

Why have a cerebellum? What does it do? Cerebellar lesions produce a variety of clinical findings: an inability to stand in one place, an extremely wobbly walk, jerky movements of the limbs, nystagmus (directional beating of the eyes), a lost ability to accurately throw a baseball. Currently much interest has focused on non-motor functions of the cerebellum, particularly its role in cognition. We also know a great deal about the cerebellum's elegant structure, its wiring, and its basic operation. Linking these two levels of knowledge, the basic and the clinical, remains incomplete, but generally the cerebellum modulates an output (motor, cognitive), based on inputs (environmental sensations, cerebral cortex) and the march of time. To pick up a cup requires seeing the cup and judging its location, knowing where your hand and joints are now, calculating the trajectory to reach the cup, activating the motor program to follow that trajectory, and finally modifying the movements from environmental cues as it is executed. Your cerebellum helps coordinates your eye movements (vestibuloocular reflex), continuously receives joint and muscle information during movements, and modulates motor output, smoothing the motion. The velocity of a movement, not just how fast the hand reaches the cup but also at what rate to activate a muscle and at what angular speed to rotate a joint, requires exquisite timing, which is another role for the cerebellum. The cerebellum also learns from the past, so then next time you reach for that cup, toss a spear at a mastodon, or beat out a complex rhythm, you do it better. The cerebellum allows you to better do what you do.

Anatomic Divisions

As you have seen in previous chapters, the cerebellum lies in the posterior fossa, dorsal to the brainstem. Over the centuries it has been divided in many ways into multiple substructures. Some sound almost poetic, like declive and uvula. However, ignorance of these names will in no way impede your knowledge of neurology. In this laboratory we will consider only a few major structures, as detailed in Figure 10.1.

Cerebellar Histology

The cerebellum is the most beautiful site in the brain (see Fig. 10.2). Its well-named dominant structure is its *folia* (leaves), which is the dendritic arborization of its cortex. Deep to the folia lie the cerebellar's output nuclei, the most prominent of which is the *dentate nucleus.*

The folia comprise three cell layers: internal granular, Purkinje, and molecular (see Fig. 10.3). Distributed over these layers are five cell types. *Purkinje neuron* dendrites contact the ascending axons of the internal granular neuron parallel fibers in the outer *molecular layer.* This outer layer has a few inhibitory *basket* and *stellate* neurons embedded in its neuropil, which modify and focus the Purkinje projections. Purkinje cells are among the largest neurons in the brain. Their proximal dendrites receive select signals from the *climbing fibers* of the contralateral *inferior olivary nucleus.* The Purkinje cells lie in their own layer between the molecular layer and the *internal granular layer.* This latter layer has *granular neurons* (5×10^{10}) but also a smaller population of larger inhibitory neurons, the Golgi cells, that modify the granular cell output. Excluding the olivary input, this layer is the input region to the cerebellar cortex, and receives *mossy fibers* from the spinal cord, medulla, and pons. One useful bit of trivia is that the granular layer has nearly as many neurons as the rest of the brain combined. The Purkinje cells provide the neural output from the cortex, supplying exclusively inhibitory input to the deep output nuclei (5×10^5 neurons).

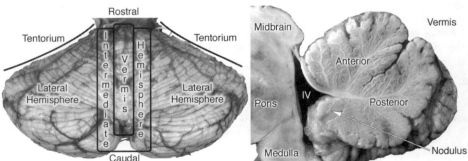

FIGURE 10.1. Cerebellar anatomic divisions.

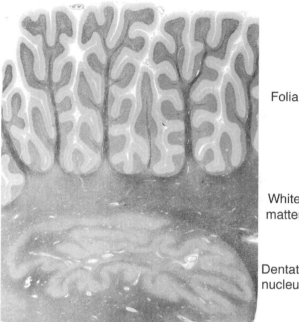

Folia

White matter

Dentate nucleus

FIGURE 10.2. Histology of the cerebellum, H&E/LFB stain.

Extrinsic Cerebellar Connections

Only three main roads lead into or out of the cerebellum; the inferior cerebellar peduncle (also known as the restiform or "rope-like" body), middle cerebellar peduncle (or brachium pontis), and the superior cerebellar peduncle (or brachium conjunctivum). These divisions correspond the cerebellum's connections with the brainstem: the inferior cerebellar peduncle connects to the medulla, the middle connects to the pons, and the superior connects to the midbrain (see Fig. 10.4).

Generally, peripheral information about the body enters the cerebellum through the inferior peduncle, higher cortical information enters via the middle peduncle, and processed output travels through the superior peduncle. An important exception is the vestibular system, which has its own pathways and nuclei.

Cerebellar Inputs

Sensory information about muscle length, tension, and limb position ascends in the spinal cord and projects to the cerebellum. The primary fibers, like all of the other spinal sensory fibers, have their cell bodies in the dorsal root ganglia. In contrast to the dorsal column system, these pathways synapse at their level of entrance in the spinal cord. Their target is *Clarke's nuclear column,* which lies at the base

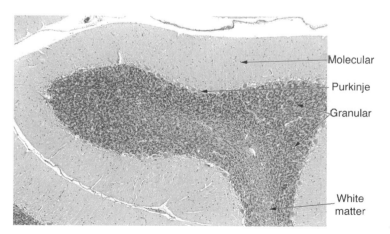

Molecular

Purkinje

Granular

White matter

FIGURE 10.3. Cerebellar cortex.

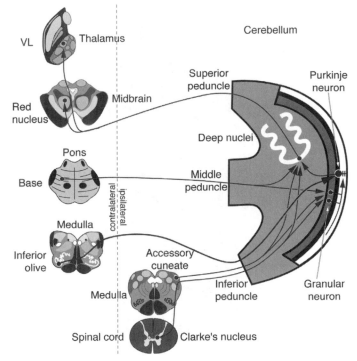

FIGURE 10.4. *Cerebellar inputs and outputs.*

of the dorsal horn in the thoracic and upper lumbar regions. Fibers from its large neurons ascend in the ipsilateral dorsolateral perimeter of the cord in the ***dorsal spinocerebellar tract*** and project to the ipsilateral cerebellar nuclei and cortex. The equivalent of Clarke's nucleus for the arms and head is the accessory or ***lateral cuneate nucleus*** in the medulla. Other cerebellar fibers synapse in the posterior horn and double cross before reaching the ipsilateral cerebellum; their function remains enigmatic. See Table 10.1. In contrast to the contralateral projections of other sensory systems, cerebellar sensory information projects to the ipsilateral cerebellum. These sensory axons are termed mossy fibers, as their large bulbous ends in the internal granular layer have a grainy appearance like moss (see Fig. 10.4).

All of the information carried in these spinocerebellar tracts remains unconscious; we are never aware of it. Yet it contributes importantly to coordinated movement. When these tracts degenerate, as they do in some hereditary diseases, severe ataxia is the result.

An older cerebellar sensory system processes vestibular information. Direct connections from the vestibular apparatus and second-order vestibular nuclei neurons project to select parts of the cerebellum, including the ***flocculus*** and ***nodulus,*** via a fiber bundle adjacent to the inferior peduncle (juxtarestiform body). These convey information about the head's acceleration and position in space, key data for head and eye movements.

In addition to peripheral sensory data, the cerebellum also receives feedback information from the cerebral cortex. Since our cerebral hemispheres concentrate on contralateral signals, while our cerebellum processes ipsilateral data, the cortical information must cross before reaching the folia.

TABLE 10.1. Major Sensory Cerebellar Tracts

Tract	Cell Origin	Crossed?	Information Carried
Dorsal spinocerebellar	Clarke's nucleus	No	mostly proprioceptive, from trunk and legs
Ventral spinocerebellar	Dorsal horn	Yes, double-crossed! (cord and superior cerebellar peduncle)	
Cuneocerebellar	Lateral cuneate in medulla	No	Same, from arms

Cortex projects to ipsilateral neurons in the base of the pons, which in turn send their axons across the midline to the contralateral cerebellum.

Unlike the sensory and pontine information entering the cerebellum as mossy fibers, the inferior olivary inputs project as climbing fibers. As in the pontine tracts, these projections are contralateral. The functions of the inferior olive remain elusive, but it probably plays a role in cerebellar learning and timing.

Outputs

The output from the cerebellum originates from its deep nuclei. These neurons receive excitatory signals from various cerebellar inputs and negative signals from Purkinje neurons. They in turn project out of the cerebellum, principally to the contralateral red nucleus and thalamus (ventral lateral motor thalamus). From these neurons, signals transmit both to the cerebral cortex and to the lower brainstem and spinal cord. Vestibular signals follow a different course, using brainstem vestibular nuclei as its output nuclei and communicating through the juxtarestiform body.

Cerebellar Circuitry and Function

Figure 10.5 shows a simplified version of cerebellar neuron interconnections. The cerebellum receives sensory inputs (Clarke's nucleus in the spinal cord and the accessory cuneate nucleus) and cortical inputs (base of the pons). These neurons project excitatory *glutamatergic* signals to both the deep cerebellar nuclei and the cerebellar cortex (internal granular layer). Unique among the cerebellar inputs is information from the inferior olivary nucleus, each of whose climbing fibers has a cozy excitatory projection to only a few Purkinje neurons. Within the cerebellar cortex, the mossy fibers make contact with many internal granular neurons, which in turn synapse on the distal dendrites of hundreds of Purkinje neurons. In contrast, a Purkinje neuron receives a projection from only one climbing fiber, and a climbing fiber targets (or climbs around) only a handful of Purkinje neurons on their proximal dendrites. The output from the cerebellar cortex comes exclusively from the inhibitory, *GABAergic* Purkinje neurons. Final cerebellar output from its deep nuclei represents a balance of inputs from inhibitory Purkinje neurons, excitatory mossy fibers, and cerebellar cortical modulation of inhibitory inputs by both mossy and climbing fibers.

The cerebellum is a humbling example of the failure of simple reductionism: while we know a great deal about the interconnections of cerebellar cells, we are still in our infancy in understanding how they work together to support the structure's functions.

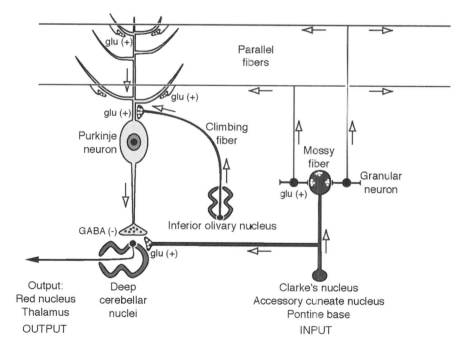

FIGURE 10.5. *Intrinsic cerebellar circuitry.*

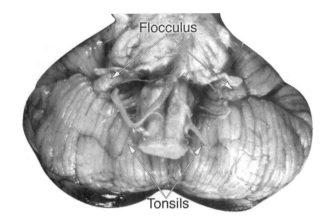

Flocculus

Tonsils

FIGURE 10.6. Flocculus.

Cerebellar Functional Divisions

Like a flower, the cerebellum unfolds in evolution and in function from medial to lateral. The most medial structure is the midline vermis, then the intermediate hemispheres, and finally the lateral hemispheres (see Fig. 10.1). The lowest folia of the *vermis,* the nodulus, interconnects with flocculus (see Fig. 10.6) to form the flocculonodular lobe. These anatomic divisions correspond to the cerebellum's functional divisions. Most of the vermis regulates posture, the intermediate hemispheres control limb movements, the flocculonocular lobe controls eye movements and balance, and the lateral hemispheres have roles in planning and cognition.

From the *Homo sapiens* point of view, the oldest and most primitive region of the cerebellum is the *vestibulocerebellum.* Although this region occupies only a small portion of the cerebellum, it is essential for the control of balance and eye movements. Its components, principally the flocculus and nodulus, receive input from the vestibular system. Its output Purkinje cells project back upon these neurons. As mentioned above, this circuitry bypasses the classic cerebellar nuclei. The vestibulocerebellum provides essential information for the vestibulospinal tracts and inputs into eye muscle nuclei.

Most of the vermis and intermediate lobe subsume the spinocerebellum. This is the part we most associate with the cerebellum and is important for such things as axial stability, tracking movements (finger to nose testing), and control of fine movements. More medial regions of cerebellum (vermis) control more medial regions of the body, while the paravermal or *intermediate hemispheres* control the limbs. The *spinocerebellum* receives major inputs from the spinal cord and accessory cuneate nucleus, and in turn modifies the output to lower motor neurons. After leaving the deep nuclei (interposed or globose and emboliform) through the superior cerebellar peduncle, these fibers cross and synapse on the neurons of the red nucleus. From there, the information crosses again to the descending rubrospinal tract. Fibers also project to the ventral lateral thalamic nucleus, and then on to motor regions of the cerebral cortex. In a pattern seen in other brain systems, probably originating from our days as limbless mudsuckers, axial or midline control derives mostly from the brainstem. For the cerebellum the vermis projects to the fastigial nuclei, which then project bilaterally to brainstem nuclei that influence posture.

As humans we are most proud of the cerebellar hemispheres, the cerebrocerebellum, since this is most developed in our species. It receives input from the cerebral cortex via relay neurons in the base of the pons and sends its output through the dentate nucleus to both the red nucleus and thalamus. We don't fully understand the functions of these hemispheres. However, over the last decade, reports from patients with lesions exclusively in the cerebellum indicate that it has a role in cognition. Infarcts, hemorrhage, and other pathology involving the cerebellum lead to deficits such as perseveration, visuospatial difficulties, and personality changes. The deficits are greatest when the damage also involves the vermis. These lesional studies complement functional neuroimaging reports showing cerebellar activation during specific cognitive tasks. It is perhaps reassuring that an advanced part of our brain has more to do than moving your finger from your nose to an examiner's finger.

Clinical Aspects and Diseases of Cerebellum

Many of the clinical aspects of the cerebellum relate directly to the functional site involved in pathology. The superior vermis is especially vulnerable to toxins, most notably alcohol. These toxins produce the clinical scenario that opened the introduction, a drunk with axial ataxia and a wide-based gait. Like the rest of the brain, the cerebellum is also subject to infarcts, tumors, and hemorrhages. These may have special manifestations, including eye movement abnormalities like nystagmus. Some cerebellar infarcts may be clinically "silent," or may be overshadowed by associated nearby lesions, as in the in the case of the lateral medullary syndrome. The cerebellum has its own unique selection of tumors and rare primary degenerative diseases.

As will be emphasized throughout the chapter, most clinical symptomatology of cerebellar lesions is ipsilateral to the site of the pathology. While you may think this makes your life easier, in fact this superficial simplicity is a result of the double crossing of most of the cerebellar circuitry. Your bliss will soon be shattered by complex, crossing wiring diagrams that will make you think you had majored in electrical engineering.

Schedule (2.5 hours)
15   Cerebellar clinical examination
30   Cerebellar dissection
15   Cerebellar histology
60   Cerebellar connections
30   Clinical cases

CLINICAL INTRODUCTION TO THE CEREBELLUM

One way to get an idea about what the cerebellum accomplishes is to understand the clinical tests that attempt to isolate some cerebellar functions. Be careful to remember, however, that just because a clinical test is abnormal does not mean that the cerebellum is necessarily the problem. For example, similar clinical manifestations can happen when the pathways that feed into the cerebellum are dysfunctional.

Q10.1. Select a partner and try the following. Person A holds her finger out; Person B places his finger close to Person A's without touching it. Person A moves her finger to a different location; Person B moves his finger to that new position, again without touching the finger (as if facing a mirror). Try some reverse engineering; what do you need to track accurately? What are the peripheral components of this activity? Be as specific as you can. What are the central components? In particular, consider sensory, motor, and processing systems. From your readings, what functional divisions of the cerebellum are utilized?

A10.1. *You can break the problem down into inputs, processing, and outputs. Inputs include not only your vision but all of the muscle spindles, Golgi tendon organs, and other sensory modalities that tell you where your finger, arm, and eyes are. Outputs include the muscles of your shoulder girdle and arm, extraocular muscles, and fine muscles within the spindle sensory complex.*

The processing center is that lovely organ in your skull. Sensory systems include vision and ascending spinocerebellar fibers. Motor outputs come from motor neurons in the spinal cord and precentral gyrus. These are integrated and fine-tuned by multiple areas, especially the cerebellum, red nucleus, thalamus, basal ganglia, and regions of the cortex in front of the motor strip.

You use all of the main cerebellar systems for this task: vestibulocerebellum (eye movements), spinocerebellum (axial control), and cerebrocerebellum (appendicular fine control).

Q10.2. To get a sense of cerebellar function without the input of the visual system, have your partner hold out his arms and hands in front of him with eyes closed. Then ask that person to touch his own nose with eyes closed. Again, analyze the role of the cerebellum in this task. Aside from cerebellar pathology, how might this test fail?

A10.2. *Such a test becomes difficult to interpret when the inputs and outputs fail, such as may happen with a severe sensory neuropathy or a profound muscle weakness. Finer neurologic testing should localize the deficits to either central or peripheral components. Remember cerebellar function can be completely masked by lesions elsewhere in the brain, such as a corticospinal tract infarct in the internal capsule.*

Q10.3. Illustrating vestibulocerebellar activity requires a brave volunteer with a strong stomach. If anyone is so gullible, have the volunteer rapidly spin in place for a while and then sit down. Make sure they don't fall. Have them fixate on a spot and then carefully watch their eyes. What do you see? Which way do they beat, toward or away from the direction of spinning? What is this called? What sensory organs have been fooled by this action?

A10.3. *Provided the person doesn't vomit, you should be able to see the eyes beating to one side. This is called* **nystagmus.** *By spinning for a while, you have fooled your middle ear organs, specifically your semicircular canals, into believing you are still spinning. When you try to fixate, your cerebellum gets inaccurate information, and its modulation of eye movements during fixation produces nystagmus.*

Nystagmus is a huge topic, but certain aspects can be emphasized here. Clinicians should be careful about attributing eye movement abnormalities specifically to cerebellar damage, since many syndromes involve destruction of brainstem as well as cerebellar loci. Nevertheless, midline lesions (especially those that involve deep cerebellar nuclei) are associated with dysmetria, generally a hypermetria or overshoot of visual targets. Lesions of the flocculonodular lobe are associated with gaze-evoked nystagmus. Gaze-evoked nystagmus occurs when the eyes are held in an eccentric position; a slow and fast phase are observed, with the latter more obvious to the naked eye than the former. Certain parts of the cerebellum are involved in coordinating eye movements to hold an image steady upon the retina.

CEREBELLAR DISSECTION AND REGIONAL ANATOMY

Q10.4. Study the intact brain. Notice how the superior surface of the cerebellum is juxtaposed to the base of the temporal and occipital lobes. What structure would lie in this space? What vascular channel lies in this structure?

A10.4. *The tentorium separates the cerebellum from the temporal and occipital lobes. Venous blood from the center of the brain drains from the internal cerebral veins and inferior sagittal sinus into the upper fold of the tentorium as the straight sinus. This blood meets up with venous drainage from the superior sagittal sinus at the torcula in the back of the dura.*

Q10.5. You should have available from a previous lab a half cerebellum attached to the brainstem. On the anatomic specimen and in Figure 10.7, review the location of some important landmarks:
- Midbrain, including the tectum, tegmentum, peduncles, and red nucleus
- Aqueduct
- Fourth ventricle
- Pons
- Medulla

Examine the relationship between the cerebellum and the brainstem. How is the cerebellum connected with the brainstem? Using your atlas, identify these structures:
- Superior cerebellar peduncle or brachium conjunctivum
- Middle cerebellar peduncle or brachium pontis
- Inferior cerebellar peduncle or restiform body

A10.5. *See Figure 10.8. Note that most signals travel up into the cerebellum through the inferior peduncle, travel more or less out of the paper through the middle peduncle, and travel up from the deep cerebellar nuclei through the superior peduncle.*

Q10.6. Now focus your inspection on the cerebellum itself. On the vermis, note the incredible arborization of the folia. Notice how the gray matter of the cortex completely sheathes the thin white matter beneath. Conceptually divide the cerebellum into vertical stripes. Use your atlas to identify the vermis and intermediate lobes. To which functional division do these structures correspond? Locate the hemispheres

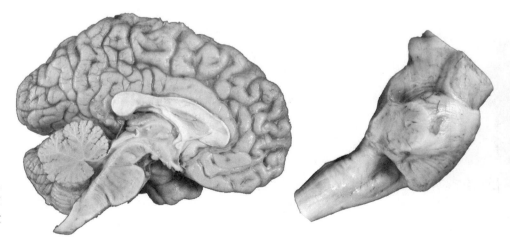

FIGURE 10.7. *Sagittal section through cerebellum and brainstem and close-up of brainstem after removing the cerebellum.*

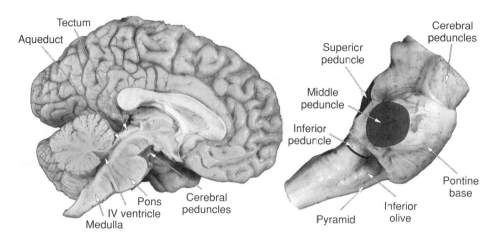

FIGURE 10.8. *Cerebellar peduncles.*

and indicate their functional category. Finally try to find the flocculus and nodulus. If you start at the rostral-most part of the vermis, where it attaches to the superior medullary velum, and move around the outer border, the nodulus is the farthest lobule away, lying at the caudal-ventral surface. The flocculus looks like an excrescence of cerebellar folia lateral to the nodulus, in the posterolateral fissure. Depending on the preservation of the specimen, the flocculus is occasionally difficult to identify. To which functional division do these two parts belong?

A10.6. *Most of the vermis and intermediate lobe (or paravermis) correspond to the spinocerebellum. The hemispheres subsume the cerebrocerebellum, and the flocculonodular lobe houses the vestibulocerebellum. Toxic lesions especially involving the vermis lead to truncal ataxia, small lesions in the flocculus or nodulus produce nystagmus, while occasionally significant infarcts involving only the hemispheres may not come to clinical attention.*

Q10.7. Hold the cerebellum with its rounded base in your right hand. Place your left hand on the flatter tentorial surface. The superior cerebellar artery (SCA) feeds the tissue under your left hand, the posterior inferior cerebellar artery (PICA) nourishes the tissue in your right hand, and the basilar and its penetrating arteries, including the anterior inferior cerebellar artery (AICA) feeds the more ventral structures. Review the vasculature in your atlas and separately shade the three main territories in Figure 10.9.

A10.7. *See Figure 10.10. As in all of these exercises, these figures are approximate.*

Q10.8. Figure 10.11 shows an old cerebellar infarct. In what vascular territory was the ischemic injury?

A10.8. *This lesion is in the inferolateral portion of the left cerebellar hemisphere. It is a typical AICA infarct.*

Q10.9. Figure 10.12 shows a medial view of the cerebellar vermis with an acute infarct. What is the vascular territory?

A10.9. *Superior cerebellar artery.*

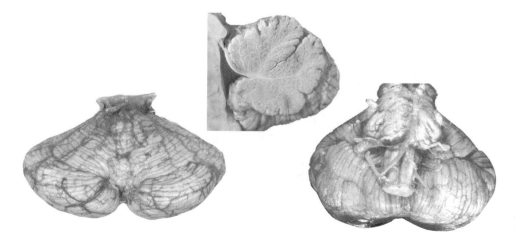

FIGURE 10.9. *Cerebellum vascular territory worksheet.*

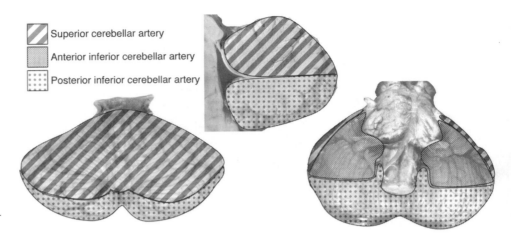

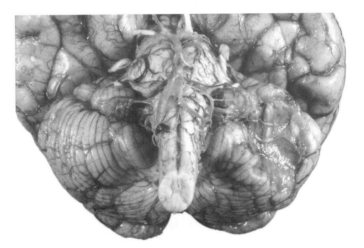

FIGURE 10.10. *Main vascular territories of the cerebellum.*

FIGURE 10.11. *Remote cerebellar infarct.*

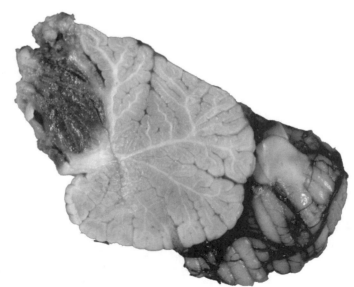

FIGURE 10.12. *Acute cerebellar infarct in midline vermis.*

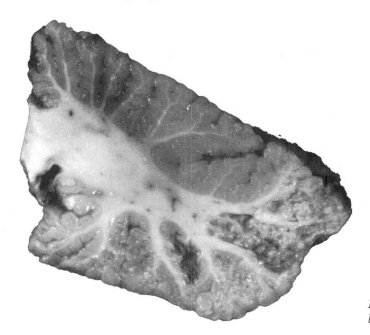

FIGURE 10.13. *Organizing cerebellar infarct, several weeks old.*

Q10.10. Figure 10.13 shows an infarct at a later stage. What is the vascular territory?

A10.10. PICA.

Q10.11. Finally carefully dissect the half cerebellum with the brainstem attached by finely slicing it transversely, more or less perpendicular to the brainstem. Compare the quantity of white matter in the hemispheres with that in the vermis. Locate the dentate nucleus. Identify its outflow tract, the superior cerebellar peduncle. Find the decussation of the superior cerebellar peduncle in the midbrain. What nucleus lies above this decussation? What major brain division lies immediately above it? To answer this, you may have to compare the slices with the intact hemisphere.

A10.11. The superior cerebellar peduncle outflow tracts cross as they come into the midbrain. Many of the fibers synapse on the immediately rostral red nucleus, while others will go on to the next way station in the motor thalamus (VL), which endows them with their name: the dentatorubrothalamic tract. The thalamus lies rostral to the midbrain, above the red nucleus. Some red nucleus neurons also project to thalamus, while others cross and project caudally to the spinal cord in the rubrospinal tract or descend to the ipsilateral inferior olivary nucleus in the central tegmental tract.

CEREBELLAR HISTOLOGY

Q10.12. As a review from the histology chapter, re-examine the microscopic slide of the cerebellum (see Fig. 10.14). Focus first on the cortex. How many distinct layers can you identify? Describe the cellularity as you move from outside to the white matter. Describe how the neuronal size changes as you move down these different layers.

A10.12. The adult cerebellar cortex is traditionally divided into three layers: an outer molecular layer (M in Fig. 10.14), a single neuron thick layer having the large Purkinje cells (P), and a densely cellular internal granular layer (G). Fetuses and young infants have an additional external granular layer, which you will encounter in a later chapter.

The pink molecular layer is where the central action happens. Remember that pink = neuropil = action, the site of synapses. The Purkinje cells are the output from the cerebellar cortex. The granular layer is the complex processing center for most cerebellar input.

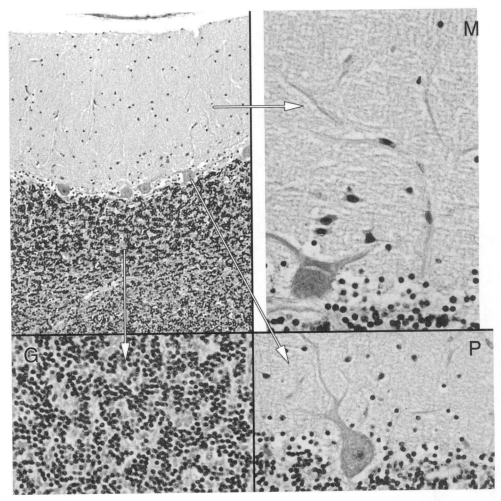

FIGURE 10.14. *Histology of the cerebellum.*

Q10.13. The introduction discussed the different neuronal types in the cerebellum. On the glass slide or in Figure 10.14, see if you can find:
- Basket neurons
- Stellate neurons
- Purkinje neurons
- Granule neurons
- Golgi neurons

A10.13. *You may sometimes see the proximal portions of the Purkinje cell dendrites as they extend up into the proximal parts of the molecular layer (see Fig. 10.14, P).*

While the Purkinje cells and internal granular neurons are easy to see, the Golgi neurons are more difficult. They are slightly larger cells within the internal granular layer and form the core of the layer's substructure. The basket cells and stellate cells are nearly impossible to distinguish from other cells in the molecular layer in this simple H&E preparation. The few dark cells above the Purkinje cell in panel M of Figure 10.14 are probably basket neurons.

Many of the cerebellar neuronal connections were well-illustrated by Ramón y Cajal at the turn of the 19th century. Figure 10.15 is one such figure. It shows the dense arborization of the Purkinje neuron dendrites (top neuron), the basket (*b*) and stellate neurons (*c*) of the molecular layer (*A*), and granular neurons (*s*). It also illustrates the different ascending inputs into the cortex, including climbing fibers (*n*).

Q10.14. Now focus on the white matter in the center of the cerebellum (see Fig. 10.16). Find the deep neurons (depends on the cut). Knowing that early neuroanatomists were

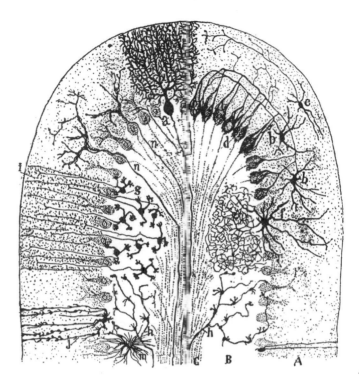

FIGURE 10.15. Cerebellar folia, Golgi stain, as drawn by Ramón y Cajal. (Modified from Ramón y Cajal, Histology of the Nervous System, volume II, reissued by Oxford University Press, © 1995, New York, figure 11, page 13.

obsessed with their stomachs, suggest some names for the large nucleus. Although it may require hallucinogens, try to imagine how information flows into and out of this nucleus. Can you identify exit fibers?

A10.14. *While an olive or raisin may be good names, the early neuroanatomists settled on teeth as the description, and so named it the* **dentate nucleus** *(D in Fig. 10.16). Its neurons receive information from Purkinje cells in the lateral hemispheres and transmit signals through the superior cerebellar peduncle. Like the hemispheres, the dentate nucleus is the most developed of the output nuclei and most developed in humans.*

The other nuclei indicated in the figure relate to other functional divisions of the cerebellum. E and G (emboliform and globose) relate to the limb aspects of the spinocerebellum, while F (fastigial) transmits axial information. If you expect you will remember these names, you are probably delusional. Sometimes Fat Guys/Gals Eat Donuts helps. However, the names are not that important (ask most neurologists for these names and they will groan in relived agony). What is key is not the wonderful sounding names, but the concept that the functional output from the cerebellum is via these deep nuclei, as modulated by corresponding functional divisions of the cerebellar cortex.

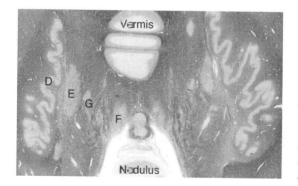

FIGURE 10.16. Deep cerebellar nuclei histology. This is from a lucky transverse section through the entire cerebellum that happened to cross all of the nuclei. The dentate nucleus is large, the others are small.

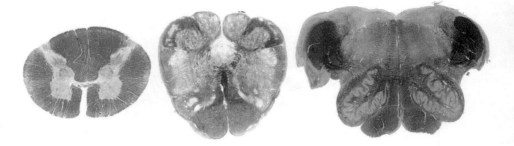

FIGURE 10.17. Cerebellar sensory fiber worksheet.

CEREBELLAR CONNECTIONS

Q10.15. In the three diagrams of Figure 10.17, showing the thoracic spinal cord and medulla, identify and label the following input structures:
  • Clarke's nucleus or column (receives input from dorsal root ganglion; origin of dorsal spinocerebellar tract)
  • Dorsal spinocerebellar tract
  • Accessory or lateral cuneate nucleus (equivalent to Clarke's column for the arms and head)
  • Inferior olivary complex
  • Vestibular nuclear complex
  • Inferior cerebellar peduncle (caudal input to cerebellum)

A10.15. *See Figure 10.18*

One important aspect of the main cerebellar sensory inputs is that they are uncrossed. A secondary system of tracts, the ***ventral spinocerebellar tract*** and an analogous tract in the brain stem do cross, but cross back before terminating in cerebellum. These are then double-crossed and hence act like they are uncrossed.

Q10.16. Figure 10.19 shows major output targets of the cerebellum. Identify and label these structures:
  • Red nucleus
  • Thalamus (ventral lateral nucleus)
  • Cerebral cortex
  • Reticular formation (pons and medulla)
  • Vestibular nuclei

A10.16. *See Figure 10.20.*

Q10.17. Figure 10.21 is a dissection of the major cerebellar white matter output tracts. Label the following structures and tracts:
  • Dentate nucleus
  • Interposed nuclei (globose and emboliform)
  • Fastigial nucleus
  • Superior cerebellar peduncle
  • Decussation of cerebellar peduncles
  • Red nucleus
  • Rubrothalamic and dentatothalamic fibers

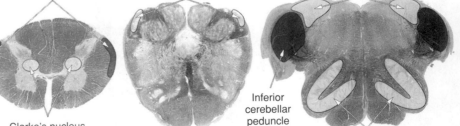

FIGURE 10.18. Cerebellar sensory tracts and nuclei.

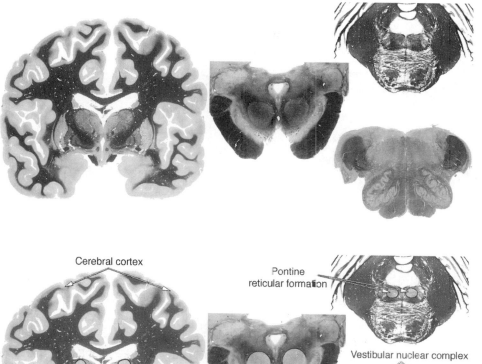

FIGURE 10.19. Cerebellar output worksheet.

Cerebral cortex

Pontine reticular formation

Vestibular nuclear complex

Red nucleus

Thalamus VL

Medullary reticular formation

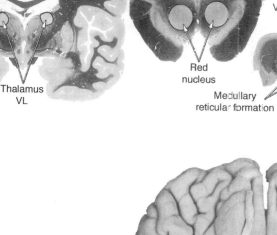

FIGURE 10.20. Major cerebellar output targets.

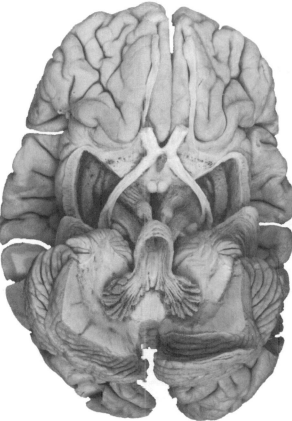

FIGURE 10.21. Cerebellar white matter tract dissection worksheet. (Modified from Gluhbegovic and Williams, The Human Brain, © 1980, Harper & Row, New York, figure 5-23, page 145.)

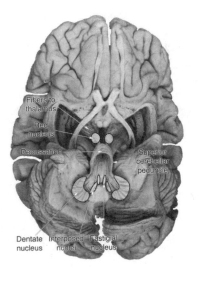

FIGURE 10.22. *Cerebellar white matter tract dissection worksheet. (Modified from Gluhbegovic and Williams, The Human Brain, © 1980, Harper & Row, New York, figure 5-23, page 145.)*

A10.17. See Figure 10.22.

Q10.18. Finally it is time to connect these components together. First, in Figure 10.23, connect the major components of the cerebrocerebellum:
  • Lateral cerebellar hemispheres
  • Dentate nucleus
  • Red nucleus
  • Thalamus
  • Cerebral cortex
  • Base of pons

A10.18. See Figure 10.24. Contralateral cerebral inputs to the cerebellum synapse in the base of the pons. The lateral hemisphere and dentate nucleus are the major parts of the cerebrocerebellum. Output projections include the red nucleus and thalamus.

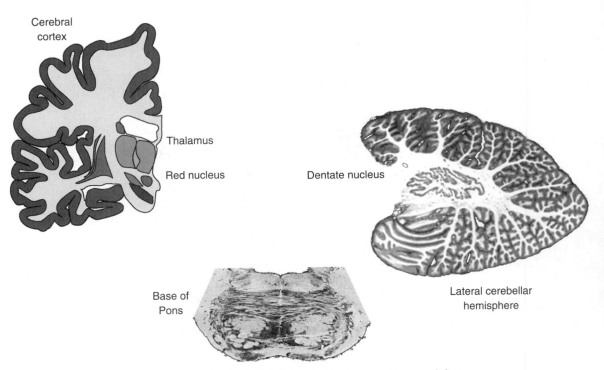

FIGURE 10.23. *Cerebrocerebellum worksheet.*

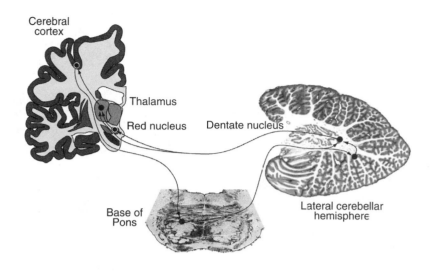

FIGURE 10.24. Cerebrocerebellar connections.

Q10.19. The **spinocerebellum** has two subdivisions: the vermis and the intermediate hemisphere. The medial vermis regulates medial axial stability, while the more lateral intermediate hemisphere modulates the movement of the limbs. In Figure 10.25 first label the ascending sensory inputs (e.g., Golgi tendon organs, muscle spindles):
- Clarke's nucleus and its brainstem equivalent, the accessory cuneate nucleus
- Dorsal spinocerebellar tract
- Inferior cerebellar peduncle
- Vermis and intermediate hemisphere targets

Next show the outputs from the (medial) vermis (these become bilateral, since they concern axial muscles):
- Medial (fastigial) nucleus
- Reticular formation (only the medulla is shown here, but signals also go to pons)
- Reticulospinal tracts

Finally show the outputs from the (more lateral) intermediate hemisphere:
- Output nuclei (interposed)
- Red nucleus (Where do the fibers cross?)
- Rubrospinal tract
- Lower motor neuron

Axial information and other signals that need to be bilaterally coordinated typically utilize interneurons to coordinate their actions. This is true of the axial information from the vermis, which projects via the reticular formation and then through interneurons in the spinal cord before reaching the lower motor neurons in the ventral horns. You saw this in the spinal reflex arc and will see this several times again, especially in some of the cranial nerves.

A10.19. *See Figure 10.26. Note that in this figure the thalamic and cortical connections have been supressed. The reticulospinal axons synapse on interneurons, which then project to the motor neurons. Remember, vermis is axial, intermediate hemisphere is limbs; vermis allows you to wiggle like a worm, the intermediate hemisphere allows you to crawl out of the mud.*

Q10.20. While the concept of the vestibular system is simple, coordinating the head with the body and eyes, its connections quickly becomes very complex and difficult. Figure 10.27 presents some of the components controlling eye movements. You will investigate eye movements in a later chapter (only the abducens and oculomotor nuclei are shown). Here, focus on the vestibular circuitry controlling eye movements. Draw the axonal projections, starting in the vestibular labyrinth. The vestibular apparatus sends axons to the cerebellum both directly and indirectly through the vestibular nuclei. The vestibular nuclei act as the deep cerebellar nuclei, since they receive the output directly from the cerebellar cortex.

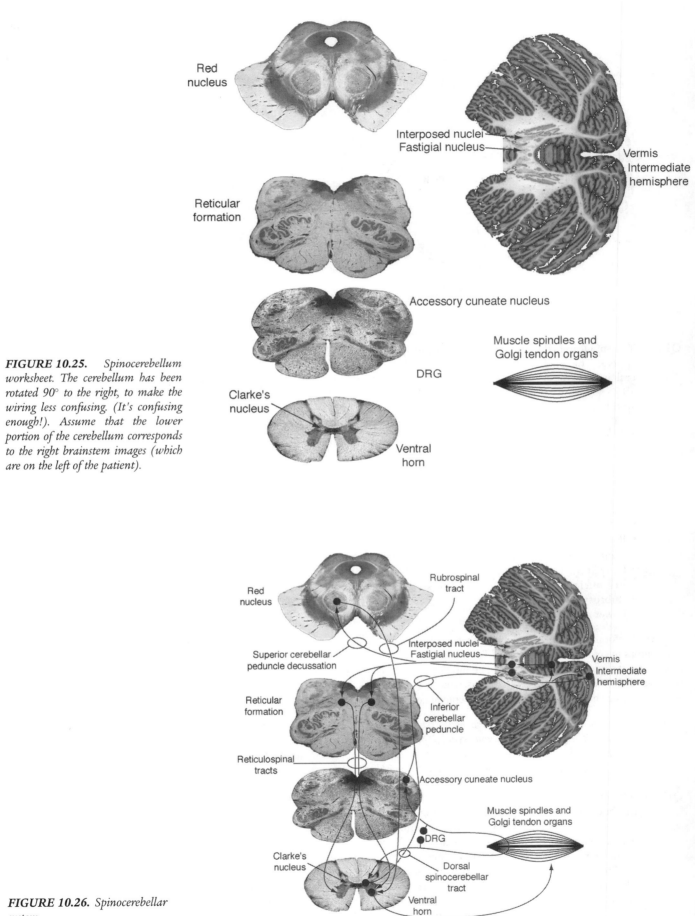

Red
nucleus

Interposed nuclei
Fastigial nucleus

Vermis
Intermediate
hemisphere

Reticular
formation

Accessory cuneate nucleus

Muscle spindles and
Golgi tendon organs

DRG

Clarke's
nucleus

Ventral
horn

FIGURE 10.25. *Spinocerebellum worksheet. The cerebellum has been rotated 90° to the right, to make the wiring less confusing. (It's confusing enough!). Assume that the lower portion of the cerebellum corresponds to the right brainstem images (which are on the left of the patient).*

Red
nucleus

Rubrospinal
tract

Interposed nuclei
Fastigial nucleus

Vermis
Intermediate
hemisphere

Superior cerebellar
peduncle decussation

Reticular
formation

Inferior
cerebellar
peduncle

Reticulospinal
tracts

Accessory cuneate nucleus

Muscle spindles and
Golgi tendon organs

DRG

Clarke's
nucleus

Dorsal
spinocerebellar
tract

Ventral
horn

FIGURE 10.26. *Spinocerebellar system.*

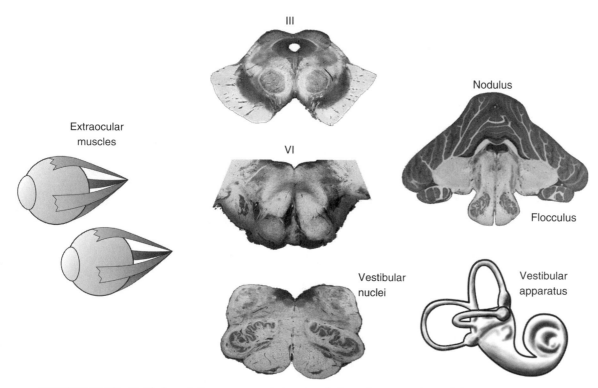

FIGURE 10.27. *Vestibulocerebellar system worksheet (vestibulo-ocular connections only).*

A10.20. See Figure 10.28. You should probably feel "Uhhhh! This is absurd!" These wiring diagrams quickly become ridiculously complicated. Figure 10.28 is really a very simplified view (real anatomists are probably shuddering at its inaccuracies). The essence here is that a small region of the cerebellum is essential for eye movements and balance.

Similar to other parts of the nervous system that require bilateral coordination, vestibular projections regulating eye movements use interneurons and gaze control centers in the pons and midbrain to control the extraocular muscles.

Q10.21. As the final wiring diagram (Fig. 10.29), show the interconnections of the olivocerebellar system. This system is presented separately, since different parts of the

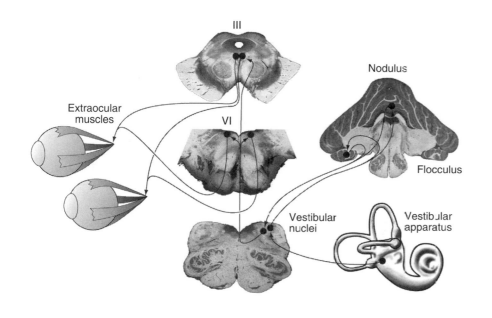

FIGURE 10.28. *Vestibulocerebellar system, showing only simplified vestibulo-ocular connections.*

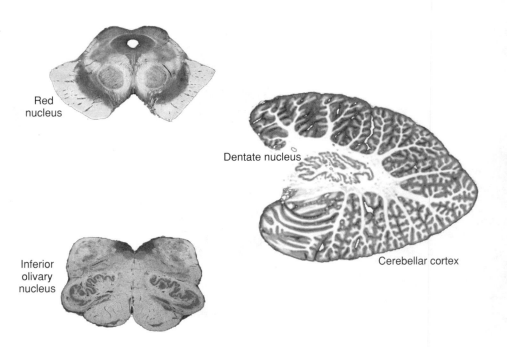

FIGURE 10.29. *Olivocerebellum worksheet.*

inferior olivary complex regulate the different functional divisions of the cerebellum. At least in this figure, it is simpler than the others! However, remember that the olivary neurons have a unique and cozy relationship with the cerebellar cortical output Purkinje neurons.

A10.21. See Figure 10.30. This "triangle" (Mollaret's triangle) is at least simpler than the other circuits. It is sobering to realize that we don't understand what the inferior olive does, although evidence points to a role in cerebellar learning and timing.

Q10.22. What important tract lies just medial to the dorsal spinocerebellar tract in the spinal cord? Why is this clinically relevant?

A10.22 The corticospinal tract is just medial to the spinocerebellar tract. Since nearly all conceivable injuries to the spinocerebellar tract would also involve the corticospinal system, the pyramidal symptomatology would overwhelm any clinical cerebellar deficit.

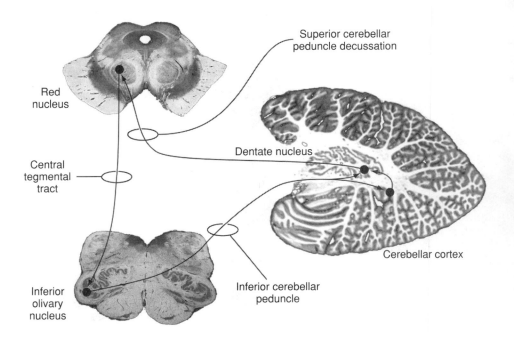

FIGURE 10.30. *Olivocerebellar connections.*

It is very unusual for any specific disease process to pick one of these tracts in isolation. For example, most injuries that would affect the ascending dorsal spinocerebellar tract would also affect the descending corticospinal tract; the latter would clinically dominate. Therefore we do not hear much about the spinocerebellar tracts clinically despite their importance in maintaining coordination of movement.

HIGHER COGNITIVE FUNCTIONS

We have emphasized the cerebellum's involvement in the control of posture and movement, but it is important to realize that it also makes less well understood contributions to several cognitive aspects of behavior. These "higher order" roles of the cerebellum are an active area of brain research. Consider two examples that we present below. The first is a case of a patient with a cerebellar hemispheric lesion, and the second is an fMRI study of subjects performing cognitive tasks.

Case 1: Cerebellar Hemispheric Infarction

(Reported by J. A. Fiez et al., Brain, 115: 155–78, 1992)

The patient was a 49-year-old lawyer with a history of hypertension, who presented with a sudden onset of nausea, vomiting, and vertigo, in addition to a loss of motor control. On neurological exam he had diminished tone of the right arm and was ataxic for finger to nose touching on the right. In addition the right pupil was smaller than the left.

Q10.23. Examine the image shown in Figure 10.31. Where is the lesion? Be specific as to side and functional regions.

A10.23. *The lesion is primarily on the right, involving both the hemisphere and some vermis and intermediate lobe regions. The largest area involved is the cerebrocerebellum (hemispheres), although spinocerebellum and vestibulocerebellum are also involved (clinically and neuroanatomically!)*

Q10.24. What vascular territory does the lesion represent?

A10.24. *The lesion is in the distribution of the right posterior inferior cerebellar artery (PICA).*

Six months after his stroke, the patient had largely recovered from his major motor deficits and the vertigo. Both he and his wife noticed that his speech included semantic paraphasic errors ("slips of the tongue"). Cognitive testing revealed that while he displayed excellent intelligence, memory and language skills, he had significant deficits in practice-related learning, and in detecting errors in his performance on tests.

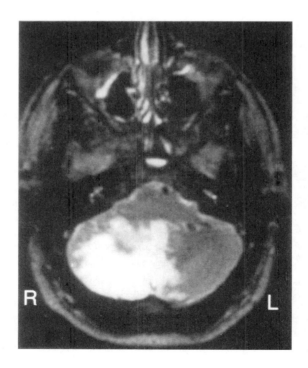

FIGURE 10.31. *MRI of patient. (Modified from Fiez et al., 1992. Brain, 115: 155–178).*

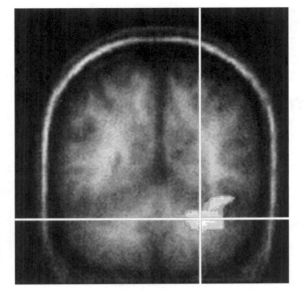

FIGURE 10.32. *Averaged responses for fMRI on 8 subjects doing tasks involving changes in timing. The demarcated gray-to-white area in the cerebellum represents the averaged signals, with white the highest intensity (converted from original color data). (Modified from The roles of the cerebellum and basal ganglia in timing and error prediction, Dreher, J.-C. and Grafman, J., 2002. European Journal of Neuroscience 16: 1609–1619.)*

Case 2: Cerebellar Activation during Timing Tasks

(Reported in J.C. Dreher and J. Grafman, Eur. J. Neurosci., 16: 1609–1619, 2002)

Q10.25. Examine the fMRI imge shown in Figure 10.32. This represents the average change in neural activity for a group of subjects who were performing simple cognitive tasks. In this case the subjects performed two tasks involving letters. In one task they had to determine if a letter was a consonant or vowel, and in the other, whether the letter was upper or lower case. The different tasks were presented to the subjects either in a predictable order or in a random fashion, and the timing between presentation of each new letter was either uniform or irregular. First, where do you see signal?

A10.25. *The signal is present in the left dentate nucleus and cerebellar hemisphere. Some also seems to spread into the adjacent occipital lobe.*

Q10.26. The authors found that the posterior cerebellar hemisphere and dentate nucleus were activated specifically when the timing between tasks was irregular. What does this suggest about the role of the cerebellum?

A10.26. *The authors suggested that the cerebrocerebellum was involved in functions requiring timing adjustments during the cognitive tests.*

CLINICAL CASES

Case 1: Epilepsy and Phenytoin

Q10.27. A 47-year-old woman had severe mental retardation and seizures since childhood. She had been on phenytoin therapy for many years, and occasionally had developed toxicity from the drug. Figure 10.33 shows a portion of her cerebellum. Where is the pathology? Compare this with Figure 10.1, if necessary. Suggest what symptoms she may have had.

A10.27. *The patient's inferior cerebellum is whiter, more sclerotic, than her superior portion. Microscopically it contained no Purkinje neurons and the molecular layer was shrunken. This atrophy extends into the vermis medially, although the nodulus (most medial part, beneath the dentate nucleus) seems to be spared. The patient required a walker to ambulate. When tested, her gait was wide-based. She also has some limb ataxia, although detailed testing could not be done because of her severe mental retardation.*

Case 2: Alcoholism

The patient was a 52-year-old man who had been institutionalized for uncontrolled behavior. He had been an alcoholic and had symptoms of Wernicke-Korsakoff's syndrome. In addition to his behavioral problems (pulling fire alarms, abusing nurses), he also had a wide-based gait and marked limb ataxia.

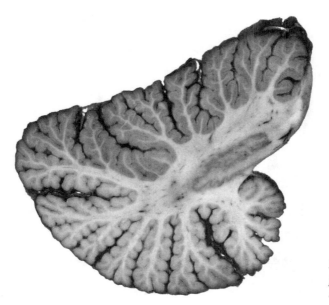

FIGURE 10.33. *Cerebellum from a patient with epilepsy since childhood and chronic phenytoin therapy.*

Q10.28. Where is the most prominent pathology in Figure 10.34? How can you tell? What signs developed from just this pathology?

A10.28. The patient's cerebellar vermis is atrophic, especially the rostral or anterior vermis. The folia are more separated in this region, indicating loss of cells and neuropil. This region of the cerebellum helps control axial stability. Lesions here produce a wide-based gait and postural instability.

Case 3: Cerebellar Hemorrhage

The patient is a 55-year-old woman. She called her doctor to report a sense of dizziness and nausea. She found that as she looks rightward objects appeared to become vertically separated. For example, when she was driving she saw two trucks come into view when they approached from the right side. When she closed her eyes while standing she found herself falling toward the right.

On examination, she had nystagmus on right gaze, slight vertical separation of the visual axes on the right, and some numbness on the left face on testing with light touch. Her gait was unsteady. On finger-to-nose testing her right arm was unsteady.

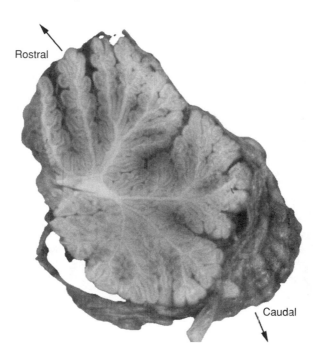

Rostral

Caudal

FIGURE 10.34. *Alcoholic cerebellar degeneration.*

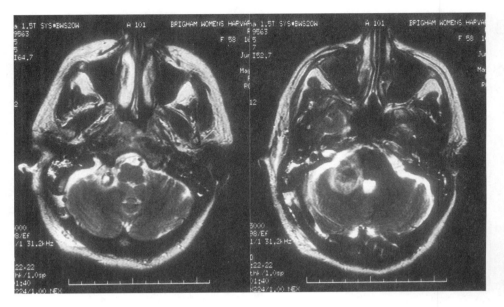

FIGURE 10.35. *Case axial MRI scans.*

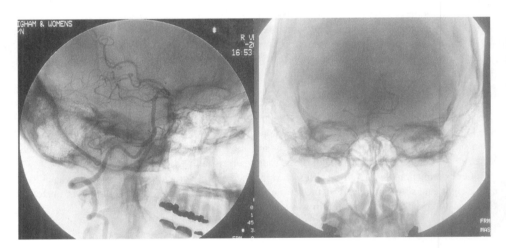

FIGURE 10.36. *Nonsubtracted posterior circulation angiograms. Left is lateral and right is anterior-posterior.*

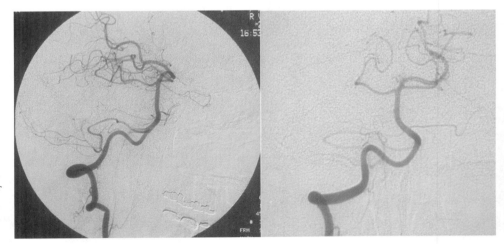

FIGURE 10.37. *Angiogram of posterior circulation following injection of the right vertebral artery. The left image is a lateral view, while the right is an anterior-posterior view.*

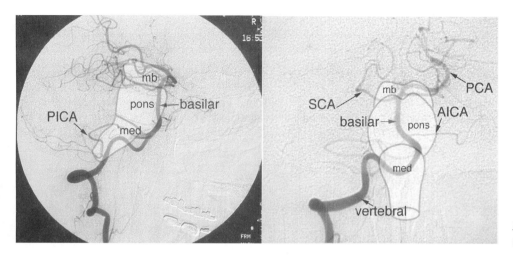

FIGURE 10.38. *Posterior circulation and brainstem regions.*

Q10.29. Examine her brain MRI in Figure 10.35. Try to predict where the abnormality was located, left or right? Above the tentorium or below? If below, is it within the nervous system or outside causing external compression? Are any cranial nerves affected?

A10.29. *The scan shows a complex lesion of the right lateral cerebellum, very near the cerebellopontine angle. It is intra-axial (within the brain parenchyma), rounded, and hemorrhagic. Nerves arising from this site include the facial, vestibular, and cochlear nerves. The trigeminal nerve also arises from the body of the pons.*

The appearance suggested an aneurysm coming off the posterior inferior cerebellar artery (PICA), so an angiogram was performed by injecting one vertebral artery with contrast. Figure 10.36 is the raw data, without surrounding structures subtracted away. This is to orient you.

Q10.30. Figure 10.37 illustrates the posterior circulation. The image on the left is a lateral view, while the image on the right is an anterior-posterior view. Try to locate the following structures:
- Vertebral artery
- Basilar artery
- Posterior cerebral arteries
- Branches off the basilar; which are they?

Based on their vascular supply, also find where the following structures lie in Figure 10.37:
- Medulla
- Pons
- Midbrain

Do any of the vessels supply the cerebellum?

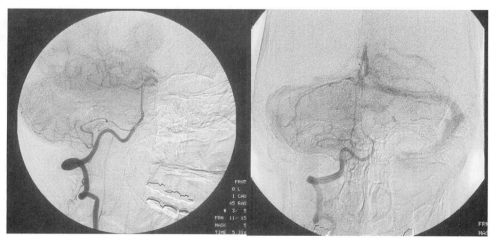

FIGURE 10.39. *Angiogram at a later time point than in Figure 10.38.*

A10.30. The major arteries and parts of the brainstem are indicated in Figure 10.38. Figure 10.39 is similar to Figure 10.38, except that the dye has had a longer time to distribute. You can now see that the cerebellum is supplied by the vessels, since it is outlined by the blush of contrast.

The patient underwent an operation. At surgery the meninges were stained a yellowish-brown color, indicating old hemorrhage. Within the cerebellum was a plum-colored recent hemorrhage, which was evacuated. The patient did well. This hemorrhage likely was the result of a small cavernous vascular anomaly. The lesion did not fill with contrast during the angiogram, which is typical of this malformation.

Chapter 11—BRAINSTEM AND CONTROL SYSTEMS

As a mud-sucking, early vertebrate, life was simple. You basically had to keep your mouth down and your simple eyes up. All you really needed was a brainstem. You needed a vestibular system to tell you if you were pointed the right way. No need to move your eyes too much, since they just pointed upward in the murky water, looking for possible threats to your life. Now, you are a land vertebrate, walking, bending over to look for food, fighting over your mate, swinging through trees, and reading from neuroanatomy texts. Eye movements, balance, blood pressure regulation, respiration, and many other functions have all become much more complicated. You really don't want to either miss the branch and fall to the leopard or swing into the tree as you glide through the forest. However, the control system of eye movements and other basic body functions evolved from that simple fishlike organism, and much of these control systems remain in your original brain, the brainstem.

The subject of these next two laboratories is the most complicated anatomic area for the budding neurologist. In the brainstem lie structures vital to your existence, packed together with little extra room. What is confusing to the novice about the brainstem is its apparent disregard for any logical organization. For example, pain fibers from the face enter the middle of the brainstem in the pons and then descend down into the upper cervical cord, while those for proprioception remain in the pons. Nearby the extremely important "spinal trigeminal" area is the most aesthetic area of the brainstem, the inferior olivary nucleus, wonderfully developed in humans but with little known clinical significance. Although this city and seaport of the brain does indeed have a structure, to appreciate it, like string theory in physics, requires a lifetime of study.

In this chapter you will initially review the external anatomy and circulation of the brainstem, and then study a few specific systems operating in its divisions. In the next chapter you will focus on brainstem structure, and then, like Humpty Dumpty, try to put it back together again by investigating the cranial nerves.

Know that the purpose of examining histologic sections is not to make you neuroanatomists, but to help you remember what these areas of brain do and a bit how they all fit together.

Functional Neuroanatomy: An Interactive Text and Manual, by Jeffrey T. Joseph and David L. Cardozo
ISBN 0-471-44437-5 Copyright © 2004 John Wiley & Sons, Inc.

LEARNING OBJECTIVES

- Correlate the macroscopic anatomy of the brainstem to its adjacent bone and brain structures.
- Detail the salient aspects of the brainstem circulation.
- Recognize main levels of the brainstem and important structures at those levels.
- Describe brainstem controls of eye movements.
- Discuss the diffuse systems within the brainstem.

INTRODUCTION

Divisions of the Brainstem

The three main rostrocaudal regions of the brainstem are the midbrain, pons, and medulla. Cranial nerves are associated with each part. Also each part is associated with one of the three cerebellar peduncles: superior (midbrain), middle (pons), and inferior (medulla). These three regions of the brainstem have a ventral base, a surface (or integument) dorsal to the base termed the tegmentum, and in the midbrain, a roof named the tectum. The long tracts connecting the cerebral hemispheres and spinal cord generally run in the ventral layer and the cranial nerve nuclei are found in the tegmentum. The tectum (or roof), which is dorsal to the aqueduct, contains the paired superior and inferior colliculi.

Relationship to the Skull

Over half a billion years of evolution we have taken our simple body plan and created confusion, which you must learn. Exits of the cranial nerves from the skull are examples of this process (see Fig. 11.1). There is, however, some logic to it: The olfactory bulbs, overlying the olfactory nerves, lie on top of the cribriform plate. The optic nerves exit through the optic canal. Cranial nerves 3, 4, and 6, which regulate eye movement, and the first division of 5 (the ophthalmic division of the trigeminal) all go through the superior orbital fissure. The second and third divisions of the trigeminal exit more posteriorly, through the foramen rotundum and foramen ovale, respectively. Cranial nerves 7 (facial) and 8 (vestibular and cochlear) exit through the internal auditory meatus and travel through the petrous bone. Cranial nerves 9, 10 (swallowing and neck muscles and parasympathetic fibers), and 11 (outer neck muscles) go through the jugular foramen (the accessory nerve, cranial nerve 11, having first entered the skull through the foramen magnum). Finally, cranial nerve 12 regulating the tongue exits via the hypoglossal foramen. Thus successively lower groups of cranial nerves exit at successively more caudal locations in the skull. The spinal cord exits through the foramen magnum.

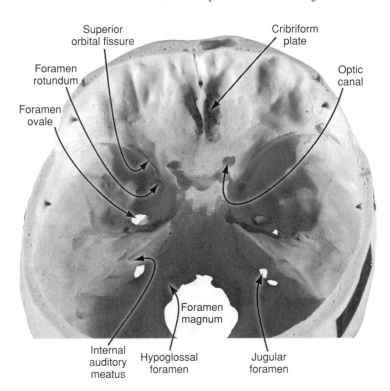

FIGURE 11.1. Base of skull.

Summary of Brainstem Functions

Below is a summary of clinically important brainstem functions, listed by region. These will be reviewed extensively during this and subsequent chapters. The short summary is to get you oriented.

Midbrain

- Cranial nerve 3 (including parasympathetics) Pupillary constriction; adduction, elevation, and depression of the eyes; eyelid elevation; control of vertical gaze.
- Parts of the reticular "activating" system, essential for consciousness.
- Parts of the motor system, including the red nucleus and the substantia nigra.

Pons

- Cranial nerve 6 and horizontal gaze centers.
- Corneal reflexes (cranial nerves 5, 7) (corneal reflexes also affected by descending tract of cranial nerve 5 in medulla).
- Motor functions of jaw (cranial nerve 5) and face (cranial nerve 7).
- Touch sensation on face (cranial nerve 5, main sensory nucleus).

Medulla

- Vestibular function (important for control of eye movements while moving head).
- Hearing functions (cranial nerve 8, near pontomedullary junction).
- Pain/temperature on face (descending tract and nucleus of cranial nerve 5).
- Pharyngeal and laryngeal functions (cranial nerves 9 and 10).
- Motor functions of tongue (cranial nerve 12).

Diffuse Systems

The term "diffuse systems" applies to several neurotransmitter networks that project diffusely throughout the brain. Usually, only the small neurotransmitters dopamine, norepinepherine, serotonin, histamine, and acetylcholine are included in this concept, although certainly other, larger peptides such as metenkephalin can also have more "diffuse" projections.

The major origins and projections for the diffuse systems are well understood; however, the actual functions of a given system are more subtle. For example, you have witnessed the importance of dopamine in the control of movement. But the actions of this transmitter are not so simple; a major side effect of drugs used to treat Parkinson's disease is psychosis. Dopamine is important for addictive behaviors. These examples point to the more diffuse actions of dopamine, actions that are not well explained by a simplified basal ganglia wiring diagram. In addition to having widespread projections, the diffuse systems also have multifaceted functions.

Details about these transmitters are important since they are major drug targets. Aside from monosodium glutamate (MSG), few agents are designed to interact with glutaminergic transmission. In contrast, medications created to modify serotonin transmission have alleviated depression in many people and enriched drug company shareholders. Yet because of the other roles of serotonin, these medication often have "side effects," such as sleepiness. At times the side effects themselves may also be useful.

You will encounter these transmitter systems multiple times throughout your career. This laboratory will scratch the surface. Its purpose is to impart a sense for their neuroanatomic basis and functions.

Vasculature

The brainstem derives its circulation from the vertebral artery system. These two arteries, arising off the subclavian arteries, follow a tortuous path through the transverse foramina of the cervical vertebral column and then travel through the foramen magnum. Before they join, they give off the long and vulnerable *posterior-inferior cerebellar arteries* (PICA), which supply the rostral dorsolateral medulla and inferior cerebellum. At their confluence near the pontomedullary junction, they form the *basilar artery.* This unpaired artery gives off a series of vessels that either penetrate the brainstem directly or travel around it some distance before entering its substance. The largest of these circumferential arteries is the *anterior-inferior cerebellar artery* (AICA), which feeds the dorsolateral pons and ventral portions of the cerebellum. Around the pontomesencephalic (pons-midbrain) junction, the basilar feeds the superior cerebellar arteries shortly before ending at the origin of the

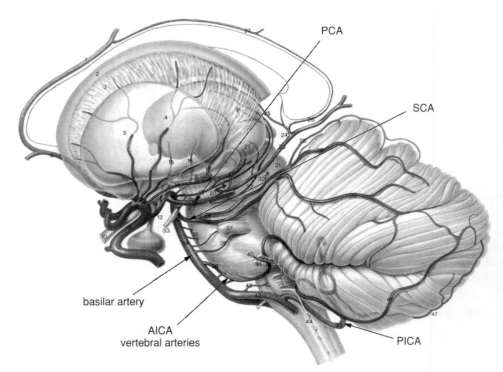

FIGURE 11.2. Posterior fossa circulation. (Modified from Nieuwenhuys, Voogd, van Huijzen, The Human Central Nervous System. A Synopsis and Atlas. 3rd edition. © 1988. Springer-Verlag, Berlin, figure 40, page 44.)

posterior cerebral arteries at the top of the brainstem. As you can imagine, these vessels are clinically extremely important and also lend themselves to many questions for students. See Figure 11.2.

Schedule (2.5 hours)
20 Regional anatomy
20 Macroscopic anatomy
10 Vasculature
30 Histology
30 Eye movements
30 Diffuse systems
10 Case: Multiple sclerosis

REGIONAL ANATOMY

Q11.1. Examine the gross brainstem specimen and Figure 11.3. Try to identify the following structures:
- Basilar artery
- Inferior olivary nucleus
- Pyramids
- Superior colliculus
- Inferior colliculus
- Superior, middle, and inferior cerebellar peduncles
- IVth ventricle

Also identify external cranial nerves:
- Oculomotor nerve (III)
- Trochlear nerve (IV)
- Trigeminal nerve (V)
- Abducens nerve (VI)
- Facial nerve (VII)
- Vestibulocochlear nerve (VIII)
- Glossopharyngeal nerve (IX) and vagus nerve (X)
- Hypoglossal nerve (XII)

A11.1. See Figure 11.4.

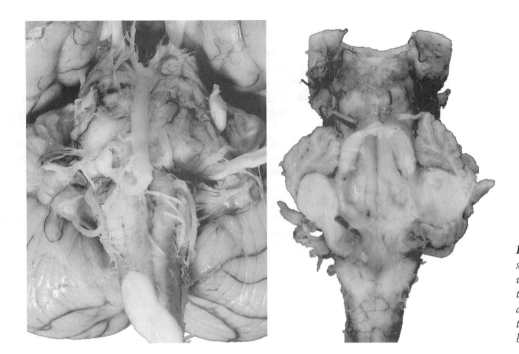

FIGURE 11.3. Brainstem worksheet. The left panel is a ventral view with the brainstem still attached to the cerebellum and brain. To view the dorsal brainstem in the right panel, the cerebrum and cerebellum have been removed.

External Features

Q11.2. If it is available, turn to a model of the brainstem. You should be able to figure out front from back. Locate the midbrain, pons, and medulla, then find their corresponding cerebellar connections. Also find the pyramids and inferior olivary nuclear bulge on the surface of the medulla and the cerebral peduncles (aliases include crux cerebri and pedunculus cerebri) in the midbrain. Next identify the cranial nerve roots. Use your atlas as a guide. Describe where the oculomotor nerves exit the brain. Compare these to the abducens and trochlear nerves. Anything unusual? Notice the size and location of the trigeminal nerve.

A11.2. The **oculomotor nerves** exit the bottom of the midbrain just medial to the cerebral peduncles. These nerves, along with the **abducens** and **trochlear,** all exit just off of midline. However, the trochlear nerve, just to trick students, is located on the dorsal rather than the ventral surface and has the second distinction of crossing before exiting.

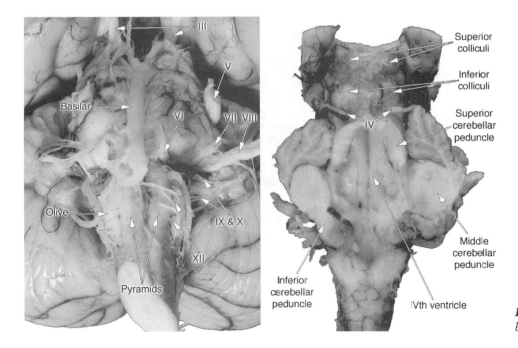

FIGURE 11.4. Salient external brainstem structures.

Q11.3. Distinguish the facial, vestibular, and cochlear nerves? What is the site called where they exit the brain?

A11.3. *The seventh and eighth nerves exit the brainstem as a bundle off the* **cerebellopontine angle** *(CPA). While textbooks usually illustrate them as easily distinguishable, reality is more difficult, especially when you consider that this complex actually contains four nerves:* **facial nerve, nervus intermedius** *(taste),* **vestibular nerve,** *and* **cochlear nerve.** *The facial/intermediate nerve occupies a position slightly more medial and superior than the vestibulocochlear complex.*

Q11.4. Compare the exit of the *hypoglossal nerve* with that of the *vagus* and *glossopharyngeal* nerves. What structure lies between them? From where does the spinal accessory nerve originate? Use Figure 11.5 to guide you.

A11.4. *The glossopharyngeal and vagus nerves exit the brainstem lateral to the inferior olivary nucleus bulge on the rostral medulla, while the hypoglossal exits between the olive and the pyramid column. The accessory nerve originates in the upper cervical spinal cord, travels through the foramen magnum, and then catches up and exits with the ninth and tenth nerves.*

Q11.5. Now that you have sharpened your skills on plastic, try the real thing. Locate as many cranial nerve roots on a human brain as you can. Available brains will have been removed with varying levels of skill, and so will show variation in what remains of the cranial nerves. Try to locate on a brain the glossopharyngeal and vagus nerves. Notice how fine they are. How well can you distinguish between them?

A11.5. *The glossopharyngeal and vagus nerves both arise lateral to the inferior olivary nucleus as multiple fine fibers. Really the only way to distinguish them is to note that the glossopharyngeal nerve lies rostral to the vagal complex.*

Appreciate on the real specimen just how compact the brainstem is. You can later contrast this compactness with the luxurious estate that is the cerebral cortex.

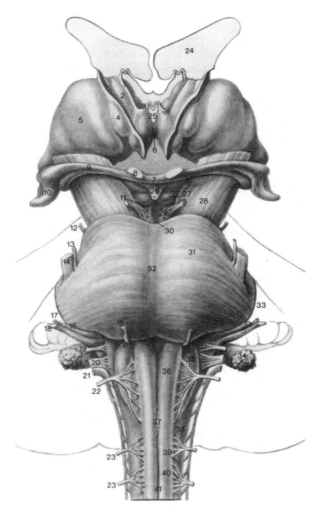

FIGURE 11.5. *Ventral brainstem and thalamus. (Modified from Nieuwenhuys, Voogd, van Huijzen, The Human Central Nervous System. A Synopsis and Atlas. 3rd edition. © 1988. Springer-Verlag, Berlin, figure 17, page 22.)*

Relationship to Skull

Q11.6. Using the human brain and human skull, locate the exit foramina of the cranial nerves (whether they are on the brain or not). Name the exit sites for the different cranial nerves. Carefully insert a pipe cleaner through the holes to determine the exit holes. (Some sections of skull are paper thin and can easily be punctured or fractured by a vigorous pipe cleaner.) Complete Table 11.1. Give at least one function or activity of the cranial nerve.

A11.6. *See Table 11.2. The additional information that you may not yet know will be useful later and in the next laboratory.*

MACROSCOPIC ANATOMY

Q11.7. Cut the half brainstem from the previous laboratory into close (every 3–4 mm) transverse sections. Using an atlas for assistance, identify grossly and in Figure 11.6:
- Inferior olivary nucleus
- Pyramids and their decussation
- Inferior cerebellar peduncle
- Basis pontis
- Pontine tegmentum
- Exit of cranial nerve V
- Exit of cranial nerve III
- Middle cerebellar peduncle

TABLE 11.1. Cranial Nerve and Skull Worksheet

Nerve Number	Name	Exit	Function
1			
2			
3			
4			
5a part			
5b part			
5c part			
6			
7			
8v part			
8c part			
9			
10			
11			
12			

TABLE 11.2. Cranial Nerve Exits and Functions

Nerve Number	Name	Exit	Additional Information (Afferent and Efferent)
1	Olfactory nerve and tract	Cribriform plate	Afferent olfactory (nerve only travels from sinus to bulb; olfactory tract is what you see on the brain)
2	Optic nerve	Optic canal	Afferent visual from retina (not a nerve at all, but an extension of the brain)
3	Oculomotor	Superior orbital fissure	Efferent motor to eye (medial, superior, and inferior rectus muscles and inferior oblique muscle, levator palpebrae) Efferent parasympathetic to eye (pupillary constriction)
4	Trochlear	Superior orbital fissure	Efferent motor to superior oblique muscle
5a	Ophthalmic branch	Superior orbital fissure	Afferent sensory from upper face, including cornea (forehead, upper eyelid, cornea, conjunctiva, dorsum of nose, nasal membranes)
5b	Maxillary branch	Foramen rotundum	Afferent sensory from middle portion of face and upper jaw (upper lip, lateral nose, upper cheek, anterior temple, membranes of nose, upper jaw and teeth, roof of mouth)
5c	Mandibular branch	Foramen ovale	Efferent motor to muscles of mastication Afferent sensory to lower face and jaw (lower lip, chin, posterior cheek, temple, external ear, lower jaw and teeth, cheeks, floor of mouth, anterior two thirds of tongue)
6	Abducens	Superior orbital fissure	Efferent motor to lateral rectus
7	Facial	Internal auditory meatus	Efferent motor to superficial facial muscles and stapedius (also posterior belly of digastric muscle) Efferent parasympathetic fibers (lacrimal and salivary glands) Afferent gustatory (taste) from anterior tongue Afferent sensory from portion of external ear skin
8v	Vestibular nerve	Internal auditory meatus	Afferent vestibular information from labyrinth
8c	Cochlear nerve	Internal auditory meatus	Afferent auditory information from cochlea
9	Glossopharyngeal nerve	Jugular foramen	Efferent motor to pharynx skeletal muscle Efferent parasympathetic fibers to parotid gland Afferent sensory from portion of external ear skin Afferent sensory from pharynx, middle ear, carotid body and sinus Afferent gustatory from posterior tongue
10	Vagus nerve	Jugular foramen	Efferent motor to striated muscle of palate, pharynx, larynx Efferent parasympathetic fibers to viscera Afferent sensory from portion of external ear skin, meninges Afferent sensory from larynx, trachea, gut, aortic arch Afferent taste from larynx
11	Accessory nerve	Jugular foramen	Efferent motor to sternocleidomastoid and trapezius
12	Hypoglossal	Hypoglossal canal	Efferent motor to tongue (intrinsic and extrinsic)

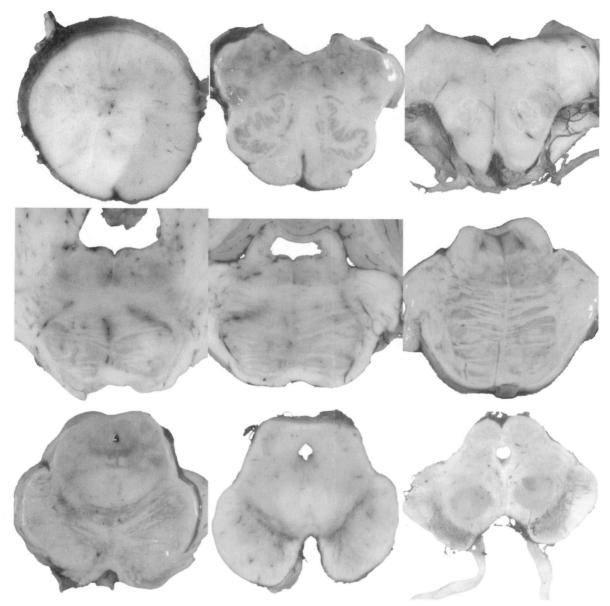

FIGURE 11.6. *Gross brainstem worksheet. These are not drawn to scale and do not all come from the same brain.*

- Superior cerebellar peduncle and its decussation
- Cerebral peduncles
- Cerebral aqueduct
- Locus ceruleus
- Substantia nigra
- Red nucleus

A11.7. *See Figure 11.7.*

VASCULATURE

Q11.8. The Figure 11.8 is an angiogram of the posterior circulation, taken at two time points. In this figure, label:
- Vertebral artery
- Basilar artery
- Posterior inferior cerebellar (PICA)

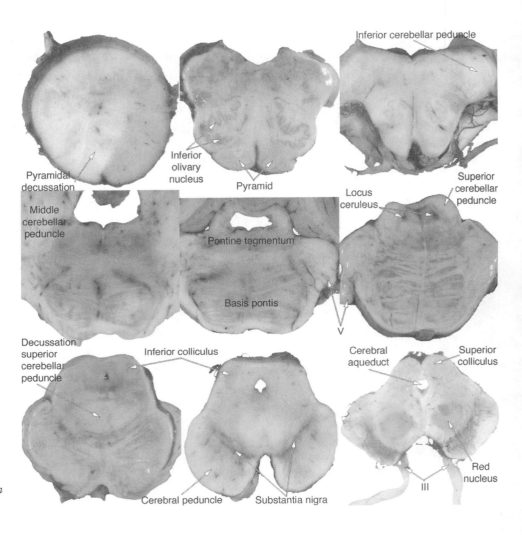

FIGURE 11.7. *Salient structures in gross brainstem dissection.*

- Anterior inferior cerebellar (AICA)
- Superior cerebellar (SCA)
- Posterior cerebral arteries

What is happening at the large arrowhead? Why do you only see one vertebral artery?

A11.8. See Figure 11.9. *The vertebral artery leaves the intervertebral foramen and curves medially at the arrow before entering the foramen magnum. Only one vertebral artery is imaged, since*

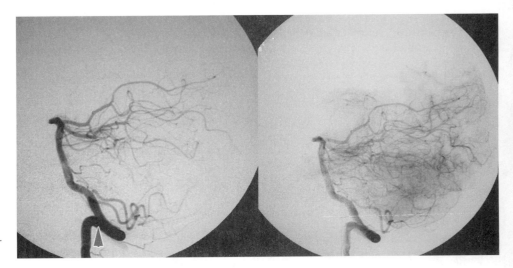

FIGURE 11.8. *Vertebral artery angiogram at two points in time.*

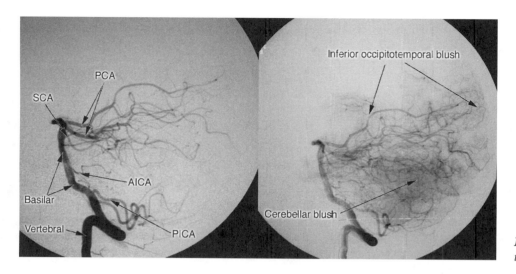

FIGURE 11.9. Posterior circulation.

it was the only one injected! The flow travels upward from the heart, so you don t see the other vertebral artery. The cerebellar blush is derived principally from the PICA and SCA, with some contribution of the AICA. The inferior temporal and occipital lobe blush is derived from the PCA.

In some circumstances, especially with a blockage of the artery below (proximal), you may see retrograde flow into the opposite vertebral artery.

BRAINSTEM HISTOLOGY

INST In the next set of exercises, use histologic slides of the brainstem (medulla, pons, midbrain) and Figure 11.10 to identify and trace components of different neuroanatomic systems. You may want to use different color pencils on the figure to separate each system. Note that many of these sites occur at only a restricted level of the brainstem, and may not be present on your particular histologic slides (although they are present in Fig. 11.10). You will, however, remember them better if you first suffer with the glass slides!

Q11.9. In Figure 11.10, find the components of the medial lemniscal system:
- Gracilis and cuneatus nuclei
- Arcuate fibers
- Medial lemniscus in all sections
- Trigeminal principal sensory nucleus (restricted level)

A11.9. *See Figure 11.11.*

Q11.10. Similarly, find the major components of the auditory system:
- Cochlear nuclei (restricted level)
- Superior olivary nucleus
- Lateral lemniscus
- Inferior colliculus (restricted level)

A11.10. *See Figure 11.12.*

Q11.11. Find brainstem components associated with the cerebellum:
- Inferior, middle, and superior cerebellar peduncles
- Inferior olivary nucleus
- Accessory cuneate nucleus (restricted level)
- Vestibular nuclei
- Basis pontis
- Decussation of superior cerebellar peduncle (restricted level)
- Red nucleus (restricted level)

A11.11. *See Figure 11.13.*

Q11.12. Find brainstem components controlling neck and face muscles:
- Hypoglossal nucleus and exit fibers
- Nucleus ambiguus (well-named)

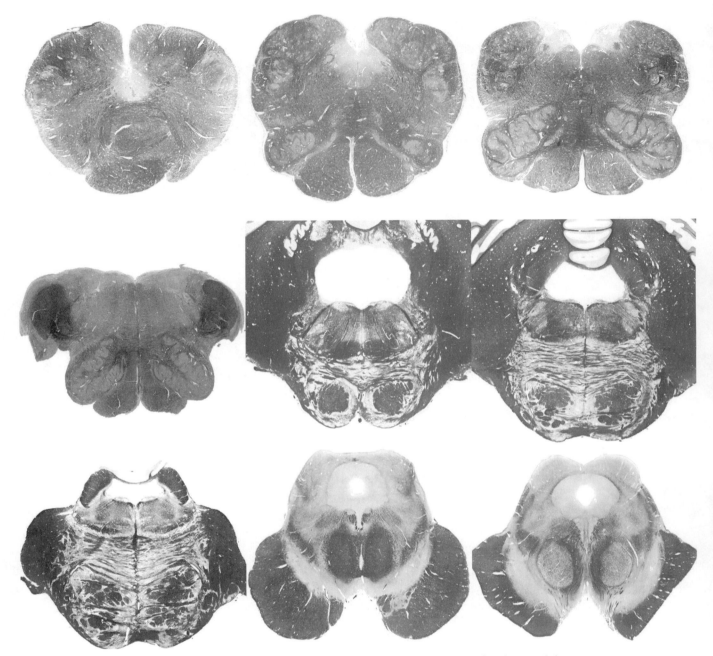

FIGURE 11.10. *Brainstem histology worksheet.*

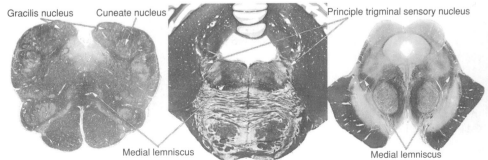

FIGURE 11.11. *Medial lemniscal system.*

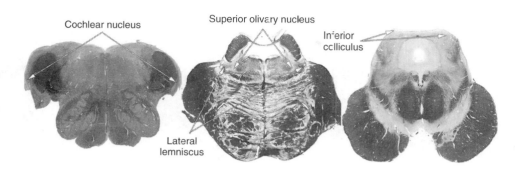

Cochlear nucleus

Superior olivary nucleus

Inferior colliculus

Lateral lemniscus

FIGURE 11.12. *Brainstem audi-tory system.*

- Facial nucleus and its fibers (restricted level)
- Trigeminal motor nucleus (restricted level)

A11.12. See Figure 11.14.

Q11.13. Find brainstem components involved in controlling eye movements:
- Medial longitudinal fasciculus (mlf) in all levels
- Vestibular nuclear complex
- Abducens nucleus (VI) and paramedian pontine reticular formation (PPRF, basi-cally the neurons just medial to the VI nucleus, restricted level)
- Trochlear nucleus (IV, restricted level)
- Oculomotor nucleus (III)
- Superior colliculus (restricted level)
- Posterior commissure (present only in the highest sections of midbrain; best seen on sagittal sections of brain, just below the pineal)

A11.13. See Figure 11.15.

Q11.14. Use your atlas to identify components of the anterolateral pain and temperature system:
- Ascending fibers throughout the medulla
- Spinal trigeminal tract
- Spinal trigeminal nucleus
- Periaqueductal gray

A11.14. See Figure 11.16.

Q11.15. Find some of the components of the autonomic control systems:
- Solitary tract and nucleus
- Lateral medullary reticular formation

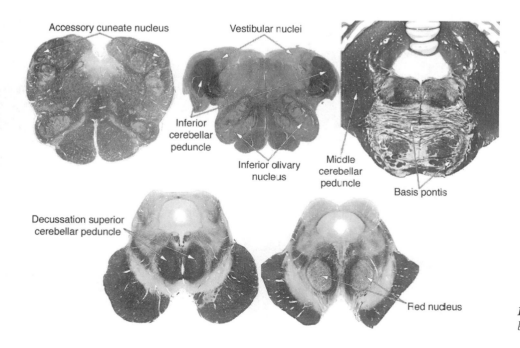

Accessory cuneate nucleus

Vestibular nuclei

Inferior cerebellar peduncle

Inferior olivary nucleus

Middle cerebellar peduncle

Basis pontis

Decussation superior cerebellar peduncle

Red nucleus

FIGURE 11.13. *Brainstem cere-bellar components.*

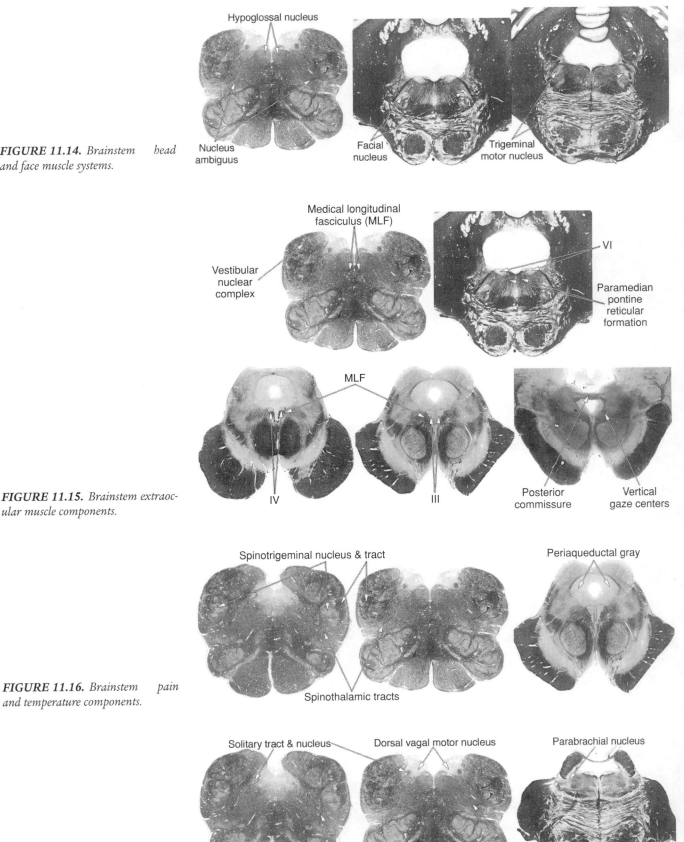

FIGURE 11.14. *Brainstem head and face muscle systems.*

FIGURE 11.15. *Brainstem extraocular muscle components.*

FIGURE 11.16. *Brainstem pain and temperature components.*

FIGURE 11.17. *Brainstem autonomic centers.*

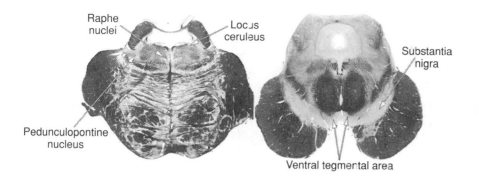

FIGURE 11.18. Brainstem diffuse projection systems.

- Dorsal motor nucleus of the vagus (X)
- Parabrachial nucleus (in pons, medial to the brachium conjunctivum or superior cerebellar peduncle)

A11.15. *See Figure 11.17.*

Q11.16. Last but not least, identify four components of the diffusely projecting systems:
- Locus ceruleus ("blue locus") (norepinepherine)
- Raphe nucleus (serotonin) (midline in the medulla and pons)
- Substantia nigra (dopamine)
- Pedunculopontine nucleus (acetylcholine) (this one is hard; it is in the highest pons, around the base of the superior cerebellar peduncle—don't look too long!)

A11.16. *See Figure 11.18.*

CONTROL SYSTEMS

This chapter discusses two control systems involving the brainstem: the extraocular muscle system and two diffuse systems. Other chapters will discuss the brainstem autonomic controls and other diffuse systems. All of these systems have important interactions with and connections to other brain regions. However, it is in the brainstem that much of their activity originates.

Eye Movements

INST   Hold up this manual and begin to read this text. Slowly start to move your head from side to side, keeping the manual stationary. Do this more rapidly until you can't read, then stop. Now repeat the same exercise, but instead keep your head stationary and move the paper (or have a classmate to this for you). In which activity is it easier to keep your eye on the text and be able to read it?

Q11.17. To begin studying eye movements, you will need to refresh your knowledge of the extraocular muscles. In Figure 11.19 is a diagram of the eye with its musculature. The left figure is drawn from above, after removing the bones over the orbits. Label the indicated structures. Note where they insert on the eye. Beneath the name, indicate which cranial nerve controls that muscle.

A11.17. *See Figure 11.20.*

   If our eyes always looked directly forward, and their muscles inserted directly from behind, understanding eye movements would be easy. The superior rectus would raise the globe, the lateral rectus pull it to the side. As Figure 11.19 shows, the eye muscles instead insert off to the medial side of the forward direction and our eye balls are often not looking directly forward. For these reasons the effect of the extraocular muscles is complex. For example, if the right eye is adducted (pointing inward), then contraction of the superior rectus muscle will cause the globe to rotate counterclockwise. But if the eye is abducted (pointed outward), the same muscle will cause the globe to point upward.

Q11.18. Three brainstem motor nuclei control the six extraocular muscles. Two muscles, the superior oblique and the lateral rectus (find them in Figure 11.20) have their own nerves and nuclei (IV or trochlear and VI or abducens, respectively), while the remainder are all controlled by the large oculomotor complex in the midbrain. Understanding why we have such an arrangement would require about 500 million years to explain; just accept it. Find these extraocular motor nuclei in Figure 11.21.

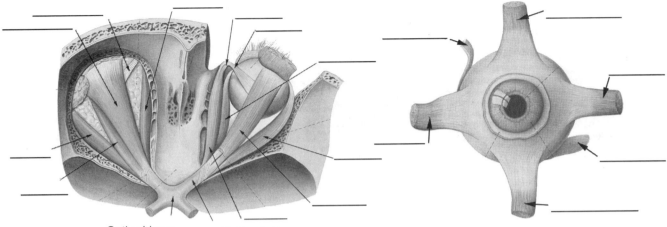

Optic chiasm Optic nerve

FIGURE 11.19. *Extraocular muscle worksheet. The left drawing is a view down into the front of the skull base after the bones over the eyes have been removed. The right drawing shows the right eye. (Adapted from Clemente Anatomy, 3rd edition, © 1987, Urban & Schwarzenberg, Baltimore-Munich, left panel from figure 668 and right panel from figure 665.)*

A11.18. See Figure 11.22. Notice the VIIth nerve coming out laterally to the abducens nucleus (dark fiber band); this nerve sweeps around the VIth nucleus as the facial colliculus and exits laterally. The three paired extraocular nerves all exit medially, III and VI ventrally and IV dorsally.

Q11.19. The extraocular motor nuclei consist mainly of lower motor neurons that innervate extraocular muscles. Unlike your fingers, which you want to move independently, your eye movements are coordinated. The area just medial to the lowest extraocular nucleus, known as the ***paramedian pontine reticular formation*** or PPRF, organizes horizontal gaze. At the other end of the extraocular nuclear chain, lateral and superior to the oculomotor nuclei, lie the vertical gaze and vergence control centers. Find the PPRF and vertical gaze control centers in Figure 11.23. If you are reading this manual, then you have probably spent a good deal of your life using your vergence center. This region of the upper midbrain controls the convergence of your eyes and constriction of your lens so you can pick lice off your mate or read the printed page. Convergence requires bilateral eye muscle cooperation; necessary information crosses in the posterior commissure. Find this commissure in Figure 11.23.

A11.19. See Figure 11.24.

Q11.20. Convergence also requires that you constrict your pupil. For camera buffs, this increases the f-ratio of your lens. For everyone else, constricting the iris increases your visual depth-of-field; at close range, more things are in focus. Pupillary constriction is a parasympathetic function. The parasympathetic nucleus controlling your

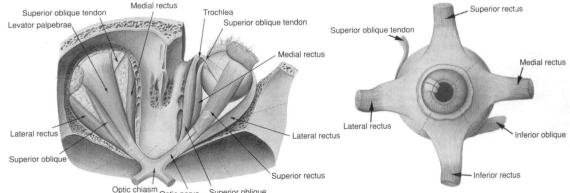

FIGURE 11.20. *Extraocular muscle worksheet. The left drawing is a view down into the front of the skull base after the bones over the eyes have been removed. The right drawing shows the right eye. (Adapted from Clemente Anatomy, 3rd edition, © 1987, Urban & Schwarzenberg, Baltimore-Munich, left panel from figure 668 and right panel from figure 665.)*

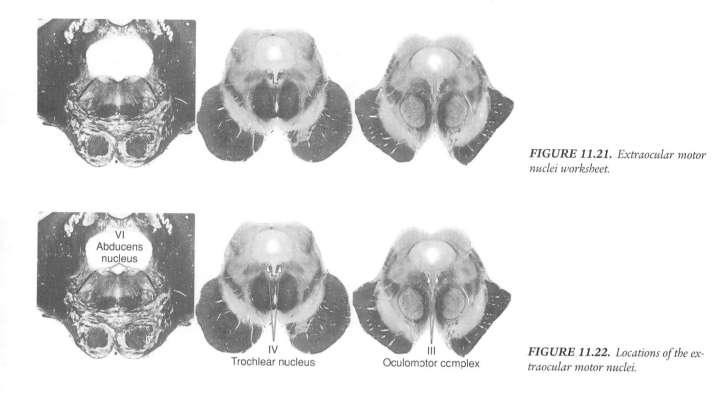

FIGURE 11.21. *Extraocular motor nuclei worksheet.*

VI
Abducens
nucleus

IV
Trochlear nucleus

III
Oculomotor complex

FIGURE 11.22. *Locations of the extraocular motor nuclei.*

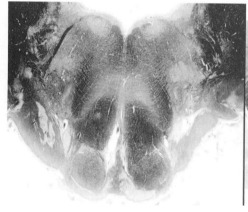
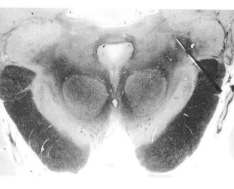

FIGURE 11.23. *Brainstem control centers for eye movements worksheet.*

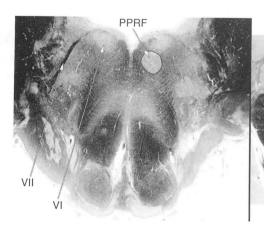
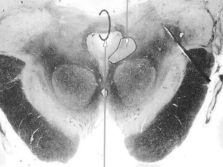

PPRF

Vertical and vergence centers

VII

VI

Posterior commissure

FIGURE 11.24. *Brainstem eye movements control centers.*

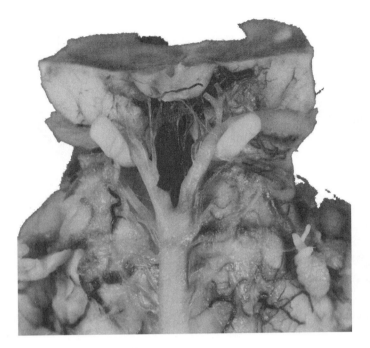

FIGURE 11.25. *Close-up of brainstem at exit of the oculomotor nerve.*

pupils lives exactly where it should, just on top of the oculomotor complex near the vergence centers. The parasympathetic information travels with the third nerve. Look at Figure 11.25 and re-find the oculomotor nerves (you did this in the first exercise). What vessel lies immediately above this nerve? Which one lies below it? Predict what you would see in a patient suffering from downward compression of the brainstem (uncal herniation) on the right side over relatively fixed vessels.

A11.20. *The first portion of the posterior cerebral artery lies immediately rostral to the oculomotor nerve, while the superior cerebellar lies just caudal. In uncal herniation the third nerve would be crushed between these two vessels. On the right side, the patient's right eye would be fixed outward (unopposed action of the abducens nerve) and dilated (unopposed sympathetic dilatation of the iris). A "blown pupil" is an ominous emergency room finding.*

Q11.21. The control of your eye movement in the context of continuously changing body and head position has evolved to a fine degree in vertebrates. As a review from the cerebellum chapter, which sensory organs identify changes in head position? How and where does this information enter the brain? Find this site on an actual brainstem, a brainstem model, or in left panel of Figure 11.26. In the right panel of Figure 11.26, identify the ***vestibular nuclear complex*** (you did this in the last chapter!). This is a large and diverse collection of neurons in the rostral dorsolateral medulla, just medial to the inferior cerebellar peduncle. Since the head is attached to the body via the neck, all of which move, suggest other types of sensory information that contribute to control of eye movements.

A11.21. *See Figure 11.27. The vestibular nuclei provide the principal sensory information about changing head positions. The semilunar canals indicate angular acceleration and the utricle and sacculus sense linear acceleration. Their encoded information enters the brainstem at the lateral pontomedullary junction. The eyes also respond to sensation from stretch and position receptors in the neck and torso.*

Q11.22. We have seen several eye movement integration centers in the pons and midbrain. We also know that vestibular information has its major nuclei in the medulla, and that eye movements also require other sensory inputs from the neck and elsewhere. To put these all together requires the ***medial longitudinal fasciculus,*** or more commonly, just the MLF. In Figure 11.28, find the medial longitudinal fasciculus in all of the panels. Remember, it is more or less where it should be, surrounding the primary cranial nerve extraocular motor nuclei. How far rostrally and caudally should it travel? Give reasons for your answer.

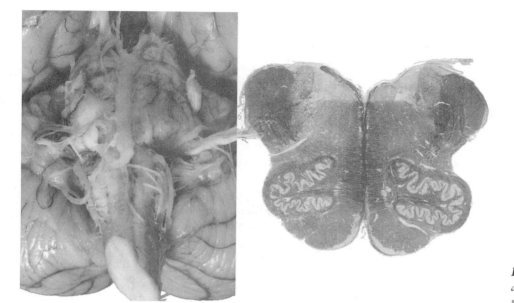

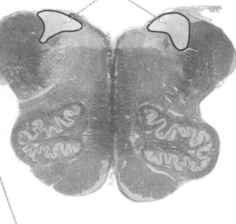

FIGURE 11.26. *Brainstem close-up and histologic section of the upper medulla.*

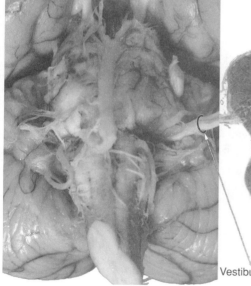

Vestibular nuclear complex

Vestibulocochlear nerve (VIII)

FIGURE 11.27. *Vestibular nerve entering brainstem and vestibular nuclei in upper medulla.*

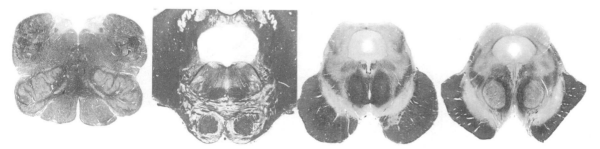

FIGURE 11.28. *Medial longitudinal fasciculus worksheet.*

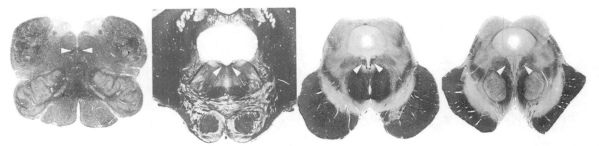

FIGURE 11.29. *Medial longitudinal fasciculus. The arrowheads show its location in the medulla, pons, and midbrain.*

A11.22. See Figure 11.29. The medial longitudinal fasciculus interconnects all of the essential eye movement centers in the brainstem. To coordinate actual eye movements, it connects the oculomotor complex and the trochlear nucleus in midbrain with the abducens nucleus in the lower pons. Starting most rostrally it begins above the oculomotor nucleus in the upper midbrain, at the vertical gaze center. These control both vertical gaze, accommodation, and convergence. Information crosses in the posterior commissure, conveniently located nearby. To regulate horizontal gaze, the medial longitudinal fasciculus also connects the paramedian pontine reticular formation in the lower pons. This fasciculus also receives projections from the vestibular nuclear complex in the medulla and descends down into the upper cervical cord to convey neck and body position information.

So far the chapter has discussed only the elementary aspects of eye movements. Details of how the cortex controls visual fixation on a target and how it directs the eyes in smooth pursuit and saccades is beyond the scope of this textbook. However, certain anatomic sites of the system are important clinically. The ***frontal eye fields,*** lying around the middle the lateral frontal cortex, just anterior to the premotor cortex, are important for the volitional movement of our eyes. The ***parietal eye fields,*** behind the primary sensory cortex in the lateral parietal lobe, help us attend to what we see. These aspects are different: you can attend to an object without looking at it, and you can look at an object without attending to it. Patients with lesions in the frontal eye fields have trouble suppressing eye movements generated by our attention. In these patients it seems that the attentive parietal lobes direct the eyes, independent of the will of our executive function. These cortical control centers send signals to the superior colliculus, which in turn controls saccadic eye movements via gaze centers in the brainstem.

Q11.23. On Figure 11.30, locate three of the important sites involved in the cortical control of eye movements:
- Frontal eye fields
- Parietal eye fields
- Superior colliculus
- For good measure, find the medial longitudinal fasciculus in the brainstem

A11.23. See Figure 11.31.

Clinical Extraocular Muscle Testing

INST For the following exercise, find a partner. Face this person and instruct them not to move their head. Using a pen with a tip or just your finger, have your partner follow the target with their eyes

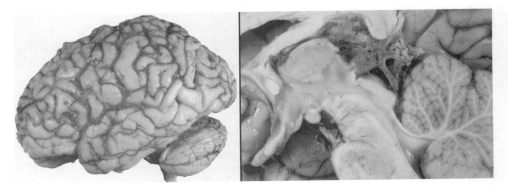

FIGURE 11.30. *Control of eye movement worksheet.*

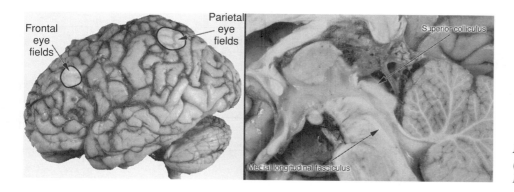

FIGURE 11.31. MRI of patient. (Modified from Fiez et al., 1992. Brain, 115: 155–178).

only, as you move it around. Have them track the target with their eyes as you trace a large "H" in the air. Watch each eye. Do they move in conjugate? Any beating? A little nystagmus is common at extreme end-gaze. See Figure 11.32.

Q11.24. With the target at their left horizontal line, what extraocular motor nuclei and muscles in the left eye are active? How about for the right eye?

A11.24. *Left abducens nucleus in the lower pons and left lateral rectus muscle. Right oculomotor nucleus in the midbrain and right medial rectus muscle.*

Q11.25. While you have their eyes pointed to the left, move your target to the top of the "H." Now what is active for the left eye? The right eye is more complex in this position. If the right eye is turned inward (adducted) what muscle and nucleus will raise it upward?

A11.25. *The left superior rectus will raise the left eye in the lateral position. The right superior rectus will be at nearly a right angle to the motion when the right globe is raised, so it is essentially useless for this task (see Fig. 11.20). Instead, raising the right eye requires that you contract the right inferior oblique muscle, which receives its commands from the right oculomotor complex.*

Q11.26. So as not to discriminate against the right, have your partner move her eyes to the right and down to the bottom of the "H." Now which muscles and nuclei produce this motion in the right eye? Left eye?

A11.26 *For the right eye pointing right, analogously to the last question, the inferior rectus, controlled by the IIIrd nerve nucleus, will drop the globe. The left eye now needs to be pulled down and inward. A perfect job for the superior oblique muscle and the left trochlear (IVth) nucleus.*

Q11.27. Finally, while looking directly at you, have your partner rotate their head slightly upward to one side. Watch the globes carefully. What happens to the eyes?

A11.27. *They rotate!* **Intort** *and* **extort** *are the professional terms, meaning to rotate inward or outward.*

Q11.28. Using the right eye as an example, complete Table 11.3. Indicate the action of each muscle when the right eye is in the three different positions.

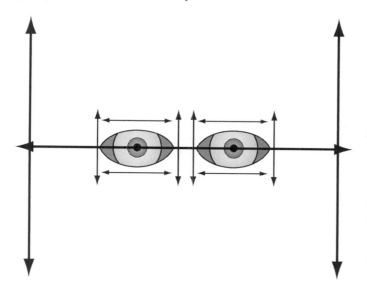

FIGURE 11.32. Averaged responses for fMRI on 8 subjects doing tasks involving changes in timing. The demarcated gray-to-white area in the cerebellum represents the averaged signals, with white the highest intensity (converted from original color data). (Modified from The roles of the cerebellum and basal ganglia in timing and error prediction, Dreher, J.-C. and Grafman, J., 2002. European Journal of Neuroscience 16: 1609–1619.)

TABLE 11.3. Extraocular Muscle Action Worksheet

Muscle	Neutral or Forward	Adducted	Abducted
Lateral rectus			
Medial rectus			
Superior rectus			
Inferior rectus			
Superior oblique			
Inferior oblique			

The Eye Movement Web site (*http://cim.ucdavis.edu/EyeRelease/Interface/TopFrame.htm*) from the University of California, Davis (developed by Rick Lasslo, Gary Henderson, and John Keltner) is a great tool to use to learn about eye movements. You can make virtual lesions to the muscles or nerves and determine what happens to the eye movement.

A11.28. See Table 11.4.

If you can imagine a more complex (typical) human with multiple eye movement abnormalities, you'll appreciate why the world needs neuro-ophthalmologists who specialize in understanding these actions.

Diffuse Systems

We examined the dopamine system in the basal ganglia chapter and will examine the cholinergic projections in the limbic system chapter. Here we will touch on the other brainstem diffuse systems.

Locus ceruleus   Located in the rostral pons, ventrolateral to the IVth ventricle and periaqueductal gray, this nucleus utilizes norepinepherine as a neurotransmitter. It is the largest such nucleus and projects diffusely to the forebrain as well as the lower brainstem and spinal cord.

Norepinepherine System

Q11.29. Look at the microscopic slide from the upper pons. Locate the ***locus ceruleus.*** What color are its neurons on the slide or on a slice of pons? Do you think they are blue ("blue locus")? What fluid-filled space is above the locus? What gray matter lies dorsal to the locus? What is the great white matter tract around the lateral edge of the locus?

A11.29. *Although the locus ceruleus was named the "blue locus," we've never found anything blue about it. The brown pigment is histologically identical to that found in the substantia nigra (which at least was better named). This pigment ("neuromelanin") is a nonenzymatic adduct of catecholamines, which translates as a brown substance that accumulates with age in neurons producing norepinepherine and dopamine.*

The locus ceruleus lives in the lateral aspect of the fourth ventricle, just beneath the periaqueductal or central gray. In this region the superior cerebellar peduncle has left the deep

TABLE 11.4. Extraocular Muscle Actions

Muscle	Neutral or Forward	Adducted	Abducted
Lateral rectus	Abduct	Abduct	Abduct
Medial rectus	Adduct	Adduct	Adduct
Superior rectus	Elevate (plus adduct and intort)	Intort	Elevate
Inferior rectus	Depress (plus adduct and extort)	Extort	Depress
Superior oblique	Depress (plus intort and adduct)	Depress	Intort
Inferior oblique	Elevate (plus extort and adduct)	Elevate	Extort

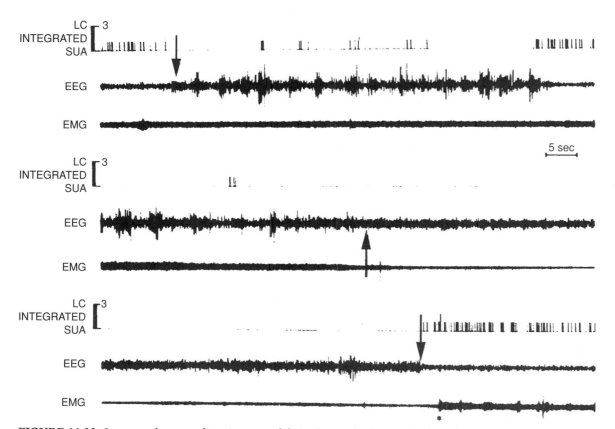

FIGURE 11.33. *Locus ceruleus recordings in a rat while in sleep and when awakening. The upper trace is neuronal activity from the locus ceruleus, the middle trace is the EEG, and the lower trace is an EMG. Just as the recording starts in the upper panel, the animal "passes" from waking to slow-wave sleep (down arrow). In the middle panel, the animal transitions from slow-wave sleep to desynchronized sleep (up arrow). The bottom panel presents the onset of waking (down arrow). (Modified from Aston-Jones, G. and Bloom, F. E. Activity of norepinepherine-containing locus coeruleus neurons in behaving rats anticipates fluctuation in the sleep-waking cycle. 1981. J. Neurosci 1: 887–900.)*

cerebellar nuclei, and its arms, which wrap around lateral to the locus, are headed for a decussation in the midbrain.

Q11.30. Examine the recordings from the locus ceruleus in a rat in Figure 11.33. Inspect the trace from the locus ceruleus ("integrated SUA"). What happens to the neuronal activity during wakefulness? Slow-wave sleep? Desynchronized sleep? Compare the locus ceruleus and EMG at onset of wakefulness in the lower panel. What possible conclusions can be reached about this tiny nucleus and the sleep-wake cycle?

A11.30. *While the animal is awake, the locus ceruleus is active. Although not directly presented on these traces, locus ceruleus activity increases when the animal is attentive (e.g., when you pinch it) compared to when it is just hanging out. At the onset of wakefulness in the lower panel, activity in the locus begins before movement, indicating the animal is "awake" for a brief period before they realize it! As the animal delves deeper into sleep, ceruleus activity progressively decreases.*

From the data presented here, one can only conclude that the locus is hushed in slow-wave sleep and silenced in desynchronized sleep.

The locus ceruleus is currently thought to play a major role in attentiveness. Medications such as Ritalin are postulated to influence the central norepinepherine system (and the dopamine system as well). The ceruleus decreased firing in sleep is considered secondary to an active inhibitory influence from other portions of the pontine reticular formation. Its silencing may be necessary to "permit" sleep to happen.

Serotonin System

Q11.31. Using the microscopic section of pons and Figure 11.34, find the **raphe nucleus.** The raphe are actually a series of nuclei extending from the medulla into the midbrain.

Raphe nucleus *A group of nuclei located throughout the brainstem have their neurons clustered just off the midline ("raphe" is Greek for seam). Large neurons in these nuclei utilize serotonin as a neurotransmitter and also project diffusely both rostrally and caudally. A major projection goes to the cholinergic pedunculopontine nucleus in the upper pons, which in turn helps regulate sleep-wake states.*

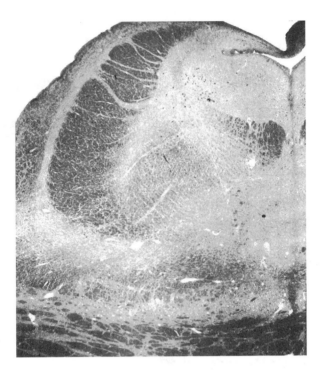

FIGURE 11.34. *Rostral pons worksheet.*

Unlike the locus ceruleus and substantia nigra, the neurons have no pigment to mark them.

A11.31. *See Figure 11.35. The raphe nuclei are paramedian in the pontine tegmentum. They live immediately lateral to the midline white matter fibers, at the edge of the pontine reticular formation. Additional raphe neurons spill out into the periaqueductal gray above the medial longitudinal fasciculus.*

Q11.32. Now examine Figure 11.36 of a rat brain immunostained with antibodies against the 5-hydroxytryptamine 2A receptor. The nuclei are labeled on the left side. What

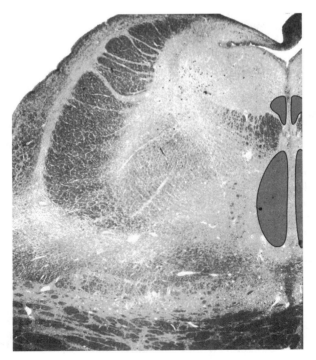

FIGURE 11.35. *Raphe nuclei in the rostral pons.*

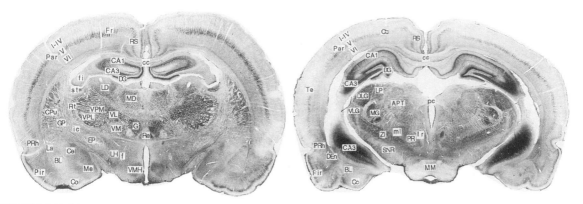

FIGURE 11.36. *Serotonin 2A receptors in a rat brain. Brain slices were immunostained with antibodies against the 5-hydroxytryptamine 2A receptor (5-HT2A-R) (Modified from Cornea-Hebert, V., Riad, M., Wu, C., Singh, S. K., Descarries, L. Cellular and subcellular distribution of the serotonin 5-HT2a receptor in the central nervous system of adult rat. J Comp Neurology 409: 187–209, 1999.)*

sites are staining (dark coloration)? What specific cortical lamina? Areas of thalamus? The hippocampus (to be encountered in laboratory 13) is divided into CA1, CA3, and dentate gyrus. Which stains most intensely?

A11.32. *Most important, do not attempt to learn the details here! It is the general principle that this system has diffuse but specific projections that is important.*

The sites of immunostaining for 5-HT2A-R include layer V of the frontal and parietal cortices, CA1/CA3 in the hippocampus, and ventral posterior medial and lateral of thalamus (which relay what type of information?). Other selective sites are also stained in the images.

Q11.33. Briefly (don't spend more than a minute on this) contrast the in situ hybridization pattern of the 5-HT1A, 5-HT1C, and 5-HT2 receptors in Figure 11.37. List some of the drugs you know that affect the serotonergic system. Discuss some of the difficulties in trying to interpret drug-binding studies and correlating the binding with neuroanatomic function, especially when the agents are only "relatively" selective for receptor type.

A11.33. *Figure 11.37 emphasizes the differences in the regional distribution of these receptor subtypes. The 5-HT1A, receptor mRNA is mostly localized in the hippocampus, while the 5-HT1C, mRNA lies mostly in the amygdala, and at this level little 5-HT2 mRNA is detectable.*

These types of studies indicate several facts. Foremost is that the serotonin system is diffuse and involves many areas of the brain. Remember, although receptors and projections are widespread, the transmitter comes only from neurons restricted to midline regions of the brainstem. Alteration of serotonin action predictably should have multiple effects on the nervous system. To understand the functions of the serotonin system requires a deeper understanding of the neuroanatomic distribution of the receptors receiving this transmitter.

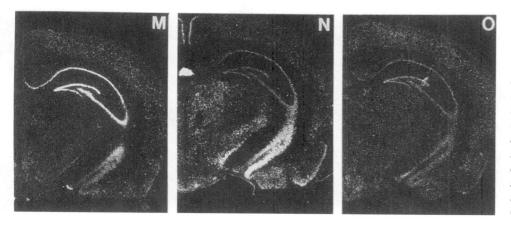

FIGURE 11.37. *Serotonin receptor in situ hybridization in a rat. The in situ hybridization shows transcription of 5-HT1A (M), 5-HT1C (N), and 5-HT2 (O) receptor genes. (Modified from figure 2, Wright, D. E., et al. Comparative localization of serotonin-1A, 1C, and 2 receptor subtype mRNAs in rat brain. 1995. J Comp Neurol 351: 357–373.)*

Finally, although many extremely useful drugs act on the serotonin system, either by binding to receptors or blocking reuptake, understanding their complete mechanism of action is complicated by the overwhelming forest of receptor subtypes that they may effect in addition to their unique but overlapping anatomic distributions.

CLINICAL CASE: MULTIPLE SCLEROSIS

Q11.34. A 38-year-old man presented with difficulties of balance and "visual problems." He then developed tingling in his hands. A lumbar puncture demonstrated an increased number of lymphocytes in his cerebrospinal fluid. Examine of his MRI scan in Figure 11.38. Are the lesions in the white matter or gray matter? Do they form masses or is the involved brain diminished? In what general location are most of the lesions? What structure lies just medial to the lesions at area 1 and why is this important? What great projection would be compromised by the lesions in area 2? In what structure does lesion area 3 reside? How do the scans help?

A11.34. *The scans show multiple lesions, which have a predilection for the periventricular white matter. Rather than forming masses, at this time the involved brain is partially shrunken. The corpus callosum lies just medial to area 1 and is severely affected. Little interhemispheric information would be able to traverse this region. Note, in particular, the dark waves extending away from the corpus callosum, which are known as "Dawson's fingers." The optic radiation flows around the occipital horns of the lateral ventricles and would be affected by the lesions demarcated by area 2. Area 3 is the anterior limb of the internal capsule.*

The scans demonstrate the classic findings of multiple sclerosis: white matter plaques predominantly located in the periventricular region.

Near the end of the patient's life, he developed seizures. He had several severe falls, one of which produced brain trauma necessitating insertion of a ventricular drain. He died of an aspiration pneumonia following a seizure.

Q11.35. Examine the photographs of the coronal brain sections in Figure 11.39. What structure is identified in area 2? Why is it thin? Note the dark plaques in areas 3 and 4. How would you describe their locations? What important white matter tracts lie near the lesion in area 4? What signs would you expect? What is area 1?

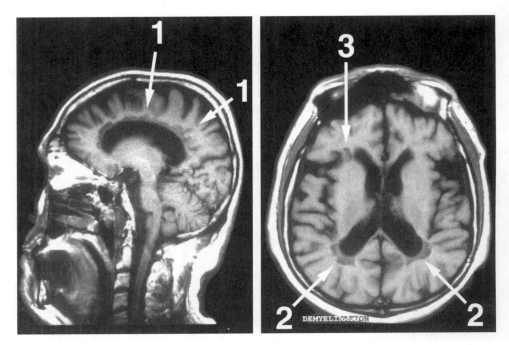

FIGURE 11.38. *MRI scan of patient.*

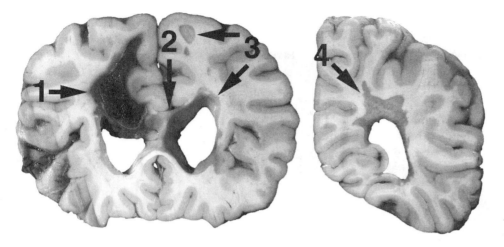

FIGURE 11.39. Coronal sections through patient's brain.

A11.35. *Area 2 is the corpus callosum, which is demyelinated and thin. Although multiple sclerosis is an inflammatory disease of white matter, loss of myelin-producing oligodendrocytes leads to secondary loss of axons. The thin corpus callosum at this site is secondary to three pathologies: loss of myelin from his multiple sclerosis, Wallerian degeneration of the crossing fibers injured by more lateral plaques (as in area 3), and Wallerian degeneration produced by the hemorrhage in area 1.*

The classic white matter plaques in multiple sclerosis are similar to those in area 4, namely in the periventricular white matter. Although classic, the plaques are by no means restricted to that region. They may be found in any white matter, including in subcortical white matter (as in area 3) and even in myelinated axons within the gray matter. Multiple sclerosis is an inflammatory disease of oligodendrocyte myelin, not white matter per se.

The optic radiation skirts around the lateral portion of the occipital horn and was partially involved by the plaque designated area 4. Lesions in the right optic radiation would produce a left partial hemianopia, although in this patient, his demyelinated plaques were bilateral.

Area 1 represents hemorrhage around his ventriculostomy site. This may have been secondary to his falls that occurred after it was inserted.

Q11.36. Now examine the photographs of the patient's brainstem lesions in Figure 11.40. Where are the demyelinated plaques? Be as specific as possible; assume that right is on the right. What type of eye movement disorder would you predict from this lesion? What is this called?

A11.36. *The irregular dark area in the medial pontine tegmentum is the plaque. One of his demyelinated plaques involves the medial longitudinal fasciculus in the pons. Only rarely do such lesions inactivate just one side of the medial longitudinal fasciculus. More typically, as in this case, they involve a portion of one or portions of both, giving a more complex* **internuclear**

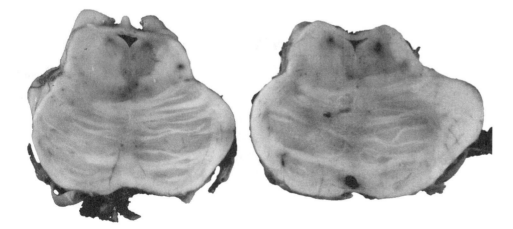

FIGURE 11.40. Transverse sections through the patient's brainstem.

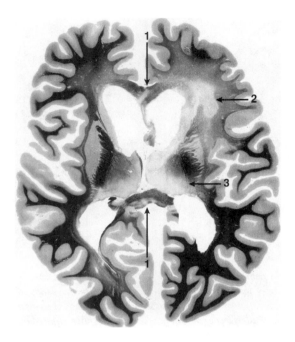

FIGURE 11.41. *Giant section through brain of a patient who suffered from multiple sclerosis.*

ophthalmoplegia. *You might expect to see some form of this anomalous eye movement pattern, showing a palsy of right medial rectus function on left lateral gaze and nystagmus produced by the contralateral lateral rectus. Convergence by both medial rectus muscles should be preserved, if the lesion were restricted to this level.*

Q11.37. Figure 11.41 illustrates another patient with multiple sclerosis. The giant section has been stained for myelin using LFB and PAS. What is the structure in area 1; describe the lesion. What structure is identified in area 2, and what signs may be present because of this plaque. What structure is identified in area 3? What would be the clinical manifestations of lesions in this structure?

A11.37. *Area 1 points to both the genu and splenium of the corpus callosum. The linear streaks of demyelination are, again, known as "Dawson's fingers," and are a characteristic finding in patient's with multiple sclerosis. The patient also had a large demyelinated plaque in his corona radiata and internal capsule, labeled area 2. While the exact signs depend on where the internal capsule has been affected, major findings of internal capsule damage include pyramidal tract signs, including hemiparesis and spasticity, sensory changes and in this patient, frontal lobe dysfunction. The thalamic lesion in area 3 is in the more posterior portions of thalamus, including the pulvinar and probably the ventral posterior medial and lateral nuclei. Lesions in the latter nuclei would produce loss of sensation in the contralateral face and body. Since neurons are typically spared and axons are partially injured, the clinical findings of a plaque in a predominantly gray matter structure may be more complex.*

APPENDIX: BRAINSTEM TRANSVERSE HISTOLOGY

The histologic sections in Figures 11.42 and 11.43 are transverse sections through the entire brainstem that have been stained for myelin.

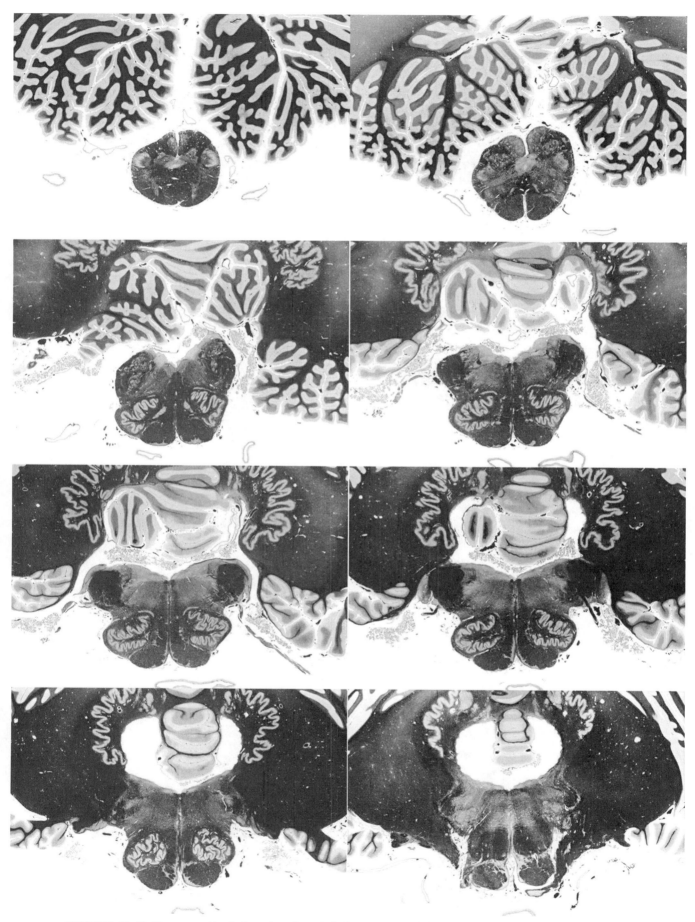

FIGURE 11.42. *Transverse histologic sections through the brainstem, caudal.*

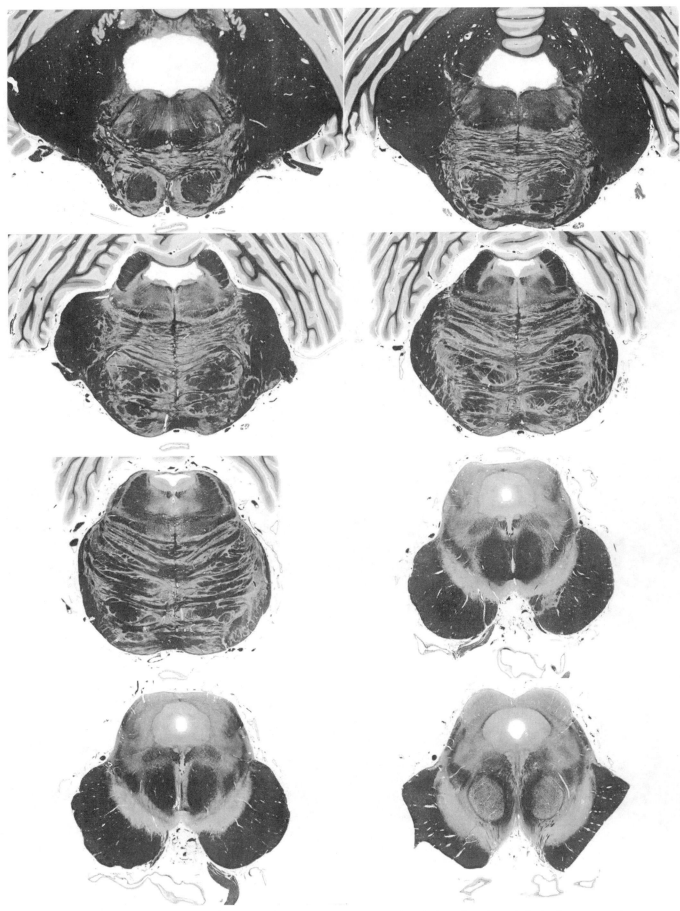

FIGURE 11.43. *Transverse histologic sections through the brainstem, rostral.*

Chapter 12—CRANIAL NERVES

In this second laboratory on the brainstem, you will focus on its structure. While you most likely won't become a brainstem neuroanatomist, this region does interact with many aspects of the body that will interest you in the future. Cardiologists, gastroenterologists, and even urologists treat systems influenced by the brainstem.

One key to understanding deficits produced by brainstem lesions is to know the location of the lesion and what lives in that spot. Another key is to know what traffic passes through that region. Today's laboratory will take you through some of the most important anatomy. At the end of the laboratory, you will use your knowledge to "build" the cranial nerves.

Remember, the goal is not to learn a lot of obscure terminology, but to learn the functional anatomy of the brainstem.

LEARNING OBJECTIVES

- Trace different neuroanatomic systems throughout the brainstem, identifying their major nuclei and white matter tracts.
- Correlate brainstem lesions with clinical findings.
- Identify the location and principal functions of the brainstem cranial nerves.

INTRODUCTION

The cranial nerves are typically first described in an ideal vertebrate brainstem and then by discussing how similar our brainstem is to this ideal. For example, in Figure 12.1, cranial nerve function is divided into an ideal structure with six divisions: somatic motor (Sm), branchial motor (B), autonomic (A), visceral sensory (Vi), somatic sensory (Ss), and special sensory (Sp). While such diagrams help those who already have an understanding of the brainstem, novices are left wondering "What is branchial motor?" or "Why is hearing special sensory but vision is not?" Also, if you happen to pick up a histologic slide of the medulla, you will gain little clarity from the diagram. To compound these problems, an entirely

Functional Neuroanatomy: An Interactive Text and Manual, by Jeffrey T. Joseph and David L. Cardozo
ISBN 0-471-44437-5 Copyright © 2004 John Wiley & Sons, Inc.

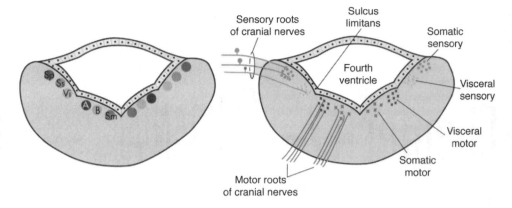

FIGURE 12.1. *Organization of the brainstem nuclei. (Adapted from The Human Brain: An Introduction to Its Functional Anatomy, Fourth Edition, by John Nolte © 1999, Mosby, Inc. St. Louis, figure 12-1, page 284.)*

new use of vocabulary emerges, where muscles of mastication are termed "special visceral efferent" ("Why visceral?"), yet extraocular muscles are called "general somatic efferent" ("Why aren't these special?"), and parasympathetic fibers are called "general visceral efferent" ("Why general?"). Such terms are quickly forgotten. Just ask your laboratory instructors or any clinician.

While the ideal vertebrate approach may become mired in terminology, it does try to create order in the seeming chaos of the brainstem. Below is an alternative, semi-evolutionary attempt to explain the cranial nerves. It is not standard, so feel free to resort to other texts that discuss brainstem organization. The objective is to explain how we evolved from an orderly segmented creature to our current form.

Before embarking, we need to briefly discuss the first two cranial nerves. The ***olfactory nerve*** is really a short nerve that connects olfactory receptors in the nasal epithelium, through the cribriform plate, to the olfactory bulb. The large tract on the surface of the brain is not a nerve at all, but an extension of the central nervous system. The eye is also an extension of the brain, as it develops from the diencephalon. While we speak of the ***optic nerve,*** like the olfactory tract, it is also an extension of brain tissue. Since both of these senses are discussed in other laboratories and neither is associated with the brainstem, they will not be further discussed here.

Key Concepts

Several key concepts will help you better understand the structure of the brainstem.

The first concept is that the nervous system originated as a series "primitive" segments, each containing both a ventral root and a dorsal root. From your knowledge of the spinal cord, this should not be a surprise. The dorsal component had both sensory and motor functions, the latter of which was lost in the spinal cord. As you know, in the spinal cord both roots merge just distal the dorsal root ganglion to form a mixed nerve.

The second concept is that the head retained two primitive traits: the dorsal and ventral roots failed to merge and the dorsal root retained its motor functions. Because of the failure to merge and the subsequent explosive evolution of our large heads, the dorsal and ventral components of a segment have become isolated from each other. For example, the abducens and facial nerves are ventral-dorsal pairs. Being a dorsal nerve, the facial nerve has also retained motor functions, in particular those innervating facial muscles. Chewing muscles and those that make you smile are not derived from myotomes (and hence have been termed "special viscera") and are innervated by the archaic dorsal roots rather than ventral roots. Our advanced head essentially has retained an earlier state of evolution.

The third concept goes back to our origins as fish-like creatures with gill slits (see Fig. 12.2). Each of the head segments had an associated gill slit, which determined the general structures of each dorsal branchial arch segment. Each idealized dorsal root would have a motor and several sensory branches, as depicted in Figure 12.3. The "pretrematic" branch of each root carried ventral surface sensations. Visceral sensations of the pharynx, notably taste, traveled in the pharyngeal branch. The "post-trematic" branches transmitted both motor efferents and sensations. Dorsal sensations from the skin were carried in the dorsal branch. Each of the dorsal branchial nerve roots had a corresponding ventral, purely motor root.

The final useful concept is that the nuclei controlling a similar function all lie in the same column within the brainstem. For example, the ventral motor nuclei innervating myotome-derived

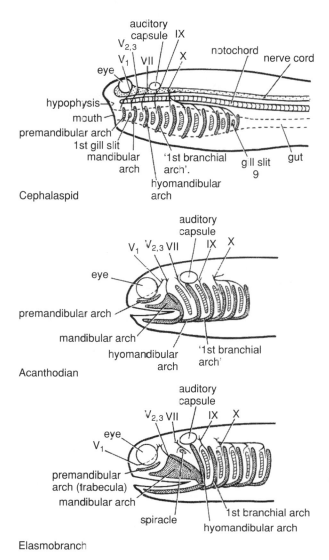

FIGURE 12.2. *Cranial nerves and branchial arches in a primitive vertebrate. (Modified from J. Z. Young, The Life of Vertebrates, third edition, © 1981, Oxford University Press, Oxford, figure 5.16, page 127.)*

muscle all reside in the medial and dorsal parts of the brainstem, while motor nuclei of the branchial nerves innervating non-myotome muscles all line up laterally. This helps explain why the pain and temperature sensations from the facial area derived from four cranial nerves all project to the single longitudinal spinal trigeminal nucleus. Similarly, all of the autonomic information coming from three cranial nerves (VI, IX, and X), including baroreceptors, chemoreceptors, and taste, all end up in the solitary nucleus or its rostral extension, the gustatory nucleus.

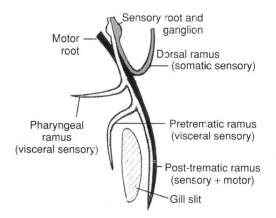

FIGURE 12.3. *Idealized branchial arch components. (Modified from A. S. Romer and T. S. Parsons, The Vertebrate Body, fifth edition, © 1977, Saunders College Publishing, Philadelphia, figure 397, page 510.)*

The functional divisions of a regular spinal nerve are:

- Motor projections to striated muscles derived from myotomes (general somatic efferent)
- Motor output to autonomic targets (general visceral efferent)
- Somatosensory input (general somatic afferent)
- Autonomic sensory information, like pressure receptors (general visceral afferent)

The ideal segment in the head has these activities, but also has unique branchial functions:

- Taste (special visceral afferent)
- Motor innervation of non-myotome musculature (special visceral efferent)

Hearing and vestibular sensations have a unique place in evolution, having displaced several other segments and lost the usual segmental operations. Rather superficially, these sensations are classified as "special somatic afferents." Vision is usually included as a special somatic afferent while smell is lumped into special visceral afferents. However, since these two "nerves" are not really nerves at all, such inclusion can only be a result of tradition rather than analysis.

Specific Cranial Nerves

Our heads are no longer segmented, except during development, and the nice order of the branchial arches has been distorted. Portions of different nerves have been lost, others have migrated away from their origin, and yet others have been pushed aside as different structures have mushroomed around them. We have lost our first cranial nerve (terminal nerve). The fifth nerve is really a combination of two arch nerves, the ophthalmicus profundus nerve, which becomes V1 or the ophthalmic division, and the trigeminal nerve proper, which forms V2 and V3. The facial, glossopharyngeal, and vagus nerves all contain mixtures of the components that differ from their ideal dorsal branchial nerves.

The first three ventral roots became cranial nerves III (oculomotor), IV (trochlear), and VI (abducens). These innervated the myotomes that evolved to form the extraocular muscles. The eye's superior oblique muscle came to lie in a dorsal position, so its nerve from the trochlear nucleus traveled dorsally in the brainstem to innervate it. The last "segment", the hypoglossal nerve, is also a pure motor ventral root, and like the first three segments, has no sensory component. However its muscles originated dorsally and later migrated to their ventral position in the mouth.

The oculomotor nerve and ophthalmicus profundus were the ventral dorsal roots corresponding to the first segment. The ophthalmicus represents only the dorsal ramus of the branchial nerve (see Fig. 12.3), as it innervates the skin of the forehead. Its fibers have joined the remainder of the trigeminal nerve as V1, the ophthalmic division.

The second segment had a ventral trochlear root and a corresponding dorsal root that now subsumes the remainder of the trigeminal nerve. V2 (maxillary branch) and V3 (mandibular branch) are equivalent to the pre- and post-trematic rami, respectively, and so contain sensory and sensory plus motor function. The trigeminal nerve is intimately associated with the mouth and especially the jaws. In fossils of jawless fish (see Figure 12.4) the fifth nerve, especially its V3 component, has not yet evolved into its massive proportions in later vertebrates. This nerve has lost its autonomic visceral afferent and efferent fibers.

The third segment had the abducens nerve as its ventral root and the facial nerve as the dorsal root. The pharyngeal arm of the facial nerve contains visceral taste sensations from the front of the tongue ("special visceral afferent"). Its post-trematic horn sends "special visceral motor" fibers to the muscles of facial expression and "general visceral motor" parasympathetic efferents to the lacrimal glands and some salivatory glands. The facial nerve also receives superficial sensations from the external ear.

The eighth cranial nerve itself associates with the receptors that detect sound and accelerations of the body. In early vertebrates, the vestibular and auditory apparatuses occupied a large portion of the brain case (see the jawless bony fish in Fig. 12.4). The structure of their original segments has been obscured over a half billion years of evolution. It has lost all but its unique "special somatic afferent" functions.

Remaining segments were caudal to the developing ear. The dorsal glossopharyngeal branchial root lost its corresponding ventral root. Segments from several arches joined together to form the branchial vagus nerve dorsally and hypoglossal nerve ventrally, hence giving these nerves their various rootlets arising from the medulla. Like other branchial nerves, the glossopharyngeal and vagal nerves transmit several types of information. Both have taste (special visceral), cutaneous (general somatic), and autonomic (general visceral) afferent fibers as well as parasympathetic (general visceral) and

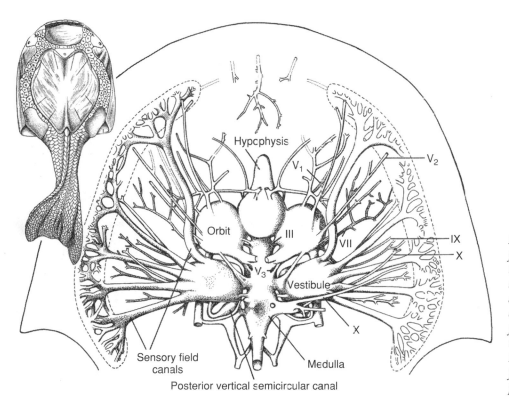

FIGURE 12.4. *Fossil jawless fish from the Devonian period, about 380 million years ago. The inset in the upper left shows the external appearance, while the main figure shows the organism's cranial nerves. (Modified from R. L. Carroll, Vertebrate Paleontology and Evolution, © 1988, W. H. Freeman and Company, New York, figure 3-9, page 33, and figure 3-14, page 37.)*

branchial (special visceral) efferent fibers. Their targets are mostly the muscles and sensory receptors in pharynx and visceral receptors in the body.

One area of potential confusion is "How did these dorsal gill slit muscles end up in the face and mouth?" During evolution, recapitulated during development, the muscles do originate dorsally, but then migrate ventrally to their final position either in the mouth as muscles of mastication (trigeminal), more superficially as muscles of "expression" (facial), or into the pharynx where you might expect gill-slits (glossopharyngeal and vagus).

The view of an embryonic shark head in Figure 12.5 recapitulates a more "primitive" state of the cranial nerves (from Young).

We now return to our original diagram (see Fig. 12.1). During the laboratory, when you investigate the positions of the cranial nerve nuclei, keep this diagram in mind. See how well or how poorly reality matches the ideal situation.

Long Tracts in the Brainstem

As if the cranial nuclei and cranial nerves were not enough, the brainstem is also a conduit of major long white matter tracts. These include the descending tracts from the cerebral cortex (corticospinal and corticobulbar), descending tracts from the brainstem itself (rubrospinal and tectospinal), ascending sensory tracts from the cord (spinothalamic, spinocerebellar), and ascending tracts with nuclei in the brainstem (medial lemniscus, diffuse system projections).

Several of the long tracts of greatest clinical importance cross in the brainstem, including the corticospinal and corticobulbar tracts and the dorsal column/medial lemniscal tracts (vibration, conscious joint position sense, and light touch). The corticobulbar tracts cross rostral to the motor nuclei at which they will synapse. The corticospinal tracts cross in the decussation of the pyramids in the caudal medulla. The ascending second-order neuronal fibers that originated in the dorsal column nuclei (gracilis and cuneatus) cross as the internal arcuate fibers in the lower medulla to enter the medial lemniscus. In contrast, the spinothalamic fibers cross in the spinal cord, prior to their ascent through the brainstem.

As in the spinal cord, the cell bodies of the first-order sensory neurons of the cranial nerves lie outside the brainstem, in ipsilateral sensory ganglia (with, of course, one exception, the mesencephalic nucleus of the trigeminal nerve). The fibers of these ganglia will synapse onto second-order neurons and cross more rostrally in the brainstem on their way to the contralateral side of the thalamus.

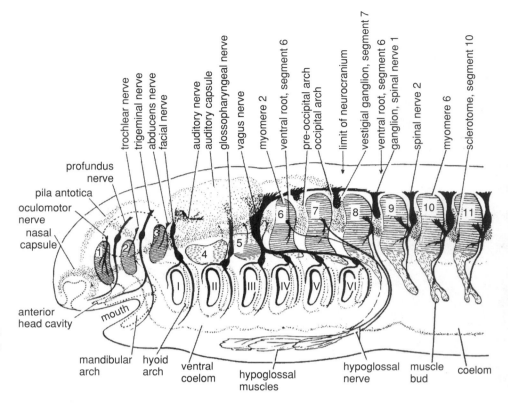

FIGURE 12.5. *Embryonic shark head. (Modified from J. Z. Young, The Life of Vertebrates, third edition, © 1981, Oxford University Press, Oxford, figure 5.17, page 128.)*

Clinical Tidbits

Several important bits of knowledge may help guide you through this complex area:

As in the spinal cord, weakness, sensory loss, and certain reflex changes may be suprasegmental (supranuclear, long tract, or cortical) rather than segmental. Therefore, before using a neurologic symptom or sign to establish a level, be sure that it is truly segmental, for example, that it has lower motor neuron or dermatome/peripheral nerve attributes. Inability to move your eyes down may be caused by a third nerve palsy, but it may also indicate disease in your vertical gaze centers or cortical eye fields.

A "crossed pattern" of a deficit involving a cranial nerve function on one side and arm and leg weakness on the other side usually implicates the brainstem. The reason for this is that the main corticospinal tract and the posterior column/medial lemniscal sensory pathways cross in the caudal medulla, while all the cranial nerves themselves (save CN 4) are uncrossed. This is probably the most important single vignette to derive from this laboratory.

Deficits in cranial nerve functions may be due to either intra-axial (within the brainstem) or extra-axial lesions. Associated long-tract signs produced by the same lesion as the cranial nerve signs would usually indicate an intra-axial lesion, although external compression could affect the long tracts.

In Figure 12.6 is a summary diagram from the Netter *Nervous System* text of the most clinically important gray matter sites of the brainstem.

> **Schedule (2.5 hours)**
> 90   Building a brainstem
> 15   Case reviews
> 30   Cranial nerves
> 15   Clincal case

BUILDING A BRAINSTEM

The next exercise is designed to make you more aware of the three-dimensional anatomy of the brainstem. See appendix V for the materials you will need. In these exercises you will arrange a set of brainstem images in ascending order, and then connect together with yarn the different

Cranial Nerves: Nerves and Nuclei Viewed in Phantom From Behind

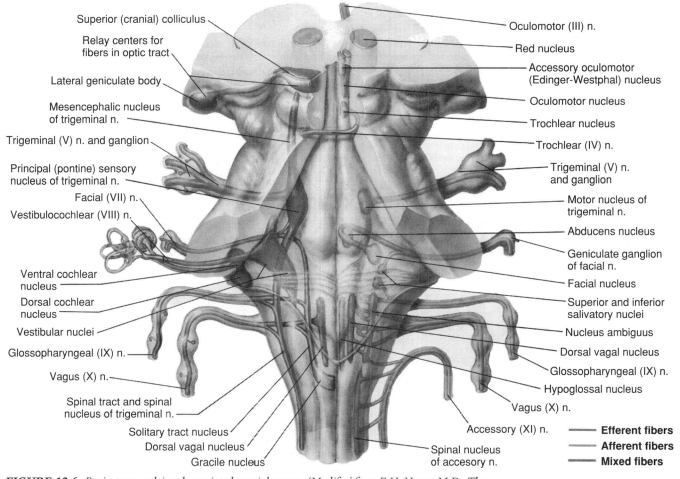

FIGURE 12.6. Brainstem nuclei and associated cranial nerves. (Modified from F. H. Netter, M.D., The Ciba Collection of Medical Illustrations, Volume 1, Nervous system, Part I, Anatomy and Physiology, © 1991, CIBA-Geigy, Summit, New Jersey, plate 2, section V, page 92.)

nuclei belonging to select systems. You'll trace the longer tracts through the multiple sections of the brainstem.

INST   To begin, photocopy onto nine sheets of overhead transparency film images of the brainstem using Figures 12.50 through 12.58 in the appendix of this chapter. Arrange them in ascending order across the laboratory table. Make sure the order is correct, and that you haven't mixed up dorsal and ventral. It may help to remember that the ventricle is always dorsal. While you can't tell the side from the slice, once you decide what is left, keep it left. Punch holes in the top corners of each sheet and hang them in order on a rack (*e.g.* file cabinet rack) using large rings. Thread your needles and yarns through the sheets. *See appendix V.*

SENSORY SYSTEMS

Somatosensory System (orange)

Medial Lemniscus

INST   Label the gracilis (GN) and cuneate nuclei (CN) in orange on the medulla. Tie a knot in the orange yarn. Insert this through the card in one gracilis (or cuneatus) nucleus. This begins the medial lemniscus. Drag the orange yarn around the arcuate fibers to the contralateral medial lemniscus, thread the yard through this site. Then thread it through each of the remaining cards at the appropriate site and side. Leave extra yarn at the end so you don't pull it out.

Trigeminal Primary Sensory Nucleus and Tracts

INST   You will add the face onto the medial lemniscus. First find, delineate, and label in orange the primary sensory nucleus of the trigeminal (1°V). Remember, the sensory nucleus is lateral to the already lateral branchial motor nucleus. Take a second orange thread, tie a knot to anchor it, and pass this through the nucleus, then follow it up through the brainstem. Remember, these fibers get tacked onto the medial lemniscus in the pons, such that the homunculus is a person lying down, feet pointed lateral. Also remember the fibers cross before ascending, although not as elegantly as the arcuate fibers in the medulla.

Anterolateral System (red for heat and pain)
Spinothalamic Tracts

INST   These tracts ascend through the brainstem, while giving off fibers to the reticular formation and periaqueductal gray. We won't get too elaborate here. Take a red thread and pass it through this tract each of the levels of the brainstem at the appropriate site on one side. Remember from which side of the body this information comes! Notice in your various references that this "tract" is less distinct than the posterior column–medial lemniscal system; it sends many collateral fibers to multiple levels of the brainstem and spinal cord before reaching thalamus or your conscious mind. Pain requires a visceral as well as an intellectual response.

Spinal Trigeminal Tract and Nucleus

While the distribution of the spinothalamic portion of the anterolateral system is relatively straightforward, adding the facial pain and temperature sensations is not. This information enters the pons in the trigeminal nerve, but needs to be processed in the medullary reticular formation before it ascends to thalamus.

INST   First find, delineate, and label in red the spinal trigeminal nucleus (SV). It stretches out over most levels of the medulla. Now take your red yarn, thread it through the entrance site of the trigeminal nerve, and thread it down to some level of the spinal trigeminal nucleus. Tie a knot at its terminus to indicate that here the axons synapse. Tie another knot at its origin in the nucleus and then thread it all of the way back up the brainstem. Remember where it decussates! Note its relationship to the medial lemniscus at higher levels. Like the spinothalamic tracts, the trigeminothalamic tracts send branches into the medullary reticular formation and to other levels of the brainstem.

Auditory System (white)

INST   On the appropriate sheet, outline in black the cochlear nucleus. It lies on the outer rim of the inferior cerebellar peduncle. Also bilaterally outline the superior olivary complex in the pons, the lateral lemniscus, and the inferior colliculus. Thread the white yarn between the cochlear nucleus on one side to both superior olivary nuclei. You'll need two threads, one for each side, since the information is bilaterally represented. Then thread these two fragments of yarn among the different levels of the brainstem along the pathway of the lateral lemniscus to the inferior colliculus in the midbrain. From the inferior colliculus the projections leave the brainstem, synapse in the medial geniculate nucleus, and finally end in the primary auditory cortex.

MOTOR SYSTEMS
Pyramidal Tracts (green for go)

INST   These tracts are easy. On BOTH sides thread green yarn through the entire brainstem in the descending corticospinal tracts. Think of these as an anchor for your other tracts. Make sure you attend to the decussation in the lowest medulla. Notice that the tracts break up a bit in the pons before reforming into the compact pyramids. For this exercise, ignore the 10% of the fibers that don't cross in the decussation.

Eye Movements (blue)

INST   You reviewed the eye movement system in the previous laboratory. Now you want to figure out where its components lie. With the blue pen, outline and label the three main eye movement lower motor neuron nuclei on both sides: oculomotor (III), trochlear (IV), and abducens (VI). Remember, these are derived from the ventral roots of the original three segments, and so lie the most medial. Make solid blue the medial longitudinal lemniscus, which is the important white matter bundle that interconnects them. (No one says medial longitudinal fasciculus, they just say the "MLF.") Now use the blue yarn to interconnect these nuclei via the MLF in the different levels. Start at the midbrain and move down. But don't stop at the abducens; find this tract in the medulla and extend the yarn down into the lower brainstem.

If you wonder why the MLF drops all the way into the medulla and beyond, just remember that your head, hopefully, is attached to your shoulders. Coordination of your eye movements requires this information, as well as positional and acceleration data from the medullary vestibular system.

Movements of the Head and Face Muscles (purple)
Mastication

INST Outline and label (V) in purple the main nucleus controlling the muscles of mastication. With the purple pen, trace its pathway from the nucleus to its exit from the brainstem. This will give you something to chew!

Facial Movements

INST By this point in the laboratory, you should be either laughing or crying. Either way, your facial expression should have changed. Outline and label (VII) in purple the nucleus responsible for your expression. Since the nerve usually lies mostly in one level, use the purple pen to highlight its path. Note its circuitous course around the abducens nucleus. This bulge is referred to as the facial colliculus. Remember where the facial nerve exits from the brainstem. With the column diagram from the introduction in mind, compare the positions of the trigeminal and facial branchial motor nuclei.

Tongue

INST Stick your tongue out at your instructor. This action, like all motion, requires contraction of a muscle. Here the muscles are in the base of the tongue, and their contraction propels the tongue forward. Outline and label (XII) in purple the hypoglossal (beneath the tongue) nucleus and its nerve twigs traveling through the medulla. Stimulating the right nucleus contracts the right muscles. If the left nucleus is injured, figure out which way would the tongue then point ("points toward side with the lesion").

AUTONOMIC SYSTEMS (BROWN)

INFO The hypothalamus and brainstem are important autonomic nervous system control centers (along with the amygdala, which will be discussed in a later laboratory). While some of the involved nuclei and tracts are difficult to find and less neurologically useful, several are clinically important.

Solitary Tract and Nucleus

INST Use the brown pen to outline the solitary nucleus and fill in the solitary tract. This tract is well-named. The solitary nucleus is the main central sensory nucleus of the autonomic system. While we don't usually think of the autonomic system as having a sensory arm, systemic data like blood pressure and blood oxygen content do represent sensory data relevant to both the sympathetic and parasympathetic efferent systems. Use the brown pen to outline the input fibers to the solitary nucleus, the glossopharyngeal (IX) and vagus (X) nerves. The main taste fibers enter via the facial nerve, and some data also enter via the trigeminal and glossopharyngeal nerves. You can try to thread the brown yarn from the input nerves to this nucleus, but your model will become quite tangled!

Vagus Nucleus

INST A major integration center for the autonomic nervous system resides in the lateral medulla. Just accept this, since it is not straightforward to outline. These neurons process some of the sensory information from the solitary nucleus and control autonomic output. You should find, outline, and label the major parasympathetic motor nucleus in the medulla, the dorsal motor nucleus of the vagus (X), which receives input from this lateral medullary reticular formation control center. More difficult to find, but clinically relevant are the descending sympathetic control fibers. These travel in the lateral medulla, close to the ascending spinothalamic fibers, ventral to the spinal trigeminal nucleus. Place a vague brown circle near the ascending spinothalamic fibers to recognize this.

Remember, sympathetic information leaves the nervous system only in the thoracic and upper lumbar cord. Fibers from the hypothalamus and medullary reticular formation travel in the lateral medulla and descend to the intermediolateral cell column of the spinal cord. The fibers are clinically important since they may be infarcted in a relatively common brainstem stroke. Such lesions are loved by neurologists, who call them a "Wallenberg stroke." You will encounter this stroke both in this course and probably in some of your patients.

INST Review the pathway from the lateral medulla, to the intermediolateral cell column, to the sympathetic ganglia, and finally to the eye. The lack of sympathetic input to the ipsilateral eye would produce a Horner's syndrome: a contracted pupil (unopposed parasympathetics) and a droopy eyelid (as well as a decreased ability to sweat on that side of the face).

CEREBELLAR SYSTEMS (YELLOW)

INST The cerebellum is interwoven with the brainstem in a complex fashion, so this part of the excercise will leave your model a bit confusing. First find, outline, and label in yellow the main players:

- Inferior cerebellar peduncle (ICP)
- Middle cerebellar peduncle (MCP)
- Superior cerebellar peduncle (SCP)
- Inferior olivary nucleus (ION)
- Basis pontis (PONS)
- Red nucleus (RN)
- Accessory cuneate nucleus (ACN)
- Dorsal spinocerebellar tract (DST)

INST The inferior cerebellar peduncle contains fibers from the ipsilateral dorsal spinocerebellar tract, the ipsilateral accessory cuneate nucleus, and the contralateral inferior olivary nucleus (and some other fibers that we won't illustrate here). Thread yellow yarn from the dorsal spinocerebellar tract in the lowest section of medulla up to the exit of the inferior cerebellar peduncle (e.g., on the left side). Remember, these fibers originate in the ipsilateral Clarke's nucleus. Although quite an aesthetic nucleus, adding the inferior olivary nucleus fibers will create an unaesthetic model. Add the contralateral projection from the olive anyway.

INST The middle cerebellar peduncle contains fibers from the large neurons in the contralateral basis pontis. These neurons receive information from the ipsilateral cerebral cortex. Notice how the pyramidal tract also passes through this region. Thread some yellow yarn from one side of the pontine base, across the midline, into the contralateral middle cerebellar peduncle. This region of the brain is quite large, since it is the principal site whereby cortical motor information reaches the cerebellum to control fine motions. Show the cortical inputs by threading yellow yarn down through the ventral cerebral peduncle in the midbrain to your pontine base neuron.

INST The superior cerebellar peduncle derives most of its fibers from the dentate nucleus in the cerebellum, which is not present on the acetates. However, you can weave a fragment of yellow yarn from where you first encounter this tract in the upper pontine tegmentum, past its site of decussation in the lowest midbrain (the great decussation of the superior cerebellar peduncle) to one of its termination sites in the red nucleus. Remember, it sends it major projection on to the ventral lateral nucleus of the thalamus.

INST You are almost done. The red nucleus has several projections. Take another fragment of yellow yarn and thread it from the red nucleus, have it immediately decussate, and then have it descend in the lateral part of the tegmentum throughout the brainstem. It eventually lies just medial to the

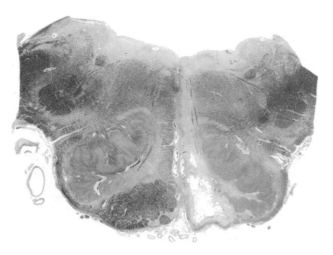

FIGURE 12.7. *Medial   medullary infarct histology.*

descending lateral cortical spinal tract in the spinal cord. Notice the information from the cerebellum to the spinal cord is double-crossed: a right-sided cerebellar lesion will produce a right-sided clinical ataxia. Finally add the ipsilateral projection from the red nucleus to the inferior olivary nucleus via the central tegmental tract.

This model only gives you a sense of how complex the brainstem is. It is worthwhile remembering that brainstem lesions don't cause madness, but recreating its tracts does.

CASE REVIEW

INST   Below is a set of cases (both histology and gross pictures) in which lesions are present in a part of the brainstem. Identify the anatomic sites involved. Predict the clinical outcome of each lesion. Assume that the right side of the image is on the right side of the patient.

Q12.1. The patient had several embolic infarcts to his brain and other vital organs. Figure 12.7 shows the major infarct in his medial medulla.

A12.1. *The infarct involves the entire right pyramid, the right hypoglossal nerve as it exits the medulla, the right medial lemniscus, and a small portion of the inferior olivary nucleus.*

The patient would have an alternating hypoglossal hemiplegia. Translating this into English, the patient would have a contralateral (left) hemiplegia from involvement of the corticospinal tract in the pyramids and an ipsilateral (right) tongue paralysis from the infarction of the right hypoglossal nerve. He should also have contralateral loss of somatosensory sensations from the body, but not the head. Note: Any possible cerebellar effects from the right olivary lesion would be overshadowed by the pyramidal tract lesion. Think about why.

Q12.2. The patient with the histology shown in Figure 12.8 had a small medullary infarct. (In this image, tissue in the upper left portion of the specimen was lost in processing. This is not the lesion!)

A12.2. *The infarct is in the lateral medulla but spares the spinal trigeminal nucleus and tract as well as the vestibular nuclei. It does involve the descending sympathetic and ascending spinothalamic fibers, as well as portions of the lateral medulla, including the nucleus ambiguus.*

This patient's main problem was a severe swallowing disorder. The infarct extends up to and partially involves the nucleus ambiguus, which produced hemiparesis of bulbar musculature necessary for swallowing. The patient actually died as a result of this small lesion, since he aspirated and developed a subsequent pneumonia (aspiration pneumonia).

You might predict as well that the patient would have an incomplete Wallenberg syndrome. The infarct lies in the region of the descending sympathetic fibers and ascending spinothalamic fibers. Consequently you would predict that the patient had an ipsilateral (right) Horner's syndrome (right eye miosis or a small pupil from an inability to dilate the eye, right ptosis or a droopy right eye lid from loss of innervation to the tarsal muscle (assists the levator palpebrae), and right-sided anhidrosis or loss of sweating) and a contralateral (left) anesthesia to pain and temperature.

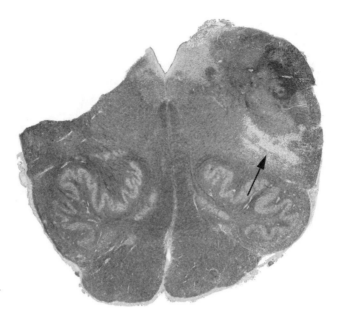

FIGURE 12.8. *Lateral medulla infarct histology.*

Q12.3. The pons pictured in Figure 12.9 is from a young boy who developed a glioblastoma in his brainstem. These are frequently called "pontine gliomas." Based on just this slice, which contains necrotic tumor, what deficits might you predict?

A12.3. *The necrosis involves the descending corticospinal tracts and corticobulbar tracts. In addition pontine base neurons projecting to the contralateral cerebellum are destroyed. Less apparent is the involvement of the trigeminal fibers exiting from the lateral pons, just below this level.*

On just this slice, you would expect the patient to have a dense right hemiplegia. A left trigeminal palsy would also be expected.

Patients with brainstem gliomas develop multifocal cranial nerve palsies, based on sites of tumor necrosis, infiltration, and pressure on nearby peripheral nerves.

Q12.4. The lacunar infarcts in Figure 12.10 are near some major structures. In contrast to the other images, suggest why the patient did not have major sensory or motor findings.

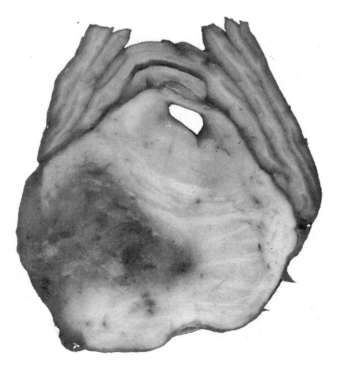

FIGURE 12.9. *Gross pathology from a boy with a brainstem glioblastoma.*

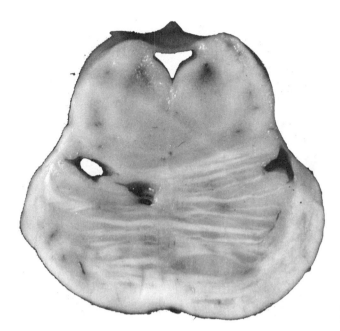

FIGURE 12.10. *Lacunar infarcts in the pons.*

A12.4. *These lacunar infarcts are in the dorsal part of the pontine base. This is dorsal to the sites of the major descending corticospinal and corticobulbar fibers and just ventral to the medial lemniscus, spinothalamic fibers, and lateral lemniscus.*

While the patient had several pontine infarcts, he had no reported symptoms or signs (although he also had no careful neurologic examination). You may have predicted some right-sided cerebellar signs and perhaps some right-sided pyramidal signs (weakness and spasticity).

Q12.5. Figure 12.11 is from a man who developed a thrombus at the bifurcation of his basilar artery, which produced a complex "top of the basilar" infarct.

A12.5. *Both oculomotor nuclei and nerves are infarcted, along with the medial longitudinal fasciculus. In addition other central regions are necrotic, including portions of the periaqueductal gray, portions of the red nuclei, and the dentatothalamic tracts that runs just medial to the red nuclei. The corticospinal tracts, medial lemniscus, and anterolateral system have all been spared.*

As you might predict, the patient would have a complete, bilateral third nerve palsy. Since the abducens nerve is in the lower pons and uninvolved by the lesion, the patient's eyes would both be fixed looking lateral. The third nerve also carries parasympathetic inputs to contract the eye. The patient would initially have "blown pupils" from the unopposed sympathetic input to the iris. While you may also guess that the patient would have severe cerebellar signs, you would not be able to elicit them, since his entire reticular activating system, traveling medially to the cerebrum, was severed and left him in a deep coma.

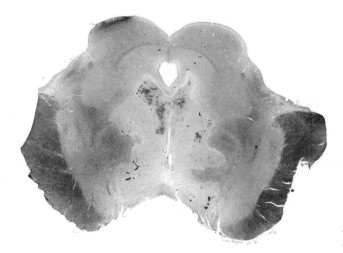

FIGURE 12.11. *Top of the basilar infarct histology.*

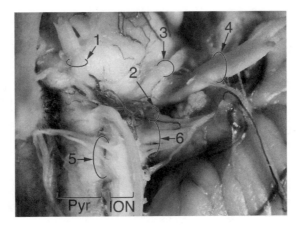

FIGURE 12.12. *Cranial nerve worksheet. Close-up of the cerebellopontine angle.*

QUICK REVIEW

Q12.6. Figure 12.12 is a close-up of the brainstem shown in the previous chapter. It shows only one-half of the upper medulla and lower pons. The pyramid (Pyr) and inferior olivary nuclei are labeled. Refresh your memory by identifying the indicated cranial nerves:

12.6.1 _____

12.6.2 _____

12.6.3 _____

12.6.4 _____

12.6.5 _____

12.6.6 _____

A12.6. 12.6.1. *Abducens*
12.6.2. *Glossopharyngeal*
12.6.3. *Facial*
12.6.4. *Vestibulocochlear*
12.6.5. *Hypoglossal*
12.6.6. *Vagus*

BUILDING THE CRANIAL NERVES

In this section you will build the cranial nerves that are attached to the brainstem. Figures 12.49 and 12.50 at the end of the chapter contain 18 images of different brainstem levels, each with a single nucleus highlighted. You'll cut these out and use them to indicate which nuclei correspond to each cranial nerve. You may want to photocopy these figures and cut the copies.

INST   First, on Figures 12.49 and 12.50 label each nucleus that is highlighted in the designated level. Note that some nuclei are repeated. This is because they are associated with more than one cranial nerve. Then cut out each square. For each nerve, follow the instructions, including pasting the appropriate site with its cranial nerve and labeling the nerve in the brainstem figure from the Nieuwenhuys atlas (R. Nieuwenhuys, J. Voogd, and Chr. van Huijzen, *The Human Central Nervous System. A Synopsis and Atlas,* 3rd rev. ed., © 1988, Springer-Verlag, New York).

Oculomotor Nerve (III)

Q12.7. This nerve contains two distinct types of efferent signals. Name them and what they do. Highlight where this nerve exits the brainstem in Figure 12.13 and paste the associated nuclei into Figure 12.14.

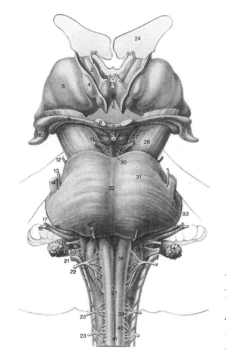

FIGURE 12.13. *Modified from Nieuwenhuys, Voogd, van Huijzen, The Human Central Nervous System. A Synopsis and Atlas. 3rd edition. © 1988. Springer-Verlag, Berlin, figure 17, page 22.*

A12.7. *Efferent signals: motor neuron input to the extraocular muscles (medial, inferior, and superior rectus muscles and inferior oblique) and parasympathetic input to iris and lens. From the discussion in the introduction, the parasympathetics don't belong here. You may either think of them as displaced from the trigeminal nerve or just accept reality.*
      See Figures 12.15 and 12.16

Trochlear Nerve (IV)

Q12.8. Although having relatively simple function, the trochlear nerve has a complex course. Describe its function and its course. Paste its nucleus in Figure 12.18 and highlight it on the model in Figure 12.17 (notice the model is different from others in this series).

A12.8. *Surprise! This nerve innervates the trochlear or superior oblique intrinsic eye muscle, that intorts and depresses the globe. Its course is more interesting. The lower motor neurons lie in the ventral, caudal midbrain, at the level of the decussation of the superior cerebellar peduncle. The trochlear nucleus lies buried in the medial longitudinal fasciculus. Its fibers descend, move dorsally, cross at the dorsal side of the periaqueductal gray, and exit from the posterior (hence the posterior view of the brainstem, after the cerebellum has been removed). After that, they move ventrally around the brainstem, eventually join up with VI and III, and exit through the superior orbital fissure.*
      See Figures 12.19 and 12.20

FIGURE 12.14. *IIIrd nerve nuclei histology worksheet.*

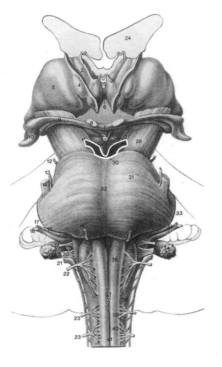

FIGURE 12.15. Modified from Nieuwenhuys, Voogd, van Huijzen, The Human Central Nervous System. A Synopsis and Atlas. 3rd edition. © 1988. Springer-Verlag, Berlin, figure 17, page 22.

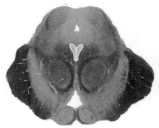 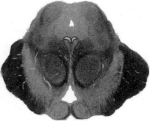

FIGURE 12.16. IIIrd nerve nuclei in midbrain.

oculomotor nucleus   Edinger-Westphal nucleus

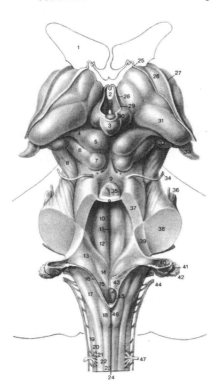

FIGURE 12.17. Trochlear nerve worksheet. (Modified from Nieuwenhuys, Voogd, van Huijzen, The Human Central Nervous System. A Synopsis and Atlas. 3rd edition. © 1988. Springer-Verlag, Berlin, figure 15, page 20).

FIGURE 12.18. Trochlear nucleus worksheet.

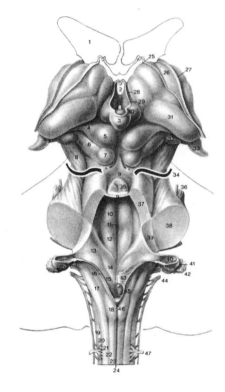

FIGURE 12.19. Trochlear nerve worksheet. (Modified from Nieuwenhuys, Voogd, van Huijzen, The Human Central Nervous System. A Synopsis and Atlas. 3rd edition. © 1988. Springer-Verlag, Berlin, figure 15, page 20).

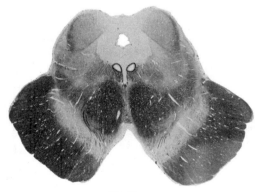

trochlear

FIGURE 12.20. Trochlear nucleus in the caudal midbrain.

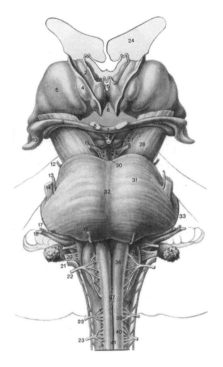

FIGURE 12.21. *Modified from Nieuwenhuys, Voogd, van Huijzen, The Human Central Nervous System. A Synopsis and Atlas. 3rd edition. © 1988. Springer-Verlag, Berlin, figure17, page 22.*

Trigeminal Nerve (V)

Q12.9. This most massive cranial nerve controls two major functions, one sensory and one motor. What are its sensory divisions? Its motor functions? Mark its position on the brainstem in Figure 12.21 and describe its peripheral ganglion. Name and paste its associated nuclei in Figure 12.22. Discuss the level of the brainstem and the functional aspects of each nucleus.

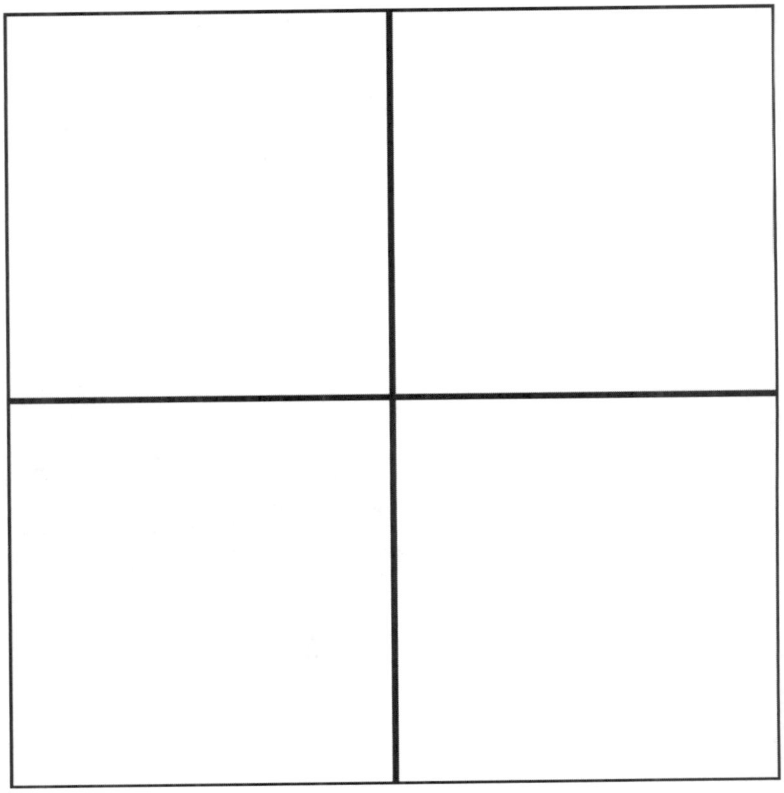

FIGURE 12.22. *Nuclear worksheet for the trigeminal nerve.*

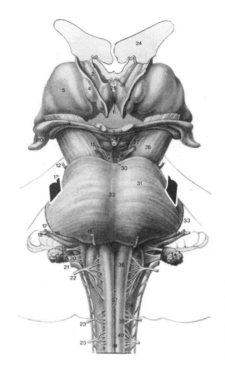

FIGURE 12.23. *Modified from Nieuwenhuys, Voogd, van Huijzen, The Human Central Nervous System. A Synopsis and Atlas. 3rd edition. © 1988. Springer-Verlag, Berlin, figure 17, page 22.*

A12.9. *The trigeminal nerve has both sensory and motor functions. Its ganglion lies outside the dura at the base of the brain. Because of its importance it has been given three different names: trigeminal, semilunar, and Gasserian ganglion (depending on whether you like to view it from below, above, or historically). Like three fingers poking through the skull, its three divisions travel through three foramen: superior orbital fissure for the ophthalmic division (sensation above the midline of the eyes), the foramen rotundum for the maxillary division (sensation below the midline eye to the jaw), and the foramen ovale for the mandibular division (jaw sensation and motor function). See a sensory dermatome map for specifics. Remember from the introduction that VI, the profundus nerve, was originally associated with III, which may explain why they leave the skull together.*

    The pain and temperature fibers from the face descend from their entry in the pons down into the medulla and upper spinal cord, ending in the spinal trigeminal nucleus. This is true not only for trigeminal nerve fibers but for pain sensations traveling into the brain through other cranial nerves as well. The information crosses and ascends to join the spinothalamic fibers.

    Proprioceptive information is processed in the principle trigeminal sensory nucleus, immediately lateral to the trigeminal motor nucleus. Remember, the branchial nuclei are all lateral, but their motor fibers lie more medial than the sensory fibers. This information also crosses and joins the medial lemniscal fibers.

    A special set of sensory fibers derived from the muscles of mastication have their dorsal root ganglion neurons in the brainstem itself, in the trigeminal mesencephalic nucleus. These are involved in the jaw jerk reflex, presumably to protect your teeth in the age before processed foods.

    From an evolutionary perspective, the trigeminal controls among the most important motor functions in the body: eating. Grabbing food and munching on it has been around at least since the jawed bony fishes in the Silurian. Fibers project from the trigeminal motor nucleus, through the mandibular division, to the muscles of mastication.

    See Figures 12.23 and 12.24.

Abducens Nerve (VI)

Q12.10. This simple cranial nerve is nevertheless clinically relevant. Show its exit from the brainstem in Figure 12.25 and paste its nucleus in Figure 12.26. What is its function? Give two possible reasons why this nerve is is particularly susceptible to disease.

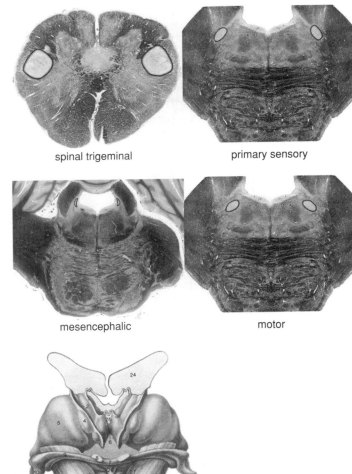

spinal trigeminal

primary sensory

mesencephalic

motor

FIGURE 12.24. *Spinal trigeminal nucleus in medulla, primary trigeminal sensory nucleus in pons, mesencephalic nucleus in upper pons, and trigeminal motor nucleus in pons.*

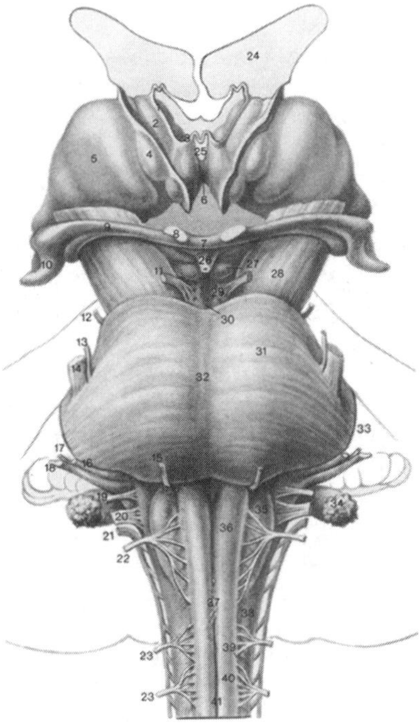

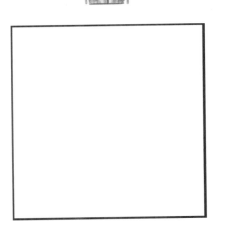

FIGURE 12.25. *Modified from Nieuwenhuys, Voogd, van Huijzen, The Human Central Nervous System. A Synopsis and Atlas. 3rd edition. © 1988. Springer-Verlag, Berlin, figure 17, page 22.*

FIGURE 12.26. *Abducens nucleus worksheet.*

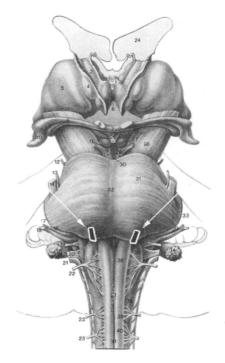

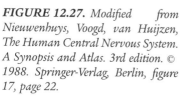

FIGURE 12.27. *Modified from Nieuwenhuys, Voogd, van Huijzen, The Human Central Nervous System. A Synopsis and Atlas. 3rd edition. © 1988. Springer-Verlag, Berlin, figure 17, page 22.*

A12.10. The abducens nerve controls the lateral rectus muscle, and thus abducts the eye. While apparently simple, it does travel far from the base of the pons to the eye muscles, and in its course may be subject to the slings and arrows of diseases such as diabetes. Its nucleus also lies at the other end of the pons from its siblings in the midbrain; their connection, the medial longitudinal fasciculus, is long and also may be injured by diseases such as multiple sclerosis.
See Figures 12.27 and 12.28.

Facial Nerve (VII)

Q12.11. This nerve has four components, both sensory and motor. Somatic sensory information from the external ear travel through this nerve but ends up in brainstem trigeminal sensory nuclei. It also contains parasympathetic fibers innervating salivary and lacrimal glands. However, it has two much more important and interesting functions. Name its other motor and "visceral" sensory functions. Paste their associated nuclei in Figure 12.30. Indicate the facial nerve's exit on the brainstem model in Figure 12.29.

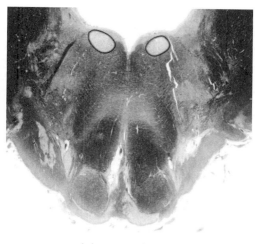

abducens nucleus

FIGURE 12.28. *Abducens nucleus in lower pons.*

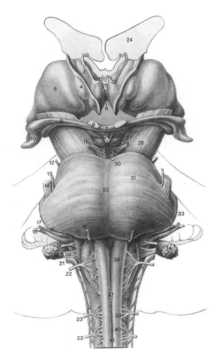

FIGURE 12.29. *Modified from Nieuwenhuys, Voogd, van Huijzen, The Human Central Nervous System. A Synopsis and Atlas. 3rd edition. © 1988. Springer-Verlag, Berlin, figure 17, page 22.*

A12.11. *The head really has two sets of muscles, those deep muscles of mastication and the superficial muscles controlling facial expression. The facial nerve, from its motor nucleus in the lowest pons, controls the superficial muscles. These not only express your feelings, but control your cheeks and blinking. Your taste sensations from most of your tongue travel through the chorda tympani, through the nervous intermedius (tacked onto and included in the facial nerve) to the rostral solitary nucleus. Notice how these nuclei, like the trigeminal, are lateral.*
    See Figures 12.31 and 12.32.

Vestibulocochlear Nerve (VIII)

Q12.12. This nerve is really two. Show their entry into the brainstem in Figure 12.33. What are their peripheral sensory organs? Paste their nuclei into Figure 12.34. Schwannomas, a tumor of Schwann cells, have a penchant to form on the vestibular nerve at its exit from the skull, and crush both nerves. What might be your first guess as to such an afflicted patient's symptoms? What really happens? What happens if you perturb this system quickly, say by putting cold water in one ear canal?

A12.12. *The semicircular canals, saccule, and utricle send their circular and linear acceleration information to the vestibular nuclei (four of them, not further distinguished here), and the cochlea transmits its auditory signals to the cochlear nuclei (dorsal and two ventral, again, not distinguished here).*
    See Figures 12.35 and 12.36.

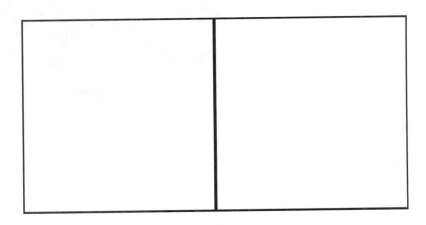

FIGURE 12.30. *Brainstem nuclei of facial nerve.*

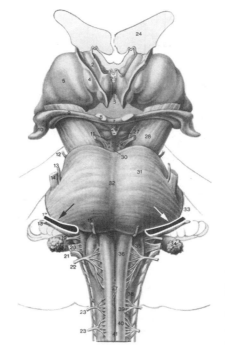

FIGURE 12.31. *Modified from Nieuwenhuys, Voogd, van Huijzen, The Human Central Nervous System. A Synopsis and Atlas. 3rd edition. © 1988. Springer-Verlag, Berlin, figure 17, page 22.*

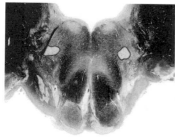

facial nucleus   solitary nucleus

FIGURE 12.32. *Facial motor nucleus in the caudal pons and the solitary nucleus in the dorsal medulla.*

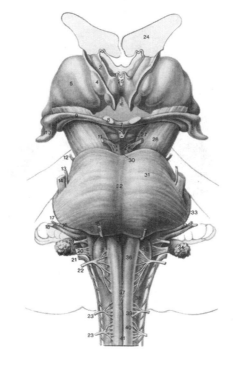

FIGURE 12.33. *Modified from Nieuwenhuys, Voogd, van Huijzen, The Human Central Nervous System. A Synopsis and Atlas. 3rd edition. © 1988. Springer-Verlag, Berlin, figure 17, page 22.*

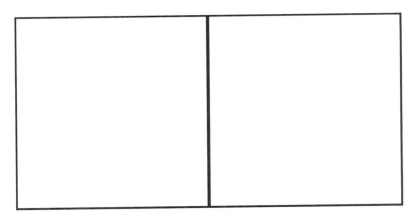

FIGURE 12.34. *Vestibular and cochlear nuclei worksheets.*

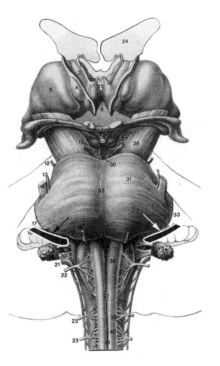

FIGURE 12.35. *Modified from Nieuwenhuys, Voogd, van Huijzen, The Human Central Nervous System. A Synopsis and Atlas. 3rd edition. © 1988. Springer-Verlag, Berlin, figure 17, page 22.*

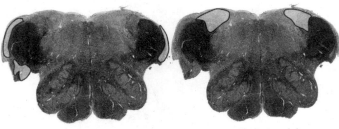

cochlear nuclei   vestibular nuclei

FIGURE 12.36. *Location of the cochlear nuclei and vestibular nuclear complex in the rostral medulla.*

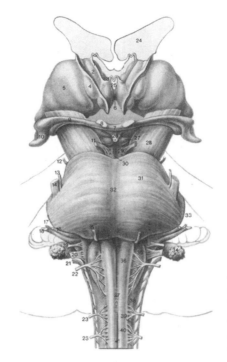

FIGURE 12.37. Modified from *Nieuwenhuys, Voogd, van Huijzen, The Human Central Nervous System. A Synopsis and Atlas. 3rd edition.* © *1988. Springer-Verlag, Berlin, figure 17, page 22.*

You may at first expect a tumor crushing both of these nerves would lead to complaints of deafness and vertigo. However, these often go unnoticed until the facial nerve also becomes compressed. Some patients may notice a unilateral hearing loss when using the telephone. Because hearing is bilaterally represented in the brain, people frequently fail to notice unilateral loss. The vestibular system is highly adaptive and can accommodate a slowly growing tumor like a Schwannoma. An acute change, such as placing cool or warm water in the external auditory meatus, will produce nystagmus and vertigo. This is a test of brainstem function in an unconscious patient (but not your friends!).

Glossopharyngeal Nerve (IX)

Q12.13. This nerve is like the runt of a litter, diminished compared to its siblings the facial and vagus nerves. Like the facial nerve, it transmits taste sensation, but only from the back of the tongue. It also sends parasympathetic impulses to the parotid gland (from a salivatory nucleus). Like the vagus, it controls a muscle of the pharynx, but only one. The glossopharyngeal nerve, however, does transmit two important types of information: special autonomic sensory receptors in the neck (which ones?) and general afferent sensory from the pharynx, palate, and other parts from the back of the mouth. Mark the glossopharyngeal nerve on Figure 12.37 and paste its autonomic sensory and motor nuclei in Figure 12.38.

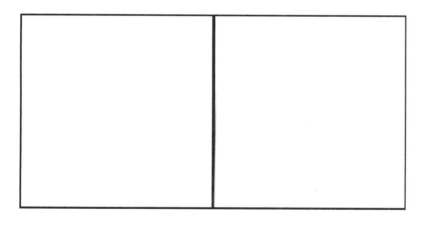

FIGURE 12.38. Nuclear components of the glossopharyngeal nerve.

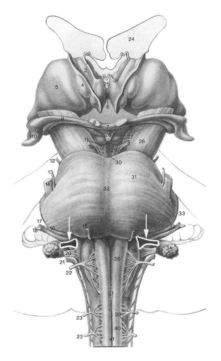

FIGURE 12.39. *Modified from Nieuwenhuys, Voogd, van Huijzen, The Human Central Nervous System. A Synopsis and Atlas. 3rd edition. © 1988. Springer-Verlag, Berlin, figure 17, page 22.*

A12.13. The special sensory receptors are in the carotid body (chemosensory) and carotid sinus (pressure). This information, along with taste from the back of the tongue, ends up in the solitary nucleus. The pharyngeal sensory fibers end up in the trigeminal sensory nuclei. The stylopharyngeal muscles are innervated by motor neurons in the nucleus ambiguus.

  The sensory portion of the gag reflex derives from glossopharyngeal receptors in the mouth, while most of the motor component originates from ambiguus nucleus and travels in the vagus nerve.

  See Figures 12.39 and 12.40.

Vagus Nerve (X)

Q12.14. You have encountered several of the main functions of this nerve. List them. Also paste their associated nuclei in Figure 12.42 and mark the nerve's exit on Figure 12.41.

  The vagus has several other functions. Just as it transmits autonomic efferent information to the body, it also receives autonomic or visceral afferent sensations from the body. Sites include parts of the pharynx and larynx, the trachea, and from the abdominal and thoracic contents. As in the facial and glossopharyngeal nerves, name the associated brainstem nucleus, and paste this nucleus in Figure 12.42.

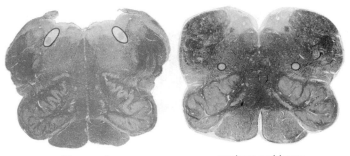

solitary nucleus   nucleus ambiguus

FIGURE 12.40. *Solitary nucleus and nucleus ambiguus in medulla.*

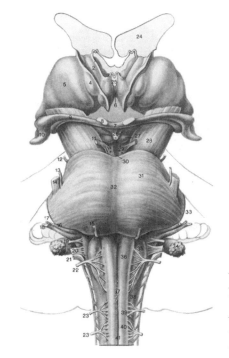

FIGURE 12.41. *Modified from Nieuwenhuys, Voogd, van Huijzen, The Human Central Nervous System. A Synopsis and Atlas. 3rd edition. © 1988. Springer-Verlag, Berlin, figure 17, page 22.*

Not to be left out, the vagus also transmits some taste sensation from the epiglottis, which is not generally considered when you swirl wine in your mouth. Finally, somatic sensations from a bit of the ear and the external auditory meatus also travel in the vagus nerve and project to trigeminal sensory nuclei.

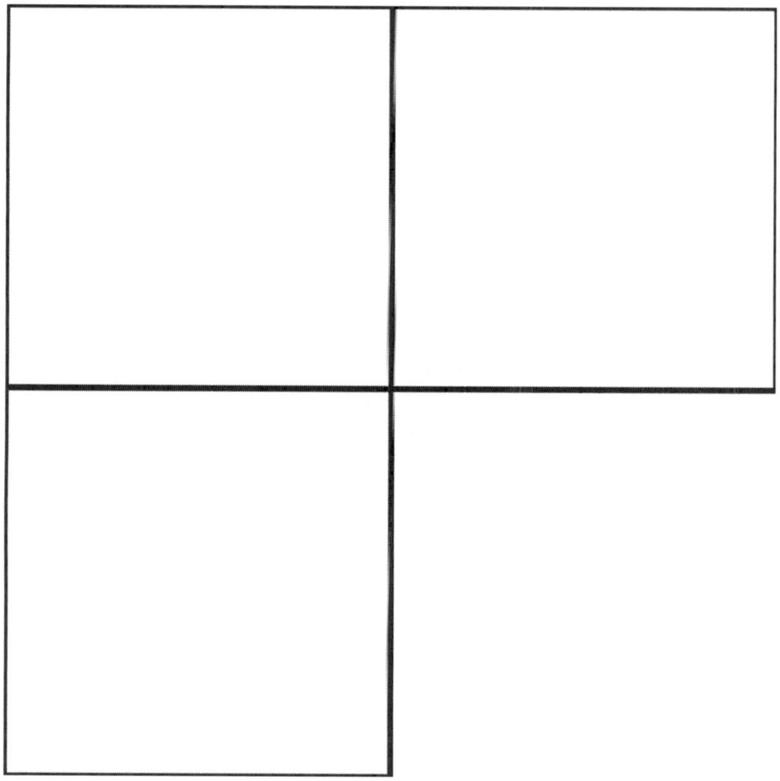

FIGURE 12.42. *Vagal nuclei worksheet.*

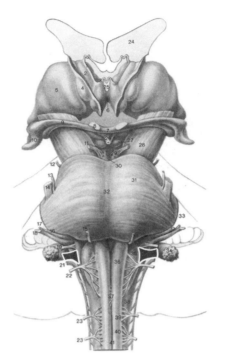

FIGURE 12.43. *Modified from Nieuwenhuys, Voogd, van Huijzen, The Human Central Nervous System. A Synopsis and Atlas. 3rd edition. © 1988. Springer-Verlag, Berlin, figure 17, page 22.*

A12.14. For the practicing clinician, the two major functions of the vagus are providing preganglionic parasympathetic motor fibers to most of the body and supplying motor control over swallowing and your vocal cords. The parasympathetic fibers originate from the dorsal motor nucleus of the vagus, while the pharyngeal muscle lower motor neurons reside in the nucleus ambiguus. The autonomic sensations, like all autonomic sensations, pass to the solitary nucleus.
   See Figures 12.43 and 12.44.

Hypoglossal Nerve (XII)

Q12.15. You may feel relieved that you're finishing with this nerve. It only innervates one muscle function and has a large, distinct nucleus. Paste the nucleus in Figure 12.46 and highlight the nerve's exit from the brainstem in Figure 12.45.

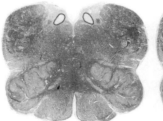

dorsal motor nucleus of vagus   nucleus ambiguus

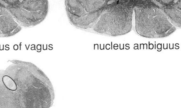

FIGURE 12.44. *Nuclear components of the vagus nerve.*

solitary nucleus

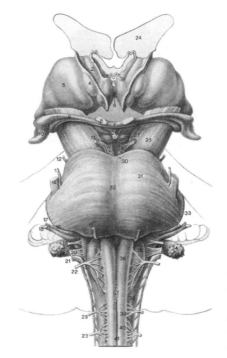

FIGURE 12.45. Modified from Nieuwenhuys, Voogd, van Huijzen, The Human Central Nervous System. A Synopsis and Atlas. 3rd edition. © 1988. Springer-Verlag, Berlin, figure 17, page 22.

FIGURE 12.46. Hypoglossal nucleus worksheet.

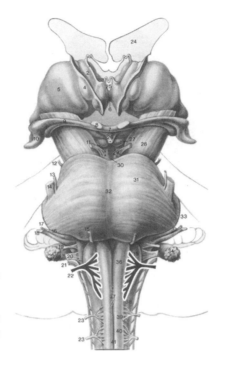

FIGURE 12.47. Modified from Nieuwenhuys, Voogd, van Huijzen, The Human Central Nervous System. A Synopsis and Atlas. 3rd edition. © 1988. Springer-Verlag, Berlin, figure 17, page 22.

The main source of confusion about the hypoglossal nerve is that it makes the tongue protrude by contracting a muscle. Discuss the clinical manifestation of a patient having a left hypoglossal nerve palsy.

A12.15. *The hypoglossal nerve innervates muscles in the base of the tongue. Contracting both sides causes the tongue to protrude directly out, while contracting the left side makes the tongue move right. Should you ask a patient with a left hypoglossal nerve palsy to "stick out their tongue," only the right side will contract, and their tongue will point left or toward the side of the lesion.*

See Figures 12.47 and 12.48.

As humans, we put a lot of faith in our tongue. It helps us eat and articulate our speech. It can be an effective tool of social discontent. It is surprising therefore to find out it derives in evolution from muscles in the back of the skull. The hypoglossal nerve is not even present in some fish!

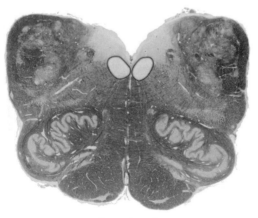

FIGURE 12.48. Hypoglossal nucleus in the medulla.

hypoglossal

APPENDIX: SECTIONS FOR BRAINSTEM EXERCISES

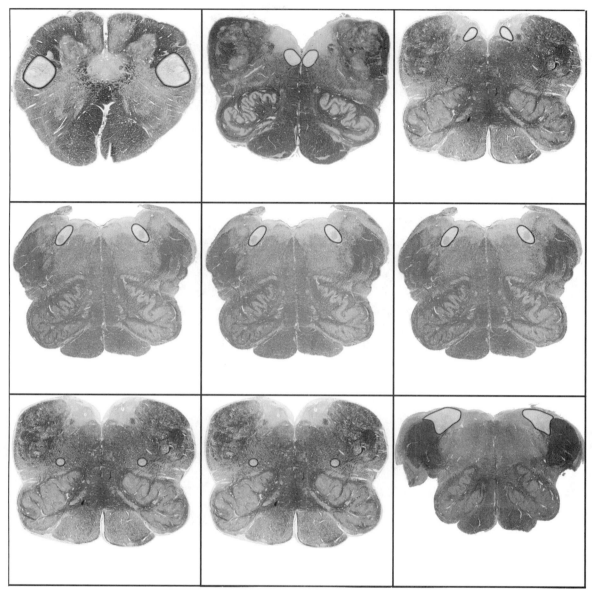

FIGURE 12.49. *Cut these out and use them in the previous set of exercises.*

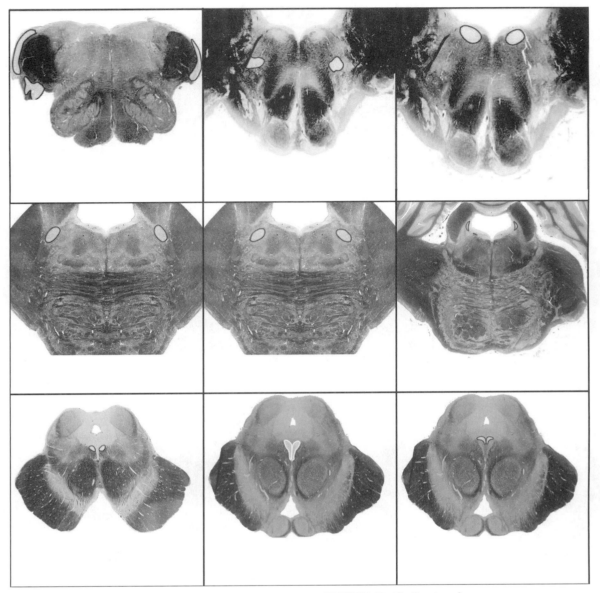

FIGURE 12.49. *Continued.*

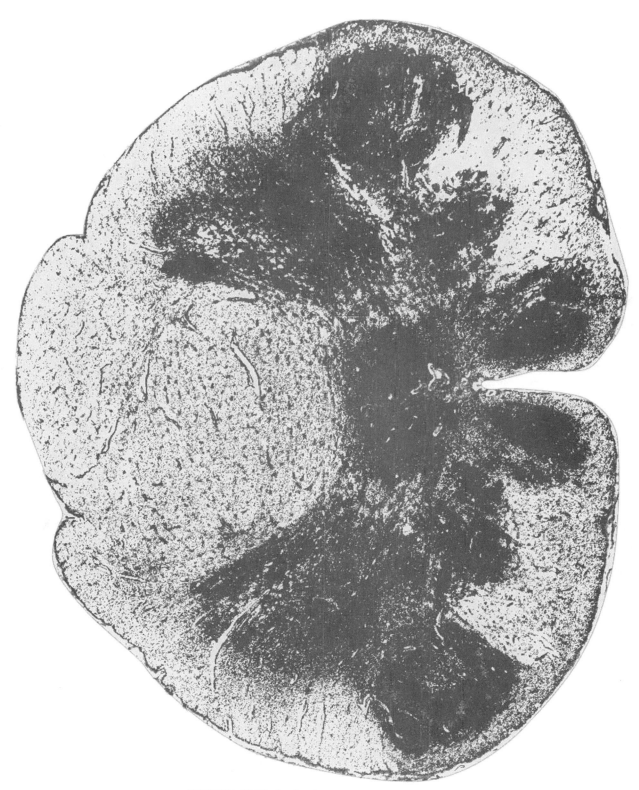

FIGURE 12.50. *Section 1.*

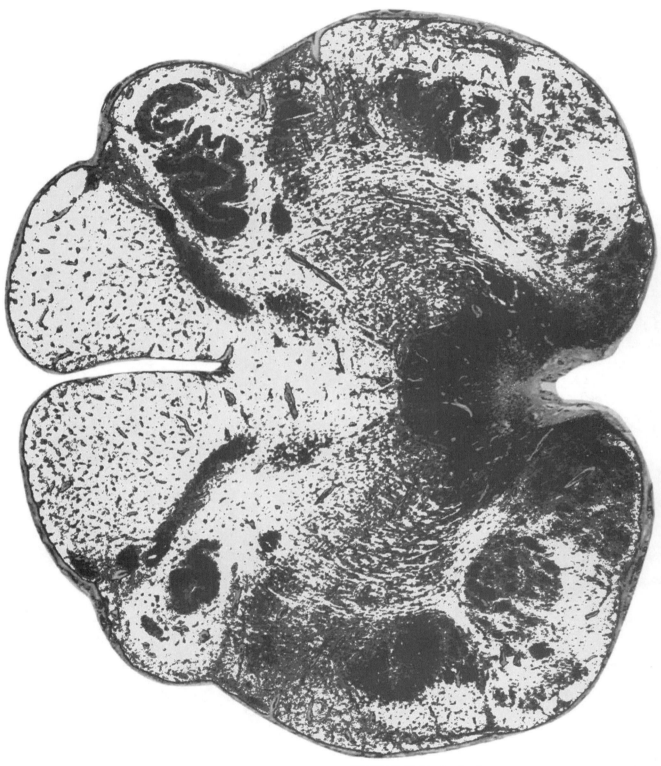

FIGURE 12.51. *Section 2.*

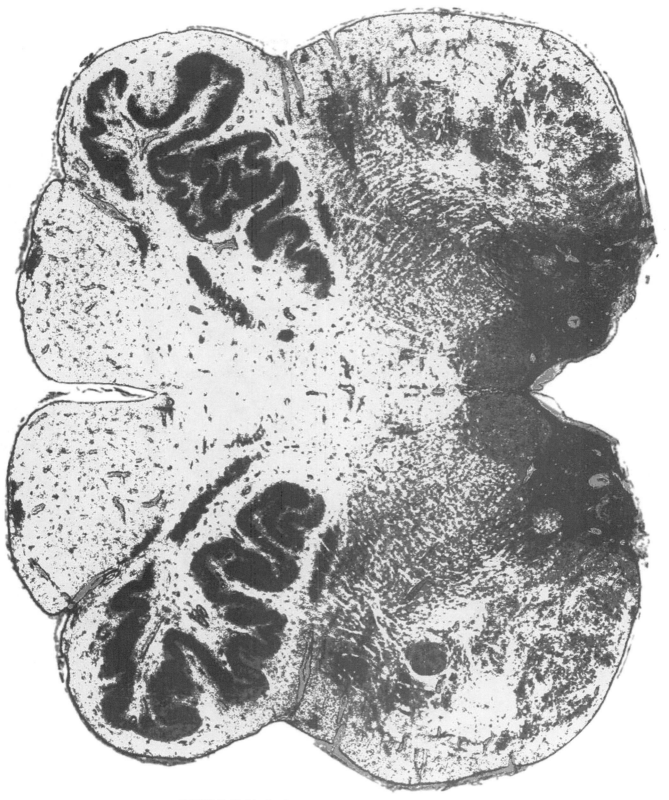

FIGURE 12.52. *Section 3.*

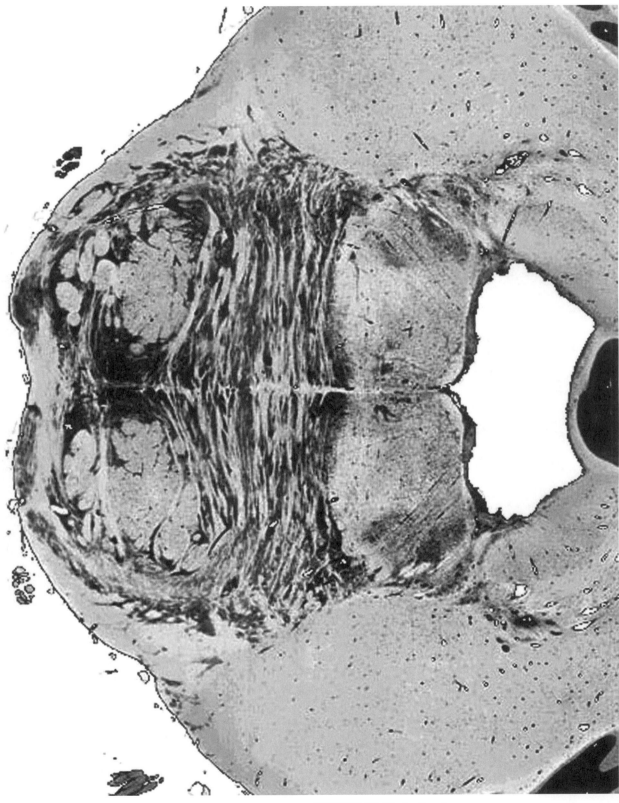

FIGURE 12.53. *Section 4.*

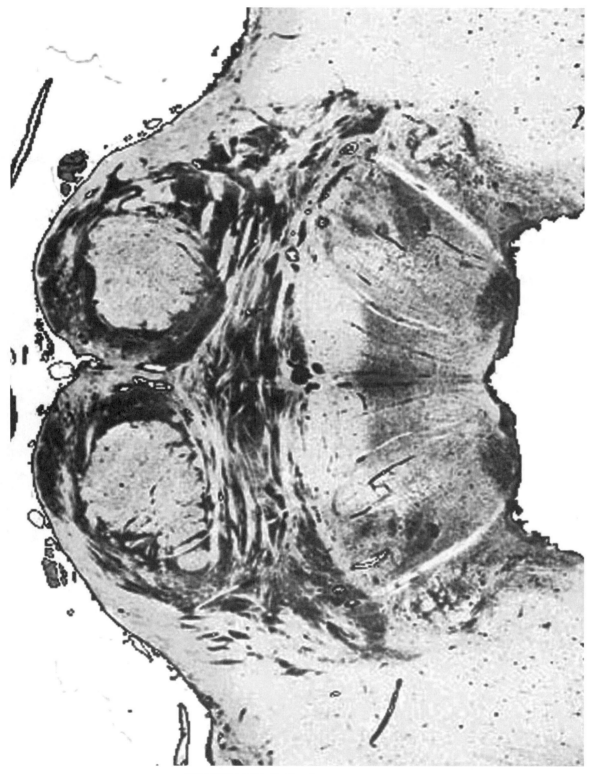

FIGURE 12.54. Section 5.

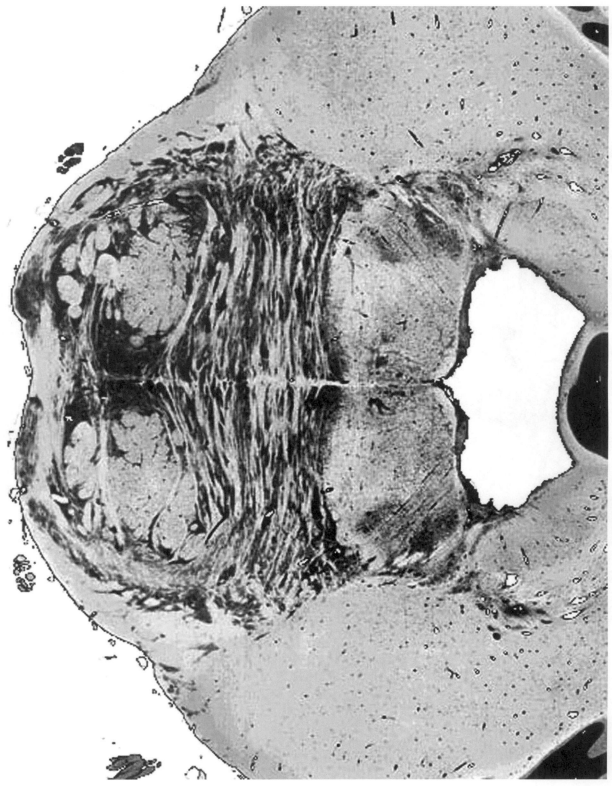

FIGURE 12.55. Section 6.

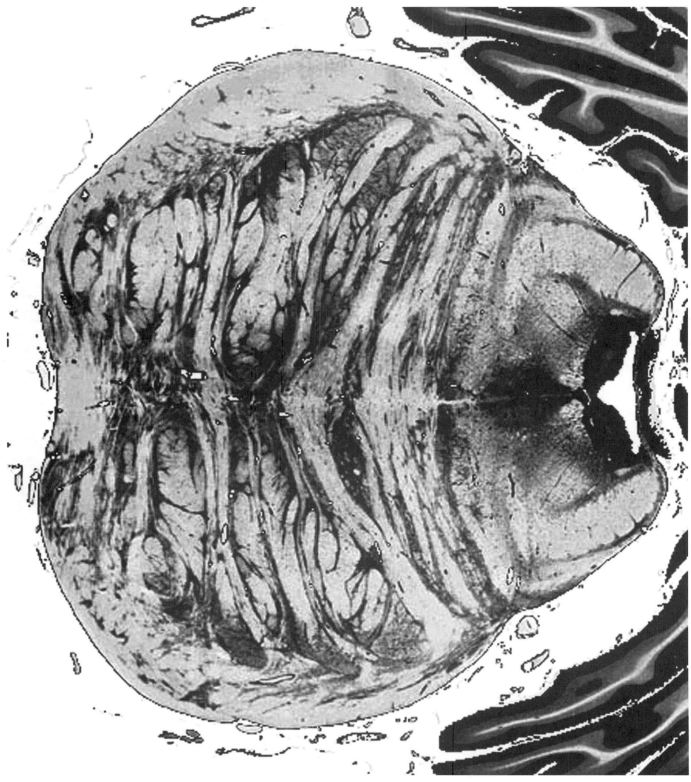

FIGURE 12.56. *Section 7.*

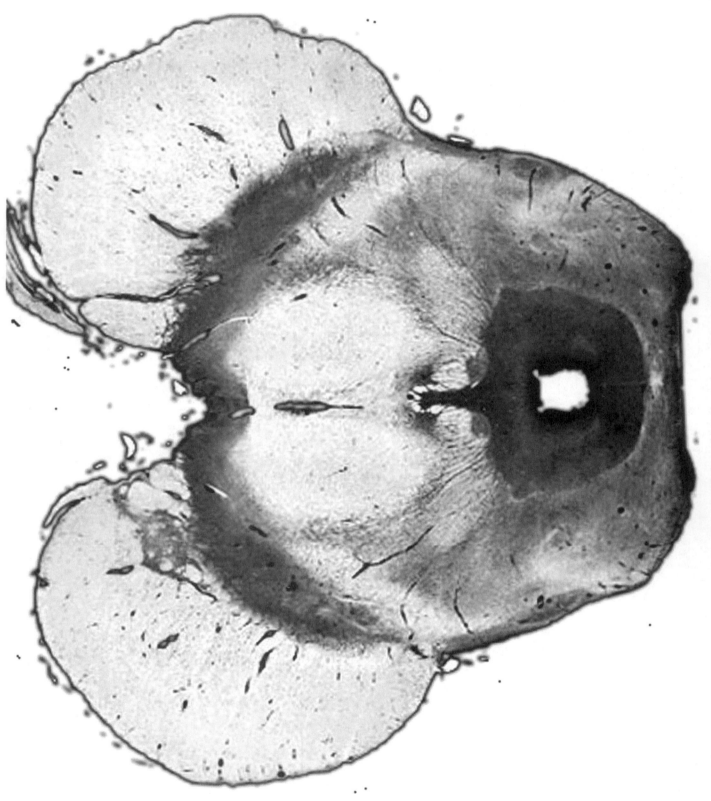

FIGURE 12.57. Section 8.

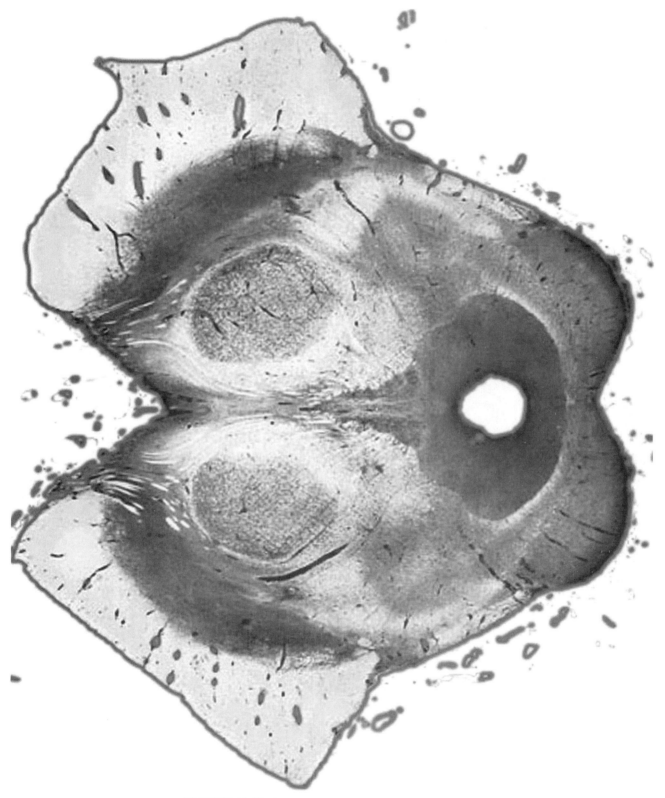

FIGURE 12.58. *Section 9.*

Chapter 13——HYPOTHALAMUS

ou had fallen in a hole in the snow bank. The mitten your Mommy had helped you put on had come off, and your hand felt the cold. Two of your now former friends were at the top of the hole, throwing snowballs at you. What a fix. How to get out? That hand was tingling. Snow pelted your sides. No way out. Then the greatest injustice, a snow ball to the face. That was it. Your hand stopped hurting, although you didn't realize it. Rational thought had ceased. You were now warm, your eyes dilated, your senses tweaked. Somehow, you climbed out of that hole, sent one of your schoolmates into it, and sent the other home crying for his mother. Nice to have a flight-or-fight mechanism built into your brain.

LEARNING OBJECTIVES

- Identify and describe functions of important neuroanatomic structures near the hypothalamus.
- Describe the major functions of the hypothalamus, including autonomic, hormonal, and behavioral regulation.
- Detail the hypothalamic-pituitary axis, including the anterior and posterior hypophyseal control mechanisms and the hormones involved.
- Describe some of the special techniques required to study the brain, including immunoperoxidase staining.

INTRODUCTION

The hypothalamus is critically important for homeostasis. It receives information from the internal environment and operates directly on the internal environment, regulating many vital functions, including temperature control, heart rate, blood pressure, blood osmolarity, water and food intake, energy metabolism, stress responses, and reproductive behaviors. In its central integrative role, it has widespread connections with and acts through three major systems: the limbic system and other forebrain structures, including the neural substrates for motivation and drive, the pituitary gland and endocrine system, and the autonomic nervous system. The limbic system gives that flight-or-fight signal and the hypothalamus has a major role in executing it.

Functional Neuroanatomy: An Interactive Text and Manual, by Jeffrey T. Joseph and David L. Cardozo
ISBN 0-471-44437-5 Copyright © 2004 John Wiley & Sons, Inc.

Hypothalamic Interactions

The hypothalamus regulates the endocrine system by two distinct mechanisms, both of which involve the master endocrine gland, the pituitary. One pathway is direct: two hypothalamic nuclei produce vasopressin and oxytocin, which is transported down their axons and released in the posterior pituitary lobe or neurohypophysis. The other pathway is indirect. Several nuclei secrete "releasing" polypeptide hormones into the local portal venous system of the median eminence, which in turn drains into the vessels of the anterior pituitary. Note that although most hypothalamic input to the adenohypophysis releases the target hormones, the dopamine input inhibits prolactin secretion.

The hypothalamus acts as "head ganglion" of the autonomic nervous system, integrating various inputs into a well-organized, coherent, and appropriate set of autonomic and somatic responses. Its cells are inferred to possess a wide range of receptors for neuroactive hormones and cytokines that mediate eating, drinking, sexual and other behaviors. The recently described leptin receptor on certain hypothalamic neurons, involving them intimately in food intake and fat metabolism, would seem to be just the "tip of the iceberg." This head ganglion has major caudal outputs to the brainstem (parasympathetic nuclei) and intermediolateral cell column of the spinal cord (sympathetic). These major outputs are carried in several (bidirectional) fiber systems: the medial forebrain bundle, the mammillotegmental tract, and the dorsal longitudinal fasciculus.

Higher cortical centers communicate with the hypothalamus via the limbic system. This allows thought, perception, and emotion to influence hypothalamic regulation. Limbic system inputs to the hypothalamus include a portion of the hippocampal formation known as the *subiculum* that projects fibers through the fornix to the *mammillary bodies* of the posterior hypothalamus, the *amygdala* that transmits information to the hypothalamus via the arching *stria terminalis* (which lies just medial to the caudate nucleus) as well as via a more direct *amygdalofugal pathway* traveling in the basal forebrain, and the cingulate gyrus that also has direct projections to the hypothalamus via the *medial forebrain bundle.* Hypothalamic outputs to the limbic system and other forebrain structures include relays through the *mammillothalamic tract* to the anterior thalamic nucleus and then to the cingulate gyrus, the hippocampal formation through the fornix, and the amygdala via the stria terminalis.

Finally, the hypothalamus has several intrinsic systems concerned with the regulation of sleep, feeding, and other behaviors. For example, the ventrolateral preoptic hypothalamic-to-tuberomammillary hypothalamic pathway is involved in sleep and arousal.

Hypothalamic Inputs and Outputs

As indicated above, several distinct systems send information to the hypothalamus. The hypothalamus receives visual information to its *suprachiasmatic nucleus,* enabling it to regulate the day/night cycle. It also receives visceral, pain, and olfactory sensory information. The hypothalamus receives some systemic information directly through hormones and other humoral factors. While the blood-brain barrier isolates most of the brain from such effects, this shield is weakened in specific midline areas of the brain. These so-called *circumventricular organs* include the *organ vasculosum of the lamina terminalis* (OVLT), which provides the hypothalamus with humoral data, and the *area postrema,* which informs the medullary vomiting centers that tissue injury has happened somewhere in the body. The latter suggests a possible toxic cause and the necessity for cleaning the gastrointestinal tract.

Hypothalamic neurons participate in several classes of reflexes, based on the type of input and output:

- Neural input and neural output, for example, the flight or fight reaction.
- Neural input and humoral output, for example, milk ejection and uterine contraction regulated by oxytocin.
- Humoral input and humoral output, including short feedback loops (e.g., pituitary hormones feedback to modulate the hypothalamic releasing factors) and long feedback loops (e.g., corticosteroid release by the adrenal gland feeds back onto both the anterior pituitary and the brain).
- Humoral input and neural output, for example, the binding of androgens to motor neurons, thereby increasing muscle bulk and strength.

Regional Anatomy

While few diseases produce primary hypothalamic dysfunction, this lowly region is situated in a high-rent district. It lies immediately above the optic chiasm, behind which it drops its pituitary stalk. The circle of Willis makes its path beneath the hypothalamus, sending penetrating vessels into its substance. The third ventricle separates the two halves of hypothalamus. Above the hypothalamus lies the thalamus, while just caudal to it is the midbrain. During development, the neural tube ends at the lamina terminalis, and it is from this region that the cerebrum derives. The organ vasculosum of the lamina terminalis lies within this structure.

The hypothalamus may be divided up into workable regions. From front to back are the anterior and posterior hypothalamus and the mammillary bodies. The fornix divides the medial and lateral parts. Within the medial regions are most of the pituitary control sites, the suprachiasmatic nucleus, and some of the autonomic centers. The lateral hypothalamus has connections with the medial regions, and regulates sleep-wake, feeding, and other visceral functions. It also has long projections to the brainstem, spinal cord, and cortex.

Comprehending the anatomy of the numerous hypothalamic nuclei is not a goal of this text; memorizing their locations and even their specific functions would largely be lost by the time you walk out of the examination room. However, it is important that you retain the main functions and interconnections of the hypothalamus, since these you will encounter in your medical careers.

Autonomic Nervous System

We all learn of the autonomic nervous system early in our lives. We have "adrenaline" rushes. Most of us have heard of people allergic to bees who need to keep "adrenaline" on hand. And we perhaps have seen the trembling side effects of asthma medications. In your prior studies you may have already examined the autonomic system in relationship to the cardiovascular system and its effects on bronchioles. It's your poor, neglected brain, however, that regulates the system.

The central autonomic system has two effector branches: the sympathetic and parasympathetic. These are tightly coordinated by several different nuclei within the brain. These nuclei need to receive information about the body before they can act. Much like the ascending pain, temperature, and proprioceptive sensory systems you have encountered previously, the autonomic system has its own sensory pathways. The sensory organs include baroreceptors and chemoreceptors. The major autonomic input station in the brain is the *solitary nucleus* in the medulla. Here information from your cardiovascular system arrives via the vagus and glossopharyngeal nerves. The most meaningful sensory data also come into the upper parts of the solitary nucleus from wonderful taste chemoreceptors on your tongue and pharynx. These essential sensations stop over in the ventral posterior medial nucleus of thalamus and end up in the *insular cortex* for digestion.

Autonomic information is routed to and processed at several levels throughout the nervous system. Much happens just in the medulla. Near the solitary nucleus in the ventrolateral medulla is a major autonomic control site, which regulates your heart and breathing rates, and coordinates both sympathetic output via the spinal cord and parasympathetic impulses from the vagus. In essence, this is the only part of your brain you need to stay alive. Destroy the lower medulla and you are dead. However, we all know that our autonomic nervous system goes into high gear during emotional situations. Embarrassment, aggression, and pleasure all have their autonomic responses. After ascending through several other nuclei, autonomic information reaches thalamus and then cortex. The insular cortex has a major control on autonomic output. The central integrator for our autonomic responses is the hypothalamus. It receives inputs from the amygdala, limbic system, insular cortex, and many other areas of brain, and in turn projects directly and indirectly down into the brainstem and spinal cord to parasympathetic and sympathetic control centers.

After the autonomic data have been integrated and processed, the control signals need to leave the nervous system. The parasympathetic nervous system is often called the craniosacral system, while the sympathetic system is termed thoracolumbar. In this laboratory you will see firsthand the origin of these designations. The various pathways and targets for these two complementary systems are best demonstrated in the somewhat bizarre diagrams presented in many textbooks, which have a spinal cord on one side and various floating organ on the other.

Diseases

Several disease processes may affect the hypothalamus, including tumors (hamartomas, pituitary adenomas) and inflammatory diseases (tuberculosis, sarcoidosis). As you will see, the hypothalamus is bilateral and has a rich vascular network, so infarcts rarely present clinically. If global brain disease mechanically impinges on the hypothalamus, as may happen in catastrophic hemorrhages or massive infarcts, the clinical manifestation is usually death. Diabetes insipidus, caused by a deficiency of vasopressin, may occur in isolation or secondary to tumors, granulomas, or trauma.

Many processes affect the autonomic nervous system. Diabetes mellitus can affect autonomic sensory input. Some neurodegenerative diseases, notably Parkinson's disease (Lewy body disease) and multiple system atrophy, can also affect these control system. However, the greatest effect on the autonomic nervous system is iatrogenic. Many of our current medications either are designed to modulate specific aspects of the sympathetic or parasympathetic nervous systems or produce significant side effects via their unintended autonomic interactions.

Schedule (2.5 hours)
30 Regional anatomy
30 Microscopic anatomy
30 Hormones and transmitters
30 Autonomic nervous system central control
30 Clinical cases

REGIONAL ANATOMY

Q13.1. Examine the gross brain specimen and Figure 13.1. Try to identify the following structures:
- Internal carotid artery
- Optic nerve
- Optic chiasm
- Infundibulum, stalk, and pituitary

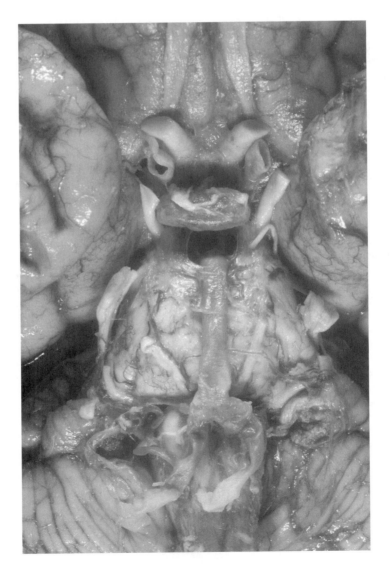

FIGURE 13.1. Base of brain.

- Uncus
- Olfactory tracts

As a quick review, identify some brainstem structures:
- Basilar artery
- Abducens nerve
- Oculomotor nerve
- Trochlear nerve
- Trigeminal nerve
- Pons base

A13.1. See Figure 13.2. The hypothalamus sits just in front of the brainstem. Both are "beneath" the thalamus. You can't really see the hypothalamus in Figure 13.2, but the stalk protrudes from the infundibulum, which is the base of the hypothalamus. The mammillary bodies lie in the space between the pituitary and the top of the basilar artery.

Q13.2. Now examine the classic circle of Willis drawing in Figure 13.3, illustrating the vasculature to the hypothalamus. Which circulation supplies the hypothalamus (anterior or posterior)? Try to identify the major vessels and other structures in the figure. Based on the picture and your neuroanatomic knowledge, suggest why strokes do not commonly present in the hypothalamus.

A13.2. See Figure 13.4. The hypothalamus receives blood from both the anterior and posterior circulations, in multiple fine vessels coming off the circle of Willis. Since no single large end vessel supplies this region, it is more resistant to selective infarcts. Clinically, most significant stokes to the hypothalamus usually involve large areas of additional brain, for example, in the entire middle cerebral artery circulation. Also hypothalamic functions are represented bilaterally. (Ever have unilateral hunger?) Thus small lesions tend to go unnoticed clinically, and large lesions are dominated by other massive neurologic deficits like coma and death.

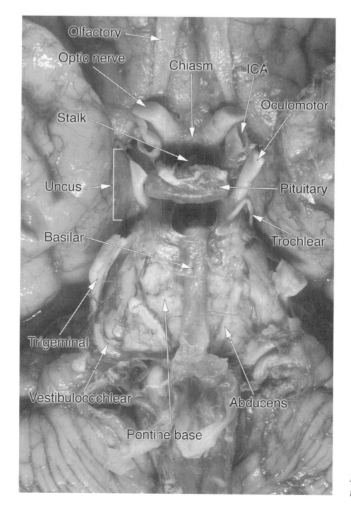

FIGURE 13.2. *Salient structures on the base of the brain.*

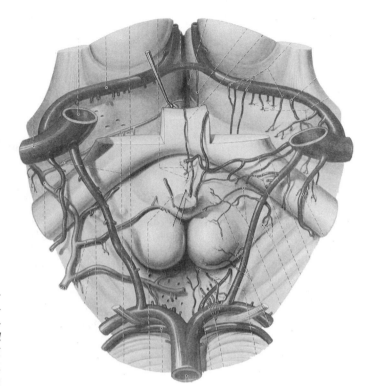

FIGURE 13.3. *Hypothalamic circulation and the circle of Willis. (Adapted from an original drawing belonging to Dr. Clifford Saper produced for The Hypothalamus, edited by W. Haymaker, E. Anderson, and W. J. H. Nauta, Thomas, Springfield, Illinois.)*

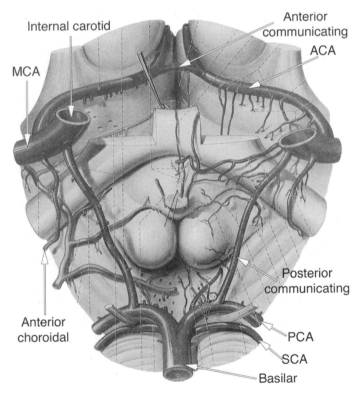

FIGURE 13.4. *Hypothalamic circulation and the circle of Willis. (Adapted from an original drawing belonging to Dr. Clifford Saper produced for The Hypothalamus, edited by W. Haymaker, E. Anderson, and W. J. H. Nauta, Thomas, Springfield, Illinois.)*

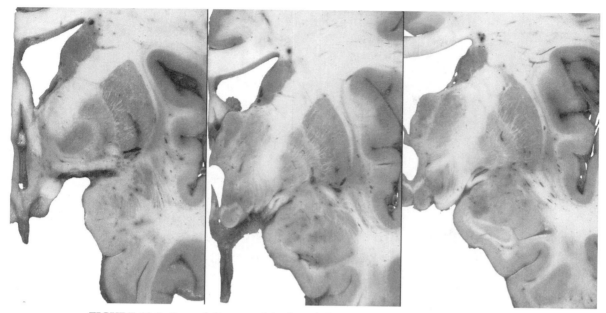

FIGURE 13.5. *Coronal slices containing hypothalamic structures.*

Q13.3. Review your coronal slices from previous laboratories and select the sections containing hypothalamus. Most likely these will be thick and irregularly sliced. Carefully cut them into thinner sections. Using the available atlases, identify the following in these slices, or if you are desperate, in Figure 13.5:
- Optic chiasm and tract
- Fornix columns and fornix
- Anterior commissure
- Internal capsule
- III ventricle (iii)
- Infundibulum and infundibular stalk
- Mammillary bodies and mammillothalamic tract
- Amygdala
- Where stria terminalis would lie
- Where pituitary should have been
- Thalamus, including anterior nucleus
- Caudate nucleus, putamen, and globus pallidus

A13.3. *See Figure 13.6. The mammillothalamic tract is better seen in the slightly different coronal dissection shown in Figure 13.7.*

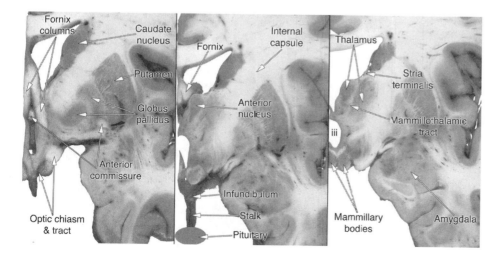

FIGURE 13.6. *Salient hypothalamic structures on coronal brain sections.*

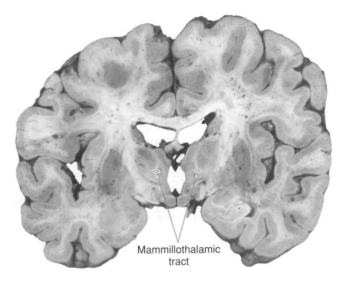

FIGURE 13.7. *Mammillothalamic tract.*

Mammillothalamic tract

Q13.4. The hypothalamus is important but small. To gain a sense of its size, roughly calculate its volume and compare it with the entire brain. The height goes from the base of the brain to the anterior commissure, the width from the third ventricle to the globus pallidus edge, and the length from in front of the optic chiasm to the back of the mammillary bodies. Assuming the brain has an approximate volume of 1200 milliliters, what proportion is occupied by the hypothalamus?

A13.4. *When calculated using more accurate anatomic landmarks, the hypothalamus normally weighs about 4 grams, indicating it represents only about 0.3% of the entire brain.*

MICROSCOPIC ANATOMY

Q13.5. Examine the microscopic slide of the pituitary (see also Fig. 13.8, although an H&E slide would be much better). Notice the two major divisions of the pituitary. The anterior pituitary or adenohypophysis is composed of large cells with abundant cytoplasm, while the posterior pituitary or neurohypophysis has a fibrillary background and spindle cells. Hematoxylin is blue and stains basic proteins, while eosin is red and stains acidic proteins. Describe the overall structure of the anterior

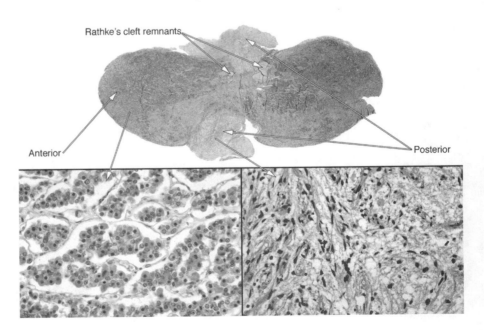

Rathke's cleft remnants

Anterior

Posterior

FIGURE 13.8. *Pituitary histology. The field coronal view slices through two portions of the posterior pituitary. In the head, the neurohypophysis is one continuous structure at the posterior end of the pituitary.*

pituitary. How are the cells structured? Sheets, nests, rosettes? Describe the colors of the cells in the adenohypophysis and what they indicate about the cells' contents. What does this mean? What lies between the adenohypophysis and neurohypophysis? From what you know of the mechanics and function of the posterior pituitary, what structures should be present? Can you see them?

A13.5. *The anterior pituitary has various cell types, each containing one of the six types of hormone (adrenocorticotrophic hormone, thyroid stimulating hormone, FSH, LH, growth hormone, prolactin). The hormones have characteristic pH properties and so stain differently with H&E. These cells are arranged in small nests, usually with several cell types in a single nest. They are distributed throughout the adenohypophysis, although different regions have a greater predominance of one cell type. Each cell responds to one of the releasing factors added to the portal circulation from the hypothalamus.*

Between the anterior and posterior pituitaries are often some small lakes of fluid enclosed by an epithelial lining. These "Rathke's cleft" remnants originated from the roof of the mouth, as the adenohypophysis fused with the neurohypophysis during development. The anterior pituitary did not originate from and is not really part of the central nervous system, but rather is a unique endocrine gland.

Unlike the esthetic colors of the anterior pituitary, the neurohypophysis has a bland, fibrillary appearance, devoid of secretory cells or neurons. Instead, it contains specialized glial cells (pituicytes) that regulate the release of posterior pituitary hormones. The specialized structures you may have expected are the nerve endings terminating upon blood vessels. Although these are present (eosinophilic, slightly grainy bodies), they are difficult to see on routine stains. So don't flog yourself trying to find them; just appreciate that they are there.

Q13.6. Next, look at the H&E/LFB microscopic section of the hypothalamus or Figure 13.9. Locate the third ventricle on one side, lined by cuboidal ependymal cells.

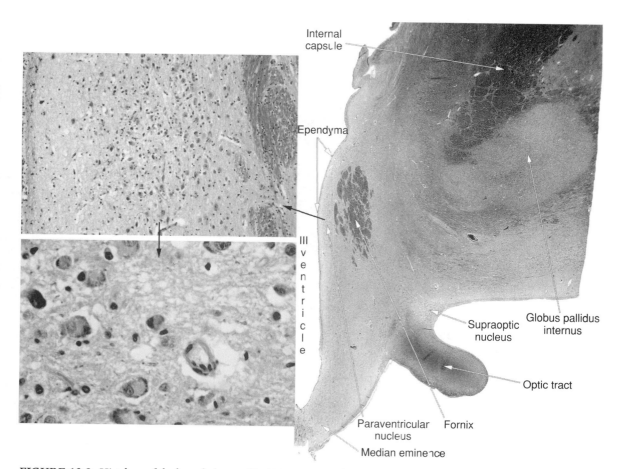

FIGURE 13.9. *Histology of the hypothalamus, H&E/LFB stain. The left two panels are increasingly higher microscopic views from the paraventricular hypothalamic nucleus.*

Find the optic tract (homogeneous white matter tract at the base of the brain). Hypothalamic slides may have the fornix descending on their way to the mammillary bodies. How does the fornix compare with the optic tract? Notice how the neuron size changes. Where do you see the largest neurons? Can you identify all of the nuclei within the hypothalamus?

A13.6. *If you can identify more than several of the many hypothalamic nuclei, you should become a neuroanatomist. On regular H&E stains, only the paraventricular, supraoptic, and mammillary (not in the figure) nuclei are "easy" to see. Others, like the arcuate nuclei, are less distinct but may also be visible. However, special staining or other histologic techniques are necessary to fully appreciate the hypothalamic nuclei. The supraoptic and paraventricular nuclei contain the largest neurons. These produce systemic hormones, as compared to many hypothalamic neurons that produce only releasing hormones for the anterior pituitary.*

The fornix looks like a complex braid of yarn, while the optic tract has a much more organized structure. Perhaps emotions are more complicated and less organized than vision!

Q13.7. Peptide hormones cannot normally cross the blood-brain barrier. However, the brain does receive such systemic hormonal and other humoral information through specialized sites termed the "circumventricular organs." In the hypothalamus, for example, leptin and angiotensin II cross the blood-brain barrier in the organ vasculosum of lamina terminalis (OVLT). The "vomiting center" in the medulla, termed the area postrema, is another example of a circumventricular organ. Examine the low-power photograph in Figure 13.10 of the organ vasculosum of the lamina terminalis on the left (which also includes another circumventricular organ, the subfornical organ, SFO) and a higher power photomicrograph of the area postrema on the right. Describe their appearance. Especially contrast the structure of their vessels and tissue with those elsewhere in the brain.

A13.7. *While examination of the actual blood-brain barrier (formed by extensive endothelial tight junctions) requires electron microscopy, you can gain a "feel" for the looseness of the circumventricular organs by their microscopic appearance. In contrast to other sites in the brain, the vessels in these organs are more haphazardly arranged and are intermixed with "loose" neural and glial elements. The hypothalamus receives complex systemic information via the*

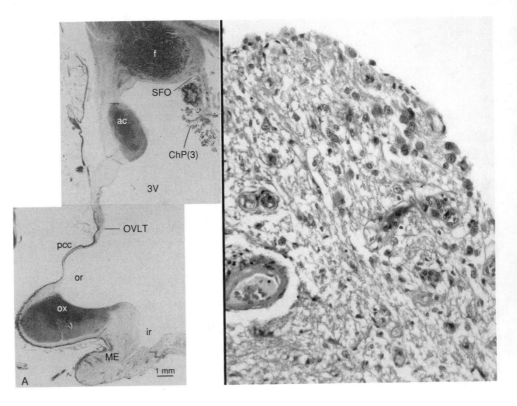

FIGURE 13.10. *Circumventricular organs. The left panel is a sagittal histologic section through the optic chiasm (ox), anterior commissure (ac) and fornix (f), which shows the organ vasculosum of the lamina terminalis (OVLT) and the subfornical organ (SFO). (Adapted from M. J. McKinley and B. J. Oldfield,* Circumventricular Organs in The Human Nervous System, *edited by G. Paxinos, © 1990, Academic Press, San Diego.) The right panel shows a higher-power H&E section through the area postrema in the medulla.*

circulation through the organ vasculosum of the lamina terminalis and the subfornical organ. If you think you will remember the actual names of these circumventricular organs (they number seven, for the obsessive-compulsive), you are delusional. What is important to remember is that the brain receives humoral information about the body via sites without a blood-brain barrier.

HORMONES AND TRANSMITTERS

Q13.8. Examine Figure 13.11, which shows two views of the hypothalamus immunostained for vasopressin. The paraventricular hypothalamic nucleus (PVH) is located just adjacent to the ventricle, and the supraoptic nucleus (SO) is just above and medial to the optic tract. What size are the main neurons? To where do the large fibers project? Suggest why they may be so large and have such prominent Nissl substance (basophilic or blue staining on H&E).

A13.8. *Unlike the H&E, the vasopressin staining clearly defines the neurons containing this hormone/transmitter. The most prominent staining is in the large (magnocellular) neurons in both the paraventricular hypothalamic nucleus and supraoptic nucleus. The axons from both nuclei project down the hypophyseal stalk into the posterior pituitary. It is their endings that terminate upon blood vessels and release vasopressin into the systemic circulation. Their large size and prominent Nissl substance indicate they are metabolically active and synthetic. A similar type of staining pattern would be seen had the section been stained with oxytocin, rather than vasopressin. The cell types and projections of these two hormones are comparable.*

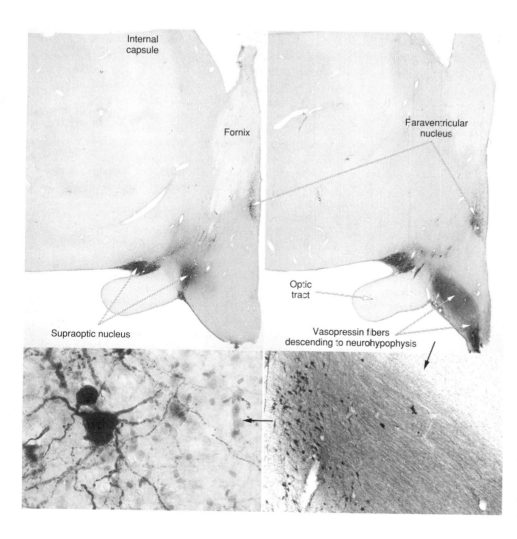

FIGURE 13.11. *Hypothalamus immunostained for vasopressin. The upper two figures are from different coronal levels of the hypothalamus, while the lower figures are increasingly higher power views from near the supraoptic nucleus.*

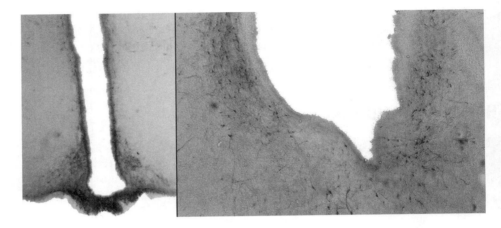

FIGURE 13.12. *Dopamine-containing neurons in the arcuate nucleus of the hypothalamus, immunostained for tyrosine hydroxylase. The left panel is from the rat, while the right shows the human hypothalamus.*

Q13.9. Another, smaller population of neurons also stain with vasopressin. Where are they on the microscopic slide? Are these neurons also producing hormones (think of their size)?

A13.9. *The brain is both a spendthrift and a penny-pinscher; while it has a plethora of receptors, receptor subtypes, and receptor sub-subtypes, the brain also may use a single peptide for several different functions. In the hypothalamus, both oxytocin and vasopressin are used as circulatory hormones from the neurohypophysis as well as neurotransmitters to autonomic centers in the brainstem and spinal cord. The parvocellular (parvo: Latin parvus for small) autonomic neurons lie medial to the magnocellular (large cell) hormone-producing neurons in the paraventricular nucleus. They contain less vasopressin compared to their bigger cousins, and so are more difficult to identify. Vasopressin and oxytocin parvocellular neurons project to medullary and spinal cord autonomic centers. These smaller neurons use vasopressin and oxytocin as neurotransmitters, rather than as hormones like the magnocellular neurons.*

Q13.10. Now examine Figure 13.12 showing the dopamine neurons in the arcuate nucleus of the hypothalamus. The dopamine-producing neurons are highlighted by antibodies to tyrosine hydroxylase (TH), which is a critical enzyme in the biosynthesis of dopamine. The left image is from a rat arcuate nucleus, while the right is a higher power view of the human. Do these neurons form a tight grouping, or are they more diffuse? Contrast the two species. Based on your knowledge of how dopamine acts in the hypothalamus-pituitary axis, predict the qualitative changes in hypophyseal hormones after transection of the pituitary stalk

A13.10. *Studying (and teaching) the hypothalamus is difficult, in part because of the many closely packed nuclei and in part because of the special techniques required to tease functions apart. The photograph illustrates but one small region in the hypothalamus where dopamine neurons live. These TH-staining neurons are actually scattered over a much wider region and can only be studied properly by examining many sections. In the rat the tyrosine hydroxylase staining dopamine neurons are more densely packed and form a more compact nucleus than in the human. The higher power version in the human illustrates the individual neuronal cell bodies as well as their processes.*

Dopamine from the hypothalamus, including the arcuate nucleus, inhibits the release of prolactin by the adenohypophysis. The other releasing factors all promote the discharge of their hormones into the circulation. As a consequence of a stalk transection or compression, prolactin levels tend to increase (disinhibition), while the other anterior and posterior pituitary hormones decrease (producing panhypopituitarism).

Q13.11. Next, examine Figure 13.13 of anterior pituitary immunostained with antibodies to prolactin. How are the positive cells distributed?

A13.11. *Although routine H&E examination of the pituitary gland is esthetically pleasing, fully understanding its physiology requires the use of special staining techniques. Before the advent of immunostaining, determining the hormonal content of a given cell required examining its staining characteristics and ultrastructure. These techniques have been supplanted by the more definitive and much less expensive use of immunoperoxidase staining.*

The prolactin producing cells are intermixed with adenohypophyseal cells producing other hormones. These cells are all arranged in small nests within the anterior pituitary.

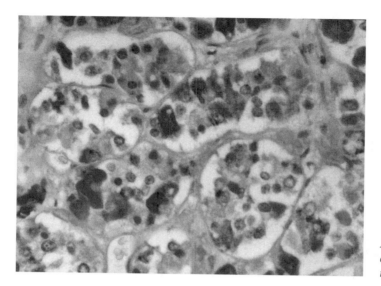

FIGURE 13.13. *High-power view of the adenohypophysis, immunostained for prolactin.*

    Adenohypophyseal hormones are not randomly distributed throughout the gland, they tend to cluster into regions within the gland. Adenomas arising within different sectors of the adenohypophysis tend to secrete the hormone normally produced by that sector. Nevertheless, some cells producing each hormone may be found outside their designated sites. Each of the small nests of cells usually contain more than one and often several different hormones, a fact appreciated just from the H&E stains.

Q13.12. In Figure 13.14, a coronal section of brain has been immunostained with antibodies against melanin-concentrating hormone (MCH) (don't worry about why this hormone has this name). Melanin-concentrating hormone neurons, along with the orexins, neuropeptide Y (NPY), leptin, and several other transmitters, are part of the complex circuitry that controls food intake and metabolism. Injection of this peptide will promote increased energy intake, while melanin-concentrating hormone knockout mice have reduced food intake and are lean. The small dark dots are individual neurons that contain melanin-concentrating hormone. Where are these neurons? Be as specific as you can. What is the rounded structure below the staining cells? What is the clear space on the left of the staining cells?

A13.12. *MCH cells lie near but not at the third ventricle (the clear space on the left) and overlie the mammillary body beneath. They extend out into the more lateral aspects of the hypothalamus and are considered a component of the lateral hypothalamus.*

    The hypothalamus has many such peptides expressed in its neurons; it is their detailed electrical circuitry and receptors for systemic indicators (like leptin) that determine the ultimate behavioral and regulatory response elicited by this small region of brain.

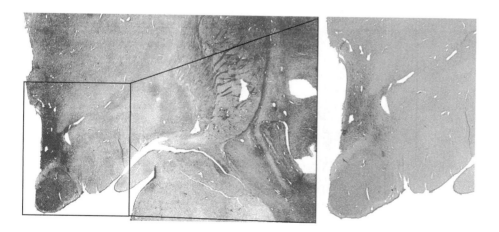

FIGURE 13.14. *Coronal section of hypothalamic region immunostained for melanin-concentrating hormone (MCH). The left panel has been highly processed to display the regional anatomy, while the right is more what the actual data look like.*

AUTONOMIC SYSTEM

In addition to its roles in transducing cerebral signals into hormone production and behavioral regulation of basic bodily functions, the hypothalamus is the foreman of the autonomic nervous system. As you saw earlier, the hypothalamus sends autonomic regulatory information to brainstem control centers.

Similar to other major systems in the brain, the autonomic nervous system is regulated at multiple levels. Some of our most basic bodily functions, which we either try to ignore (e.g., micturition, defecation) or seek (orgasm) are in part regulated by the spinal cord. For example, in a patient with an upper spinal cord injury, the bladder will sense its fullness and periodically empty in response to signals from the lower cord alone. However, several hundred million years of evolution have thankfully modified the purely spinal control.

The next level of control, and one essential for life, resides in the medulla. The first step in any affector-effector system requires peripheral sensory information. For the autonomic system, this sensory data relates not to the external environment, but to the body's internal milieu.

Q13.13. Name some peripheral sites that sense autonomic information.

A13.13. *The list includes baroreceptors (carotid sinus, aortic arch), oxygen chemoreceptors (carotid body, aorta), pH and carbon dioxide chemoreceptors (built into the medulla), and the food chemoreceptors, our tastebuds (taste is processed similarly to other autonomic information, it just happens to be one we like). Other sensations come from the gastrointestinal system. This latter system is a brain onto itself, and contains more neurons than the entire spinal cord.*

Q13.14. Through which cranial nerves does most of this information come?

A13.14. *Glossopharyngeal (IX) and vagus (X) nerves plus the facial (VII) for purely taste.*

Q13.15. Now again find the solitary nucleus on your slide of the medulla or in Figure 13.15. This most important sensory center receives autonomic information from several cranial nerves. The essential sensations (heart rate, oxygenation, blood pressure, etc.) are processed at caudal levels, and the good stuff (taste) is processed rostrally. Not only is the solitary nucleus a sensory nucleus, it also integrates some of the visceral data and sends projections to major autonomic effector nuclei.

A13.15. *See Figure 13.16.*

Q13.16. What major autonomic nucleus lies just medial to the solitary tract/nucleus? From its name, suggest what type of neurons it contains.

A13.16. *The dorsal motor nucleus of the vagus nerve contains the parasympathetic preganglionic neurons. It projects not only through the vagus nerve but also through the glossopharyngeal nerve. (As mentioned previously, the brainstem evolved as columns of neurons. In the same column, just rostral to dorsal motor nucleus of the vagus, are neurons that project preganglionic*

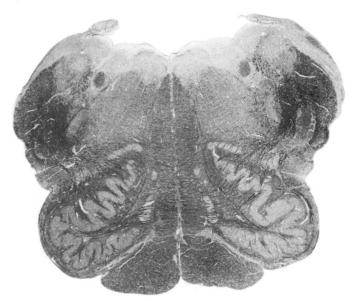

FIGURE 13.15. *Medulla solitary nucleus worksheet.*

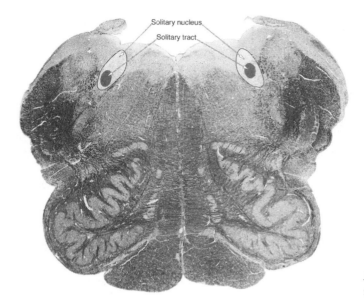

Solitary nucleus

Solitary tract

FIGURE 13.16. *Solitary tract and nucleus.*

parasympathetic efferents from the superior salivatory nucleus to salivatory and lacrimal glands.)

Q13.17. Identify on your glass slide or in Figure 13.17 the spinal trigeminal nucleus and tract. Ventral and medial to this nucleus are descending sympathetic fibers traveling to the preganglionic sympathetic neurons in the intermediolateral cell column of the spinal cord. What region more or less lies between the vagus and solitary nucleus and this descending tract?

A13.17. *See Figure 13.18. The exact location of the descending sympathetic fibers is not well delineated, especially on any given slide. The fibers travel in the dorsolateral portions of the brainstem tegmentum. In the medulla they lie somewhere ventral and medial to the spinal trigeminal nucleus.*

Lateral and ventral to the motor vagus and solitary nucleus, and near to the descending sympathetic fibers, is the part of the reticular formation that integrates much of the essential autonomic information. It is in this region that your respiratory, heart rate, and blood pressure control centers lie. These centers are close together for a reason! Fibers from the immediately adjacent neurons in the reticular formation descend in the loose sympathetic tract to the sympathetic spinal neurons.

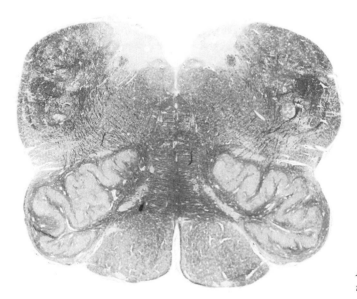

FIGURE 13.17. *Medulla autonomic worksheet.*

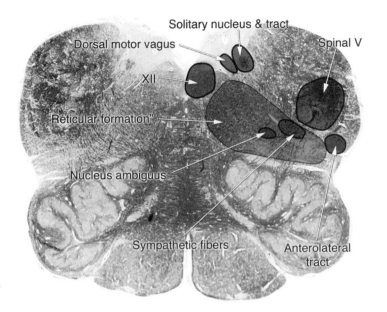

FIGURE 13.18. *Medullary autonomic centers.*

Details of the reticular formation anatomy are difficult, and if not used frequently, are quickly forgotten. Even the position of labels in this figure should be considered approximate, not gospel. What is important to remember is that a major function of the medullary reticular formation is the control of visceral functions. It is this area of the medulla that is essential for life.

Q13.18. Although it is not strictly part of the laboratory, find the intermediolateral cell column in the spinal cord histologic slide or in Figure 13.19. At what levels should you find this column of neurons? What is their function? Transmitter?

A13.18. *See Figure 13.20. The intermediolateral cell column receives signals from the descending adrenergic fibers that you saw in the medulla. Its neurons are the preganglionic sympathetic neurons of the sympathetic nervous system. Remember, the axons from these neurons travel to peripheral sympathetic ganglia (e.g. sympathetic trunk in the thorax), release acetylcholine, and trigger the post-ganglionic sympathetic neurons.*

Q13.19. Several other brainstem nuclei participate in controlling the autonomic nervous system. Find the superior cerebellar peduncle in you slide of the pons or in Figure 13.21. Around the superior cerebellar peduncle in the rostral pons are the parabrachial nuclei. These nuclei transmit visceral sensations (taste and cardiorespiratory) to higher centers in the periaqueductal gray, hypothalamus and amygdala. Using Figure 13.21, or better your glass slides, try to find some neurons medial to the superior cerebellar peduncles, a bit ventrolateral to the locus ceruleus. This is

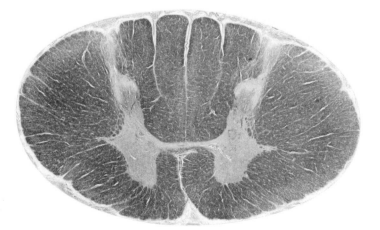

FIGURE 13.19. *Spinal cord autonomic worksheet.*

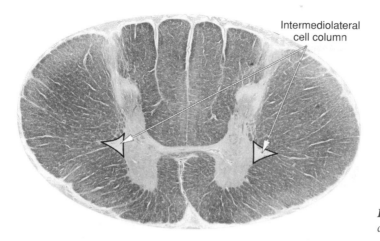

FIGURE 13.20. *Intermediolateral cell column.*

the medial parabrachial nucleus. These nuclei never have many neurons, so don't look too hard for them!

A13.19. *See Figure 13.22.*

Q13.20. Pain produces autonomic responses. Just think what happens to your heart rate when you burn yourself on a hot stove. On the midbrain slide in Figure 13.23, find the periaqueductal gray. This region receives ascending pain and visceral inputs, which in turn modulate autonomic responses in the lateral medulla. The periaqueductal gray also influences the autonomic effects of fight-or-flight responses, based on signals from higher centers.

A13.20. *See Figure 13.24.*

As discussed earlier, the hypothalamus integrates numerous humoral and neural signals and sends projections to several brainstem autonomic centers. Recall from above the location of the hypothalamic centers in the paraventricular nucleus that project to brainstem autonomic centers.

Several cortical and subcortical sites also regulate the autonomic nervous system. The amygdala receives visceral information from the brainstem autonomic relay nuclei, integrates these data with cortical inputs, and projects to the autonomic centers in the hypothalamus. The amygdala will be discussed in more detail in the limbic system laboratory.

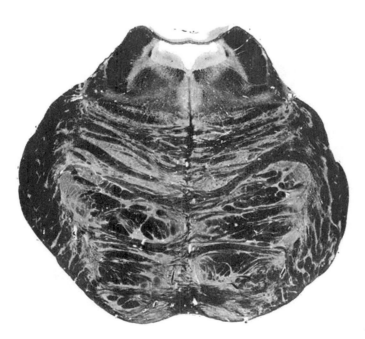

FIGURE 13.21. *Pons worksheet.*

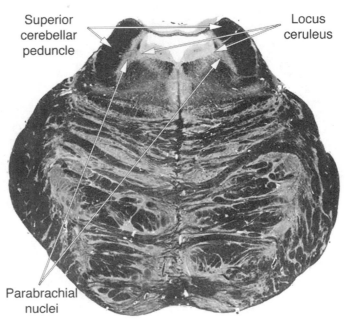

FIGURE 13.22. *Pons autonomic centers.*

CLINICAL CASES

Case 1: Hypothalamic Tumor

The patient is a 21-year-old man with excessive sleepiness.

In high school he had very delayed development of pubic hair and was 8 inches shorter than his classmates. Tests during his first year in college demonstrated he was hypogonadotropic. Further evaluation disclosed a large craniopharyngioma in the suprasellar region, extending posteriorly beyond the mammillary bodies. The patient underwent a total resection of the tumor.

Following surgery he remained comatose for a month, and was very slow to wake up. Over the subsequent several years he has slowly become more alert. Only after several years did he have relatively normal waking periods.

His current medications include hydrocortisone, testosterone, thyroid hormone, growth hormone, and DDAVP. He now has a relatively stable body temperature, serum sodium and endocrine status. While he was a bright student in high school, he currently requires 24-hour care. He is able to dress and feed himself, but has such poor memory function that he cannot be left alone. He has grown 8 inches since the surgery, and has an adult hair pattern.

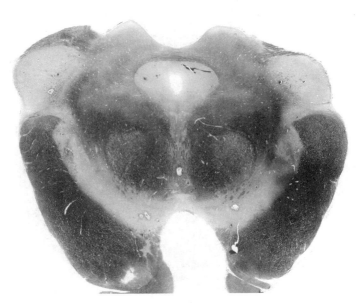

FIGURE 13.23. *Midbrain pain and autonomic center worksheet.*

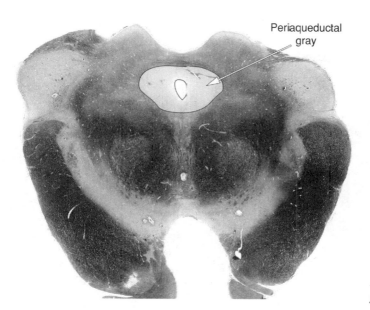

Periaqueductal
gray

FIGURE 13.24. *Periaqueductal gray.*

He exhibits excessive daytime sleepiness and cataplexy. He often takes a two-hour nap in the afternoon, and also easily dozes off in the evening. After hearing a good joke or being surprised, he may suddenly develop weakness, including neck muscles, dysarthria, and occasionally may drop something from his hand.

Examination showed him to be somewhat overweight, lacking facial hair, and walking with a shambling gait. His speech was slurred. His memory was impaired (one object after five minutes). He had a left homonymous temporal field defect and a smaller right temporal defect peripherally. Neither eye could be elevated or depressed, and the right eye was exodeviated, with a deficit in adduction.

Q13.21. Review the patient's MRI scans in Figure 13.25. As accurately as you can, using your atlases to assist, try to determine the location of his postsurgical infarct. What portion of his hypothalamus is preserved? What other structures are involved, aside from the hypothalamus?

A13.21. *The scans demonstrate loss of tissue bilaterally in the hypothalamus, which is greater on the left. The lesion covers much of the left medial and lateral hypothalamus from behind the optic chiasm into the rostral midbrain, including the ventral surface. Preserved is the lateral portion of the right hypothalamus and the preoptic area bilaterally. Other structures involved are the left amygdala, left thalamus, portions of the rostral midbrain, some of the left accumbens, and a segment of the anterior limb of the internal capsule.*

Q13.22. Correlate the following clinical deficits with the neuroimaging results:
- Initial coma
- Narcolepsy
- Panhypopituitarism
- Overweight
- Memory impairment
- Left homonymous hemianopsia
- Vertical gaze palsy

A13.22. *See Table 13.1.*

Q13.23. Explain how his temperature control has remained stable. What other deficits might you have predicted, based on the bilateral loss of his medial hypothalamus? What hormones are missing from his replacement therapy?

A13.23. *Temperature control and aspects of dietary control reside in the lateral hypothalamus, which were preserved on the right side. Also running through this region is the medial forebrain bundle. Preservation of some of the ascending fibers in this bundle from the brainstem reticular activating system (locus ceruleus, raphe nucleus, cholinergic fibers, and other reticular formation neurons) probably allowed him to slowly come out of his coma. Since much of his medial hypothalamus was infarcted, you may have expected him to have autonomic dysfunction. In fact, he does, but this only manifests as intermittent hand flushing. The anterior pituitary hormones that are not being replaced are prolactin, FSH, and LH. He also receives no oxytocin.*

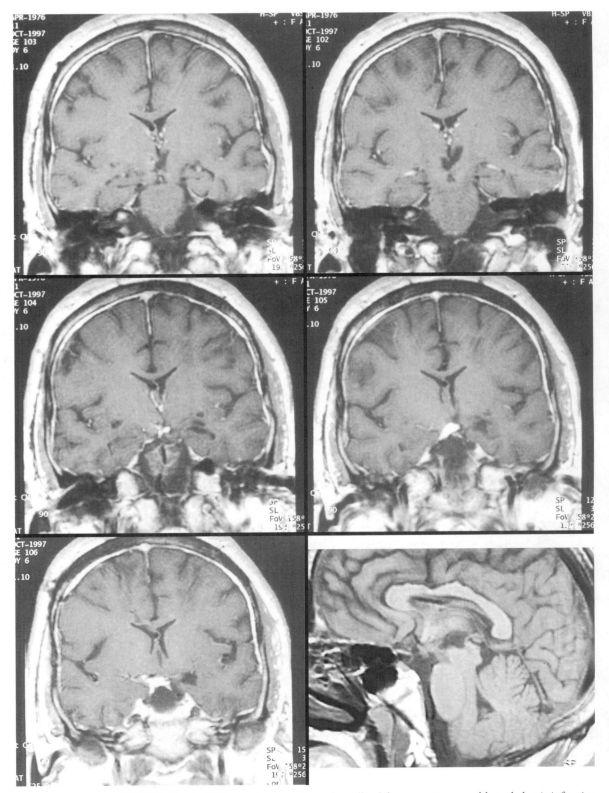

FIGURE 13.25. *MRI scans in the patient who suffered from vasospasm and hypothalamic infarction following surgery to remove a craniopharyngioma.*

TABLE 13.1. Correlation of Clinical Findings with Anatomic Lesion

Clinical Finding	Neuroanatomic Deficit
Initial coma	Interruption of medial forebrain bundle connecting midbrain reticular activating system to thalamus
Narcolepsy	Injury to orexin neurons in lateral hypothalamus
Panhypopituitarism	Loss of most of medial hypothalamus and possibly pituitary itself
Mild obesity	Loss of lateral hypothalamus combined with lesion in ventral medial hypothalamus leptin binding region (arcuate nucleus)
Memory impairment	Loss of medial temporal lobe structures
Left homonymous hemianopsia	Optic tract infarct
Vertical gaze palsy	Rostral midbrain infarct, probably involving vertical gaze centers

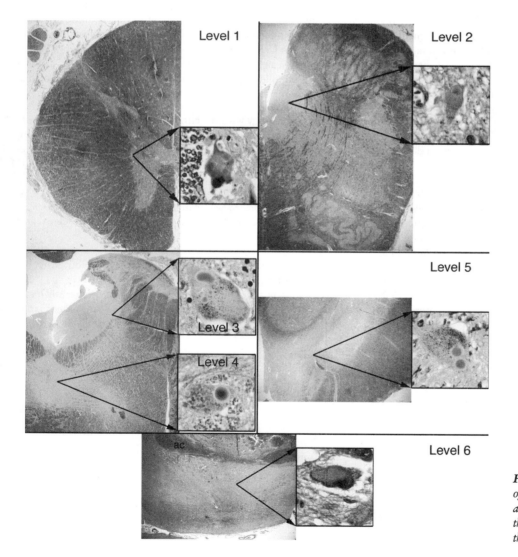

FIGURE 13.26. *Montage of pathology at different levels of the neural axis. Each level shows a field view of the structure and a high-power view of the pathology.*

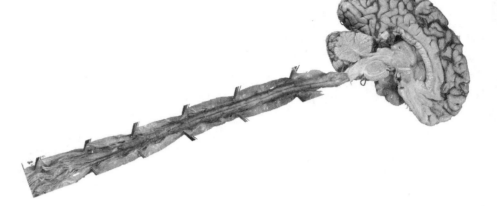

FIGURE 13.27. *Neuraxis   level worksheet.*

Case 2: Lewy Body Disease

The patient was a 75-year-old retired English professor with a history of progressive cognitive de-cline, hallucinations/perceptual disturbances, and parkinsonism. He was first noted to be symptomatic approximately 13 years ago when he had trouble finding his way while in familiar settings. Over the intervening years he became more withdrawn and developed shaking of his hands, difficulty walk-ing, increasing memory problems, and intermittent hallucinations/visual perceptual disturbances. In follow-up several years later he continued to have problems with hallucinations and abnormal gait. He had developed problems with hypotension and syncope, and was noted to have had long-standing bladder and erectile dysfunction. He expired following complications from a large, acute myocardial infarction.

Q13.24. Try to correlate the patient's pathology with his clinical findings. The photographic montage in Figure 13.26 presents the low-power view from several areas in the brain, with demarcated areas that are then displayed at high power. Figure 13.27 is a some-what sagittal diagram of the nervous system (the spinal cord has been "grafted" onto the sagittal brain). In the latter figure, draw a line to indicate approximately the location of each level in Figure 13.26. What is the pathology?

A13.24. *The neuronal inclusions you see are Lewy bodies. See Figure 13.28 for the levels of the neuroaxis.*

Q13.25. Complete Table 13.2; indicate the level of the neural axis, the involved nucleus, and the system that is affected.

A13.25. *See Table 13.3.*

Q13.26. Abnormalities in which of the sites of Figure 13.26 may have contributed to his cognitive decline? His movement disorder? His orthostatic hypotension?

A13.26. *See Table 13.3. The nucleus basalis is involved in attention and cognitive functions, and the lo-cus ceruleus participates in alertness. Dysfunction of these systems is suspected of contributing to the cognitive decline in Lewy body disease. Other probably more important sites are also*

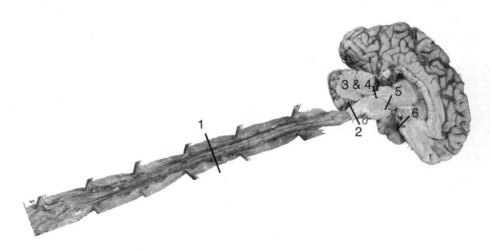

FIGURE 13.28. *Levels where Lewy bodies are found in Lewy body disease.*

TABLE 13.2. Lewy Body Disease Sites and Systems

Number	Level	Nucleus	System
1			
2			
3			
4			
5			
6			

involved, including portions of cortex and especially limbic cortex, which may be more important in causing this decline. You will investigate these structures further in the limbic and cortex laboratories.

The substantia nigra is a major nucleus in the extrapyramidal system, which is involved in controlling the initiation of movement. As has been discussed elsewhere in this book, it probably plays a seminal role in the patient's parkinsonian movement disorder.

Finally, the patient has Lewy bodies in several autonomic centers, including the dorsal motor nucleus of the vagus and the intermediolateral cell column. Pathology in these sites has been linked to orthostatic hypotension, both in this and in other neurodegenerative diseases.

TABLE 13.3. Functional Pathology in Lewy Body Disease

Number	Level	Nucleus	System	Outputs	Drugs (Many)	Clinical
1	Thoracic spinal cord	Intermediolateral cell column	Sympathetic	Sympathetic ganglia	Clonidine ($\alpha 2$), phenylephrine ($\alpha 1$), many others	Autonomic instability (hypotension, syncope)
2	Medulla	Dorsal motor nucleus of vagus	Parasympathetic	Vagus nerve and ganglia within end organs	Atropine, others	Autonomic instability (hypotension, syncope)
3	Pons	Locus ceruleus	Norepinepherine	Diffuse to most areas of brain	Desipramine, other tricyclic antidepressants	Decreased attentiveness
4	Pons	Raphe nucleus	Serotonin	Diffuse to most areas of brain	Fluoxetine, other "new" antidepressants	Sleep, depression, nociceptive modulation
5	Midbrain	Substantia nigra	Dopamine	Striatum	l-Dopa, Sinemet, many antipsychotics	Movement disorder
6	Basal forebrain	Basal nucleus of Meynert	Cholinergic	Diffuse to cortex	Tacrine (Cognex), donepezil (Aricept)	Decreased vigilance

Chapter 14—LIMBIC SYSTEM

The night on the porch had been chilly. Eight years old, you had snuggled with your doll deeply under your covers. As you came downstairs in the morning and opened the kitchen door, you felt the warmth of the wood stove. A light odor of burning wood intermingled with the essence of the blueberry pie your grandmother was just removing from the oven. Many years later, when you fumble to roll out a crust, you imagine you can almost taste her pie.

Memories, smells, hunger, love, curling up in the cold; these are all connected with your limbic system. In the previous laboratory you investigated the control of visceral functions by the hypothalamus, while in the next session you will reach our most advanced cognitive domain, the neocortex. In this laboratory you will be introduced to the limbic system, a loosely related group of structures that in part connects these domains and drives our lives. You will identify its various components, their connectivity and anatomical organization, and some of their functional affiliations.

LEARNING OBJECTIVES

- Identify the components and review the organization of the limbic system.
- Study the intrinsic and extrinsic connections of limbic system with particular emphasis on the relationship between core limbic structures, paralimbic cortex, the rest of the cerebral cortex, and hypothalamus.
- Review some of the major functional affiliations of limbic system structures.
- Use the pathophysiology and clinical features of Alzheimer's disease to reinforce understanding of the connectivity and functions of some of the limbic system structures.

INTRODUCTION

The term *limbic,* which means "bordering," was first used by Pierre Paul Broca to designate a continuous ring of cortical gyri found on the medial rim of the cerebral hemisphere. The anatomical structures identified by Broca, along with several other anatomically and functionally related areas, make up what in current terminology is called the limbic system.

The limbic system has several distinct characteristics. First, many components of the limbic system are parts of the cerebral cortex. The limbic cortical zones are considered "primitive," because they are phylogenetically the oldest cortical areas and exhibit relatively poor laminar differentiation. Second, limbic system structures are intimately interconnected with the hypothalamus, on the one

Functional Neuroanatomy: An Interactive Text and Manual, by Jeffrey T. Joseph and David L. Cardozo
ISBN 0-471-44437-5 Copyright © 2004 John Wiley & Sons, Inc.

hand, and with neocortex (particularly association cortex), on the other. Third, and as a result of this pattern of connectivity, the functional affiliations of the limbic system include those related to the cognitive domain (e.g., memory), which are a specialty of the cerebral cortex, and those related to the internal milieu (e.g., autonomic function), which is under direct control of the "head ganglion," the hypothalamus. Fourth, the limbic system is the only major route through which the hypothalamus can have access to the neocortex, and therefore to the external environment. Conversely, information processed in the cerebral cortex and potentially bound for the hypothalamus is conveyed primarily through limbic system structures. Thus the limbic system is in a perfect position to allow satisfaction of basic drives and needs under the control of the hypothalamus, through execution of appropriate responses made possible by the cognitive calculations of the neocortex.

In this laboratory you will first examine the macroscopic and then the microscopic structure of the limbic system. After this, you will investigate some of its functional affiliations. As a recapitulation you will examine a case of a neurodegenerative disease that initially and prominently affects parts of the limbic system.

Anatomic Components
Limbic Lobe

You have previously met the *cingulate gyrus* on the medial surface of the brain. Its most rostral extent dives down below the corpus callosum to form the parolfactory gyrus. From here this ring of gray matter extends onto the base of the brain or the *basal forebrain.* As in so much of neuroanatomy, the basal forebrain has received several other, even more confusing names, including the substantia innominata or "nameless substance" and the anterior perforated substance (which is at least descriptive, as you will see). The basal forebrain then spreads out to the *piriform cortex* and *uncus* in the anterior-medial temporal lobe. From here the limbic ring encompasses the *parahippocampal gyrus* and finally completes the circle at the cingulate gyrus.

Cortical Components

The limbic system has a cortical core and an adjacent zone that acts as a transition to "higher" cortical areas. The core has two main divisions:

- *Primary olfactory cortex;* also known as piriform cortex. This area is located at the point of convergence of the temporal pole, insula, and posterior orbitofrontal cortices.
- *Hippocampus.* This region lies in the fold of the medial temporal lobe.

Each aspect of the core has associated paralimbic zones:

- Orbitofrontal cortex (associated with olfactory core and frontal neocortex)
- Insula (associated with olfactory core and parietal neocortex)
- Temporal pole (associated with olfactory core and temporal neocortex)
- Parahippocampal gyrus (associated with hippocampal core and temporal cortex)
- Cingulate cortex (associated with hippocampal core remnant and frontoparietal cortices)

Corticoid Components

These are surface gray matter components of the cerebrum, and thus meet one definition of "cortex." But in another sense they are not cortex: they are not layered structures—hence the term "corticoid." The main members of this class are located in the basal forebrain and the anteromedial aspects of the temporal lobe.

The septal area, diagonal band, and substantia innominata are located within the basal forebrain, at the posterior base of the frontal lobe. The *septal area* consists of a set of several small nuclei in the base of the septum pellucidum, just behind the rostrum of corpus callosum in each cerebral hemisphere. Ventrally and ventrolaterally, the septal area is continuous with the nucleus and tract of the diagonal band (also referred to as the diagonal band of Broca). This merges imperceptibly into the substantia innominata, located posterior and lateral to the diagonal band, underneath the anterior commissure. This large "unnamed" region contains the *basal nucleus of Meynert.*

The *amygdaloid complex* is an almond-shaped (amygdala means almond in Greek) structure in the anteromedial aspects of the temporal lobe. It consists of many nuclei or regions, and is situated in the uncal region of the medial temporal lobe.

Other Components

There are several other structures, which as we will see in our study of limbic system connectivity, can be considered part of the limbic system because their primary connections are with limbic system structures. Among these are several thalamic nuclei (including the habenula, anterior nucleus, dorsomedial nucleus, and midline nuclei), ventral aspects of the neostriatum and globus pallidus (olfactory tubercle, nucleus accumbens, and ventral globus pallidus, all referred to as the limbic striatum), and additional structures within the brainstem (including the interpeduncular nucleus and dorsal and ventral tegmental nuclei).

Limbic System Connections

Our knowledge of the connections of the limbic system is based, to a large extent, on studies in animals (particularly nonhuman primates). The pattern of limbic system connectivity is exceedingly complex. Here only the major connections of limbic structures will be reviewed.

Cortical Connections

The neocortex or association cortex connects to the core limbic areas via transitional areas of cortex, termed paralimbic cortex. The information flows in both directions but is greater toward the limbic system:

Neocortex (association) ↔ Paralimbic cortex ↔ Core limbic area

This pattern of connectivity is relatively strict. For example, processed information from association cortex does not pass directly to a core limbic zone. The information is first received by a paralimbic area and then relayed to a core limbic structure.

Besides the cortical limbic components, other limbic structures have connections with the cerebral cortex. As you shall see below, the thalamus serves as a relay station for many limbic projections to the cerebral cortex.

Corticoid Components

The basal forebrain corticoid structures are the septal nuclei, the horizontal and vertical limbs of the diagonal band of Broca and the substantia innominata. Within these structures are magnocellular *cholinergic* neurons that project to the entire cortical mantle. The cholinergic neurons of the medial septum and the vertical limb of the diagonal band of Broca project to the hippocampus. The horizontal limb of the diagonal band of Broca provides the cholinergic innervation of the olfactory bulb and the cholinergic neurons of the substantia innominata project to the rest of the cerebral cortex.

Papez Circuit

In 1937 James Papez (pronounced "papes") proposed the existence of a reverberating circuit made up of the limbic lobe and diencephalic structures that he considered to serve as the neural basis of emotion. Today we recognize that the set of structures delineated by Papez is too restrictive, and further, little evidence has ever been brought forth to support his idea that information reverberates around this "circuit." However, the "Papez circuit" is useful for reviewing some of the limbic system structures and their relationships.

This hypothetical circuit begins in the entorhinal cortex of the parahippocampal gyrus (see Fig. 14.1). Via the perforant pathway the information flows into the hippocampal formation. From there, signals travel in the fornix to reach the *mammillary bodies.* A short but distinct white matter tract, the *mammillothalamic tract,* connects the mammillary bodies to the *anterior nucleus* of the thalamus. From there, information flows to the cingulate gyrus then, via the cingulum bundle underneath, back to the entorhinal cortex.

Fornix and Stria Terminalis

The *fornix* is a major pathway that carries information from (and to a smaller extent to) the hippocampus. The fornix follows a complex three-dimensional path. It emanates from the fimbria of the hippocampus, ascends out of the temporal lobe in the medial wall of the ventricle, and passes forward

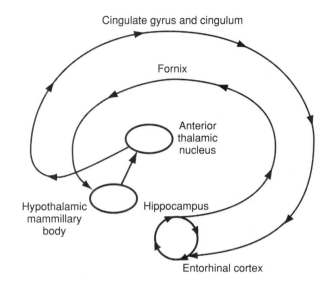

Cingulate gyrus and cingulum

Fornix

Anterior
thalamic
nucleus

Hypothalamic
mammillary
body

Hippocampus

Entorhinal cortex

FIGURE 14.1. *Papez circuit.*

under the corpus callosum. Just posterior to the anterior commissure, the fibers of the fornix branch into bundles to terminate in various structures.

The *stria terminalis* is a bundle of fibers that carries information to and from the amygdala. It emanates from the amygdala and follows a course similar to that of the fornix. In most of its course, the stria terminalis is situated next to the caudate nucleus.

Hippocampal Connections

You have already encountered some of the connections of the hippocampus. This wonderful structure has many other connections as well. Association cortex input comes via the parahippocampal gyrus (paralimbic structure) to the *dentate gyrus.* In addition the hippocampus receives cholinergic information from the septal area and the diagonal band via the fornix. Finally, it also receives projections from the hypothalamus.

Outputs from the hippocampal formation also reach the association neocortex via the parahippocampal gyrus. In addition the hippocampus also projects back to the septal nuclei via the fornix and back to the amygdala. The connection to the cingulate gyrus is part of the Papez circuit you encountered earlier, with relays in the mammillary bodies (via the fornix) and anterior thalamic nuclei.

Septal Connections

The septal nuclei, lying just off the midline at the base of the septum pellucidum, receive inputs from the hippocampus (via the fornix) and the amygdala (via the stria terminalis). They also receive information from the midbrain tegmentum and hypothalamus.

Their outputs also include the hippocampus (via the fornix; this should not be a surprise). But in addition they project to the lateral hypothalamus and midbrain tegmentum. Finally they have a wonderful large and distinct projection that travels to the habenular nucleus, interpeduncular nucleus, and finally back to the midbrain tegmentum. However, our knowledge of the function of this last projection remains poor.

Amygdaloid Connections

This gray matter structure, lying at the anterior reaches of the temporal horn, has many nuclear subdivisions, each with its own connections. This complex of nuclei receives inputs from the olfactory bulb, hypothalamus via the stria terminalis and other, more direct pathways, midline thalamic nuclei, and paralimbic cortices, especially the olfactocentric cortex. It also receives input from the adjacent hippocampus.

Its outputs include reciprocal connections to the hypothalamus, again via the stria terminalis, and paralimbic olfactocentric cortex. In addition it sends information to the septal nuclei in the stria terminalis and the prefrontal cortex via the medial dorsal nucleus of thalamus.

Piriform Olfactory Cortex

Last but not least, the limbic piriform olfactory cortex receives olfactory input from the olfactory bulb. Some of this information is then transmitted to the hypothalamus.

Major Functional Affiliations of the Limbic System

The four main types of behavior mediated by the broader limbic system, as summarized by M. Marsel Mesulam (*Principles of Behavioral and Cognitive Neurology,* 2nd ed., Oxford University Press, New York, 2000) are (1) memory and learning, (2) the channeling of emotions and affiliative behaviors, (3) the linkage of visceral state, immune responses, and endocrine balance to mental state, and (4) the perception of pain, smell, and taste. These functions reflect the intimate relationships of the limbic system with the hypothalamus. Rather than dwell on the behavioral minutia, we will review here the "major" functional affiliations of the limbic system.

Learning and Memory

One type of memory is explicit or declarative and involves learning of new experiences or remembering old ones. Explicit memory is also of two types: short-term memory, which constitutes the memory of recent experiences, and long-term memory, which designates memories that have been consolidated in permanent stores. We should keep in mind that accessing long-term memory requires the existence of a retrieval mechanism or site. While explicit memory is by definition a "conscious" memory process, a second category called implicit or procedural memory is usually nonconscious. Implicit/procedural memory involves learning and remembering motor tasks and perceptual associations. For example, an amnesic patient may develop new motor skills even though she has no conscious memory of the experiences that led to this learning. It is the laying down of explicit, long-term memories that requires the limbic system.

Emotions

Love, hate, flight, fight, rage, and aggression: these visceral emotions all have intimate associations with the limbic system. Their expression requires the coordination of the hypothalamus for autonomic and hormonal control and the cortex for executive control and planning of their motor reactions.

As an example, lesions in portions of the limbic system produce a profound lowering of a rat's rage threshold. Such animals shows signs of extreme emotional arousal if someone approaches their cage. They will scream and jump wildly if gently poked at with an object or even if disturbed with a puff of air. If someone is so foolhardy as to put a hand into the cage, the rat launches a vicious, bloody attack upon it (fight). In contrast, the same treatment in mice produces an exacerbated escape (flight) response.

Other Functions

It is important to note two additional functions of the limbic system. Because of their intimate connections with the hypothalamus, limbic system structures are intimately involved in visceral and endocrine regulation. Also the primary olfactory cortex is a core limbic structure. Therefore olfactory information is processed almost exclusively within the limbic system. The remarkable economic value of the perfume industry attests to the persistence of a close working relationship between the olfactory and limbic systems in humans.

Schedule (2.5 hours)
60 Anatomical components of the limbic system
30 Cellular and laminar organization of limbic structures
30 Major functional affiliations
10 Acetylcholine diffuse system
20 Clinical case study

ANATOMICAL COMPONENTS OF THE LIMBIC SYSTEM

The limbic lobe identified by Broca consists of many surface and deep structures. This series of exercises takes you on a trip of these structures. Although some illustrations are provided, the activity will have much greater utility if you have access to a real brain or a good model.

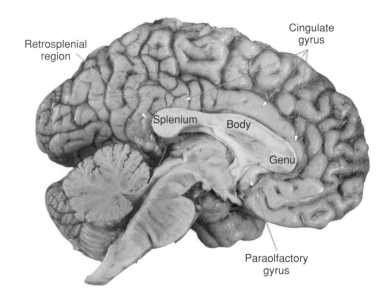

FIGURE 14.2. *Cingulate gyrus.*

Surface Components of Limbic Lobe

Inst On your hemispheric brain section (or in Fig. 14.2), track the ***cingulate gyrus*** from where it bends around the genu of the corpus callosum down and back into the parolfactory gyrus (the last bit of cortex before reaching the base of the brain). Now return to the cingulate gyrus at the genu of the corpus callosum and trace it backward over the body of the corpus callosum, to the portion that dives deep to the splenium of the corpus callosum (retrosplenial portion).

Cingulate connections follow a rough topographic order; frontal and parietal association areas relate to the anterior cingulate, occipital and temporal areas with the retrosplenial cingulate.

INST To find the ***basal forebrain*** (for confusion, also known as the substantia innominata or the anterior perforated substance), trace from the most anterior portion of the cingulate gyrus posteriorly and a bit laterally along the inferior surface of the brain. See Figure 14.3. Notice the small vessels penetrating into the tissue (hence anterior perforated substance) just posterior to the olfactory tract. This region is home to the ***basal nucleus of Meynert*** and the acetylcholine projections to the cerebral cortex. From the basal forebrain, trace caudally and a bit laterally onto the medial underside of the temporal lobe, which is the small patch of piriform cortex (where the anterior portions of the temporal pole connect to the rest of the brain) and the uncus (the bulge at the medial surface of the temporal lobe).

The ***uncus,*** as the most medial extension of the temporal lobe, actually overhangs the opening in the tentorium, between the middle and posterior cranial fossas. Any swelling of the brain tends to push the uncus over the edge, compressing the brainstem. Notice that the uncus sits very close to the course of the III (oculomotor) nerve. Uncal herniation over the tentorial edge generally compresses the

FIGURE 14.3. *Basal forebrain. The left panel shows the base of the brain after removal of the brainstem. In the right panel the inferior portion of the temporal lobes has been removed, the leptomeninges partially stripped, and the optic chiasm retracted.*

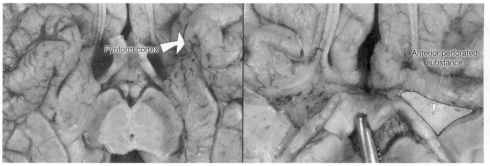

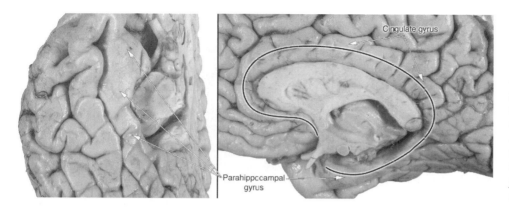

FIGURE 14.4. *Parahippocampal gyrus and limbic "circuit." The left figure is a close-up of the base of the brain after the brainstem has been removed. It is taken at a slight angle to show how the parahippocampal gyrus blends into the cingulate gyrus. The right figure is a sagittal view of the same brain.*

dorsomedial surface of the III nerve first, resulting in an enlarged pupil ipsilaterally. Further herniation will compress the midbrain.

INST Staying on the medial surface of the temporal lobe and moving caudally, you will traverse the *parahippocampal gyrus* on the medial side of the temporal lobe. Follow this around and you end up back in the retrosplenial cingulate gyrus. See Figure 14.4.

Internal Components of the Limbic System
Insula and Piriform Cortex

INST On your brain hemisphere, locate the point in the inferior aspects of the brain where the temporal pole is attached to the rest of the brain. This point also marks the most posterior aspects of the orbitofrontal cortex (the cortex at the base of the frontal lobe, sitting on top of the orbits). Now gently pry apart the lateral sulcus to expose the *insula* (the patch of cortex hidden by the lateral sulcus; see Fig. 14.5).

INST You will note that the anterior portion of the insula also ends at the point where temporal and frontal cortices meet. You are at the primary olfactory cortex. See if you can locate this point in your coronal sections (see Fig. 14.6).

At this point of convergence of the temporal pole, the insula, and the posterior orbitofrontal cortex lies the piriform olfactory cortex. The piriform olfactory cortex forms one of the two core limbic structures.

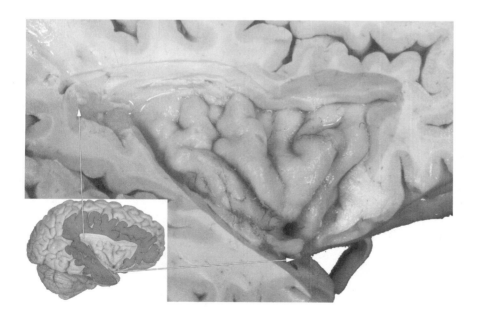

FIGURE 14.5. *Insular cortex. In the inset, portions of the frontal and temporal lobes have been dissected away (gray) to reveal the insula.*

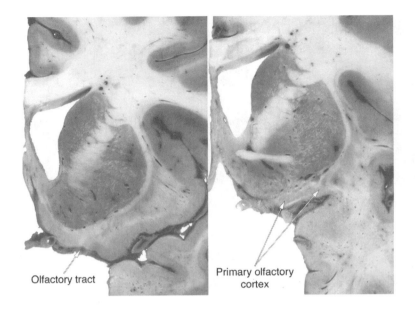

FIGURE 14.6. *Olfactory cortex on coronal sections.*

Olfactory tract

Primary olfactory cortex

INST In order to see how sensory information enters the olfactory area, return to the underneath surface of the brain. Trace the olfactory tract back from the bulb, and try to follow its course. Notice how its splits. Try to trace the lateral branch to where it merges with gray matter. Trace the medial branch as far as you can. Some of the information in the medial branch crosses in the anterior commissure. Just behind the split is the anterior perforated substance. See Figure 14.7.

Hippocampal Formation

INST The hippocampal formation forms the second core limbic structure. It is rolled inside the temporal lobe, in somewhat analogous fashion to the insula. To reveal it, pull open the fissure that lies along the most medial edge of the temporal lobe. This is the hippocampal fissure. Ordinarily it is closed, so that only the very edge of it is visible. Exposing the fissure will partially damage the specimen, so try to keep it as intact as possible. You probably won't be able to get quite the exposure presented in Figure 14.8. Use the figure to appreciate the complex and beautiful anatomy.

The term "hippocampal formation" is used generically to refer to all of the structures in this region, including the dentate gyrus, the hippocampal gyrus (which envelops the dentate gyrus), and subiculum. The term "hippocampus" sometimes is used as in hippocampal formation, while at other times is restricted to the cortex surrounding the dentate gyrus. We will use "hippocampus" to refer to the dentate gyrus and the hippocampal gyrus that surrounds it, leaving out the subiculum. Beware, these words get tossed about freely!

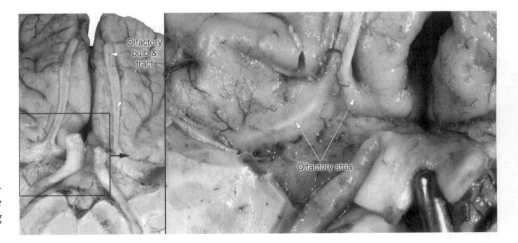

Olfactory bulb & tract

Olfactory stria

FIGURE 14.7. *Olfactory tract entering brain substance. The right figure is a close-up of the left, after retracting the optic chiasm.*

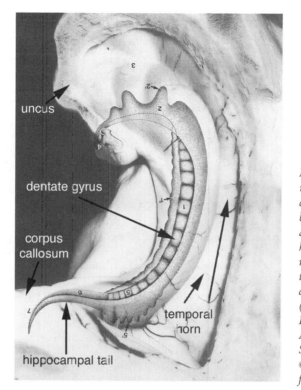

FIGURE 14.8. *Hippocampal formation viewed from above, after dissecting away superior portions of brain. The image is taken from above, after the brain tissue superior to the hippocampus and ventricle has been removed. You are looking down on the right hippocampal formation. The diagram highlights the dentate gyrus. (Adapted from H. M. Duvernoy, The Human Hippocampus. Functional Anatomy, Vascularization and Serial Sections with MRI, second edition © 1998, Springer-Verlag, Berlin, figure 22, page 47.)*

INST Retrieve the coronal slices of brain you prepared in a previous laboratory. Locate the hippocampus in these coronal slabs (see Fig. 14.9). It extends through several different slabs, from the back end of the amygdala all the way to the splenium of the corpus callosum. Notice its C-shaped structure in several slabs. Correlate these with the intact hemisphere so that you can see the position of the hippocampal fissure.

The C-shaped structure reminded earlier neuroanatomists of a horn. To them, the most famous "horn" was a gift from Ammon, King of Libia, to his mistress Amalthea. This horn was either a fertile tract of land shaped like a horn or a goat's horn from which Zeus was suckled. Either way, the term "horn of plenty" or cornucopia derives from this horn, as does "Ammon's horn" of the hippocampus. The Latin term Cornu Ammon is used to describe the histologic layers of the hippocampus (CA fields).

INST The cortex immediately surrounding the hippocampal formation is the parahippocampal gyrus. Locate the parahippocampal gyrus in the inferior aspects of the temporal lobe in your intact specimens. Most anteriorly, overlying the amygdala and the anterior tip of the hippocampus, is the portion of the parahippocampal gyrus called the ***entorhinal cortex.*** From the cortex along the medial edge of the

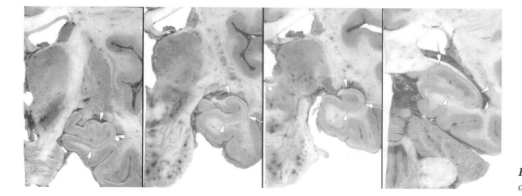

FIGURE 14.9. *Hippocampus in coronal sections.*

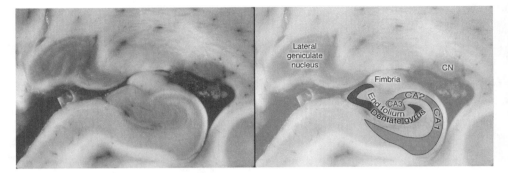

FIGURE 14.10. *Hippocampal sub-divisions.*

parahippocampal gyrus, trace the cortical ribbon back, through the subiculum and CA fields, to the dentate gyrus, using the coronal sections. See Figure 14.10.

In both panels of Figure 14.11, the lower portion of the thalamus has been removed. The right panel is from a slightly more oblique view than the left. On the right, the splenium, fimbria and anterior hippocampus have been partially removed to better reveal the dentate gyrus.

Information from the entorhinal cortex is relayed to the dentate gyrus, and from there back through a series of relays in the hippocampal CA fields.

INST   The fibers emerging from the hippocampus are called the ***fimbria*** (see Fig. 14.10). From its posterior end, you will see a ribbon of white matter fibers peeling off the hippocampus. Follow these along, from the medial aspect of the hemisphere, as they curve under the corpus callosum. These fimbria have become the ***fornix,*** which is the major hippocampal outflow pathway. Use your atlas to find the fornix on the coronal sections. It is the paired white matter bundle that lies below the corpus callosum. See Figure 14.12.

The body of the fornix follows the corpus callosum to the foramen of Monro, where the bundles separate. Some fibers drape in front of the anterior commissure to the septal nuclei (you can't see them grossly) while most descend backward to enter the hypothalamus. About half of the fibers in the fornix leave it during this segment of its course, innervating nuclei of the medial hypothalamus, while the remainder project to the mammillary bodies.

INST   Find the mammillary bodies on your coronal sections. Also find them on the horizontal sections (see Fig. 14.13). On the horizontal sections, try to trace the fornix backward (see Fig. 14.12). Differentiate between the fornix, which comes from the front to the mammillary bodies, and the mammillothalamic tract, which ascends directly from the bodies to the anterior nucleus of thalamus. Identify this structure on your coronal sections. From the anterior nucleus, the fibers project to the cingulate gyrus.

Another fiber tract, the mammillotegmental tract, also arises from the mammillary bodies and travels back to the dorsal and ventral tegmental nuclei in the brainstem.

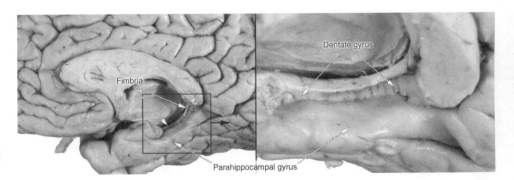

FIGURE 14.11. *Parahippocampal gyrus and dentate gyrus.*

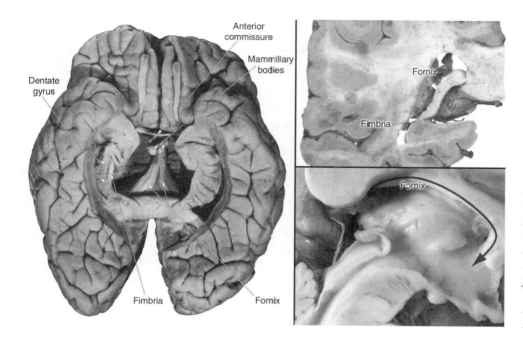

FIGURE 14.12. *Fimbria to fornix. The large figure on the left is a dissection of the limbic system from the base of the brain. The upper right image is a coronal dissection and the lower right is a sagittal section. (Left figure adapted from Gluhbegovic and Williams, The Human Brain, a Photographic Guide. © 1980, Harper & Row, figure 5-25, page 149.)*

Corticoid Components

INST Try you identify the septal area and the diagonal band in your coronal blocks. If you can't, try to make another fine coronal cut in the approximate level at which you feel these structures are located. The third basal forebrain corticoid structure, the substantia innominata, is located a bit posterior and lateral to the diagonal band. The bulk of this structure is situated underneath the crossing of the anterior commissure. Try to locate the substantia innominata in your coronal blocks (see Fig. 14.14).

In addition to other neuronal components, the basal forebrain corticoid regions contain loose clusters of cholinergic neurons that innervate the entire cortical mantle, including the hippocampus, the olfactory bulb, and the amygdala corticoid area.

INST A coronal cut at the level of the uncus (the bulge at the medial aspects of the temporal lobe) will visualize the amygdala and in some specimens, also the anterior tip of the hippocampus (the

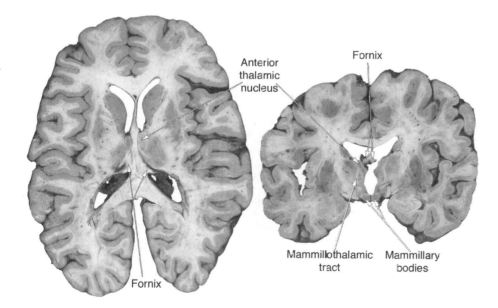

FIGURE 14.13. *Mammillary bodies and mammillothalamic tract.*

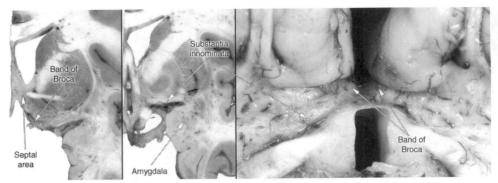

FIGURE 14.14. *Corticoid components.*

hippocampus lies just posterior and a bit inferior to the amygdala). Try to locate the amygdala in your coronal series. See Figure 14.14. On the gross specimen you may be able to distinguish several divisions of this gray matter structure. If you can't find it, make a coronal cut at the level of the uncus. Cut far enough back to enter the tip of the temporal horn of the lateral ventricle. You will see the most anterior tip of the hippocampus forming an oval mass that indents the lateral ventricle, just beneath the amygdala. Also find the amygdala on your horizontal sections. It is further down in the horizontal slices than most people realize, underlying the uncus (the bulge along the anterior medial surface of the temporal lobe). See Figure 14.15.

CELLULAR AND LAMINAR ORGANIZATION OF THE LIMBIC STRUCTURES

Q14.1. Examine microscopic slide and Figure 14.16 of the "hippocampal formation." Using your atlas and without using the microscope, identify:
- Dentate gyrus
- Hippocampal gyrus
- Subiculum
- Tail of caudate nucleus
- Fimbria
- Temporal pole of lateral ventricle
- Parahippocampal gyrus

A14.1. *See Figure 14.17.*

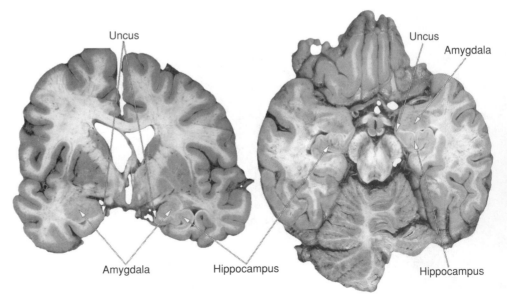

FIGURE 14.15. *Amygdala, coronal and horizontal views.*

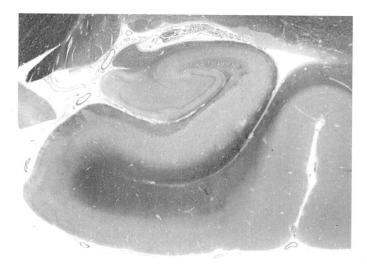

FIGURE 14.16. *Low-power histology of the hippocampal formation. H&E/LFB stain.*

Q14.2. Now using your microscope (or Fig. 14.18), identify the following components of the hippocampal formation:
- Dentate gyrus
- Neurons in the end folium
- CA3
- CA2 (compact region of pyramidal neurons)
- CA1
- Fimbria and the white matter leading to it lining the ventricle on the outside of the hippocampal gyrus

A14.2. See the schematic diagram in Figure 14.19 and Figure 14.17.

Q14.3. In Figure 14.20 locate the blade of compact small neurons (granule cells) in the dentate gyrus. How many layers can you identify in the dentate gyrus (remember to include in your count layers without visible neurons)? Now locate the neurons in Ammon's horn (cornu ammonis, or the CA field). How many layers can you identify in this region? What are the main cellular differences between the dentate gyrus and the Ammon's horn?

A14.3. *The hippocampus is a core limbic cortical structure and thus by definition is primitive cortex and poorly laminated. In general, one can identify three layers in the dentate gyrus: the obvious granular layer and the two paucicellular neuropil layers surrounding it. The hippocampal gyrus also has more-or-less three layers, a variable-width pyramidal neuron layer and the neuropil layers around it. Unlike the dentate gyrus, which is populated by granule cells, Ammon's horn or the hippocampal gyrus consists primarily of pyramidal neurons.*

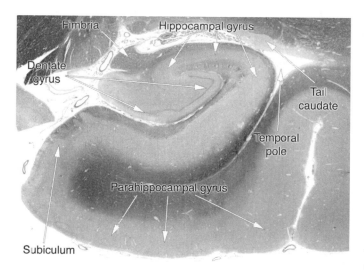

FIGURE 14.17. *Hippocampal regional anatomy.*

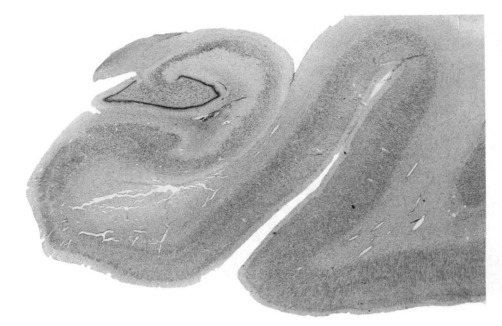

FIGURE 14.18. *Hippocampal formation Nissl-stained histology.*

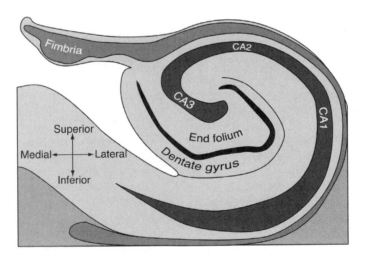

FIGURE 14.19. *Schematic diagram of hippocampal histology.*

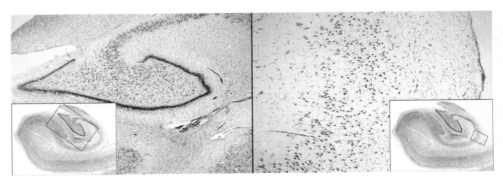

FIGURE 14.20. *Close-up Nissl histology of hippocampal formation components. The left panel shows the dentate gyrus and a portion of CA3. The right panel shows the CA1 region near the inflection of the ventricle.*

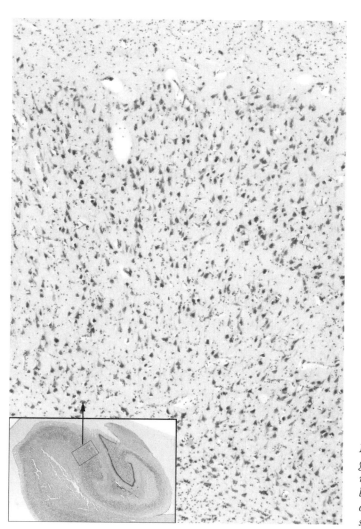

FIGURE 14.21. *Parahippocampal gyrus (presubiculum) histology. The main histology is taken from the boxed region in the presubiculum part of the gyrus, shown in the inset. Nissl stain.*

The fimbria carries axons that emanate primarily from pyramidal neurons in CA1 and the subiculum.

Q14.4. Now move through the CA fields to the parahippocampal gyrus, the cortex that is located adjacent to the hippocampal gyrus (see Fig. 14.21). How many layers can you identify in this cortex? Compare the layers to those of the hippocampus.

A14.4. *The parahippocampal gyrus is a major paralimbic cortical zone of the hippocampocentric system. By definition, paralimbic areas (including the parahippocampal gyrus) have more advanced laminar differentiation than core limbic zones. The regions of the parahippocampal gyrus closest to the hippocampus (presubiculum) have relatively poor lamination. Five to six layers are usually present. Some layers are devoid of neurons. All the neurons are large. The small granule neurons, which densely populate layers II and IV of neocortex, are conspicuously absent.*

Q14.5. Gradually move through the subiculum, down the collateral sulcus, toward temporal neocortex. Use Figure 14.22 for assistance. Can you detect any changes in the lamination (layering) of the cortex as you move closer to neocortex? If so, what changes do you see?

A14.5. *In contrast to the portions of subiculum in Figure 14.21, which are poorly laminated, those blending into temporal neocortex (at the depths of the first sulcus encountered) have six distinct layers, including layers populated by granule neurons. This layering should be easier to see in Figure 14.22.*

Q14.6. Examine Figure 14.23. Identify the core limbic structure. How many layers does it contain? As you did with the hippocampus, try to gradually move away from this core limbic structure and note changes in lamination.

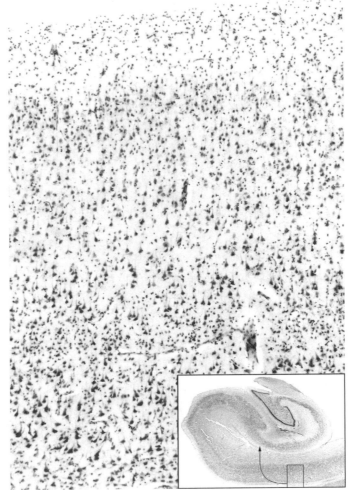

FIGURE 14.22. *Parahippocampal gyrus in collateral sulcus. The main histology is an inverted close-up view of the boxed region in the inset. Nissl stain.*

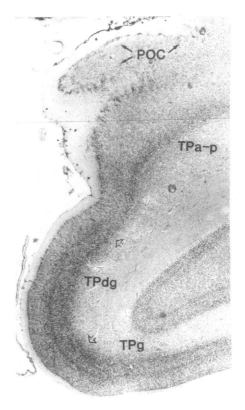

FIGURE 14.23. *Piriform olfactory cortex histology. The section is a Nissl-stained section through the anterior temporal lobe. (Abbreviations: POC, piriform olfactory cortex; TP: temporal pole; a–p: agranular-pregranular; dg: disgranular; g: granular.)*

A14.6. At the top, a fingerlike portion of the piriform olfactory cortex protrudes from the temporal pole. The POC has roughly three identifiable layers. The portions of the paralimbic temporal pole closest to POC (agranular-pregranular) also have few and irregular layers. As one moves away from the POC, more distinct layers appear, from disgranular to granular (meaning it contains a well-established layer of small neurons appearing like grains).

ACETYLCHOLINE SYSTEM

Q14.7. Examine the photographs in Figure 14.24 of the forebrain and brainstem stained with acetylcholinesterase. Using your atlas or text, identify the major sites of staining. Where do the major sites project?

A14.7. Beneath the globus pallidus and anterior commissure live the large neurons of the basal forebrain (also known as the substantia innominata or **basal nucleus of Meynert**). These provide the predominant cholinergic projection to the cerebral cortex. In the brainstem is the even more obscure pedunculopontine nucleus (lateral to the superior peduncle at the pons–midbrain junction) and the lateral dorsal tegmental nucleus (you guessed it, in the lateral dorsal tegmentum, in the gray matter around the aqueduct). These groups project to the brain stem reticular formation and the thalamus.

As in the dopamine, norepinepherine, and serotonin systems, the cholinergic neurons arise at several anatomically distinct sites, each with its own select projections and functions.

Learning the names of these nuclei is NOT an objective of this laboratory; it's the concept of an acetylcholine system that we're after. Also note the high concentration of acetylcholinesterase staining in the putamen. While this nucleus contains cholinergic neurons, the neurons only project locally and are not considered part of the diffuse cholinergic system. They represent some of the large neurons in Figure 9.8.

Q14.8. One of the many roles of acetylcholine is in rapid-eye movement (REM) sleep. In Figure 14.25, REM sleep was induced in a cat by infusing its pons with the cholinergic agonist carbachol. Cells activated by carbachol are shown as dots. The left image is a control. On the left, what nuclei are labeled LC and R? What transmitters are used by these nuclei? What other sites are activated during REM sleep? Guess the transmitter used by these other nuclei that are activated by carbachol.

A14.8. Figure 14.25 shows neurons activated during REM sleep. These include sites now familiar to you, the locus ceruleus (LC) and raphe neurons (R). The transmitters used by these are norepinephrine and serotonin (see the first brainstem chapter). The other sites activated by carbachol include the lateral dorsal tegmental area (LDT) and the pedunculopontine nucleus. Both of these nuclei use acetylcholine as a neurotransmitter. This experiment shows that activating the cholinergic system in the "reticular activating system" will induce REM sleep.

This is but one of many experiments linking the cholinergic system to REM sleep. But as you can see, several other transmitters are also involved, which suggests why so many of the medications affecting these systems also affect sleep. While the details of this experiment should not be committed to memory (you'll push out something more important), you should remember that sleep involves several different diffusely projecting brain systems.

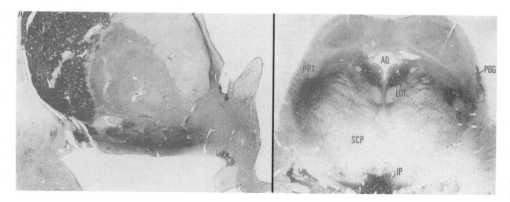

FIGURE 14.24. Forebrain (left) and caudal midbrain stained for acetylcholinesterase (Modified from C. Saper, Cholinergic System, in The Human Nervous System, ed G. Paxinos, © 1990, Academic Press, San Diego, figure 33.3, page 1101, and figure 33.8, page 1108.)

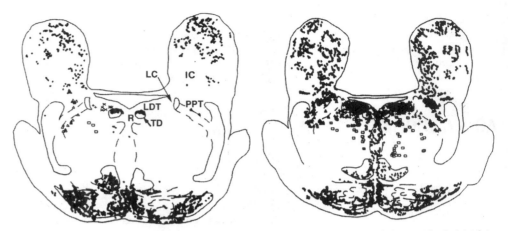

FIGURE 14.25. *Fos immunoreactivity in a cat's pons after injection of saline (left) or carbachol (right). REM sleep was induced in a cat by infusing its medial pontine reticular formation with carbachol, a cholinergic agonists. After a prolonged period of sleep, the animals were sacrificed and activated neurons were identified by their production of Fos protein. The image shows the location of neurons having Fos immunoreactivity (staining with antibodies to Fos) in the pons. (LDT, lateral dorsal tegmental nucleus; PPT, pedunculopontine tegmental nucleus.) (Modified from Shiromani, P. J., et al, 1992. Brain Res 580:351.)*

You probably use coffee to help you through neuroanatomy. Coffee is an adenosine antagonist and adenosine activates cholinergic neurons in the pedunculopontine and dorsal tegmental nuclei. Coffee keeps you awake by antagonizing the action of adenosine on these brainstem cholinergic neurons.

MAJOR FUNCTIONAL AFFILIATIONS OF THE LIMBIC SYSTEM

Learning and Memory

Patient H.M. underwent surgical resection of specific brain regions because of intractable epilepsy. Thereafter H.M. lost the ability to form new and stable memories. His short-term memory is intact, as he can converse and is pleasantly sociable. However, he fails to lay down new memories. Every time he comes to see his research examiner, he has to be reintroduced. Yet he retains memories of events prior to his surgery. When shown a picture of his wife, he can recall details of their marriage but does not remember she died after his surgery.

Q14.9. Examine the image in Figure 14.26. The left-hand column (1–3) shows T1 weighted MRI images at three coronal levels of H.M.'s brain. The right-hand column shows images from the brain of a normal individual. Where is the site of the lesion in H.M.'s brain? What specific structures are involved? What can you infer as to the specific functions of these sites?

A14.9. *The surgical resection was aimed at the medial aspects of the temporal lobe. The amygdala, hippocampus, and parahippocampal gyrus are largely removed on both sides. The hippocampus and parahippocampal gyrus have been shown to be intimately involved in the formation of new memories (learning, consolidation of short-term memories) and recall of stored memories (retrieval). It is quite likely that the extensive interconnections of the hippocampus with the cerebral cortex (and therefore access to integrated experiential information) is a strong contributor to the involvement of the hippocampus in learning and memory. (Try to review the cortical connections of the hippocampus. Which structure relays information from neocortex to hippocampus?) Indeed, humans with bilateral hippocampal and parahippocampal lesions display severe amnestic states. The site of the lesion need not be the same on the two sides, so long as the pathway is interrupted bilaterally (including lesions in structures with which the hippocampus shares a strong connection).*

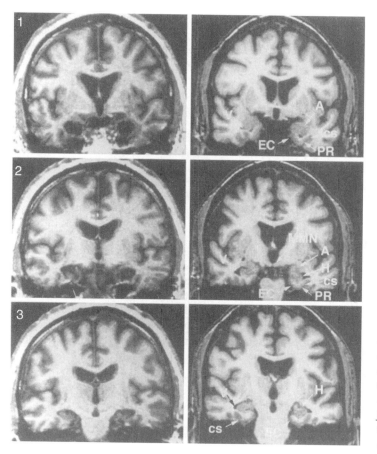

FIGURE 14.26. *MRI scans of patient HM, after he had undergone resections for intractable epilepsy. (Modified from figure 5, Corkin, S., et al. H. M.'s medial temporal lobe lesion: findings from magnetic resonance imaging. 1997. J Neuroscience 17: 3972.)*

Emotions

Q14.10. Examine the fMRI in Figure 14.27. It shows functional MRI (fMRI) images. fMRI measures blood oxygen level dependent (BOLD) magnetic signals. The brain areas activated during performance of specific behavioral tasks can be detected due to changes in the oxyhemoglobin: deoxyhemoglobin ratios as compared to the resting state. Yellow-red (here dark) indicates areas of greatest activation. In this experiment subjects were shown faces with neutral expressions (blank expression) or faces with fearful or happy (emotional) expressions. The fMRI signals were averaged over eight subjects. Those areas showing the greatest specific activation when viewing emotional faces show the greatest signal intensity.

When subjects were shown faces with neutral expressions, the area indicated by the arrow in the right MRI image was activated. Can you identify the anatomical location that is activated? Why should this site be active while the subject views faces?

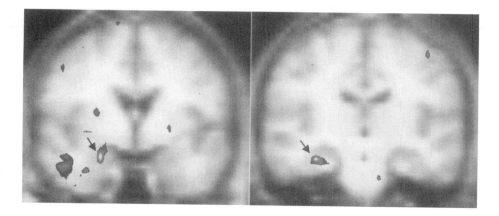

FIGURE 14.27. *fMRI showing areas specifically activated by emotional faces relative to faces have neutral expressions. The left panel shows the activation when the subject was viewing emotional expressions. The right panel, when subject was viewing faces with neutral expressions. (Data kindly supplied by Christopher Wright and Hakan Fischer)*

A14.10. *The arrow in the right image points to the hippocampus. This site is activated regardless of the emotional content of the face the subject looks at. Given the role of the hippocampus in memory, this area is most likely activated because the subjects were encoding into memory the features of the face they observed and/or were automatically attempting to identify the face they looked at. Thus the activation of the hippocampus represents the memory component of the task.*

Q14.11. When subjects were shown faces with emotional expressions, the area indicated by the arrow in the left image was activated. Can you identify the anatomical site of activation?

A14.11. *The site identified by the arrow in the left image is the amygdala. It was activated only when subjects looked at faces with emotional expression. The amygdala appears to have an important role in decoding biologically relevant stimuli such as fearful faces (which signal a threat) or happy faces (which are safety signals), and in generating an appropriate initial behavioral response. For example, freezing in the setting of danger, or approach in situations of security or reward. Patients with congenital lesions of the amygdala bilaterally often do not recognize human emotions, and particularly expressions of fear or anger.*

Q14.12. The large activated area on the lower left-hand corner of the left image was seen regardless of what type of facial expression the subject was exposed to. Try to identify the anatomical sight activated. Can you guess the behavioral significance of this site in relation to the present task?

A14.12. *The activated area on the lower left of the left image corresponds to the middle and inferior temporal gyri. These regions are an anterior extension of the visual association cortex (with which you will become more familiar in the next laboratory exercise). They have been shown to subserve visual object (and perhaps face) recognition. Hence these areas are most likely activated because of their involvement in facial feature recognition.*

Q14.13. Are the sites of interest in the two hemispheres activated to a similar extent? If not, which hemisphere contains the primary sites of activation (the image shows the brains as if the subject was facing you)? What is the functional significance of this hemispheric asymmetry?

A14.13. *The regions activated are all in the right hemisphere. Indeed, a sizable body of evidence indicates a right hemispheric specialization in processing of facial features (face recognition) as well as emotional processing. Another example of hemispheric dominance in a functional domain is the left hemispheric specialization for language.*

Rage and Aggression

Q14.14. As discussed in the introduction, lesions in the septal region (equivalent to the shaded area in Fig. 14.28) produces a profound lowering of a rat's "rage threshold." What can you conclude regarding the function of this region given the heightened emotional response of the lesioned rodents? Predict the effects of electrical stimulation of this region on emotional expression.

A14.14. *The area shaded in the figure corresponds to the septal nuclei (septal area) located at the base of the septum pellucidum. The heightened emotional response following septal lesions in the rat indicates that this region is likely to exert an inhibitory influence upon the expression of*

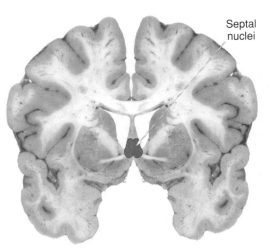

Septal
nuclei

FIGURE 14.28. *Septal nuclei on coronal section.*

emotions, particularly rage and aggression. Electrical stimulation of the septal area in rodents produces a docile and overly calm animal. It remains to be determined whether a similar function can be attributed to the human septal area.

Q14.15. The amygdala appears to exert the opposite influence upon emotional expression when compared with the site lesioned in the above mentioned rats. Try to predict the effects of lesions and electrical stimulation of the amygdala on emotional expression.

A14.15. *An intact amygdala appears to be necessary for the generation of an emotional response. Electrical stimulation of the amygdala can cause a similar (but not identical) rage response to that produced by septal lesions. Extracellular activity in the amygdala of freely moving monkeys indicates a high rate of responding during sexual and aggressive encounters. Amygdalectomy alters a monkey's position in the social hierarchy, and interferes with affective vocalizations and gestures. Depth recordings from human epileptic patients have indicated high rates of firing in association with rage attacks and the experience of other strong emotions.*

CLINICAL CASE STUDY

The patient was an 81-year-old man who was brought to a neurologist by his family with a question of what can be done to improve his memory. The patient himself had no specific complaints. When asked, he admitted that his memory may be a bit off.

His family reports that he began to have trouble 7 or 8 years ago, when he got lost several times while driving. He had to restrict his driving to local very familiar routes. Once he forgot to pick up his grandson at school, although he had been told to do so that very morning. On several occasions, he had answered the phone, went to find the person requested, but forget for whom he was looking. Despite these problems he was able to participate in family life, had no major limitations, and was unaware of the adjustments that others were making. His memory loss slowly worsened. He could not accurately recall events of the previous few days, and forgot birthdays, anniversaries, and even Christmas. He mailed out a batch of Christmas cards using Christmas seals instead of stamps. Many of his old friends no longer lived nearby; he had less contact with those that did.

In the 6 to 12 months before evaluation he had significant language problems, using sentences and words that did not make sense. He lost the ability to learn new information. His gait, coordination, hearing, and vision all seemed unaffected. He usually dressed himself without difficulty. Balance was good and there was no history of falling. He was taking no medications.

An elder brother had died with significant memory loss late in life.

Examination showed a normal gait, strength, reflexes, coordination, and cranial nerves.

He was fully alert. His speech was sparse and had little content. He could not follow complex verbal commands. He could read aloud, but with poor comprehension. Memory loss was severe. On the Mini Mental Status Examination his score was 17 (of 30).

Q14.16. What is the nature of this man's disease? You probably already know the disease; most of us know someone with it. Using your knowledge about anatomic structures important for memory, predict what the MRI scan will show.

A14.16. *This story is a typical one for Alzheimer's disease, and the likelihood of correct anatomic diagnosis in this setting is very high. Important points in the diagnosis of this neurodegenerative disease include a gradual onset and slowly progressive course over five years or more, an absence of other neurological deficits, a presentation with memory loss followed later by language deficits, including "empty" speech, and a family history of relatives with this disease.*

Other variants of Alzheimer's pose more diagnostic difficulties. Here are a few of the variants:

- *Marked behavior change—agitation, aggressiveness, severe apathy.*
- *Rapid course, a few years instead of 5 to 10.*
- *Early onset. Some of these cases have a dominant family history and may have one of the several known genetic mutations.*
- *Accompaniment by rigidity and parkinsonian features.*

Q14.17. Examine the MRI scans in Figure 14.29 of the brain from this case and the gross specimens in Figure 14.30 from similar cases. Try to find five gross structural changes in this case by comparing it to a normal brain. What do you think caused these changes? Can you relate these structural changes to the clinical deficits?

A14.17. *Both the scan and anatomic specimens show significantly enlarged ventricles and thinning of gyri (widening of sulci). This combination points to severe atrophy of the cerebral cortex, which*

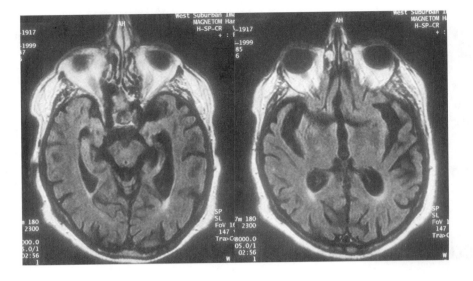

FIGURE 14.29. *MRI scan of patient.*

is caused by degeneration of cortical neurons. The generalized cortical atrophy explains the cognitive deficits in Alzheimer's disease. Specific examples of observable abnormalities include:

- *Lateral ventricles too large*
- *Third ventricle too wide*
- *Central white matter reduced in volume*
- *Too much subarachnoid space around brain—distance to skull too much*
- *Gyri small and shrunken*
- *Temporal lobes small—especially medial temporal*

Q14.18. Examine the microscope slide from a similar case, stained with a Bielschowsky silver stain (see Fig. 14.31). The stain shows two histological features characteristic of this condition (neuritic plaques and neurofibrillary tangles). Identify these features.

A14.18. *The slide shows the primary microscopic pathology of Alzheimer's disease: plaques and tangles. Two example plaques are shown in the "End CA1" and "Neocortex" panels in Figure 14.31. The former contains a "classic plaque" having a dense core of amyloid, while the latter has a "neuritic plaque," named for its dystrophic neurites. The neuritic component (a generic term for either axons or dendrites) contains haphazardly strewn irregular fragments. Some plaques have a darkly stained core (see "End CA1") composed of the* **amyloid** *β (Aβ) protein.*

In the right panels of Figure 14.31 neurons are distinctly (but not deeply) stained; the apical dendrites are clearly visible as vertically directed prolongations of the cell body. Interspersed among these normal neurons are several in which the cell body is partly or entirely filled

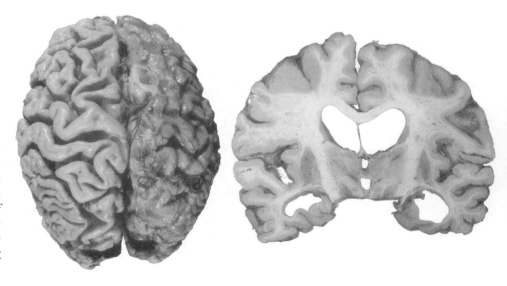

FIGURE 14.30. *Anatomic brain specimens from demented patients. In the left panel, the leptomeninges have been stripped from the left hemisphere to show the degree of atrophy. In the right panel the temporal horns of the lateral ventricles are markedly dilated, indicating tissue loss to both the hippocampus and in surrounding areas of the temporal lobe.*

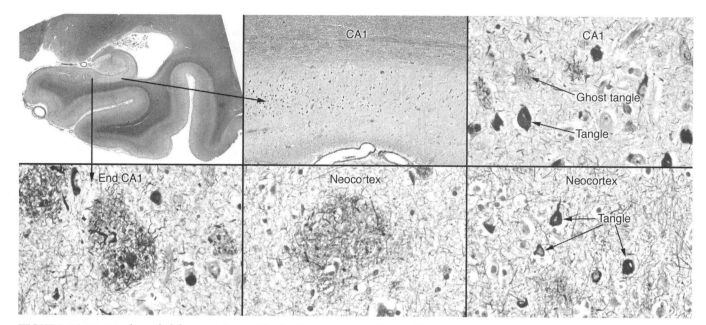

FIGURE 14.31. *Histology of Alzheimer's disease. The first figure shows a field view of the hippocampus as a reference. The two CA1 figures are at progressively higher microscopic powers. The three lower figures are all at the same power. Bielschowsky silver stain.*

with deeply stained thread- or skein-like material. Because these fibrillary deposits often have a clumped or irregularly twisted configuration (best seen under higher magnification), they are called **neurofibrillary tangles**. Many appear as empty loops; others are more like knots. Electron microscopy shows them to be made up of masses of twisted helical filaments that differ in appearance from the normal filaments of the cytoskeleton.

Q14.19. Figure 14.32 is from a section of an Alzheimer's disease patient stained immunohistochemically to visualize amyloid beta (Aβ) peptide. What do you see? Where is the staining? What type of tissue is nearly devoid of staining? Which pathologic elements are visible?

A14.19. *Aβ is the major component of plaques (the neuritic plaques mentioned above as well as a large population of plaques without neurites). A large number of Aβ-positive plaques in the cortex can be seen in this photograph. Only a few trail off into the subcortical white matter; Alzheimer's disease is a disease of gray matter.*

Aβ deposits appear first in paralimbic and limbic cortical zones and later in association cortex. Aβ deposits are found in the neuropil (extracellular space) and are gradually transformed into a neuritic plaque. Aβ is believed to exert toxic effects on neurons. The neurites in plaques may represent fragments of neurons withering as a result of such toxicity. The deposition of Aβ is a specific feature of Alzheimer's disease and occurs early in the pathologic process.

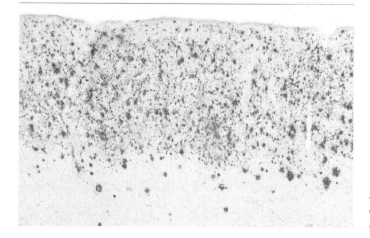

FIGURE 14.32. *Alzheimer's disease brain immunostained with antibodies against amyloid beta peptide.*

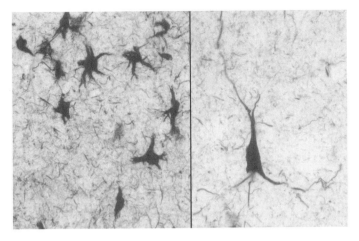

FIGURE 14.33. *Alzheimer's disease brain immunostained with antibodies against a form of phosphorylated tau protein.*

*Aβ is part of a large, transmembranous protein called the **amyloid precursor protein** (APP). APP exists in abundance in normal tissue. Aβ is cleaved out of APP through a complex set of proteolytic processes, which are under intense investigation at the present time.*

Q14.20. Figure 14.33, is from a section of an Alzheimer's disease patient stained immunohistochemically for the abnormally phosphorylated protein *tau* (PH-Tau). The left is a lower power image while the right is higher power. What do you see? What pathologic elements are visible?

A14.20. *This abnormal isoform of tau protein is present in the neuron cell bodies and their processes. These stains in some ways look similar to the classic Golgi silver stain, except of course these neurons are not healthy.*

Q14.21. Examine Figure 14.34, again from an Alzheimer's patient, and again stained for tau protein. What do you see? Where do you see tau staining?

A14.21. *In addition to the neurofibrillary tangles in the neuron cytoplasm, the tau staining discloses a dense mat of **"neuropil threads"** present in the background around the neurons. These threads are neuron processes containing abnormal tau protein.*

Tau is a microtubule-associated protein. Its abnormal phosphorylation (and/or hyperphosphorylation) leads to its aggregation in neurons as neurofibrillary tangles. PH-Tau-positive tangles can be found intra- as well as extracellularly. The latter are called "ghost" tangles, indicating that they caused the death of the neurons within which they were formed. Areas of the brain that contain a large number of tangles always display severe neuronal degeneration.

Q14.22. Does the early and most extreme pathology displayed by this disease explain the early clinical manifestations? If so, how?

A14.22. *In the early stages of the disease process, tangles are seen only in the entorhinal cortex and the immediately adjacent regions. In later stages a larger number of tangles are present in the entorhinal cortex as well as in other limbic and paralimbic areas of cortex. Only at the*

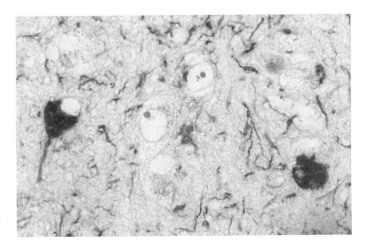

FIGURE 14.34. *Alzheimer's disease brain immunostained for tau protein.*

end-stages of the disease are substantial numbers of tangles seen in neocortical zones. Even at the end-stage of the disease process, the number of neurofibrillary tangles is significantly higher in limbic and paralimbic cortical areas as compared with neocortex.

As you saw earlier, the hippocampus is the site most intimately associated with the process of memory formation. The entorhinal cortex is the only direct access route through which the hippocampus can communicate with the cerebral cortex and thus to the external world. Formation of neurofibrillary tangles in the entorhinal cortex cuts off this route of information transfer, leading to the isolation of the hippocampus from the rest of the cortex and consequently to problems in short-term memory.

Chapter 15—CORTEX

You have at last reached the zenith of the nervous system and the body. In this laboratory you will study that area of the brain that makes us human and determines who we are.

The large expanse of the cerebral cortex in the human brain processes information relevant to many behavioral domains, including the so-called cognitive functions. Within this large expanse, specific cortical areas with relatively sharply defined borders are affiliated with distinct functions. To the unaided eye the cerebral cortex appears as a mass of homogeneous tissue rather than a mosaic of distinct zones. Microscopic examination, however, reveals definite variations in cellular composition and lamination (layering) as various cortical regions are traversed. Two general schemes have been proposed for the parcellation of the cerebral cortex into distinct identifiable zones. One scheme is based primarily on structural (cytoarchitectonic) features of the cerebral cortex. Of these maps, the one used most extensively today is that of Brodmann. The second scheme is based primarily on functional affiliations of the cerebral cortex but also uses, as a minor guide, cytoarchitectonic differences. Because of its emphasis on function rather than pure structure, this second scheme will be used for the purposes of identification of cortical regions in today's laboratory exercise.

The cerebral cortex can be divided into five major functional subtypes. These are the limbic, paralimbic, heteromodal (or multimodal) association, unimodal association, and primary sensory-motor cortices. In this laboratory exercise you will identify the specific cortical areas that belong to each of the above-mentioned functional subtypes. You will then study the cellular architecture of the cerebral cortex and the connectivity between various cortical zones as well as inputs to and outputs from cortex. Finally, you will examine the functional affiliations of a number of cortical areas with special emphasis on cognitive functions.

LEARNING OBJECTIVES

- Review the anatomical landmarks and vascular supply of the cerebral cortex: major sulci and gyri, major cortical areas and vascular territories.
- Study the regional and functional organization of the cerebral cortex, the connectivity of various cortical regions and the relationships among the neocortex, limbic structures, and the hypothalamus.
- Examine the cellular organization and lamination of the cerebral cortex and variations in this organization: neocortex, paralimbic cortex, and core limbic structures.
- Study some of the functional affiliations of individual cortical regions as well as networks of cortical areas.

Functional Neuroanatomy: An Interactive Text and Manual, by Jeffrey T. Joseph and David L. Cardozo
ISBN 0-471-44437-5 Copyright © 2004 John Wiley & Sons, Inc.

INTRODUCTION

Classifying Cortex

The cortex may be divided up in several different ways. Macroscopic divisions identify gyri and sulci, like the calcarine fissure and precentral gyrus. Under a microscope these same areas are often given new names, especially Brodmann areas. Areas 17 and 4 correspond to the two previous gyri. Another way to divide cortex is by it function. Those same regions of brain correspond to the primary visual and motor cortices. In this laboratory you will examine the cortex at these different levels.

In the first part of the lab you will identify some anatomic divisions of the cerebral cortex (e.g. precentral gyrus, calcarine fissure). Many of these gross landmarks correspond to sites where damage (e.g., stroke) reproducibly leads to specific clinical deficits. However, like fingerprints, each brain's gyral pattern is unique. The precise divisions usually represented in textbooks may seem less precise when you are finished.

While the macroscopic anatomy roughly correlates with functional divisions, the microscopic parceling has a more precise relationship to the cortical activity. For example, the Betz cells you encountered in the third laboratory are a defining feature of Brodmann area 4 (BA4); it is these cells that form the core of the corticospinal tract. However, histologic divisions have several significant drawbacks. There is no definitive parcellation of the cortical mantle. Brodmann's scheme is widely used, but other systems are better in select regions. Few studies correlate a unique histology with specific functions. In reality, most studies, particularly the current fMRI research, never correlate the function directly with the histology (who would volunteer to do such a study?). Another difficulty is practical: who can actually identify the different regions histologically? Brodmann described over 40 areas; few would be brave enough to identify the Brodmann area of random piece of cortex. Finally, histologic divisions are just impractical for most everyday clinical uses; you don't want to section your patient's brain just to find out which Brodmann area is causing her facial twitch!

It is the functional divisions that are most important in studying the human cortex. Much of the information on functional areas has previously come from "lesion" studies, from correlating a patient's clinical deficit with their underlying brain pathology. Today such lesion-and-wait studies are being supplanted by functional MRI (fMRI). As future physicians, you will want to retain the rough anatomic landmarks that correspond to the major functional divisions. It is also important that you understand the basic vascular supply to the brain and especially cortex, since this is of major clinical relevance.

Functional Types of Cortex

You have already encountered several functional divisions of the cortex: primary motor, primary somatosensory, primary visual, primary auditory, limbic, and paralimbic. Were this all to the cortex, life would be dull; what makes us human, what makes us who we are, lies in our association cortices.

In a broad view (see *Principles of Behavioral and Cognitive Neurology* by M. Mesulam for more details) the cortex may be divided into four major zones:

- Primary sensory and primary motor cortices
- Association cortex (has two main subdivisions)
- Paralimbic cortices
- Limbic cortex

Figure 15.1 shows the location of these areas of cortex, which are further discussed below.

Primary Sensory and Primary Motor Cortex

The primary sensory and motor areas are the inputs to and outputs from the cortex. But even in these areas, cortical processing is occurring. The divisions are:

- Primary motor cortex: precentral gyrus, frontal lobe.
- Primary somatosensory cortex: postcentral gyrus, parietal lobe.
- Primary auditory cortex: upper part of the superior temporal gyrus.
- Primary visual cortex: banks of the calcarine fissure, occipital lobe.
- Primary olfactory cortex: piriform olfactory cortex.
- Primary vestibular cortex: posterior depths of the Sylvian fissure where the temporal lobe joins the insula and the parietal lobe.

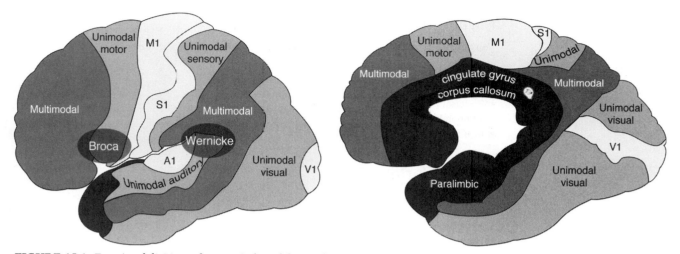

FIGURE 15.1. *Functional divisions of cortex. (Adapted from Behavioral Neuroanatomy: Large-Scale Networks, Association Cortex, Frontal Syndromes, the Limbic System, and Hemispheric Specializations, M.-Marsel Mesulam, in Principles of Behavioral and Cognitive Neurology, edited by M.-Marsel Mesulam, © 2000, Oxford University Press, Oxford.) (Abbreviations: A1 = primary auditory cortex, M1 = primary motor cortex, S1 = primary sensory cortex, V1 = primary visual cortex.)*

- Primary gustatory cortex: Located at the most inferior aspect of the postcentral gyrus, close to cortical areas encoding sensory information for the tongue, larynx, and pharynx.

Unimodal Association Cortex

Each primary sensory area is surrounded by an immediately adjacent unimodal association cortex. These association areas further process the sensory information that has been passed on by primary sensory cortex. Only one type of sensory data is processed; hence these areas are called unimodal. The unimodal association areas are:

- Visual association cortex: most of the cortex in the occipital lobe, including the cortex immediately surrounding the primary visual cortex and inferior aspects of the temporal lobe.
- Auditory association cortex: superior temporal gyrus, temporal lobe.
- Somatosensory association cortex: posterior bank of the postcentral sulcus, parietal lobe.
- Motor association cortex: anterior bank of precentral sulcus, frontal lobe.
- Gustatory association cortex: cortex surrounding primary gustatory cortex including portions of the insula.
- Olfactory association cortex: uncertain; most likely portions of the paralimbic zones of the olfactocentric system (i.e., the temporal pole, insula, and posterior orbitofrontal cortex).
- Vestibular association cortex: uncertain; most likely cortex surrounding the primary vestibular cortex, including portions of the insula.

Multimodal Association Cortex

Different modalities of processed sensory information are combined and further analyzed in multimodal association cortices. The major divisions are listed below:

- Prefrontal cortex: the mass of cortex in the frontal lobe situated anterior to motor association cortex. It extends to the medial and inferior (orbitofrontal) aspects of the frontal lobe.
- Posterior parietal cortex: consisting of the inferior parietal lobule (cortex comprising the supramarginal and angular gyri) and more superiorly, the cortex immediately posterior to somatosensory association cortex.
- Lateral temporal cortex: middle temporal gyrus.
- Medial parietooccipital and fusiform gyri.

Paralimbic Cortex

You have already met the members of this cortical group in the previous laboratory:

- Parahippocampal gyrus (entorhinal cortex)
- Cingulate gyrus (and its anterior and posterior extensions)
- Posterior orbitofrontal cortex
- Temporal pole
- Insula

Limbic Cortex

You have also studied the two members of core limbic cortical zones.

- Piriform olfactory cortex
- Hippocampus

Cortical Histology

As mentioned previously, different areas of cortex have their own specific histology. Based on subtle histologic differences, Brodmann in 1909 divided the cortex into over 40 regions, which are now known as ***Brodmann areas*** (BA). Other simpler and more complex schemes have also been devised, although Brodmann's classification is used most widely.

You have previously looked at the hippocampus and other limbic structures. These areas are considered "other cortex" (or allocortex) and corticoid, since they lack the features that define the "new cortex" (or neocortex).

Neocortex, which surrounds most of your brain and has lead to the colloquial term "gray matter" for the cortex, is divided into six layers:

- Layer 1 (molecular layer): outermost layer consisting predominantly of neuronal processes.
- Layer 2 (external granular layer): inputs from and outputs to other cortical areas.
- Layer 3 (external pyramidal layer): inputs from and outputs to other cortical areas.
- Layer 4 (internal granular layer): receives input from the thalamus.
- Layer 5 (internal pyramidal layer): large neurons projecting to the striatum, brainstem, and spinal cord.
- Layer 6: projects to thalamus.

The distinction among all of these different areas of the brain depends on the thickness and cytology of these six layers.

Thalamic Structure and Cortical Connections

Before discussing cortical connectivity in more detail, it is important to review how information enters the cortex from the body. With the exception of olfaction and primitive olfactory cortex, all sensation reaches cortex via the thalamic "gatekeeper." However, not just sensory but all regions of cortex have their own corresponding thalamic nuclei. Figure 15.2 illustrates major thalamic nuclei having extensive reciprocal connections with specific functional cortical areas. You have already met many of these in earlier chapters. The sensory relay nuclei and corresponding cortical areas are the lateral geniculate nucleus (LGN) and primary visual cortex, the medial geniculate nucleus (MGM) and primary auditory cortex, and the ventral posterior lateral (VPL) and medial nuclei (VPM), and primary somatosensory cortex. For motor functions, the thalamic nuclei and corresponding cortical areas are the ventral anterior (VA), ventral lateral (VL) nuclei, and motor areas of cortex (primary motor and supplementary motor). Limbic cortex reciprocally connects to the anterior nucleus (A) of thalamus. For multimodal cortices, the main thalamic nuclei are the medial dorsal (MD) nucleus for the prefrontal cortex (that portion anterior to the motor regions), the pulvinar (Pul) for the occipitoparietotemporal multimodal cortex, and the lateral posterior (LP) for the parietal multimodal cortex.

Note: You will never remember these nuclei or their locations! While they are reviewed here and in the exercises, the goal is not to teach you quickly lost information, but for you to remember that they exist! Clinically many classic cortical syndromes produced by large cortical strokes can be reproduced with relatively small well-placed thalamic lesions.

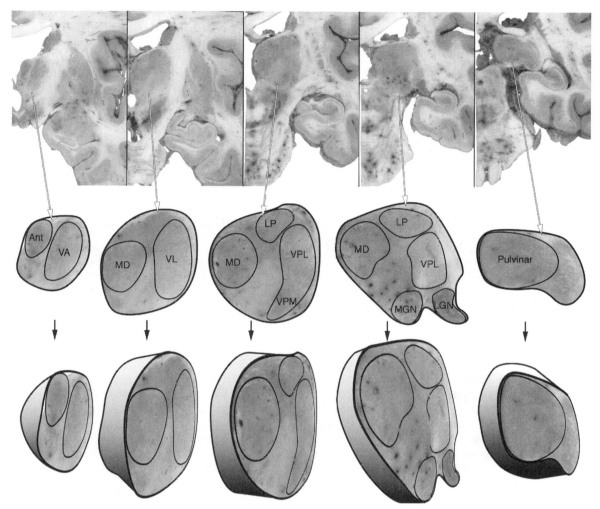

FIGURE 15.2. *Thalamic nuclei overlaid on coronal sections of thalamus.*

Cortical Connectivity

Having laid out the general functional areas of the cortex, we now must connect them.

Elucidation of cortical connectivity was a major focus of neuroscience in past decades, and continues today. Numerous techniques have been used to demonstrate neuronal projections:

- Gross dissection of the white matter bundles can dramatically show major connections, but this technique has limited usefulness today.
- Ablation studies use special silver stains to show the pathways of axonal degeneration following a focal lesion; this is also an older and somewhat crude method.
- Anterograde tracers, like PHA-L (*Phaseolus vulgaris* leukoagglutinin) and radioactive amino acids, are injected at an anatomic site, taken up by neurons, and transported to their axonal endings.
- Retrograde tracers, such as HRP (horseradish peroxidase) and some fluorescent dyes, are taken up by axonal endings and then retrogradely transported back to the cell body.
- Activation markers, notably *fos* staining, can show which neurons are activated by a given stimulus.

Three types of fibers connect various cortical areas with each other and with subcortical structures. These are association fibers, which interconnect various cortical areas with one another; commissural fibers, which interconnect cortical areas in the two hemispheres; and projection fibers, which convey impulses between cortex and subcortical structures. All of these fiber systems must travel through the massive cortical white matter to reach their destination.

Projection fibers originate in deeper layers of cortex and connect to "subcortical" structures and more distant sites. Many areas of cerebral cortex are reciprocally connected to specific thalamic nuclei. Fibers to thalamus originate in layer 6, while those from thalamus terminate in layer 4. As you saw in the basal ganglia laboratory, the cortex also has extensive connections to the striatum.

The cerebral cortex also has major connections to pons (corticopontine fibers) and hence the cerebellum, to the medulla (corticobulbar) and to the spinal cord (corticospinal).

The general pattern of connectivity within the cerebral cortex follows two basic principles:

Principle 1. In the hierarchy of cytoarchitectonic and functional groupings of cortical areas (i.e., limbic to primary sensory-motor), each group of cortical areas has major connections with groups of cortical areas at levels immediately above and below it. For example, unimodal association areas have their major connections with the primary sensory-motor areas, on the one hand, and the multimodal association areas, on the other. Unimodal association areas have only minor connections with areas that are two or more levels removed, such as the paralimbic or limbic cortices.

Principle 2. Cortical areas within functionally similar groups have extensive interconnections. For example, all paralimbic areas are intricately interconnected with each other. The only exceptions to this rule are the primary areas, which have virtually no connections with each other.

Functional Cortical Affiliations; Lateralization of Function

Each hemisphere carries out many functions that are nearly identical on the two sides—motor, sensory, and visual. The only difference being the side of the body or space that is affected. A right hemiparesis can be the mirror image of one on the left. A right-sided hemianopia is just about equivalent to a left hemianopia (except when reading, it is hard to find the start of the line with a left hemianopia). However, two major functions are particularly associated with only one hemisphere.

Left Hemisphere and Language

Language resides on the left side in over 90% of us, including virtually all right handers and approximately 70% of left handers. Details of language processing and the many types of language disorders (aphasias) are beyond the scope of this laboratory. However, a few major sites are clinically relevant. These include Broca's area in the left lateral-inferior frontal lobe, Wernicke's area in the posterior-superior temporal lobe, and an area just above Wernicke's area around the upper rim of the Sylvian fissure. Wernicke's area is important for the reception and understanding of spoken language as well as producing meaningful language. Patient's suffering from a "classic" Wernicke's aphasia seem to speak fluently, but their speech makes no sense: it is filled with nonsensical words ("phonemic paraphasias") or words substituted for other words ("semantic paraphasias"). They also fail to understand when other people speak to them. In contrast, patient's with a Broca's aphasia labor to produce speech, which seems fragmented and telegraphic (using few words without small connecting words). They understand basic conversations and only seem lost when sentences are complex. Language production is frustrating.

While many details of language may seem arcane, for practicing clinicians it is often important to realize simply that a patient suffers from a language disorder (pointing most often to the left cortex) rather than, say, from an articulation problem (suggesting posterior fossa dysfunction) or a global encephalopathy (metabolic encephalopathy or focal lesions involving the thalamus or the reticular activating system).

Right Hemisphere and Attention

As you learned in the previous laboratory session, one of the specializations of the right hemisphere is the processing of emotion. Another specialization of the right hemisphere relates to attention. Right hemispheric damage leads to the characteristic neglect syndrome. The syndrome consists of a behavior change in which the patient pays little attention to events in the world on his left side (opposite to the lesion). He will only look volitionally toward the right, pay no attention to moving objects on the left, or to sensory stimuli coming to him from that side. He may fail to move his left arm and leg, not because they are paralyzed, but because he fails to heed them. In its most extreme form the neglect syndrome can prevent a patient from even recognizing his left hand when it is held in front of him.

Schedule (2.5 hours)
- 30 Gross anatomy
- 30 Functional divisions
- 30 Cellular organization
- 15 Cortical connectivity
- 30 Functional affiliations
- 15 Clinical cases

SULCI, GYRI, AND VASCULAR SUPPLY

Review of Major Sulci and Gyri

The sulcal and gyral patterns of the cerebral cortex are used as landmarks for identification of cortical areas. As you try to identify major sulci and gyri, keep in mind that the precise location and shape of these landmarks differ considerably from one individual to the next.

Q15.1. Using whole and half brain specimens and an atlas as a guide, try to identify the following gyri and sulci on the cortical surface and in Figure 15.3:

Sulci and Fissures

- Lateral sulcus (Sylvian fissure)
- Longitudinal fissure
- Central sulcus
- Precentral sulcus
- Postcentral sulcus
- Superior frontal sulcus
- Inferior frontal sulcus
- Inferior temporal sulcus
- Superior temporal sulcus
- Cingulate sulcus
- Parieto-occipital sulcus
- Calcarine fissure
- Olfactory groove
- Collateral sulcus

Gyri

- Precentral gyrus
- Superior frontal gyrus
- Middle frontal gyrus
- Inferior frontal gyrus
- Superior temporal gyrus
- Middle temporal gyrus
- Inferior temporal gyrus
- Postcentral gyrus
- Angular gyrus
- Supramarginal gyrus
- Cingulate gyrus
- Cuneus gyrus (medial, superior occipital gyrus)
- Lingual gyrus (medial, inferior occipital gyrus)
- Parahippocampal gyrus
- Orbital gyri
- Gyrus rectus
- Occipitotemporal gyrus (fusiform gyrus)

A15.1. *See Figure 15.4.*

Vascular Supply of the Cerebral Cortex

Q15.2. With the help of an atlas, in the worksheet of Figure 15.5 shade in the portions of the cerebral cortex supplied by each of the major cortical arteries indicated below. Also try to trace back each cortical artery to its source (e.g., vertebral artery).
- Anterior cerebral artery
- Middle cerebral artery
- Posterior cerebral artery

A15.2. *See Figure 15.6*

Q15.3. Occlusion of which cerebral artery is of the greatest potential risk? Why? What larger vessel supplies this artery?

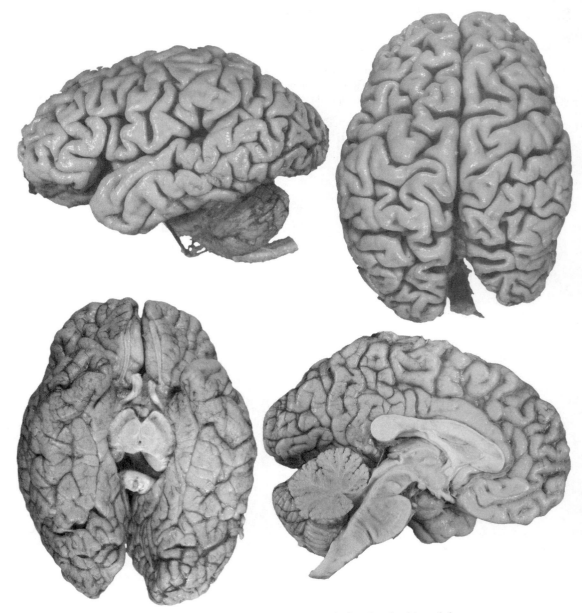

FIGURE 15.3. *Major cortical gyri and sulci worksheet.*

A15.3. *The middle cerebral artery supplies the mass of cortex on the lateral surface of the hemisphere as well as many subcortical structures. Occlusion of this artery unilaterally can lead to massive infarcts with dire consequences including unilateral paralysis and loss of sensory and cognitive functions. It is also often fatal.*

A major origin of emboli to the middle cerebral artery is from its parent vessel, the internal carotid artery. The most common site of emboli formation is at the origin of the internal carotid artery, just after the bifurcation of the common carotid arteries in the neck.

Q15.4. Which major veins drain blood away from the cortex?

A15.4. *The superior and inferior sagittal sinuses drain blood away from the cerebral cortex to the internal jugular vein via the transverse sinus.*

INST Try to locate the major cerebral arteries that are still in place in your specimens. Can you identify them? Follow their course as far as possible.

Q15.5. What is the term used to designate cortical areas situated at the border between the territories supplied by two different cerebral arteries? What is the clinical

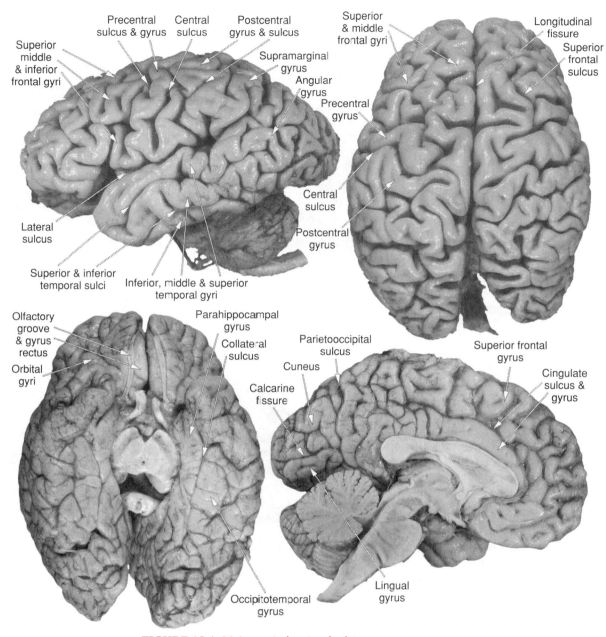

FIGURE 15.4. *Major cortical gyri and sulci.*

significance of such zones? Look at Figure 15.7. Where is the pathology in this brain? Does the cortex appear normal? If not, what do you think caused the abnormality?

A15.5. *Such border areas in the cerebral cortex are termed "border zones," or more frequently but less accurately, "watershed areas." These zones are particularly vulnerable to hypoxic/ischemic events. Figure 15.7 demonstrates two different border zone infarcts. Around the most superior sulcus on the left the cortex is thinner than nearby cortices. The patient's anoxic episode led to ischemia between the anterior and middle cerebral artery territories, which produced tissue necrosis and resorption by macrophages. Another episode of ischemia during his cardiac arrest produced a similar pattern of destruction on the right. However, this occurred shortly before the patient died, since the cortex is hemorrhagic and not sunken (see right panel in Fig. 15.7). The damage to the brain is most severe in the regions where the vascular supply is most tenuous, in the border zones between vascular territories.*

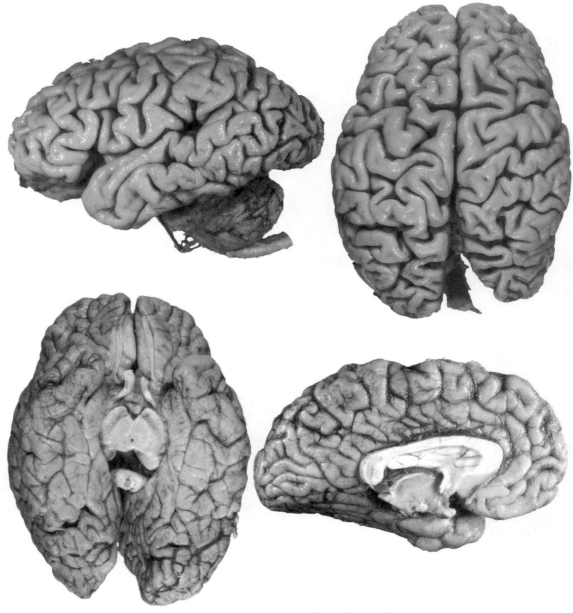

FIGURE 15.5. *Cortical vascular distribution worksheet.*

FUNCTIONALLY SIMILAR GROUPS OF CORTICAL ZONES

As we have seen, the cerebral cortex can be divided into five types of areas based on functional affiliations. On your whole, half and/or coronally cut brain specimens identify the members of each group of cortical zones listed below. Use your atlases as a guide.

Primary Sensory—Motor Cortex

Q15.6. You are already familiar with these areas of cortex. Make sure you can identify them on the gross anatomic specimens and in Figure 15.8.
- Primary motor cortex
- Primary somatosensory cortex
- Primary auditory cortex
- Primary visual cortex
- Primary olfactory cortex

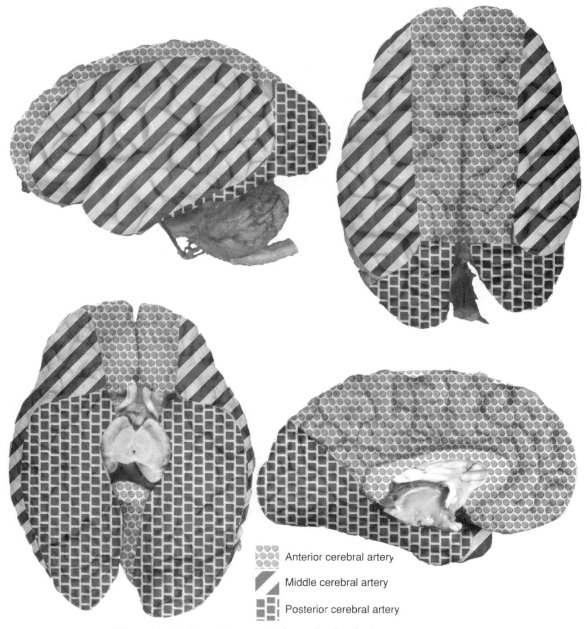

FIGURE 15.6. *Approximate cortical vascular distribution.*

Anterior cerebral artery

Middle cerebral artery

Posterior cerebral artery

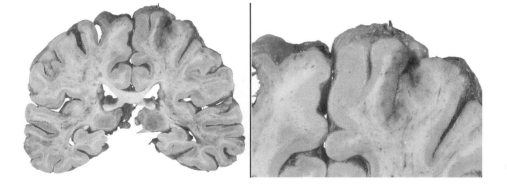

FIGURE 15.7. *Coronal brain sections from a patient who experienced a cardiorespiratory catastrophe during anesthesia for dental surgery, survived for months, and suffered from a cardiac arrest shortly before his demise.*

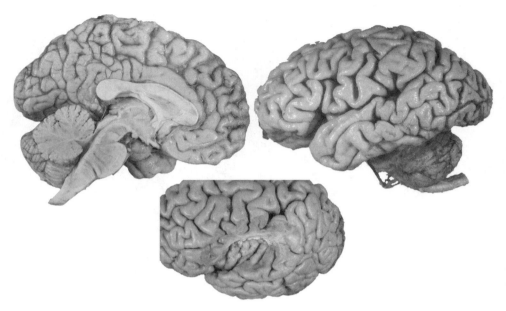

FIGURE 15.8. *Primary cortical areas worksheet. Note that a portion of the frontal and parietal lobes have been removed in the lower panel.*

Also try to identify the two other members of this family that you have not encountered in previous laboratories:
- Primary vestibular cortex (in the posterior depths of the Sylvian fissure where the temporal lobe joins the insula and the parietal lobe)
- Primary gustatory cortex (at the most inferior aspect of the postcentral gyrus, close to cortical areas encoding sensory information for the tongue, larynx, and pharynx)

A15.6. *See Figure 15.9.*

Q15.7. What are the major functions of primary sensory and motor areas? What deficit would result from damage to these areas?

A15.7. *The primary sensory and motor cortical areas provide the major channels of communication with the extrapersonal space. Lesions in each of the primary sensory areas causes nearly complete loss of function in the modality processed by that area. Damage to primary motor cortex leads to spastic paralysis as spinal reflexes take over.*

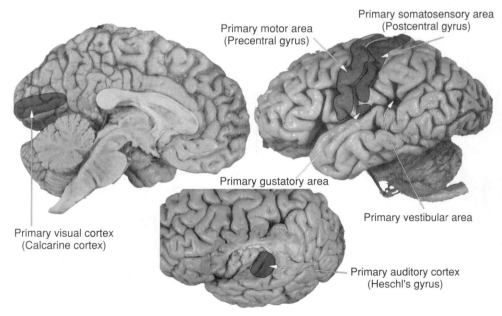

FIGURE 15.9. *Primary cortical areas.*

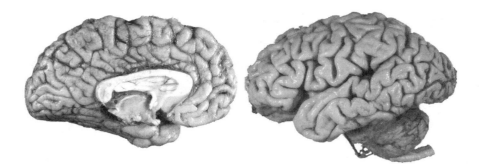

FIGURE 15.10. *Unimodal association cortex worksheet.*

Unimodal Association

Q15.8. Using the information in the introduction, also locate these unimodal association areas on your half brain or Figure 15.10:
  - Visual association cortex
  - Auditory association cortex
  - Somatosensory association cortex
  - Motor association cortex

A15.8. See Figure 15.11.

Q15.9. What are the major functions of unimodal association areas? What types of deficits would be caused by damage to these areas?

A15.9. Each unimodal association area processes and integrates information related to a single modality. Some unimodal association areas process information related to specific qualities of sensory information in regions sequentially removed from the primary areas. Such is the case with the visual association areas that process visual information related to color, motion, shape, objects, faces, words, and targets. Damage to unimodal association areas causes selective perceptual deficits in the absence of general sensory loss.

Multimodal Association

Q15.10. Try to locate the four major multimodal association cortical zones on you brain specimens or in Figure 15.12:
  - Prefrontal cortex
  - Posterior parietal cortex
  - Lateral temporal cortex
  - Fusiform gyrus (occipitotemporal gyrus)

A15.10. See Figure 15.13

Q15.11. What are the major functions of multimodal association areas? What types of deficits would be caused by damage to these areas?

A15.11. Multimodal association areas process information from two or more sensory and/or motor modalities. Damage to these areas always result in deficits that are multimodal and never confined to tasks that are under the guidance of a single modality. Damage to multimodal and some unimodal association areas often cause cognitive or personality deficits. For example, damage to the prefrontal cortex can lead to dramatic alterations in strategic thinking,

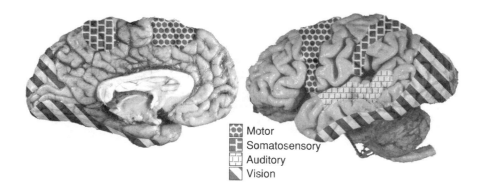

Motor
Somatosensory
Auditory
Vision

FIGURE 15.11. *Unimodal association cortices.*

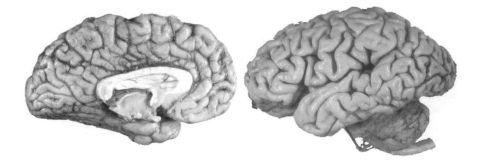

FIGURE 15.12. *Multimodal association cortical zones worksheet.*

personality, emotional integration, and comportment (conduct). Lesions of the inferior parietal lobule cause, among other things, a marked deficit in directing attention toward specific targets in the extrapersonal space.

Paralimbic Cortex

Q15.12. You have already met the members of this cortical group. Make sure you can identify them on your specimens and in Figure 15.14.
- Parahippocampal gyrus (entorhinal cortex)
- Cingulate gyrus (and its anterior and posterior extensions)
- Posterior orbitofrontal cortex
- Temporal pole
- Insula

A15.12. *See Figure 15.15*

Q15.13. What are the major structural and functional characteristics of paralimbic cortical zones?

A15.13. *Paralimbic cortical zones have relatively primitive layers. They serve as transition zones between core limbic and association cortical areas. They process and integrate information from limbic and association cortical areas.*

Limbic Cortex

Q15.14. In the last chapter you studied the two members of core limbic cortical zones. Locate them on your specimens and in Figure 15.16.
- Piriform olfactory cortex
- Hippocampus

A15.14. *See Figure 15.17*

Q15.15. What is the major structural characteristic of these cortical areas?

A15.15. *Core limbic cortical zones are the most primitive type of cortex. They are composed of few and poorly differentiated layers.*

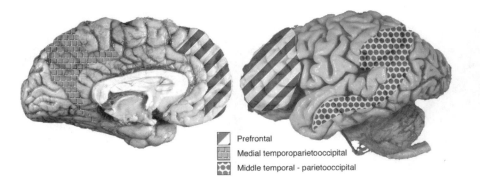

Prefrontal
Medial temporoparietooccipital
Middle temporal - parietooccipital

FIGURE 15.13. *Multimodal association cortical zones.*

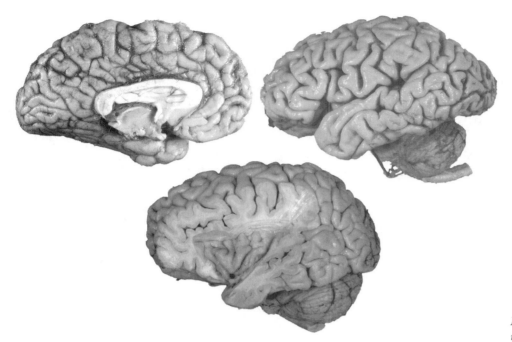

FIGURE 15.14. *Paralimbic cortex worksheet.*

CELLULAR AND LAMINAR ORGANIZATION OF THE CEREBRAL CORTEX

INST Examine the microscopic slide of association cortex (see Fig. 15.18). All nuclei stain with Nissl. However, because of their high content of cytoplasmic ribosomal RNA, larger neurons are more prominently stained.

INST The cortex in Figure 15.18 is a typical example of six-layered neocortex. Try to identify the following cortical layers in the section:

• Layer 1. The outermost neuropil layer consists primarily of neuronal processes; it contains only rare neurons.

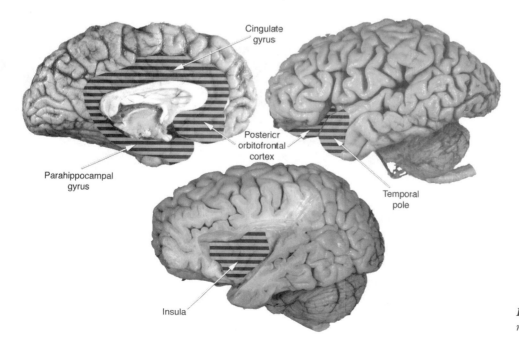

FIGURE 15.15. *Paralimbic cortical regions.*

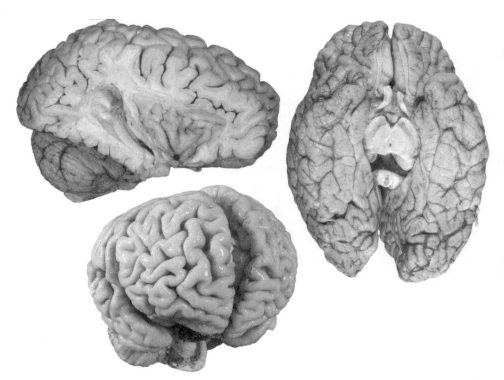

FIGURE 15.16. *Limbic cortex worksheet. In the upper left panel, the lateral cortical surfaces have been removed and a portion of the temporal lobe has been opened into the ventricle to expose the underlying structures. The lower panel is an oblique view of the front of the brain.*

- Layer 2. This layer is usually thin and consists primarily of small granular neurons (which appear as large dots).
- Layer 3. This layer is relatively thick and is composed of large pyramidal neurons (shaped like a pyramid with one dendrite directed toward the cortical surface).
- Layer 4. Like layer 2, layer 4 also consists of granular neurons. As you may recall, this layer becomes macroscopically visible as the line of Gennari in the primary visual cortex.

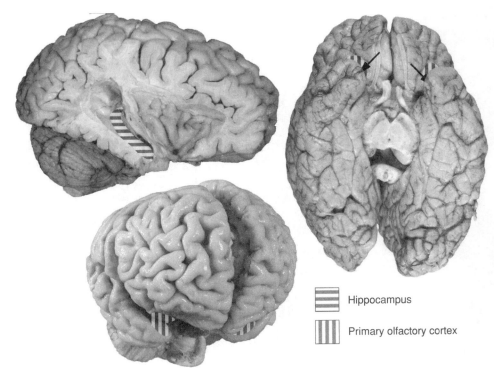

FIGURE 15.17. *Limbic cortical areas. The hippocampus cannot be seen on the surface of the brain; it lies deep in the medial temporal lobe. The upper left image shows the hippocampus from above. The primary olfactory cortex lies at the junction between the orbitofrontal and anterior temporal lobes.*

▤ Hippocampus

▥ Primary olfactory cortex

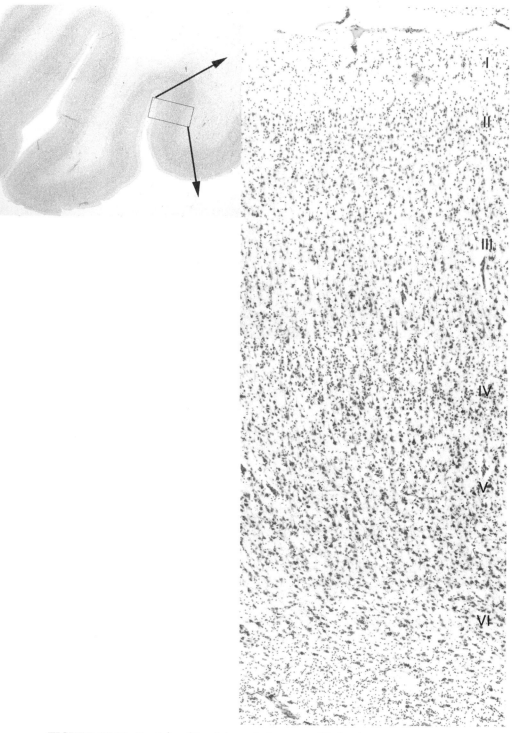

FIGURE 15.18. *Frontal multimodal association cortex, Nissl stain.*

- Layer 5. This layer consists of large pyramidal neurons and projects to subcortical structures.
- Layer 6. This layer consists of neurons of varying morphology that blend into the underlying white matter.

INST Now examine the microscopic slide of the pre- and postcentral gyri (see Fig. 15.19). This slide contains a Nissl stained section cut at a right angle to the central sulcus. Try to identify the cortical layers on each side of the central sulcus.

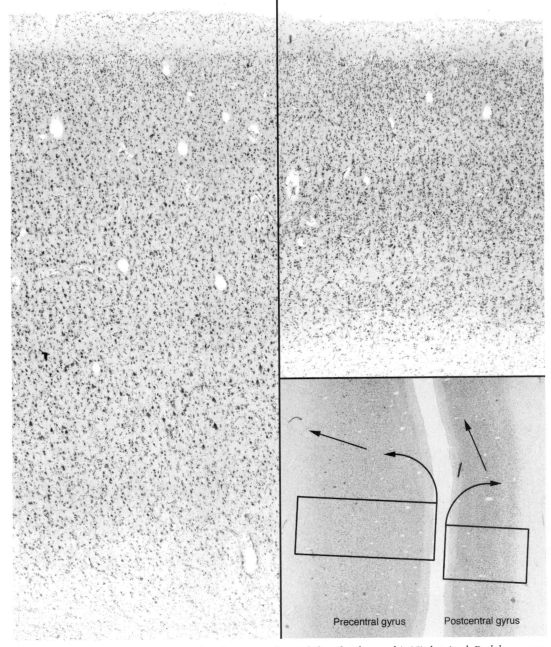

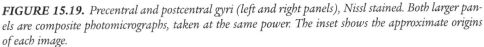

FIGURE 15.19. *Precentral and postcentral gyri (left and right panels), Nissl stained. Both larger panels are composite photomicrographs, taken at the same power. The inset shows the approximate origins of each image.*

Q15.16. Can you identify the precentral gyrus (primary motor cortex)? From your knowledge of the function of this area and connections of each cortical layer, which layer should be most prominent? Why?

A15.16. *The motor cortex sends its axons to the brainstem and spinal cord. Subcortical projections originate from pyramidal neurons in layer 5. Because of the massive nature of this projection and the long distance the axons travel, layer 5 is unusually thick and prominent in this region. Layer 5 of motor cortex contains the so-called upper motor neurons. These are very large pyramidal neurons also known as "giant Betz cells." They are the bigger black dots best seen in lower layers of the inset in Figure 15.19.*

Q15.17. Now try to identify the postcentral gyrus (primary somatosensory cortex). Which layer should be most prominent in this area? Why?

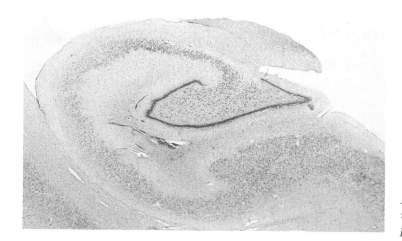

FIGURE 15.20. *Hippocampal formation, including the dentate and hippocampal gyri, Nissl stain.*

A15.17. *A major feature of the primary somatosensory cortex is the relatively large and direct input it receives from the thalamus. Layer 4 of cortex is the recipient of thalamic input. Therefore this cortical area has an unusually thick layer 4 (best seen in the upper right panel of Fig. 15.19). A prominent layer 4 is a characteristic of all primary sensory areas. Histology experts often identify sublayers within layer 4 of primary sensory areas. According to this scheme, the primary areas are even more differentiated (contain more layers) than six-layered neocortex.*

Q15.18. What are the primary laminar differences between the five functionally distinct types of cortex? Are there differences in cell types among these areas? You may want to re-examine the cytoarchitecture of the hippocampus and the parahippocampal gyrus as an aid in this process (see Fig. 15.20).

A15.18. *Limbic areas are the most primitive type of cortex. They contain very few and irregularly arranged layers. In general, they contain large (mostly pyramidal) neurons. Paralimbic areas display a range of laminar differentiation. The portions of paralimbic zones closest to core limbic areas display irregular and few layers. Laminar differentiation becomes more prominent as one moves close to neocortical zones. At the border with neocortical zones, paralimbic areas display the common characteristics of six-layered neocortex. A prominent feature of this gradual increase in laminar differentiation is the emergence of granular cells in layers 2 and 4 moving away from core limbic zones. Unimodal and multimodal association areas display typical characteristics of six-layered cortex. Finally, the primary sensory-motor cortices display a further step in laminar differentiation and contain sublamina in some layers.*

CORTICAL CONNECTIVITY

Methods for Studying Connectivity

The major methods for studying connectivity take advantage of the anterograde (away from the cell body) or retrograde (toward the cell body) transport of molecules in axons. Can you think of how these methods work?

Q15.19. Figure 15.21 shows a section from rat cerebral cortex. An investigator injected horse radish peroxidase (HRP) into a certain cortical region of the brain. Based on the granular black staining seen in these neurons, the investigator concluded that these cells project to the injected cortical target. Discuss this experiment and how it worked.

A15.19. *The major techniques for studying cortical connectivity in animals make use of anterograde and retrograde tracers. Retrograde tracers such as horseradish peroxidase (HRP) are taken up by axonal endings after injection into a circumscribed cortical region. Histochemical visualization of the tracer allows the determination of cortical sites that project to the injected site. In the animal studied in the figure, HRP was injected in the frontal cortex. The figure shows HRP-filled neurons in the corresponding cortical area in the contralateral hemisphere following retrograde transport.*

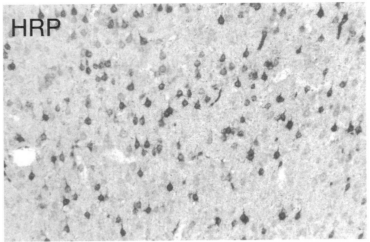
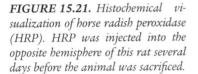

FIGURE 15.21. *Histochemical visualization of horse radish peroxidase (HRP). HRP was injected into the opposite hemisphere of this rat several days before the animal was sacrificed.*

Thalamocortical and Subcortical Connections

Q15.20. Most areas of the cerebral cortex are reciprocally connected to specific thalamic nuclei. As a refresher from the introduction, label the main (nondiffusely projecting) thalamic nuclei in Figure 15.22.

A15.20. *See Figure 15.23.*

Q15.21. Use the knowledge you gleaned about the thalamus in previous labs to indicate in Figure 15.24 the areas of cortex that are connected with the specific thalamic nuclei illustrated in Figure 15.23. This is best done using colored pencils to shade in both the thalamic nuclei below and the cortical regions above.

A15.21. *See Figure 15.25.*

Some areas of cortex show overlapping projections from thalamus, particularly the ventral anterior and medial dorsal nucleus in the frontal association areas and the lateral posterior nucleus and pulvinar in the large occipitoparietotemporal unimodal and multimodal association cortices. Each text presenting this type of information shows a slightly different pattern of interconnections!

Q15.22. The cerebral cortex projects to several other subcortical regions. Can you remember some of these projections encountered in previous labs?

A15.22. *The cerebral cortex projects to all three components of the brainstem, including the pons (corticopontine) and medulla (corticobulbar), and to the spinal cord (corticospinal). In addition widespread areas of cortex project to the striatum (caudate/putamen). The striatal output is directed toward the thalamus, which in turn projects back to the cortex.*

Q15.23. In addition to the inputs received from the thalamus, the cerebral cortex receives inputs from several diffusely projecting systems. You have met these diffusely projecting, neurotransmitter-specific systems in previous labs. Can you remember each of these systems, the neurotransmitter used, and the location of the neurons of origin?

A15.23. *Several neurotransmitter-specific groups of subcortical neurons project diffusely to the entire cortical mantle; in other words, their axons are not confined to restricted cortical areas. The*

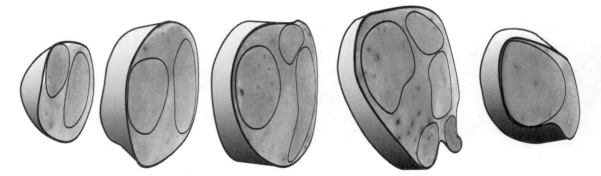

FIGURE 15.22. *Oblique view of a coronally dissected right thalamus, showing the location of major thalamic nuclei, excluding diffusely projecting nuclei.*

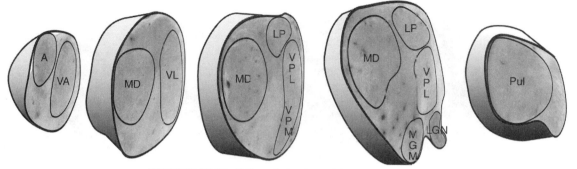

FIGURE 15.23. *Salient thalamic nuclei.*

densest of these projections is the cholinergic input that originates in the basal forebrain cholinergic neurons (located within the basal forebrain corticoid areas: septal nuclei, diagonal band of Broca, and substantia innominata). The cerebral cortex also receives diffuse noradrenergic input from the locus ceruleus, serotonergic input from the raphe nuclei, and dopaminergic input from the ventral tegmental area. Unlike activity in thalamic nuclei, which channels information to specific cortical areas, activity in the nuclei with diffuse cortical projections influences all of cortex at once and tends to "set the state" of the whole cortical mantle.

Q15.24. Where does a major convergence of cortical afferent and efferent fibers occur? Try to identify this region in your coronal specimens. What functional implications does this anatomical arrangement have when pathology is present in this area?

A15.24. Cortical afferents and efferents converge in the internal capsule. Small lesions in the capsule (usually lacunar infarcts) may affect one whole side of the body instead of just a focal area.

General Corticocortical Connections

Q15.25. Using the general principles of cortical connectivity, enter the major functional types of cortex and their major connections in Figure 15.26.

A15.25. See Figure 15.27.

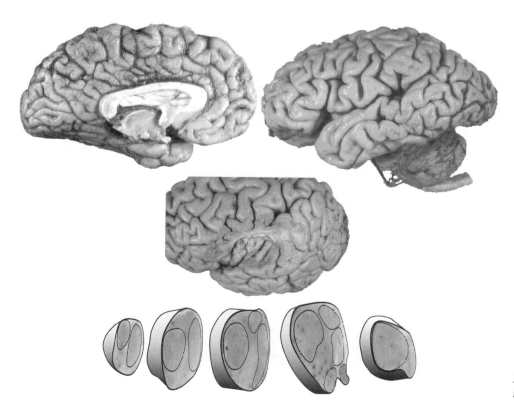

FIGURE 15.24. *Thalamocortical interconnections worksheet.*

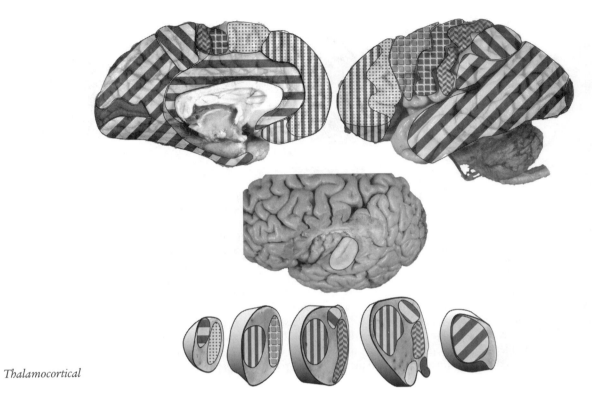

FIGURE 15.25. *Thalamocortical interrelationships.*

Extrapersonal Space

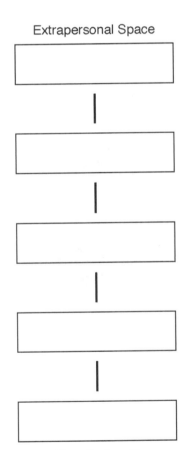

Hypothalamus
(Internal Milieu)

FIGURE 15.26. *Corticocortical connection worksheet.*

Extrapersonal Space

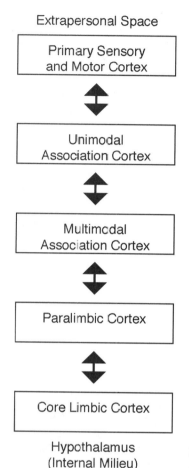

FIGURE 15.27. *Major connections among functional types of cortex.*

Commissural Connections

Q15.26. Name the major and the relatively minor pathways you have already met in previous laboratories that interconnect the two cerebral hemispheres. Try to identify these in your hemispheric specimen. What parts of the hemispheres does each pathway interconnect?

A15.26. *The corpus callosum is the major commissural pathway interconnecting most of the two cerebral hemispheres. The anterior commissure is a relatively minor commissural pathway that interconnects the anterior portions of the two temporal lobes. Similarly a hippocampal commissure underlying the splenium connects the two hippocampal regions.*

The posterior commissure interconnects rostral brainstem structures related to eye movements.

FUNCTIONAL AFFILIATIONS OF CORTICAL AREAS

Left Hemisphere and Language

Q15.27. Examine Figure 15.28. The top panel shows the lateral view of a human left cerebral hemisphere. In the lower panel are coronal MRI images at the levels indicated. Try to identify the anatomical sites depicted by the four shaded regions (try to locate each area on your whole brain specimen) and predict the language deficit that would result from damage to each site.

A15.27. **Broca's area** *is horizontally shaded in area A. It includes the foot of the precentral gyrus (also called the frontal operculum) and the area immediately anterior to it, often including the inferior frontal gyrus, or the white matter underneath it. Lesions in this area cause Broca's aphasia, or anterior aphasia. Patients have good comprehension. They can read. But they have great*

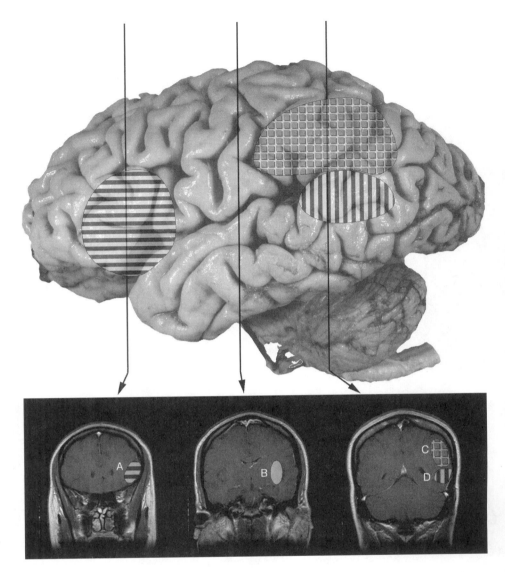

FIGURE 15.28. *Cortical areas involved in language production.*

trouble generating speech (or written language) and produce short, nongrammatical, poorly articulated speech. The patient is usually frustrated. Although they can follow commands, they cannot repeat words or sentences spoken to them.

Wernicke's area is depicted as vertical shading in D. It consists, primarily, of the portion of the superior temporal gyrus located at the posterior banks of the lateral sulcus. These areas surround the **transverse gyrus of Heschl,** home of the primary auditory cortex. Lesions in this region produce **Wernicke's aphasia,** or posterior aphasia. This is a disorder of comprehension. It is much more variable than Broca's aphasia, and there are many subtypes. Patients may be unable to read for comprehension or to follow commands. Their speech is fluent but has many errors.

The area shaded with boxes identifies the supramarginal gyrus in the inferior parietal lobule, extending inferiorly to the insula (area C). Lesions in this area cause what is known as a conduction aphasia. Simplistically, such a lesion disconnects Broca's and Wernicke's areas (which are interconnected by a bundle of association fibers called the arcuate fasciculus), so the patient can comprehend, can speak adequately, but cannot transfer spoken speech effectively from temporal to frontal lobe, and hence cannot repeat words spoken to him.

Not depicted here are language problems seen with very large lesions, usually big infarctions in much of the territory of the middle cerebral artery. Such large lesions cause global aphasia. The patient produces no useful speech and displays poor comprehension.

The loss of function in aphasia is often temporary, whether by partial recovery of the damaged area or by other areas of either hemisphere taking over some of its functions. Areas of brain that seem far distant from the primary speech areas may also less commonly produce speech and language deficits, usually incomplete. These sites include the thalamus and the medial frontal lobe. In many patients with an aphasia, compensatory mechanisms over time can help produce partial recovery of function.

Right Hemisphere and Attention

Q15.28. Examine Figure 15.29. These images show brain regions activated when the subjects were performing tasks requiring overt shifts of attention (top) or overt manual exploration of the right side of space with the right hand (bottom). Try to identify the activated anatomical sites. Can you correlate activity in each area with one of the cognitive components of attention (or can you think of the type of deficit in attention that may be caused by damage to each area)?

A15.28. *The primary sites activated are part of the precentral gyrus in the frontal lobe (F), posterior parietal cortex (P), and anterior cingulate cortex (CG). As an oversimplification, attentional processing can be broken down into three distinct components: sensory (perceptual), motor, and emotional. A person with damage to the right posterior parietal cortex will have difficulty perceiving sensory events in the left hemispace. A person with a lesion in the frontal lobe (at the position indicated by F) will have difficulty with motor manipulation of the environment on the left side. The function of the cingulate component has been difficult to ascertain. As part of the limbic system, the cingulate cortex is likely to create the motivational gradient of attention (a deficit would make the person not care about objects in the left hemisphere).*

Q15.29. The images show activation primarily in the right hemisphere, even when the subject was overtly exploring (directing attention to) the right hemispace only. However, as reviewed above, right hemisphere damage causes neglect on the left only (contralateral). Why doesn't right hemisphere damage cause neglect on both sides, despite the fact that the right hemisphere is dominant for the processing of

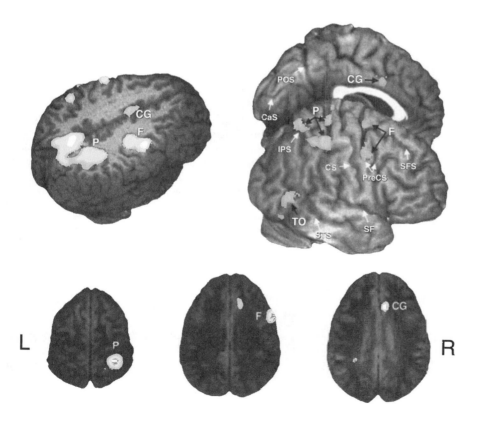

FIGURE 15.29. *MRI data (top) and PET scans (bottom) of subjects engaged in attention shifts. In the upper images, subjects performed tasks requiring overt shifts of attention, while in the lower images, they manually explored the right side of space with their right hand. Note: contrary to convention, right is on right in the lower images to match the upper ones. Whiter areas show a greater change in activity. (Figure adapted from Attentional Networks, Confusional States and Neglect Syndromes by M.-Marsel Mesulam, in Principles of Behavioral and Cognitive Neurology, edited by M.-Marsel Mesulam, © 2000, Oxford University Press, Oxford, figure 3-15, page 237.)*

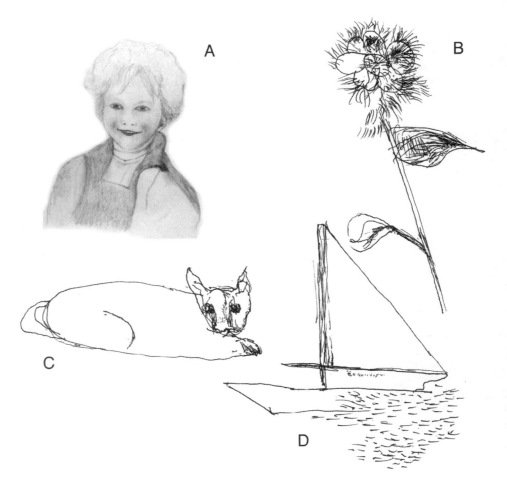

FIGURE 15.30. *Right parietal in-farct.*

attention? What do you think would happen to attentional processing as a result of damage to the left hemisphere?

A15.29. *Left hemispheric damage can also produce contralateral neglect (on the right), but this syndrome is less frequent, less severe, and not as lasting when compared with neglect caused by right hemisphere damage. Thus neglect following right hemisphere damage is more noticeable and of greater clinical and behavioral significance because of its severity and enduring quality. Furthermore, careful clinical testing reveals that damage to the right hemisphere also produces a mild syndrome of neglect ipsilaterally, which is probably masked by the severity of neglect on the left. These facts, combined with fMRI studies, have lead to the conclusion that the right hemisphere is capable of directed attention to both hemispaces (left and right) and that the left hemisphere exerts a weaker influence on attention to the right only. In such a scenario a person with right hemisphere damage would show only very mild neglect on the right because of the weak compensation by the left hemisphere.*

Q15.30. A 74-year-old left-handed man became suddenly combative and confused during a prolonged cardiac catheterization. While recovering in the hospital, a nurse later noted he had dropped his food in his lap and was unable to perform some seemingly simple tasks, like taking jam from a jar and applying it to toast. Formal testing showed a right inferior quadrantanopsia. This man had drawn extensively prior to his stroke (see panel A in Fig. 15.30). Imaging showed a moderately large right parietal infarct. A year after his stroke, he drew the objects in panels B–D in Figure 15.30. Analyze this case. What is "wrong" with the figures? How do you explain his other difficulties?

A15.30. *Each of the three objects in B–D shows more detail on the right side than on the left. Note the paucity detail in the left leaf of the flower in B, compared to the right, even though the left leaf is almost centered in the object. Water flows to the right of the sailboat in D but not on the left. Neglecting the left side is a classic deficit in patients with right parietal and superior temporal infarcts. The field cut is due to destruction of the parietal optic radiation subserving the lower visual field. This patient also has difficulties with coordinated, stereotypical sequences of movements, like buttering his toast. Such apraxias are another feature of parietal lesions.*

Neural Networks in the Cerebral Cortex

Control of various behaviors and particularly cognitive processes can rarely be attributed to a single anatomical locus within the cerebral cortex. Rather, integrated activity in a network of highly interconnected foci makes such behaviors or cognitive processes possible.

Q15.31. As an example, examine representative fMRI scans in Figure 15.31. The subjects in these experiments were presented visually with face-name pairs and asked to remember them. Some of the pairs were novel, while others were repeated (control trials). From the fMRI scans, try to identify the anatomical sites activated. Suggest the functional significance of each activated site.

A15.31. *The sites activated during task performance include the lateral frontal (prefrontal) cortex (A), the hippocampus (medial structures in B), temporal neocortex (B), primary visual cortex (banks of calcarine sulcus, medial structures in C), and visual association cortex (occipiotemporal gyrus or fusiform cortex, inferior aspects of hemisphere in C and D).*

The primary visual cortex is activated because the task is primarily a visual one. As we will see below, the fusiform cortex (visual association area) has been shown to be a cortical site for face recognition (face identification). Its activation is an indication that subjects were attempting to identify the faces they looked at. The right inferior and middle temporal neocortex is activated because, as we observed in the previous laboratory exercise, it is an extension of visual association cortex and has been shown to be responsible for object recognition. The memory component of the task (subjects were asked to remember associations) is the likely cause of activation in the hippocampus.

All of the sites above showed significant activation in both the novel and repeated components of the task when compared to the baseline. The only site that showed significantly higher activation in the novel component of the task as compared with the repeated component was

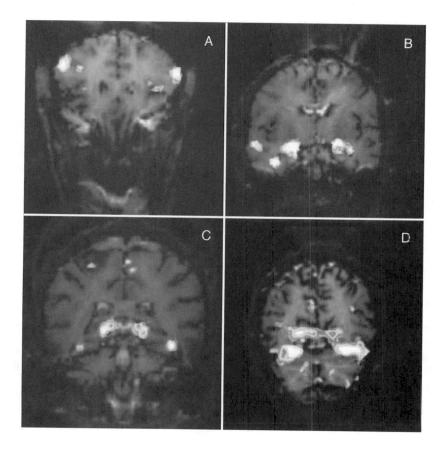

FIGURE 15.31. *fMRI images from novel versus repeated face-name association task. fMRI data from subjects remembering novel versus repeated face-name pairs. In this experiment, the subjects were engaged in a face-name association task. This task is essentially a test of recognition of novelty while performing face-name associations. At rest, subjects were asked to fixate on a blank screen. During the experimental trials, subjects were presented with novel face-name pairs and asked to remember them. Control trials consisted of repeated viewing of a few face-name pairs. (These data kindly provided by Dr. Reisa Sperling and the MGH-NMR Center, Charlestown, MA)*

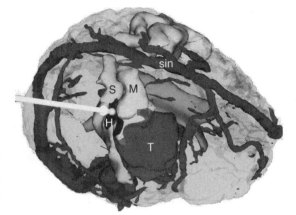

FIGURE 15.32. *3-D reconstruction of the MRI brain images from a young woman with a brain tumor. (Image courtesy of the Surgical Planning Laboratory and Reisa Sperling, Brigham and Women's Hospital, Boston)*

the lateral frontal cortex. Based on this observation, the researchers concluded that this site must function to detect or extract novelty.

Q15.32. Can you think of other cognitive processes that depend on a network of loci?

A15.32. *The concept of neural networks also applies to the cognitive processes you considered earlier (language and attention). Each of these processes is dependent on two or more highly interconnected loci.*

USE OF FUNCTIONAL MRI IN NEUROSURGERY

Q15.33. Figure 15.32 shows a 3-D reconstruction of the MRI brain images from a young woman with a brain tumor (T). Try to identify the orientation of the brain and some of the areas shown.

A15.33. *In this map, anterior is toward the right. Veins and sinuses are shown in dark gray (sin). The superior sagittal sinus is clearly visible. The cortex along the banks of the central sulcus is also visible. Precentral gyrus (motor cortex, M) and postcentral gyrus (somatosensory cortex, S) are shown in light gray. The lateral ventricle on the right is shown in slightly darker gray.*

Q15.34. The tumor, a glioma, is shown as a darker gray (T). Which hemisphere is it in? What part of cortex is it in?

A15.34. *The tumor is in the right hemisphere and infringes on the lower aspects of the precentral gyrus (motor cortex).*

Q15.35. Surgery was scheduled to remove the tumor. There was concern that in the process of resection, portions of the precentral gyrus that control hand movements may also be removed. A preoperative fMRI was conducted in which the subject moved her left hand and wrist during the scan. Can you identify the area activated as a result of the hand movements? What do you think the small circular area identified by the arrow represents?

A15.35. *The area activated as a result of hand movements in the precentral gyrus is shown in black. Stimulation of the white probe to the area during surgery produced hand movements, confirming the fMRI localization of the hand motor area.*

CLINICAL CASES

Case 1: Hemispheric Infarction

The patient is a 70-year-old man, followed in the medical clinic for multiple problems, including obesity, hypertension, smoking, and high cholesterol. Four years ago he had a major stroke. Few details are available; it is known that he did not have surgery, spent three months in a rehabilitation hospital, and made a partial recovery. He lives with his daughter and son-in-law, needs help with many activities of daily living, and is wheelchair bound.

On your exam (done for medical issues) you find that he is alert but unable to follow requests unless they are demonstrated or mimed to him. His speech consists of a few short phrases (OK, OK, or yah, yah). He has a severe spastic weakness of the right hand, which is held clenched against his body. He can forcefully extend the right leg if you demonstrate the movement to him.

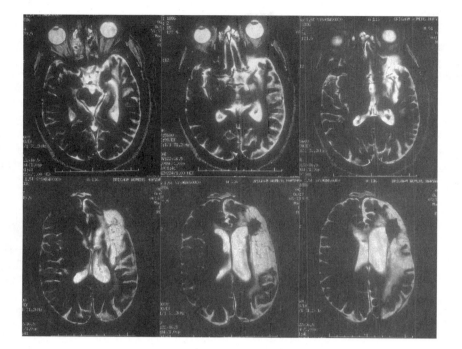

FIGURE 15.33. *MRI scan from case 1.*

Q15.36. Examine the scan in Figure 15.33. It shows the severe degree of damage. What vessel was involved? Can you see the results of atrophy in descending pathways below the area of damage? (Look in midbrain, pons, medulla). There is a large, rounded "black hole" in the patient's left frontal area. Any ideas what that might be? What type of aphasia would be predicted as a result of damage in this case?

A15.36. *Upon close examination of the scan, one can see at the level of the carotid passing through the skull base (foramen lacerum) that there is no flow void on the left side and the MCA is very much attenuated (black arrowhead in right panel in Fig. 15.34). Hence this was a case of a carotid occlusion.*

Severe atrophy is seen in the cerebral peduncle (white arrow, left panel in Fig. 15.34). Only about a third of the cerebral peduncle consists of corticospinal tract, the rest (two-thirds) are descending corticobulbar and frontopontine fibers. The lesion has affected all of these fiber systems.

The black hole is read as ectopic calcification. It looks like a CSF space but is within the damaged brain area and is actually not the same MRI intensity as CSF.

Extensive and severe damage to the left hemisphere results in global aphasia (deficit in language comprehension and production), as seen in this case.

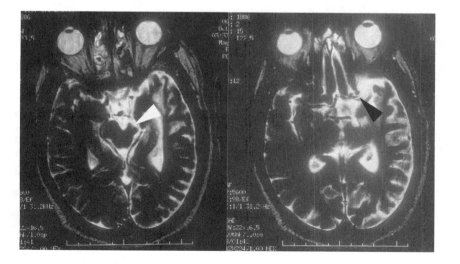

FIGURE 15.34. *Details from case 1 MRI examination.*

Case 2: Infarction in Unimodal Association Cortex

The patient is 60 years old. Two years before examination he suffered a stroke in the territory of the right posterior cerebral artery. Since that time he has had a relatively complete left homonymous hemianopsia. On the day the stroke occurred, he noted that he bumped into tables and doorways on his left side. He was not sure why this was. At work he encountered people but could not recognize their faces. (Presumably he could not see the left side of such a face by looking directly at the person, but by scanning the whole face, it could eventually be seen.) When they spoke, he could immediately tell who they were by the sound of their voices. The layout of the building also seemed very unfamiliar to him, although he had been able to follow a familiar route via bus and shuttle to his office. Simple objects such as a phone or wastebasket were easy to recognize. The defect was mainly for face recognition. He did have trouble being sure what color an object was.

Q15.37. Inspect his scan in Figure 15.35. Where is the lesion? See if you can draw out the infarction. It involves more than the primary visual area. Can you think of why the lesion caused the specific deficits?

A15.37. *The patient suffers from a condition known as* **prosopagnosia.** *It is one of a group of visual loss syndromes that can be seen with damage to the occipital lobes. By now you are familiar with hemianopsia, or loss of vision. Other patients may have visual agnosia (from the Greek, lack of knowledge), cortical blindness, or defects of eye movement control. They may be able to see, but not to form perceptual constructs, recognize familiar objects or direct their eyes to a desired target. The lesions causing these conditions are located in areas adjacent to or a few synapses away from the primary visual cortex and should be thought of as disorders of visual association cortex.*

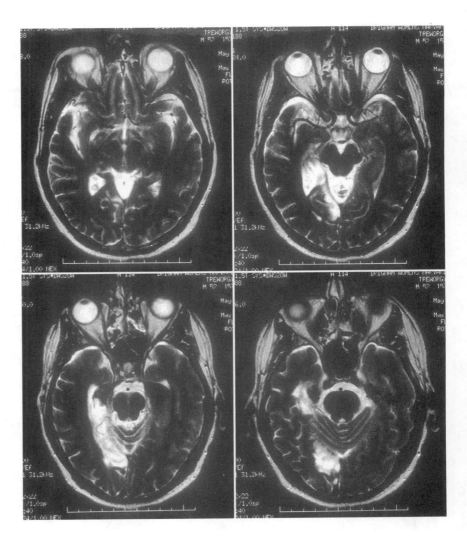

FIGURE 15.35. *MRI examination from case 2.*

Prosopagnosia is a modality-specific deficit. Patients cannot recognize faces, although they may recognize persons by voice or by known items of clothing. They may also be unable to find their own car in a parking lot. One story described a farmer with this deficit who could not recognize the cows of his milking herd. It is primarily a matter of a loss of a perceptually demanding, although commonly performed, visual task.

Patients with pure prosopagnosia, in whom the only deficit is face recognition, display bilateral lesions in the fusiform gyrus (the gyrus located inferior to the Calcarine sulcus, extending on the inferior surface of the brain into the temporal lobe). Occasional cases show unilateral right-sided lesions, involving primarily the fusiform gyrus.

Many patients have larger lesions with additional defects, especially memory loss if the lesion extends further forward (in the temporal lobe). Achromatopsia (loss of color differentiation) is often seen.

The deficit in face recognition can be tested with photos of prominent people, for example Winston Churchill, Fidel Castro, Bill Clinton or pictures of family members.

Case 3: Multimodal Association Cortex Involvement

The patient is a 78-year-old man. For three to four years he has had memory problems, found it hard to concentrate, and became confused in familiar places. One year ago he began to secretly watch pornography channels on cable TV and to tell sexually explicit jokes in front of his daughters. Once he came into the living room during a bridge party and exposed himself. These behaviors were shocking to the family, since he had previously been quite restrained and correct. He became depressed. He lost interest in his hobbies. He did not seem to care about paying bills or balancing his checkbook and his family had to take over these chores. He often paced and moved restlessly around the house. He frequently went into tantrums over minor household events. No one could trust him to carry out shopping or to answer the phone.

His mother had a similar condition in her 80s.

Examination showed a paratonic rigidity of all four limbs and tendency to a grasp reflex. Reflexes were 3+, with clonus at the ankles. The right plantar response was extensor, left was doubtful. Testing orientation, memory, and awareness of current events showed significant defects. Asked to name words beginning with the letter F, he thought of two words, and with the letter A, three words.

Q15.38. Examine the scan in Figure 15.36 from another patient with the same condition. What defects can you observe?

A15.38. *Close examination reveals severe atrophy within the frontal and temporal lobes. The gyri appear shrunken and the sulci have expanded. The MRI from the current case was unremarkable, but his SPECT scan (single photon emission spectroscopy, a measurement of metabolic activity) showed markedly reduced activity in frontal and temporal lobes bilaterally, when compared to age-matched controls.*

Q15.39. Examine the brains in Figure 15.37, which show similar but very severe cases. Where is the atrophy?

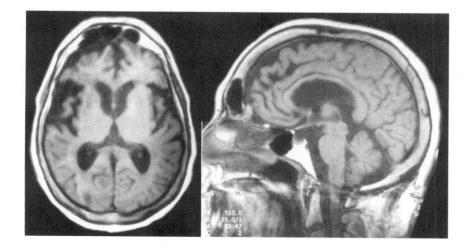

FIGURE 15.36. *MRI examination from a patient similar to case 3.*

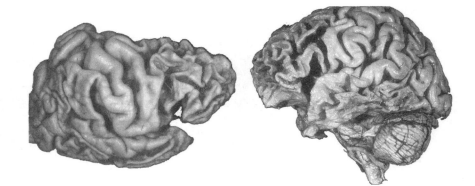

FIGURE 15.37. *Two different brains with late-stage frontotemporal dementias.*

A15.39. *This patient's condition is similar to other neurodegenerative conditions, such as Pick's disease (a rare form of dementia). Figure 15.37 shows two similar brains. Extremely severe atrophy is seen within the frontal and temporal lobes, and also within the occipital lobes (seen in very severe cases). Note that the cortex surrounding the central sulcus (pre- and postcentral gyri) is virtually intact.*

Q15.40. Can you guess the diagnosis in this case? Try to compare and contrast the clinical and pathological features of this case with the Alzheimer's case you encountered in the previous laboratory.

A15.40. *This is a case of frontotemporal dementia (FTD), a subgroup of which is genetically based (hence the dementia in his mother). The initial and most prominent clinical manifestations of FTD are abnormalities in personality, judgment, and particularly comportment (conduct). These also affect persons with other lesions affecting the frontal lobes. The degenerative process affecting the frontal lobes in FTD cases appears to be of primary clinical significance. Memory deficit is either absent in FTD or occurs later in the course of the disease. This is attributable to degeneration in temporal lobes, which eventually spreads to medial temporal lobe structures responsible for encoding and consolidation of memory (hippocampus and entorhinal cortex). In contrast, memory loss is the earliest manifestation of Alzheimer's disease (AD) and is due to early degenerative pathology in medial temporal lobe.*

A major subset of the frontotemporal dementias display significant tau pathology, either as tangles, Pick bodies, or atypical phosphorylated tau staining. The brains from these patients display different tau isoforms compared to those present in either normal brains or in Alzheimer's disease (see the left panel in Fig. 15.38). Pick's disease is another subtype of frontotemporal dementia with prominent tau pathology (Pick bodies) and has yet another tau isoform pattern. Recently, as in this patient, several reports have identified a subset of individuals with a familial history of frontotemporal dementia. Individuals in these families may have a variable clinical presentation but have prominent tau pathology. It turns out that some of these families also have mutations in the tau gene. Several of their mutations are indicated in the right panel in Figure 15.38.

FIGURE 15.38. *Alterations in the tau protein (left panel) or mutations in the tau gene (right panel) in several degenerative diseases. (Left figure modified from figure 5, Buée, L. & Delacourte, A. Comparative biochemistry of tau in progressive supranuclear palsy, corticobasal degeneration, FTDP-17 and Pick's disease. 1999. Brain Pathology 9: 681–693.)*

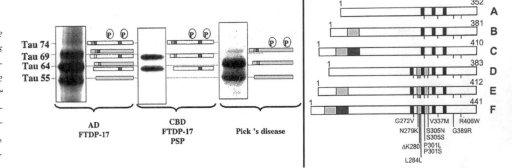

Chapter 16——DEVELOPMENT

The creation of our nervous system may superficially resemble an elaborate computer program. Such a view would be an injustice to this complex yet beautiful process; rather, development of the brain is analogous to an orchestral score with multiple instruments having harmonies, melodies, counterpoint, and rhythms, all happening in a sequence. The purpose of this laboratory is to give you a sense of this score. Hopefully the rest of the course has convinced of the brain's beauty when the score is played well. This laboratory will examine the results when the score is misplayed.

LEARNING OBJECTIVES

- Describe key features of the developing nervous system, including where most cells are born, how they arrive at their final destination, when gyri form, and when myelination occurs.
- Describe neural tube closure and identify diseases produced by failure of this closure.
- Using holoprosencephaly as a model, describe how a single gene can influence brain development. Describe major aspects of holoprosencephaly, including the timing of the insult and how the ventral pattern failure can lead to the morphologic phenotype.
- Identify important environmental agents, including folic acid and alcohol, that can influence brain development.
- Identify several types of malformations that may lead to cerebral palsy and/or seizure disorders, including encephaloclastic lesions and migrational disorders. Indicate the neuroanatomic basis for their clinical sequelae.

INTRODUCTION

As the development of the nervous system has been the primary study of many people for over a century, the field is littered with and obfuscated by obscure terminology. Whereas you have learned "midbrain" as the site of the substantia nigra, developmental neuroanatomists call it the mesencephalon. The pons, cerebellum, and medulla can somewhat confusingly be lumped together into the "hindbrain," but in order to purge all simple words from their work, neuroanatomists call this region the rhombencephalon, which they then divide into the metencephalon (pons/cerebellum) and myelencephalon (medulla). This book (and life) is too short for you to spend time learning these details. Unless you like recondite vocabulary, focus on the concepts rather than the confusion.

Functional Neuroanatomy: An Interactive Text and Manual, by Jeffrey T. Joseph and David L. Cardozo
ISBN 0-471-44437-5 Copyright © 2004 John Wiley & Sons, Inc.

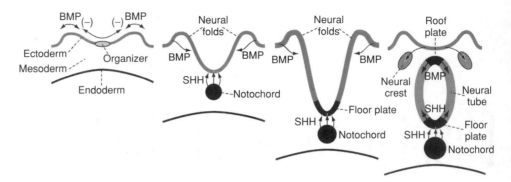

FIGURE 16.1. *Dorsal and ventral organization of the neural tube secreted factors.*

Principles of Differentiation

In general, the development of the nervous system follows a sequence of events that produce a structure of ever greater complexity. While our genes govern these events, the final product is an elaborate mixture of a genetic blueprint and the actual mortar and bricks used to construct the foundation and subsequent levels. Alteration of particular building blocks, by toxins, vitamin deficiencies, or genetic mutations, will modify the final structure. Rather than stopping construction, subsequent events will build upon the defective blocks and produce a modified morphology.

The first steps of development happen before the inception of the nervous system, and involve laying down the scaffold on which the embryo is constructed. This includes establishing the dorsal-ventral and rostral-caudal axes in the embryo. These axes are in part determined by gradients of morphogens secreted from discrete sites in the early embryo. Cellular receptors for these morphogens respond to the concentration gradients and activate a cascade of genetic programs that further regulate tissue differentiation.

Our understanding of the genetic basis for brain development is currently in its embryonic stage. A cornucopia of different genes is currently known, and these certainly represent only the vegetation on the mountain of genes to follow. The actions of specific genes in controlling development are extremely complex and incompletely understood. In your reading and in the laboratory, however, you should at least gain an appreciation for how some of these genes interact. Because of its importance, the chapter will discuss *Sonic hedgehog* in some detail.

Some of the same proteins responsible for early developmental changes are also essential later. For example, the BMP family of proteins is important for the development of the ectoderm. Their inhibition by proteins secreted from the organizer (e.g., noggin) leads to the formation of the neural plate. Later in development, their expression helps regulate dorsal differentiation of the embryonic nervous system. BMP expression in both the ectoderm and the dorsal roof plate makes topological sense, since the dorsal neural tube was previously adjacent to the ectoderm (see Fig. 16.1).

After the basic organization of the nervous system has been laid down, the fun begins. Neurons and glia must migrate to their final destination. Axons somehow must find their targets and become myelinated. Synaptic connections must be made and then modified, based on our experiences. While it is our connections that distinguish us from flies and worms, this laboratory will focus only on the gross morphological aspects of development.

Principles of Malformations

Brain malformations may be examined at many levels, including causation, phenomenology, genetics, and timing during development. Simplistically we can think of a malformation as the result of an "error" somewhere in the developmental sequences, produced by a "lesion." The lesion may occur at a specific instant during development (e.g., radiation exposure or trauma) or it may be extended or prolonged (e.g., trisomy 21). The developing fetus may also be subjected to multiple independent insults (e.g., medications or drug abuse) or by a single insult multiple times (e.g., smoking). While we tend to think of babies being finished products, any parent will tell you otherwise, and lesions producing defects certainly may happen in the young infant (e.g., "shaken baby" or radiation for a tumor). It is the timing of the lesion during the developmental sequence that determines its final form and clinical manifestations. Obviously an extended lesion early in development (e.g., folic acid deficiency) potentially will have a greater impact on the brain than a brief, isolated episode late in pregnancy.

"Lesion" is meant to be a general term. It may represent a genetic defect, a chromosomal defect, a toxin, a vitamin deficiency, an infection, or ischemia. In this laboratory we'll encounter several different types of lesions and examine the malformations they produce.

Early Events and Neurulation

The *neural plate* begins as a thickening of the ectoderm over the *notochord*. (Although neurologists may not like to admit it, basically the nervous system is just a sophisticated piece of skin.) This plate develops a midline groove (neural groove) around the middle of week three, whose walls then thicken into neural folds. It is these folds that soon fuse dorsally, forming the *neural tube* as well as the *neural crest* along its edges.

Neural tube closure is not a simple zippering up of a neural groove. The process begins at several different sites, including from the future optic area rostrally to the rostral neuropore and caudally to meet the rostrally extending closure from the rhombencephalon (hindbrain). Another site begins near the future craniospinal junction and also proceeds both rostrally and caudally.

As the neural tube closure nears completion, the tube divides into several regions. The rostral end forms three swellings, the forebrain (prosencephalon), midbrain (mesencephalon), and the hindbrain (rhombencephalon). The prosencephalon again divides into a telencephalon (the cerebral cortex and striatum) and the diencephalon (the thalamus, hypothalamus, and "epithalamus" or pineal), while the hindbrain forms the pons/cerebellum (metencephalon) and the medulla (myelencephalon). The future cortex begins as a paired swelling off the rostral end of the neural tube.

Cortical Development

Cells in the cortex largely arise from progenitors along the ventricular wall, at a site termed the *germinal matrix* or ventricular and subventricular zones. These cells migrate to their final resting place in the cortex by traveling along a previously assembled scaffolding of *radial glial fibers*. The final destination of the migrating neurons defies simple logic, since the younger cells migrate past the older cells, to take up residence in a more superficial aspect of cortex; in other words, the cortex is built inside out.

Injuries to the germinal matrix (by toxins or by intrinsic hemorrhages) can either deplete the final number of neurons or prevent the migration of already committed neurons. Developmentally abnormal brains frequently have displaced gray matter (*heterotopias*) in abnormal locations, such as within the white matter or around the periventricular region.

When we pick up a brain, what we see are the gyri and sulci. The process of cortical gyration is complex and poorly understood. It is clear, however, that normal gyration requires a previously normal development of cortex and underlying white matter. The unique buckling pattern we see in each brain arises from the strains put on the expanding cortex by their underlying axonal tethers.

Perturbations in the formation of cortex, for example, by an episode of focal ischemia, lead to abnormal cortical gyration. *Polymicrogyria,* the formation of a thin, heaped-up cortex, commonly accompanies tissue-damaging *encephaloclastic* lesions after the cortex has already been established but prior to the onset of gyration. The injured site may be hole devoid of neural tissue and covered only with meninges. Such a defect, termed a porencephalic cyst, may have polymicrogyria at its edge. When neurons fail to migrate in inverse order from the ventricular zone, the normal strains producing gyration are diminished, and the cortex may have wide, malformed gyri (*pachygyria*).

Schedule (2.5 hours)
30   Normal development
30   Neural tube defects
40   Holoprosencephaly
20   Encephaloclastic lesions
30   Case

NORMAL DEVELOPMENT

Q16.1. First examine Figure 16.2 showing the base of fetal brain from near the end of the second trimester. Name the following structures:

16.1.1 _____

16.1.2 _____

16.1.3 _____

16.1.4 _____

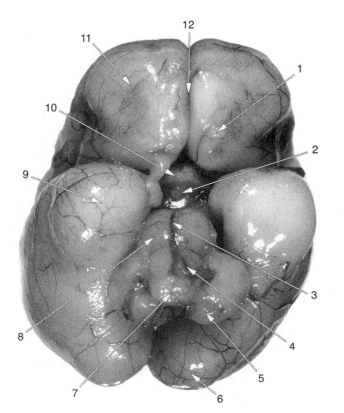

FIGURE 16.2. *Base of fetal brain. The infant died shortly after birth, at around 22 weeks gestational age.*

16.1.5 _____

16.1.6 _____

16.1.7 _____

16.1.8 _____

16.1.9 _____

16.1.10 _____

16.1.11 _____

16.1.12 _____

A16.1. 16.1.1. *Olfactory tract*
  16.1.2. *Infundibulum/pituitary stalk*
  16.1.3. *Basilar artery*
  16.1.4. *Vertebral artery*
  16.1.5. *Cerebellum*
  16.1.6. *Occipital lobe*
  16.1.7. *Medulla*
  16.1.8. *Pons*
  16.1.9. *Temporal lobe*
  16.1.10. *Optic nerve/chiasm*
  16.1.11. *Frontal lobe*
  16.1.12. *Interhemispheric fissure*

Q16.2. How does the brain differ from an adult brain? In particular, comment on the gyral pattern and the relative size of the cerebellum.

A16.2. *The fetal brain at this stage in gestation is smooth. This lack of gyration reminded earlier neuroanatomists of "lower" mammalian brains, and termed this "lissencephaly." Some gyri*

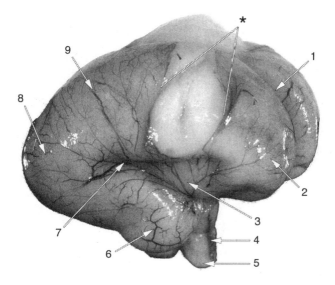

FIGURE 16.3. *Lateral view of fetal brain. This was the same brain as in Figure 16.2. The site encompassed by the lines labeled "*" is a postmortem tear of the gossamer fetal meninges.*

are present at this stage, although they are not as obvious as later. In particular, in this ventral view, a primitive gyrus rectus (in which the olfactory tract lies) has formed.

Much of the cerebellum's growth occurs after birth. At this fetal stage, it is relatively much smaller than the cerebrum. Compare the size of the cerebellum with the brainstem in this figure and in an adult brain.

Q16.3. Now examine the lateral view in Figure 16.3. Name the following structures:

16.3.1 _____

16.3.2 _____

16.3.3 _____

16.3.4 _____

16.3.5 _____

16.3.6 _____

16.3.7 _____

16.3.8 _____

16.3.9 _____

A16.3. *16.3.1. Interhemispheric fissure*
16.3.2. Frontal lobe
16.3.3. Operculum/insular cortex
16.3.4. Basilar artery
16.3.5. Medulla
16.3.6. Temporal lobe
16.3.7. Lateral (Sylvian) fissure
16.3.8. Occipital lobe
16.3.9. Parietal lobe

Q16.4. What differences can you see in this fetal brain, compared with the adult brain? What is the benefit of cortical gyration? Explain why the area designated by the star "*" is devoid of vessels.

A16.4. *As in the basal view, the lateral view shows a lissencephalic brain. Cortical gyration is a complex, poorly understood process. The final pattern is in part determined by the short and long axonal connections, and the stresses and strains they put on the developing white matter.*

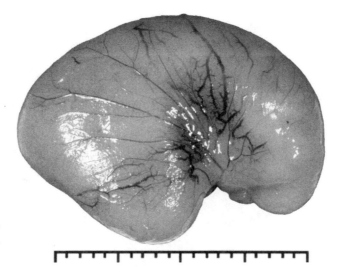

FIGURE 16.4. *Fetal brain at 18 weeks gestation. The brainstem has been removed from this specimen.*

Having gyri greatly increases the cortical area in a given volume. And most brains have a typical overall gyral pattern. Why each particular brain has a unique pattern of gyration is not clear.

Although this brain lacks the usual gyri of an adult, it does have major grooves and brain divisions. The lateral or Sylvian fissure is present, along with the interhemispheric fissure. The frontal and temporal cortices, being poorly developed, are separated, leaving the insular cortex exposed and its surrounding doorway (operculum) wide open.

Cortical vessels travel in the leptomeninges prior to feeding into the pia. The meninges over the area marked "*" slipped off at the time of autopsy, taking their vessels with them. What you are seeing is the underlying smooth, almost gelatinous fetal brain.

Q16.5. Now compare the 18-week brain in Figure 16.4 with that in Figure 16.3 (not to scale!). Generally, how do they differ?

A16.5. *The temporal lobe at 18 weeks has not ballooned around as far as at 22 weeks. The cortex has more of a C-shape than the deeper U-shape it takes on a bit later in development.*

The cerebral hemispheres basically are two balloons of tissue. They begin to bulge out at their origins near the upper sides of the hypothalamus, adjacent to the lamina terminals, and twist around into a C-shape in the confines of the skull.

Q16.6. Examine the microscopic slide with tissue from a 20 to 22 week gestation fetus at low power or even with a magnifying lens. See Figure 16.5. Try to identify all of the fragments. Can you identify any familiar structures? Anything different from an adult brain?

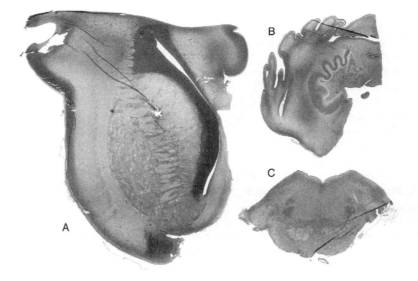

FIGURE 16.5. *Histology of fetal brain.*

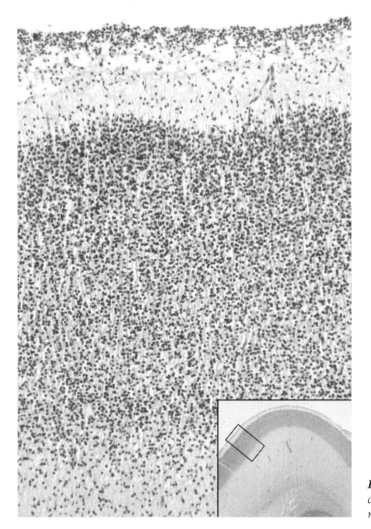

FIGURE 16.6. Histology of fetal cerebral cortex and underlying white matter.

A16.6. *Fragments on each glass slide will differ. In Figure 16.5, panel A is a coronal section through the caudate nucleus, putamen, and accumbens. Panel B is a horizontal section through the cerebellum, including the dentate nucleus. Panel C is a transverse section through the pons.*

You should be able to see the cortical ribbon (left-hand edge of panel A). Even if your stain is Luxol fast blue, you won't have myelin to help you identify structures, since the fetal brain at this age has no myelin. The dentate nucleus stands out in the cerebellar fragment in panel B. The pons in C shows the lighter tegmentum above and the more reticulated base below.

Several major differences you should be able to notice, even on low-power inspection, include the large swath of dark staining lining the lateral parts of the ventricle (right-hand side in panel A) and a dark layer on the outside surface of the cerebellum (panel B). These contain primitive germinal layers of cells. The base of the pons is also much smaller than its equivalent in adults.

Q16.7. Describe the cortex on the histologic slide or in Figure 16.6. In particular, identify the different cortical layers. Look closely at the neuronal size and differentiation. How do the neurons change over the depth of the cortex? Examine the tissue directly beneath the cortex. Describe what cell types you see. Any neurons? Oligodendroglia? Astrocytes? How about myelin? As you scan at lower power over the cortical ribbon, how does it differ from that of a mature brain? In particular, describe the pattern of gyration that you see.

A16.7. *In this immature cortex essentially all of its future neurons have been born and most have migrated to their final resting place in the cortex. All else being equal, the fetal brain would have more neurons than you. (Believe us, it's downhill from there!) However, the neurons show little evidence of differentiation; they are just small, round, blue cells. You may be able to see a hint of cortical layering: a superficial layer of immature cells, a cell-poor zone followed by a*

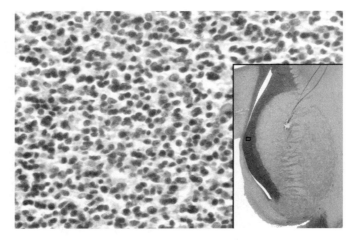

FIGURE 16.7. *Germinal matrix or ventricular zone, H&E stain. The germinal zone high-power view has been lightened to reveal more of the nuclear detail.*

cell-rich layer, then a broad region of more dispersed cells, and finally a slightly greater density of cells just before reaching the future white matter. You may also notice that many of the cells seemed to be lined-up or form columns of nuclei.

Remember, the cortex develops inside out; the deepest layers migrate first, and the superficial layers migrate past these to a more superficial position. The earliest cortical neurons to show some morphological differentiation are the pyramidal neurons in layer five. In the tissue directly beneath the cortex lies the older cortical plate. Often in this site you may see some neurons. Most but not all of these regress by apoptosis later in development.

While neurons have largely completed their migration, glia at this stage are vigorously reproducing and migrating. You may be able to discern a cell-rich zone in the midst of the future white matter; it is populated with future glia. Oligodendrocyte precursors are present, but no myelin; myelination of the telencephalon occurs largely after birth. At this stage the brain show little distinction between oligodendrocytes and astrocytes.

As you hold the slide up to the light, no gyration should be apparent. While the interhemispheric fissure and lateral fissure form early (the lateral fissure is really the brain curved over on itself), normal cortical gyration occurs after the age of this fetus. Lesions to the underlying brain prior to gyration will affect the final gyral pattern of the brain.

Q16.8. You probably already noticed the big blue area in the center of the brain. This is called the germinal matrix or the **ventricular** and **subventricular zone.** Try to distinguish this region from striatal or thalamic structures that are also on the slide (see Fig. 16.7). What is happening here? Describe the cells you see in the blue region. Can you tell what type of cells they are? What will the cells become? Where will they go?

A16.8. *Most of the cells in the central nervous system are born along the ventricles and then migrate to their final positions. The germinal matrix (named for its activity) or ventricular zone (for its location) is the site of this proliferation. This dense blue area is composed of "small round blue cells," with no evidence of differentiation. At this stage in development, the neurons have been born and moved on while the glia are still reproducing and migrating. Most of these cells will end up in the white matter as either myelin-producing oligodendrocytes or "supportive" astrocytes. Some cells will remain at this site, even in the adult. Such primordial cells represent an area of current intensive research in regeneration of tissues lost in strokes or neurodegenerative diseases.*

The primitive cells will line the ventricular system, but at this age will be thickest over the caudate nucleus. The striatal neurons, while still primitive, have much more cytoplasm than the germinal matrix cells and are arranged in a form very similar to the final adult configuration.

At an earlier stage, cells around the ventricle will migrate to cortex. Later, when the distance becomes too great, they will migrate along radial glial fibers orthogonal (perpendicular) to the cortex. Other cells born near the deep gray nuclei migrate to the cortex and move tangentially, rather than orthogonally, to their final positions. Roughly, the orthogonally migrating neurons use the excitatory transmitter glutamate while the tangentially migrating cells become inhibitory interneurons and use GABA.

Q16.9. Now look more closely at the section from the posterior fossa containing the cerebellum (see Fig. 16.8). How does the cerebellar cortex differ from an adult brain? Specifically examine the different layers: molecular, Purkinje, and granular. Where are the most immature cells?

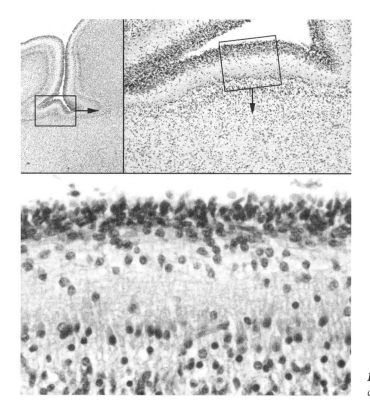

FIGURE 16.8. Histology of fetal cerebellum.

A16.9. You should be able to identify the cerebellum by its folia. In contrast to the adult brain, the fetal cerebellar cortex has a striking external layer of primitive cells, termed the external granular cell layer (which is why the adult granular cell layer is called "internal"). These are primitive precursors of the internal granular neurons. Below this layer is a thin molecular layer and then a somewhat disorganized Purkinje cell layer. Deep to the Purkinje cell layer you may see some internal granular neurons depending on the age of the fetal brain. The Purkinje cells are larger than the granular neurons but do not yet form the nice single line of cells that will eventually develop. What cannot be differentiated well on this simple stain are the **Bergmann glia**, also in the Purkinje cell layer, on whose radial glial fibers the granular neurons will travel. The granular neurons come from the lateral lip of the brainstem, migrate and replicate across the surface of the cerebellum, and then travel along the Bergmann radial glial fibers, past the Purkinje cells, to their final destination in the internal layer.

Q16.10. If available, also examine a section from the brainstem (see Fig. 16.9). Why does this section look so much different from those you have seen of adult brain? In Figure 16.9 identify the numbered structures:

16.10.1 _____

16.10.2 _____

16.10.3 _____

A16.10. The anatomy of the brainstem section will vary, depending on the level you happen to have on your slide. If you have medulla, then most likely the inferior olivary nucleus should be obvious. Other neuronal groups may stand out better than in the adult, because they are "naked," having few processes and no myelin. In Figure 16.9 the structures are:
16.10.1. Corticospinal tracts in the base
16.10.2. Superior olivary nucleus (remember, it is part of the auditory system)
16.10.3. Facial nucleus

Myelination occurs later in development, first with the most essential tracts (medial lemniscus, medial longitudinal fasciculus, cranial nerves) and last with the least essential for a baby's existence, the corticospinal tracts. Babies, after all, don't need to play the piano but do need to get food. Myelination continues into the later teenage years within the most "advanced" or human portion of

Ventricle

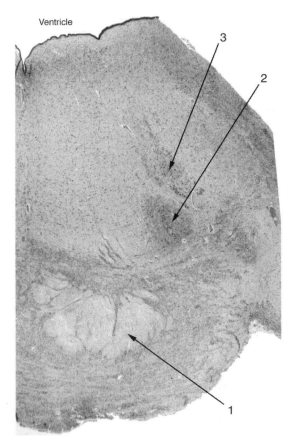

FIGURE 16.9. Fetal pontine histology, H&E stain. Only half of the pons is shown.

the brain, the frontal lobes. Maybe this is why parents lament about reckless teenager behavior; it may represent a "frontal release" sign!

NEURAL TUBE CLOSURE AND ANENCEPHALY

The next several photographs display a range of malformations generated by a failure of neural tube closure.

Q16.11. Examine Figure 16.10, which shows the faces of an ***anencephalic*** fetus. Describe what you see. What structures are present? Are they normal or abnormal? What is missing?

A16.11. *Probably the most striking finding is the fetus's large eyes. These are actually normal size, and only look prominent in relationship to the absent forehead and brain. The ears are also present, although they are diminutive. Also present are the limbs and five-fingered hands. What is missing is the brain and surrounding skull, or at least most of it.*

Q16.12. Examine Figure 16.11, which is the same fetus, viewed from above. Describe what remains of the central nervous system.

A16.12. *In place of the cranium (skull and brain) is a mass of irregular red material, which travels some distance down the back. The protuberant eyes are at the bottom of the image. Microscopically this red material is composed of abundant blood vessels and some neuroglial tissue.*

Q16.13. Finally examine Figure 16.12, which is a posterior view of a different fetus with a more extreme form of anencephaly (in this case more specifically termed craniorachischisis). The white material along the right leg is the umbilical cord. Describe what you see. What structures are present? Which are absent?

A16.13. *Essentially the entire central nervous system behind the eyes is absent in this fetus. Most of the vertebral bodies remain unfused. In the midline of the back is a light, linear structure lying in what should be spinal canal. This represents the remnant of the spinal cord. In a few sites, some light-colored strands arise from it, which are some nerve roots. The brain and most of the spinal material has degenerated into the area cerebrovasculosa.*

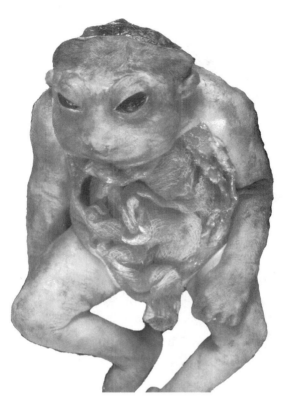

FIGURE 16.10. *Anecephalic fetus. (The picture was taken after evisceration; the material in the chest is gauze.)*

Depending on the severity of the malformation, most of the central nervous system may be missing, or only a portion of the brain. Some children are born with an intact brainstem, allowing them to perform most of the functions of a new born, including crying, responding to pain, feeding, and primitive reflex responses.

Q16.14. Based on your knowledge of neural development, try to determine when the lesion producing anencephaly may have occurred. How does the presence of normal eyes and limbs help?

A16.14. *The lesion must be around the time of neural tube closure. The presence of two normal eyes and the absence of a cleft lip indicates that ventral induction of the brain has functioned properly. Neural tube closure occurs in the fourth week of gestation, or just two weeks after the first skipped period in the mother. The presence of limbs, which depend on nervous innervation for their proper formation, indicates that the peripheral nervous system, derived from the neural*

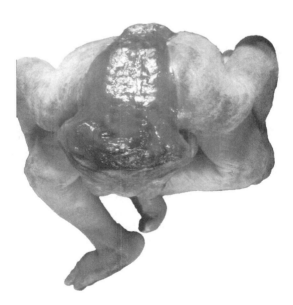

FIGURE 16.11. *Remaining neural tube tissue in anecephalic fetus.*

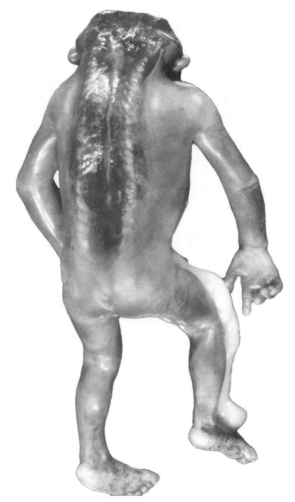

FIGURE 16.12. *Craniorachischisis; complete failure of neural tube closure.*

crest, must also have formed. In this malformation the early nervous system forms. Only later, after failing to close, do portions degenerate.

The incidence of neural tube closure malformations can be reduced by the use of folic acid during pregnancy. But since the lesion occurs early, pregnant women would have to supplement their diet immediately after (or preferably before) they know they are pregnant.

PROSENCEPHALON AND HOLOPROSENCEPHALY

Faces of Holoprosencephaly

Q16.15. Examine the series of faces in Figure 16.13 from different patients with varying degrees of holoprosencephaly. Describe how the eyes change in this spectrum of severity. How does the nose change? What is the morphologic defect that underlies all of the people in the pictures? What is "wrong" with the woman in figure *G*?

A16.15. *In A and B, the infants have a single, central eye (termed cyclopia). In B the eye seems to be separating apart, but the separation is incomplete. Above this central eye and just between the two closely spaced eyes in C is a protuberant nose with a single nostril (termed a proboscis). In D the nose/proboscis is in a more normal position, but still has a single nares. Infants E and F have a central cleft lip (not a lateral cleft lip, which is not associated with brain abnormalities) and would be missing a portion of the upper roof of their mouths. The woman in G has the most minor manifestation of this disease spectrum, with a single central incisor. All of these individuals have a defect in the midline face, where lateral structures are more closely juxtaposed than normal. More lateral and dorsal regions are less affected.*

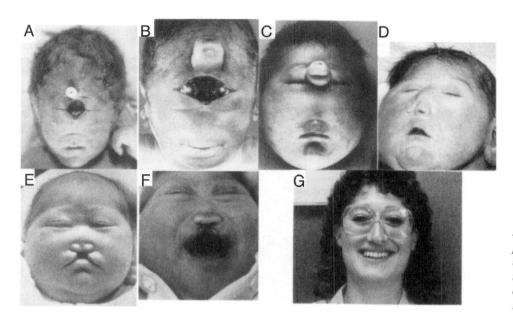

FIGURE 16.13. *Spectrum of holoprosencephaly. (Modified from figure 1, Roessler, E., et al, Mutations in the human Sonic Hedgehog gene cause holoprosencephaly. 1996. Nature Genet 14:357.)*

Holoprosencephaly Base of Fetal Brain

Q16.16. The image in Figure 16.14 is a basal view of the brain from a second trimester fetus. How does this brain differ from a normal brain?

A16.16. *The fetal brain at this age (about 20 weeks) lacks any myelin, which gives the brain its homogeneous, white, gelatinous appearance. The cortex also lacks any gyri, as we saw in the first part of the laboratory. However, this brain is different, since it also lacks an interhemispheric fissure and has no evidence of a corpus callosum. Instead, the cortex is continuous across the entire brain. Since the brain at this age has the consistency of thick Jell-O, the corpus callosum often is torn at the time of autopsy. But the horizontal fissure should still remain, along with the beginnings of the cingulate gyrus. These structures are all absent in this holoprosencephalic brain.*

Q16.17. Identify the following numbered structures:

16.17.1 _____

16.17.2 _____

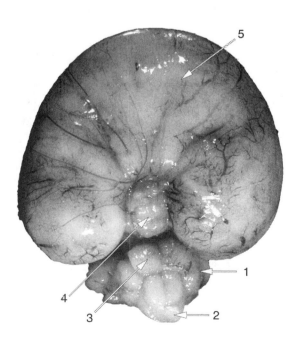

FIGURE 16.14. *Holoprosencephalic brain, basal view.*

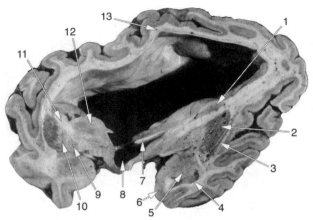
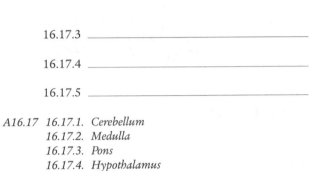
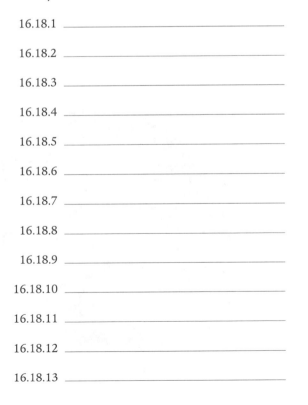

FIGURE 16.15. *Holoprosencephaly in an older child.*

16.17.3 _____

16.17.4 _____

16.17.5 _____

A16.17 16.17.1. *Cerebellum*
16.17.2. *Medulla*
16.17.3. *Pons*
16.17.4. *Hypothalamus*
16.17.5. *Holosphere (cortex)*

Holoprosencephaly, Older Child

Q16.18. The image in Figure 16.15 is a coronal section from a child with holoprosencephaly. Identify the numbered structures:

16.18.1 _____

16.18.2 _____

16.18.3 _____

16.18.4 _____

16.18.5 _____

16.18.6 _____

16.18.7 _____

16.18.8 _____

16.18.9 _____

16.18.10 _____

16.18.11 _____

16.18.12 _____

16.18.13 _____

A16.18   16.18.1. *Caudate nucleus*
        16.18.2. *Putamen*
        16.18.3. *Claustrum*
        16.18.4. *Temporal horn of lateral ventricle*
        16.18.5. *Amygdala*
        16.18.6. *Entorhinal cortex or parahippocompal gyrus*
        16.18.7. *Anterior commissure*
        16.18.8. *Third ventricle*
        16.18.9. *Globus pallidus internus*
        16.18.10. *Globus pallidus externus*
        16.18.11. *Internal capsule*
        16.18.12. *Thalamus*
        16.18.13. *No corpus callosum!*

Q16.19. What is wrong with the brain in Figure 16.15? Be as anatomically specific as you can. How does this coronal section of a child's brain differ from that of the fetus? Look especially at the cortex. What might this tell you about the timing of the injury, compared to other events in corticogenesis?

A16.19. *As in the fetal brain, this case lacks an interhemispheric fissure. No corpus callosum is present. The basal ganglia and thalamus are present and not fused. Perhaps the most striking finding is the massive dilatation of the single ventricle. The cortex and its underlying white matter are extremely thin. However, we can't assess the patency of the aqueduct to know if the dilatation is secondary to agenesis or obstruction of this channel.*

The holosphere forms its two telencephalic bulbs early in development, around five weeks gestation. Whatever the etiology of this malformation, it must have been operating around this time. Brain development after that time appears normal.

Sonic Hedgehog Expression in Neural Tube

Q16.20. Figure 16.16 is of an embryonic chick spinal cord, showing expression of the *Sonic hedgehog* gene. Name the following numbered structures:

16.20.1 _____

16.20.2 _____

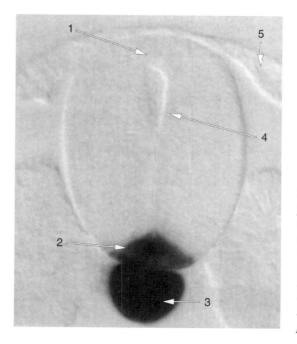

FIGURE 16.16. *Sonic hedgehog expression in an embryonic chick spinal cord. (Adapted from "The Induction and Patterning of the Nervous System" by T. M. Jessell & J. R. Sanes, in Principles of Neural Science, 4th Edition, editors. E. R. Kandel, J. H. Schwartz, & T. M Jessell, © 2000, McGraw Hill, New York, figure 52-6, page 1026.)*

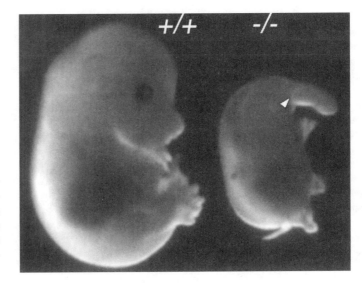

FIGURE 16.17. *Normal mouse fetus on left and Sonic hedgehog knock-out mouse on the right. (Modified from figure 2e, Chiang, C. et al. Cyclopia and defective axial patterning in mice lacking Sonic hedgehog gene function. 1996. Nature 383: 407–413.)*

16.20.3 _____

16.20.4 _____

16.20.5 _____

A16.20   16.20.1. *Roof plate*
      16.20.2. *Floor plate*
      16.20.3. *Notochord*
      16.20.4. *Ventricular zone*
      16.20.5. *Neural crest*

Q16.21. Do you think the expression in the notochord began earlier or later than that in the floor plate? Why? What main gray matter structure in the spinal cord would lie just next to the expression in the floor plate? What is the function of the cells in this site?

A16.21. *As indicated in the text, expression in the notochord induces expression in the floor plate. Secretion of a gradient of sonic hedgehog protein by both structures influences the subsequent development of more ventrolateral structures, including motor neurons. You may gain some appreciation for this based on the intensity of staining in the notochord, compared to the floor plate, although this is not a definitive determination. The main gray matter structure just lateral to the floor plate in the spinal cord would be the ventral horn, including its lower motor neurons. The gradient of sonic hedgehog expression regulates just what type of neurons their precursors will become, be it motor neurons or interneurons.*

Phenotype of SHH Knock-out Mouse

Q16.22 Figure 16.17 shows a fetal mouse who's Sonic hedgehog gene has been "knocked out." First compare the two lateral views of whole-mount embryos. Describe in as much detail as you can how the wild-type differs from the knock-out.

A16.22. *In the knock-out mouse the entire head has been reduced to a single proboscis. The triangle points to where the eye should have been. The arms and legs are also reduced in size, although the back appears largely preserved.*

Q16.23. The next pair of photographs in Figure 16.18 present an in situ hybridization of the Otx-2 gene in horizontal sections through the mouse brain. Dorsal is at the top. Much current work in developmental biology examines how expression of genes that mark or regulate development are influenced after manipulation of other genes. First, describe where you think Otx-2 is normally expressed. What do "m," "d," and "e" mean to a developmental neurobiologist? Second, describe how expression of this gene changes in the Sonic hedgehog knock-out mutant.

A16.23. *The Otx-2 gene is expressed in several sites in these embryos, including the mesencephalon (m), diencephalon (d), and primordial eye (e). Note that its expression is restricted to the dorsal*

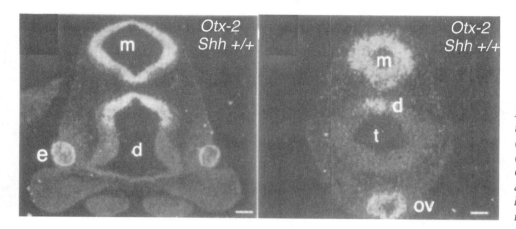

FIGURE 16.18. *In situ hybridization of the Otx-2 gene in wild-type (right) and Sonic hedgehog knock-out (left) animals. (Modified from figure 6h & 6k, Chiang, C. et al. Cyclopia and defective axial patterning in mice lacking* Sonic hedgehog *gene function. 1996. Nature 383: 407–413.)*

diencephalon (you can examine the expression well in the mesencephalon because of the plane of the cut). Also note the presence of two lateral eyes. In the sonic hedgehog knock-out mouse, the eyes are no longer separate, although this optic vesicle (ov) still expresses the Otx-2 gene. The diencephalon is now just part of the telencephalon (t), forming a single prosencephalon.

Environmental Agents Producing Holoprosencephaly

Q16.24. Pregnant ewes that consumed the corn lily *Veratrum californicum* had a high incidence of birthing cyclopean lambs. The agents in this plant that induced the malformation turned out to structurally resemble cholesterol (cyclopamine and jervine). Examine Figure 16.19, showing a series of scanning electron micrographs from different chick embryos treated with jervine. Panel *A* is an untreated embryo, while the others were all treated with the same dose of drug. Again, describe the spectrum of changes you see over this set of photographs. In particular, what happens to the optic vesicles, and what becomes of the olfactory process? Compare these with the human cases of holoprosencephaly.

A16.24. *The changes in these chick embryos closely mirror those in the holoprosencephalic infants. In the most severe phenotype, only a single central eye is present, and the nose has become a proboscis displaced above the eye. The maxilla, which normally fuses later in development, is never separate in the more severe phenotype. The cleft lip in less severe holoprosencephaly is due to a failure of the separated maxilla to fuse.*

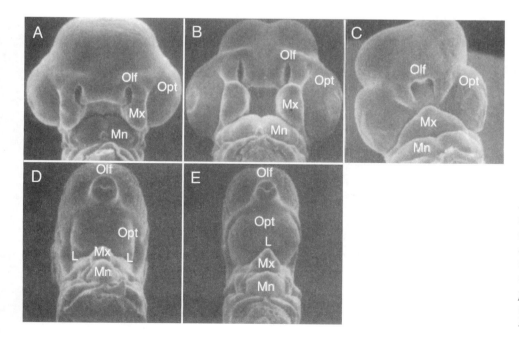

FIGURE 16.19. *Scanning electron micrographs of chick embryo heads, either without treatment (panel A) or after treatment with jervine (remaining panels). (Olf: olfactory processes; Opt: optic vesicles; Mx: maxillary process; Mn: mandibular process). (Figure slightly modified from Cooper, M. K. et al. 1998. Science 280: 1604.)*

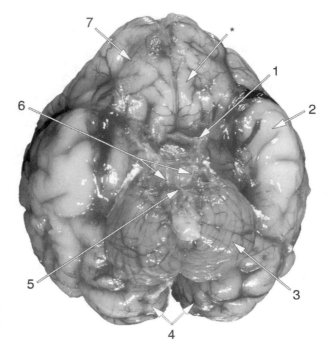

FIGURE 16.20. *Brain from a fetus aborted after determining it had trisomy 13.*

The paper from which these data were taken goes on to demonstrate that the teratogenic sterols inhibited the response of the target tissue to Sonic hedgehog.

Trisomy 13 and Holoprosencephaly

Q16.25. Figure 16.20 is from a 25-week fetus aborted after determining that it had trisomy 13. Identify the numbered structures:

16.25.1 _____

16.25.2 _____

16.25.3 _____

16.25.4 _____

16.25.5 _____

16.25.6 _____

16.25.7 _____

A16.25 16.25.1. *Optic nerve*
16.25.2. *Temporal lobe*
16.25.3. *Cerebellum*
16.25.4. *Occipital lobe*
16.25.5. *Basilar artery*
16.25.6. *Abducens nerve*
16.25.7. *Frontal lobe*

Q16.26. What is wrong with the brain? Identify the starred (*) area. What generalizations can you make about the causes of holoprosencephaly?

A16.26. *The brain has two atypical features from this angle of view: it seems to be more pointed toward the front and it lacks olfactory tracts and a gyrus rectus. The starred section is where a gyrus rectus and an olfactory tract should have been. This represents a more mild form of holoprosencephaly, which has previously been termed "arhinencephaly." Children with trisomy 13 have numerous other developmental anomalies, including neuronal migration anomalies,*

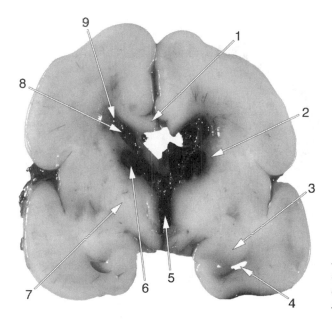

FIGURE 16.21. Coronal section of brain from a child who died soon after birth from extreme prematurity. He survived only about 20 minutes.

and usually die within the first year of life. But holoprosencephaly is a common finding, and many infants with holoprosencephaly have also been found to have trisomy 13.

While the relationship between Sonic hedgehog and holoprosencephaly makes a nice story, the malformation may be caused by several different genetic loci, as well as by complex genetic diseases like the trisomies and environmental toxins. Whether these will all eventually be related to the pathways involved in Sonic hedgehog signaling remains to be determined.

ENCEPHALOCLASTIC LESIONS

Several common pathologies related to fetal hypoxia and distress may injure the developing brain. These major injuries may participate in the development of cerebral palsy and other life-long neurologic deficits.

Hypoxic-Ischemic Hemorrhages

Q16.27. In Figure 16.21, an infant was born alive at around 26 weeks gestation and survived for only about 20 minutes. Identify the numbered structures:

16.27.1 _____

16.27.2 _____

16.27.3 _____

16.27.4 _____

16.27.5 _____

16.27.6 _____

16.27.7 _____

16.27.8 _____

16.27.9 _____

A16.27   16.27.1. *Corpus callosum*
         16.27.2. *Germinal matrix or ventricular zone*

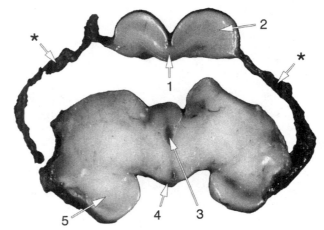

FIGURE 16.22. *Coronal section through a 23-week-gestation fetus, aborted after an ultrasound disclosed a brain malformation.*

> *16.27.3. Amygdala*
> *16.27.4. Temporal horn of lateral ventricle*
> *16.27.5. Hemorrhage in third ventricle*
> *16.27.6. Germinal matrix hemorrhage*
> *16.27.7. Globus pallidus (no myelin to help)*
> *16.27.8. Hemorrhage in lateral ventricle*
> *16.27.9. Lateral ventricle*

Q16.28. In what way will destruction of these anatomic regions affect brain development? What may be the principle clinical finding in such a person?

A16.28. *The hemorrhage lies within the germinal matrix, and is near the caudate nucleus and internal capsule. At this stage in development, all of the neurons have been born and most have migrated to the cortex. The germinal matrix is now creating the future glia, including oligodendroglial and astrocytes.*

> *Had this fetus survived, it would have a partial deficit in the number of glia. But perhaps more important, fibers from the internal capsule and portions of the striatum would have been compromised.*

Porencephaly

Q16.29. Examine the fetal brain Figure 16.22. Get your bearings by first identifying the numbered structures:

16.29.1 _____

16.29.2 _____

16.29.3 _____

16.29.4 _____

16.29.5 _____

A16.29 *16.29.1. Corpus callosum*
16.29.2. Superior frontal lobe remnant
16.29.3. Third ventricle
16.29.4. Hypothalamus
16.29.5. Temporal lobes

Q16.30. What is wrong with this brain? In what vascular territory is the starred lesion (*)? How could the upper nub of tissue remain (area 2)? What is the tissue around the outer edge of the lesion labeled "*"?

A16.30. *This type of malformation is called a "basket brain." The cerebral cortex and underlying white matter has been destroyed in the lateral hemispheres. The lesion follows the middle cerebral artery vascular territory. The anterior cerebral artery territory is preserved, as demonstrated*

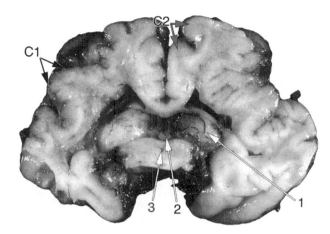

FIGURE 16.23. *Coronal section through a brain of an early third trimester fetus aborted for brain anomalies.*

by the remaining nub of tissue (the basket handle, area 2), as is the posterior territory (temporal lobe, area 5). All that remains of the lateral hemispheres is the meningeal covering (*). These meninges are in direct contact with the ventricular cerebrospinal fluid, and so would be termed porencephaly (hole in the brain).

Q16.31. A less extreme example of an encephaloclastic lesion is shown in Figure 16.23. First, identify:

16.31.1 _____

16.31.2 _____

16.31.3 _____

A16.31   16.31.1. *Pulvinar (thalamus)*
      16.31.2. *Pineal gland*
      16.31.3. *Aqueduct*

Q16.32. How does this brain (Fig. 16.23) differ from normal? What can you observe about the cortex? Specifically, contrast the cortex indicated by C1 (black arrows) and C2 (gray arrows). In what vascular distribution is the lesion?

A16.32. *The lesion is bilateral, again in the vascular territory of the middle cerebral artery. Rather than the normal cortical folds and abundant white matter that should be present in a near-term infant, the white matter is quite thin and the cortex is misshapen. At C1, it has the appearance of being "heaped up" onto itself, like an accordion. This contrasts with the more normal cortex in the anterior cerebral artery territory at C2. These small, more numerous gyri are termed* **polymicrogyria** *and are typically found at the edges of an encephaloclastic lesion. Rather than the porencephalic cysts that were present in the previous case, in no spot do the meninges reach the ventricular surface. Had this infant survived, his quality of life would have been marginal.*

Q16.33. Finally, this last case shown in Figure 16.24 is from an adult with a lifelong history of cerebral palsy, seizures, and mental retardation. The entire brain has been sectioned and stained.

First identify some major structures:

16.33.1 _____

16.33.2 _____

16.33.3 _____

16.33.4 _____

16.33.5 _____

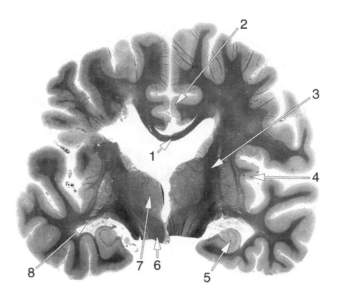

FIGURE 16.24. *Giant coronal section prepared from a chronically institutionalized adult.*

16.33.6 _____

16.33.7 _____

16.33.8 _____

A16.33 16.33.1. *Corpus callosum*
16.33.2. *Cingulate gyrus*
16.33.3. *Internal capsule*
16.33.4. *Insular cortex*
16.33.5. *Hippocampus*
16.33.6. *Red nucleus*
16.33.7. *Medial dorsal nucleus of thalamus*
16.33.8. *Tail of caudate nucleus*

Q16.34. What is wrong with the brain? Where is the lesion? Use all of your knowledge of neuroanatomy to be as specific as possible. How would you describe it? Is it unilateral or bilateral? Do you think the lesion falls within a vascular territory? At what stage of development would you place the lesion? How would you explain the patient's seizure disorder?

A16.34. *Like the other brains this case falls in the spectrum of encephaloclastic lesions. However, this is from an older individual, after the brain has undergone its full developmental programs. The lesion is unilateral, on the left side, and involves portions of the frontal lobe and insular cortex. Notice how the gray matter is also heaped up and is nearly devoid of white matter underneath. This again tells you that the lesion occurred after the neurons had been born and migrated to cortex, but before the onset of gyration or the completion of glial formation, somewhere in the middle of gestation. The cortex shows some microgyria, in a region near the motor cortex. The proximity to motor areas of the frontal lobe probably explain this patient's history of motor seizures.*

Q16.35. Compare the internal capsule on both sides. Why the difference?

A16.35. *The internal capsule on the left is pale, compared to the right (area 3 in Figure 16.24). This represents Wallerian degeneration from the left-sided cortical lesion. While much, abnormal cortex remains on the left, it has been cut off from its distant projections by the white matter lesion beneath.*

CLINICAL CASE STUDY

(The case was kindly provided by Dr. Christopher Walsh, and the radiology was prepared by Dr. Mahesh Patel).

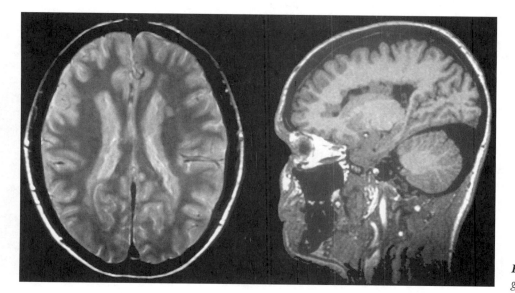

FIGURE 16.25. *Horizontal and sagittal MRI scans from case.*

An 18-year-old woman presented with generalized tonic-clonic seizures. She had two "spells" within the preceding six months. The first of these occurred while she was shopping, and was described as being transiently unresponsive. The second involved precipitous vomiting while at the dinner table that was not related to her meal.

Q16.36. What are some causes of seizures? How does the patient's age affect your opinion as to the potential etiologies?

A16.36. *Most types of insults to the gray matter can produce seizures. These would include strokes, tumors, trauma, infections, and developmental disorders. In a young patient, only strokes would be less likely (but still possible). The lack of a history of head injury and the six month course suggest that trauma and infections are unlikely. In this patient, brain tumors would be a major consideration. Many developmental disorders would be expected to produce seizures at an earlier age, since they would be present from birth. However, the brain matures all through adolescence, and these changes can unmask structural seizure foci.*

Q16.37. Examine her MRI scan in Figure 16.25. Where is the lesion? How do the MRI signal characteristics of the lesion differ from those of the overlying cortex? Do the scans explain her seizure disorder? How?

A16.37. *Around the ventricles is an abnormality with signal characteristics essentially identical to that of gray matter. In essence, the lesion is misplaced gray matter and is known as a **heterotopia**. In this patient the heterotopic gray matter is periventricular. While heterotopic gray matter per se does not offer an explanation for her seizures, it suggests her brain development was abnormal and predisposed her to epilepsy. The possibility that the signal abnormality is due to tumor can be excluded by its similar characteristics to gray matter and by its lack of enhancement.*

Q16.38. The horizontal brain slices in Figure 16.26 are from a patient with a nearly identical malformation. In the labeled figure below, name the structures numbered area 1 to 5.

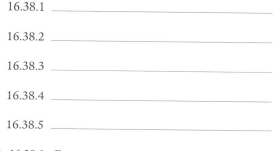

16.38.1 _____

16.38.2 _____

16.38.3 _____

16.38.4 _____

16.38.5 _____

A16.38 16.38.1. *Extra gray matter*
   16.38.2. *Caudate nucleus, head*

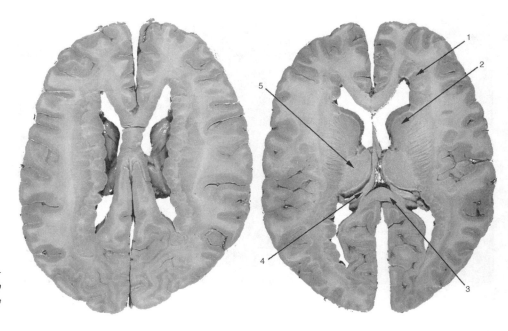

FIGURE 16.26. *Horizontal dissection of a 32-year-old woman with epilepsy who committed suicide by overdosing on acetaminophen.*

16.38.3. *Splenium, corpus callosum*

16.38.4. *Fornix*

16.38.5. *Thalamus*

Q16.39. Describe the distribution of the abnormal gray matter.

A16.39. *The periventricular nodules of heterotopic gray matter lie on the lateral surface of the lateral ventricle, more or less in the same region as the ventricular zone that gives rise to the cerebral cortex during development. In these patients the nodules carpet the entire lateral surface. Other brain structures, in particular, the deep gray nuclei, remain unperturbed.*

Q16.40. Examine Figure 16.27, showing a giant histologic section from the same case. Where are the heterotopias? Do they differ from anterior to posterior? Are they regular or irregular? Can you identify any macroscopic lesions in the overlying cortex.

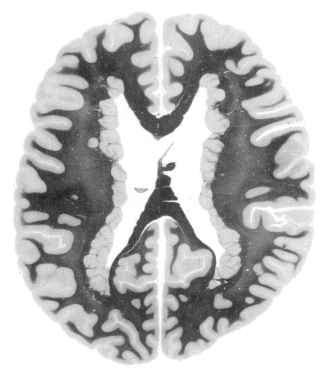

FIGURE 16.27. *Giant histologic section from the same brain as in Figure 16.26, stained with Weigert's hematoxylin (stains myelin nearly black and the neuropil only a light yellow).*

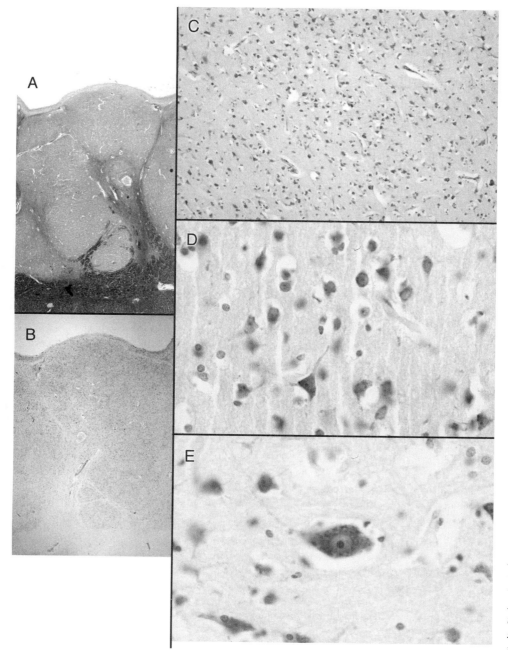

FIGURE 16.28. Histology of peri-ventricular heterotopias. Panel A is a myelin-stained section and B is the Nissl equivalent. The remaining sections from the nodules are all Nissl-stained at lower (C) and higher (D, E) powers.

A16.40. This section has been put into the lab mainly for its aesthetics. It does demonstrate several features of this type of heterotopia. They always occur on the lateral aspect of the lateral ventricles, but not around other ventricles and not medially. The nodules are irregular and partially separated by white matter strands. In the occipital poles the nodules become slightly more flagrant by dividing into a greater number of smaller nodules and having an overall increase in thickness. Finally the overlying cortex is essentially normal.

Q16.41. Examine Figure 16.28, which is histology from the autopsy case. What types of cells are in the nodules? Compare them with the overlying "normal" cortex. If necessary use figures from the cortex chapter. Notice the white matter strands surrounding the nodules, especially the orientation of the fibers immediately surrounding the gray matter.

A16.41. The figure shows large nodules of gray matter adjacent to the ventricular surface and enveloped by white matter, but with a relatively normal overlying cortex. These nodules are composed

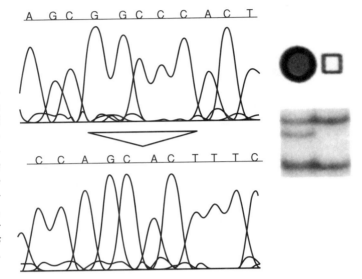

FIGURE 16.29. *DNA sequence analysis from the original patient. The sequencer produced different colored peaks for each nucleotide in the sequence. The derived nucleotide sequence is presented above the primary data. The upper figure is a normal control, while the lower is from the patient. (Adapted from Fox, J. W., et al, Mutations in filamin 1 prevent migration of cerebral cortical neurons in human periventricular heterotopia. 1998. Neuron 21, 1315–1325.)*

of different types of neurons, based on their size, shape, and Nissl substance, as well as their associated neuropil. However, unlike the cortex with its laminar organization of neurons, the neurons in the nodules appear randomly organized. While the connectivity of the neurons cannot be ascertained by this examination, the altered pattern of the myelinated fibers outside the nodules suggests their neurons have extensive connections and are not merely isolated cells. As might be expected, recent reports of depth electrodes inserted into the nodules have indicated that these neurons are active. We don't know to whom they talk.

This patient has a rare cause of epilepsy. This and similar cases have been shown to map to Xq28, and the gene has been shown to be due to mutations in filamin 1. The mutation in this patient is presented in Figure 16.29. The normal gene sequence for the coding region in exon 2 of a control is presented above, and the corresponding sequence of the patient is below. The migration of the single-stranded sequences from the involved region are presented on the gel, with the patient on the left and her unaffected brother on the right.

Q16.42. Examine the image in Figure 16.29 (originally in color). What type of mutation does this represent? How would this type of mutation in exon 2 within the coding region be expected to affect the protein? Why is it important to examine the patient's brother? Whom else might you wish to examine?

A16.42. *The sequence analysis shows the patient had a five base pair deletion in the filamin-1 gene. As a five base pair deletion would alter the reading frame, this frame shift mutation would produce a completely different protein that would most likely terminate early. In this case the deletion introduces a premature stop codon after only eight additional inappropriate amino acids.*
DNA sequence polymorphisms are common in the population. In mutational analysis it is essential to examine close relatives to avoid identifying a routine polymorphism as the cause of a disease. A similar change in the unaffected brother would also suggest that the mutation does not necessarily produce disease, or that the gene is not involved. To fully examine a patient, you would want to examine the DNA from her affected and unaffected relatives, including any children she may have.

Q16.43. Suggest why apparently half the cortical neurons don't migrate in women with this gene and why these women do not have affected male offspring.

A16.43. *The most parsimonious explanation is that approximately half of the cells express the abnormal allele because of X-chromosome inactivation, and these cells fail to migrate from their site of origin. Males who inherit the affected X chromosome die in utero.*

Filamin 1 is an actin binding protein that has been known for a long time (since 1975, during the neonatal period of molecular genetics). It encodes a protein that connects cytosolic actin to several membrane proteins. The protein has an actin binding domain, a rod connector domain, protein–protein binding domains, and is extensively regulated by phosphorylation. As is typical of many developmental gene products, filamin 1 has other important systemic functions, including roles in blood clotting and the immune system.

Over the years the patient has been managed with combinations of seizure medications. She experiences a queasy feeling as a prodrome, without other sensory phenomena, then a blank stare lasting 20 to 40 seconds. For the ensuing 20 minutes, she is fully aware, but "slow to recover," and has poor memory for the event for a short period following the spell. She has subsequently married.

Chapter 17—TRAUMA

The young man had been riding his motorbike for several hours on the interstate and was getting weary. As a car began to pull in front of him, he had to suddenly swerve to avoid some debris in the road. The action was too sudden, and he lost control. His head, with the helmet still on, struck the tree before his body. The small differences in momentum among the different components of his brain were magnified by the sudden deceleration, forcing parts to move separately from each other and his fracturing skull. Axons were sheared or severely stretched. Blood vessels were ripped from the more delicate brain, and hemorrhaged. Soft portions of his brain rode over rough surfaces of his skull, producing innumerable small surface contusions. The base of his skull fractured as his body was driven into it. He was fortunate. His brain function ceased immediately at the initial impact, and he didn't suffer.

Trauma is the leading killer of individuals in their prime, at the point in their lives when they can make the greatest contribution to society. Brain injury is a major cause of morbidity and mortality in these patients. In your careers you have already or will work with people who have suffered traumatic brain injury.

In this laboratory, you will examine some patterns of trauma. You should use this opportunity both to learn about brain trauma as well as to review your neuroanatomy.

LEARNING OBJECTIVES

- Be able to recognize some of the major patterns of central nervous system trauma, their clinical manifestations, and the types of injuries that produce them.
- Be able to distinguish among the different types of cerebral hemorrhages, their antecedent causes, and appropriate interventions.
- Correlate different sites of injury with their neurologic sequelae.
- Review neuroanatomy.

INTRODUCTION

Trauma to the nervous system can happen at all levels, including muscle contusions, wrenching of a nerve plexus, lacerating the spinal cord, and damaging the brain. Each site obviously has its own manifestations and sequelae. In modern life, trauma generally and nervous system trauma in particular is a major cause of death among young people. The cost to society from such injuries

Functional Neuroanatomy: An Interactive Text and Manual, by Jeffrey T. Joseph and David L. Cardozo
ISBN 0-471-44437-5 Copyright © 2004 John Wiley & Sons, Inc.

can be exceedingly high, not just from the injury itself but also for the long-term care these victims frequently require and the lifetime loss of productivity. Even a seemingly small injury to the frontal lobes, which produces essentially no medical deficits, can nearly totally incapacitate an individual and severely diminish his productivity.

The brain and spinal cord are housed in bone, hence any injury inducing central neurologic damage must be transmitted through bone. While sometimes the bone may deform enough to transmit injury to the brain without actually breaking, traumatic brain damage is often associated with bone fractures. The skull is not a simple sphere of bone, but rather is a complex composite of multiple smaller units, stitched together with sutures and having widely varying strengths. The type of injury (e.g., blow with sharp object versus blunt), its location (e.g., temple versus crest), and the anatomic structures beneath (e.g., artery, vein, temporal lobe) all play roles in the ensuing damage. Recognizing skull and spine fractures is important for preventing or limiting subsequent harm to the nervous system.

As for other types of tissue in the body, the brain can suffer bruises, lacerations, crush injuries, and penetrating injuries. But unlike other organs, the brain is a set of long-distance wires that may also undergo shearing injuries.

Brain contusions (bruises in Anglo-Saxon) come in two varieties: coup contusions and contrecoup contusions. When an object strikes the head or the head strikes an object, the brain directly beneath the blow may be bruised. For example, when a person hits his head on a pipe during a fall, the skull at the impact bows inward and induces a direct contusion. This more intuitive form of bruising is termed a *"coup contusion."* In contrast, some of the most massive examples of brain injury caused by accidents occur in regions nearly opposite the site of impact. By far the most common example of these is created by falls backward onto the occiput. In many cases the occipital bone has a small, hairline fracture, the cerebellum and occipital lobes remain unscathed, while the orbital surfaces of the frontal lobes and anterior temporal lobes suffer massive bruising. Such an unfortunately common process is termed a *"contrecoup contusion."*

Of course, the brain may be injured by directed, more massive trauma, as may be inflicted by baseball bats or penetrating gunshot wounds. These types of insults often lacerate (or cut) the brain and deposit foreign material (shrapnel, shards of bone, hair), which add the complicating factor of infection should the victim survive the initial insult. Bullets and other high momentum small objects of advanced civilizations, such as air gun nails, are rather flamboyantly termed missile injuries by forensic pathologists. These objects penetrate the skull and travel through the brain, wreaking extensive havoc and leaving tracts of cell death in their wake. Depending on their momentum, the skull may send the missile tumbling, or its fragments may be propelled through the brain, thus adding further injury.

Our ability to now routinely move at high speeds has blessed us with a unique type of brain injury, which twists, stretches, and otherwise wrenches our axons. Such *diffuse axonal injury (DAI)* is most frequently a sequelae of high-speed motor vehicle accidents. Sudden decelerations of the semigelatinous brain strains long axonal connections, especially at sites where fiber bundles cross each other or where they are most vulnerable to injury. For example, a major site of DAI is in the centrum semiovale, just lateral to the corpus callosum. In infants for whom cerebral myelin has just begun to form, axons are especially susceptible to shearing at the cortical-white junction.

Hemorrhage often accompanies trauma. These are especially important to recognize, since draining the blood, often a relatively minor intervention, may completely prevent subsequent major deficits, including death. Hemorrhages come in several flavors, depending on their location. Each has different etiologies, morphologies, neurological presentations, treatments, and potential sequelae. *Epidural hemorrhages* typically occur following a skull fracture that lacerates an artery. Arterial pressure blood may slowly dissect the dura from the skull, a process that may take hours. The effect is that of an expanding mass in a confined space, and is a surgical emergency. *Subdural hemorrhages,* by contrast, may occur very slowly and produce an insidious neurologic decline. Trauma, often minor in the elderly, ruptures the bridging veins and allows the slow, venous-pressure seepage of blood into the potential space between the arachnoid and dura. Chronic subdural hemorrhages frequently lead to a slow cognitive decline that may be incorrectly considered Alzheimer's disease. Because of the delicacy of the bridging veins, a subdural hemorrhage itself may induce further bleeding. These types of hemorrhage frequently recur, even after drainage. Acute subdural hematomas, by contrast, are usually associated with significant trauma. The other three types of hemorrhages, subarachnoid, intraparenchymal, and intraventricular, may be induced by trauma but also occur in other diseases that damage blood vessels. *Subarachnoid hemorrhages* originate either at the brain surface or in the meningeal vessels, and are a common sequelae of contusions, tumors, infections, ruptured aneurysms, and infarcts. *Intraparenchymal hemorrhages* may have several etiologies, including hypertensive vascular necrosis, tumors, weakening of the arterioles by amyloid deposition, infarcts, and penetrating trauma. Intraventricular hemorrhages are usually associated with intraparenchymal bleeds rupturing into the ventricles. These may leak from brainstem foramina to create subarachnoid blood around the brain base.

In contrast to the adult hemorrhages discussed above, germinal matrix and choroid plexus hemorrhages are restricted to the premature and late gestation infants, respectively. Both are associated with hypoxic-ischemic brain injury and both may be associated with intraventricular and subarachnoid hemorrhages.

The danger of mass lesions in the skull, including tumors, hemorrhages, and edema. is the lack of free space inside a rigid volume. A growing mass presses the brain, and its only exits out of the skull are through the foramen magnum or a site of fracture. Various dural sheaths around the brain further confine the brain into separate compartments. The falx separates the two cerebral hemispheres and the tentorium divides the telencephalon (hemispheres and striatum) and diencephalon (thalamus) from the posterior fossa. Brain extruded between any of these compartments is known as *herniation.* As you might guess, these come in several styles. Hemispheric masses that force the cingulate gyrus underneath the falx result in *subfalcine herniation.* Similarly extrusion of an uncus around the insertion of the tentorium gives *uncal herniation.* Bilateral cerebral swelling may press the entire diencephalon through the tentorial notch, thus generating *diencephalic herniation.* Finally posterior fossa masses and supratentorial masses large enough to compress the brainstem may propel the cerebellar tonsils around the medulla and through the foramen magnum, producing *tonsilar herniation* ("coning" in medical slang, since the skull base ends in a cone shape).

Schedule (2.5 hours)
20   Skull fractures
20   Spinal cord injuries
20   Missile injuries
20   Contusions
30   Hemorrhages
20   Herniation
20   Diffuse axonal injury

SKULL FRACTURES

Skull Examination

Q17.1. Inspect the skull again. First, review some anatomic sites. Identify the indicated structures in Figure 17.1. Indicate important structures passing through each indicated foramina.

17.1.1 _____

17.1.2 _____

17.1.3 _____

17.1.4 _____

17.1.5 _____

17.1.6 _____

17.1.7 _____

17.1.8 _____

17.1.9 _____

17.1.10 _____

17.1.11 _____

17.1.12 _____

A17.1.   *17.1.1. Frontal bone*
         17.1.2. Cribriform plate of ethmoid bone (olfactory nerve entrance)

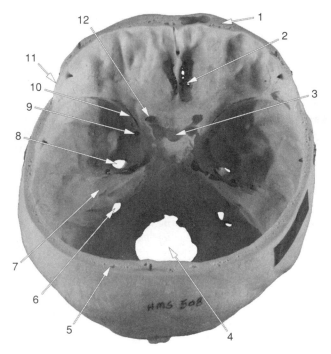

FIGURE 17.1. *Skull. The cap has been uncovered and the view is from the posterior-superior looking down. Several of the holes would normally appear black, but have been made white for emphasis.*

17.1.3. *Sella turcica or pituitary fossa (home of the pituitary gland)*
17.1.4. *Foramen magnum (spinal cord, vertebral arteries, and accessory nerve XI)*
17.1.5. *Occipital bone*
17.1.6. *Jugular foramen (jugular vein, vagus and glossopharyngeal nerves)*
17.1.7. *Petrous bone*
17.1.8. *Foramen ovale (mandibular division of trigeminal nerve)*
17.1.9. *Foramen rotundum (maxillary division of trigeminal nerve)*
17.1.10. *Superior orbital fissure (ophthalmic division of trigeminal nerve, oculomotor, trochlear, and abducens nerves)*
17.1.11. *Temporal bone*
17.1.12. *Optic canal (optic nerve)*

Q17.2. Where are the thinnest regions? Which different vascular structures lie beneath the thinnest parts of the skull? What parts of brain? What may be the manifestations of injury to these sites?

A17.2. *The skull varies widely in thickness, from the thick petrous (stonelike) bones around the ear to the eggshell thin regions around the temple and above the eyes (anterior cranial fossa beneath the frontal lobes). Overlying the temporal bones are the thick muscles of mastication, which provide some protection to the underlying thin bone. However, the middle meningeal artery lies just under the bone, so fractures can also shear the artery and produce an epidural hematoma. Overlying the orbits is the orbitofrontal surface of the brain, as well as the olfactory apparatus. As we have seen, the frontal lobes essentially define who we are and their loss, while not necessarily fatal, frequently leads to major changes in personality. For Epicureans like ourselves, the loss of smell would be devastating.*

Q17.3. Where is the skull the smoothest? The roughest? How might these textural differences contribute to the types of injuries in these sites?

A17.3 *Most of the outer skull is smooth, while the orbital surface (anterior cranial fossa), a complex of several bones, is quite rough. For the gastronomes, it is like a cheese grater. Small movements of brain over the smooth surfaces generally produce little injury to the underlying brain, while similar movements over the orbital surfaces may bruise the brain surface.*

Fractures

Q17.4. Now examine the CT scan in Figure 17.2 of a patient who was involved in a motor vehicle accident. What do you see? Can you identify the fracture? What else can you discern? What neuroanatomic sites may be involved?

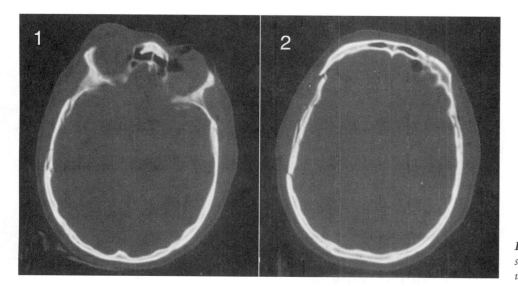

FIGURE 17.2. *Bone-window   CT scan of a patient involved in a motor vehicle accident.*

A17.4. *The fracture is where the skull bone is discontinuous, involving the right frontal and temporal bones. Beneath the fracture lies the frontal and temporal lobes. A concern in a case like this is rupture of the middle meningeal artery, which travels up underneath the thin temporal bones in the periosteal layer of the dura.*

Direct fractures of bone do not necessarily produce significant damage to the underlying brain. However, they frequently lacerate the brain and can sever important vessels.

Q17.5. Examine Figure 17.3, showing the skull base from a patient who unsuccessfully tried to kill himself by shooting himself in the head with a shotgun. Fortunately, he did not survive for more than a few days. What bones are fractured (see arrowheads)? What neuroanatomic sites would be involved?

A17.5. *This type of fracture is described as "eggshell," since the bones have fragmented into small pieces. The cribriform plate has been crushed, and the ethmoid bones and outer orbital surfaces have multiple cracks (right panel). Another crack extends over most of the left–right axis of the skull, along the lesser wing of the sphenoid bone.*

The entire brain overlying this region was hemorrhagic and necrotic, including the olfactory bulbs and tracts, gyrus rectus, major portions of the inferior frontal lobe, the hypothalamus, and the pituitary gland.

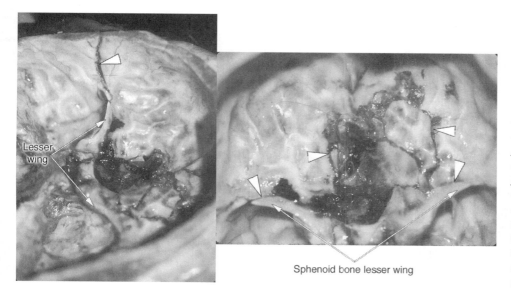

Lesser wing

Sphenoid bone lesser wing

FIGURE 17.3. *Photographs of the skull from a patient who unsuccessfully tried to kill himself by firing a shotgun under his chin and through his face. The left figure is an oblique view over the right side of his skull, after the skull cap has been removed. You are looking at the left side of his skull. The right figure is looking directly down on top of the orbitofrontal surface, with the lesser wings of the sphenoid bones in the lower portion of the figure.*

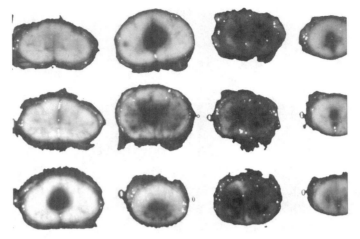

FIGURE 17.4. *Hematomyelia from spinal cord trauma. From slide files at Harvard Medical School.*

SPINAL CORD INJURY

Q17.6. Review Figure 17.4, showing a series transverse spinal cord sections from a case of acute spinal trauma. Where is the nidus of injury? What extends from this nidus? If the slices are each about a centimeter long, how long is the total extent of the injury?

A17.6. *The spinal cord has extensive hemorrhage internally. The greatest site of injury is at the thoracic level, and hemorrhage has dissected rostrally and caudally from this nidus. Traumatic hematomyelia is a further possible complication to spinal trauma. In this case the injury is about 10 cm long.*

Spinal Trauma Case

The patient is a 34-year-old construction worker. He is standing with a group of other workers, with his back turned. An inexperienced apprentice allows a power nailer to discharge three nails, at a distance of about 10 feet. Two nails penetrate him. Each is 1.0×0.2 cm. One enters the right chest below the scapula on the right side. The other enters the spinal column opposite the C7 vertebra, fractures the lamina, and comes to rest against the vertebral body. The patient falls, is taken to an emergency ward, multiple films are taken, and pain is controlled. It is found that he has partial paralysis of the legs and a right hemothorax, which requires surgery.

On examination six days post injury, he shows the following:

- The cranial nerves are normal except for pupillary asymmetry; the right pupil being 3 mm, the left 5 mm.
- The left upper extremity is normal.
- The right upper extremity demonstrates weakness of finger and thumb abduction and adduction.
- The right lower extremity is weak in all movements, approximately 3/5 (can generate weak movement against gravity)
- The left lower extremity is normal in strength.
- The sensory examination shows a loss of feeling for pinprick and cold sensation over the entire left side, up to about 2 to 3 cm below the clavicle.
- Position sense and vibration sense are markedly reduced in the right lower extremity
- The right plantar response is extensor. The left is flexor (although the patient notes he does not feel any sense of scratching on that side). The tendon reflexes are increased in the right lower extremity.

Q17.7. What section of the cord has been affected? Draw on the diagrams of spinal cord in Figure 17.5 the parts affected and those spared. Why is the right hand weak? Suggest two possible explanations. Why the pupillary asymmetry?

A17.7. *This is a Brown-Sequard syndrome, produced by a hemitransection of the cord. In this case the transection by the nail is in the C8 cord on the right side. See Figure 17.6. The loss of proprioception in the right leg comes from transection of the dorsal column. At this level it is mostly gracilis tract. The loss of left leg pain and temperature is due to interruption of the ascending contralateral spinothalamic fibers. Note that the loss is below the level of the lesion,*

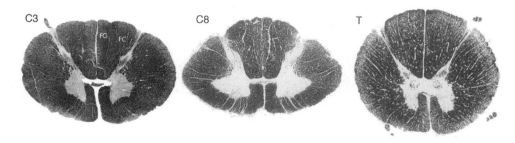

FIGURE 17.5. *Spinal cord trauma worksheet.*

Dissociated sensory loss *Loss of pain and temperature sensation on one side of the body and loss of kinesthetic and proprioceptive sensation on the opposite side. Especially if found on the trunk, it always means a location of damage in certain parts of the cord.*

around T2 instead of C8 (see dermatome map). Remember, nociceptive information ascends a few segments in Lissauer's tract before synapsing. Disruption of the lateral corticospinal tract produced the right lower leg weakness, while loss of the tract and/or loss of C8 lower motor neurons lead to the right hand weakness. Sympathetic innervation to the eye dilates the iris. Loss of these impulses caused an ipsilateral Horner's syndrome. Possible structures involved include descending ipsilateral sympathetic information from the medulla, loss of the root containing these data, and disruption of the nearby stellate ganglion.

MISSILE INJURIES

Q17.8. Review the images in Figure 17.7 from an unfortunate woman who was shot in the back of the head by her boyfriend, had a portion of the wound surgically debrided, and survived for ten years with extensive neurologic deficits. Where is the entrance wound? What clinical deficits may have ensued from just this injury? Include motor, sensory, and cognitive deficits and the side of the symptoms. In the coronal sections trace the path of the bullet through the brain, and detail the deficits produced by the injuries. What happened to the bullet at the top of the skull? Find the bullet. Contrast the final pathway of the bullet with the initial. Why might they be different?

A17.8. The bullet entered in the right parietal area and left a large wound in this site (panel 1). The patient had seizures for the remainder of her life, which may have been the cause of her final demise. Other deficits may have been a loss of sensation on the left side of her body. Neuropsychiatric testing would have found other interesting deficits as well, such as a left-sided neglect. Some of her optic fibers may also have been "clipped" by the injury, leaving her with a left inferior homonymous quadrantinopia. The bullet traveled forward and upward, destroying the internal capsule, upper putamen, a portion of the caudate nucleus, and medial high frontal lobe (panel 2). While the striatal lesions may have been expected to produce some movement difficulties, these would have been overshadowed by the spastic hemiparesis ensuing from the severing of the internal capsule. Predictably, she had a dense hemiplegia on the left side.

At the top of the brain, the bullet ricocheted off the skull, penetrated the dura again (panel 3), and ended up in the left ventricle, where it remained until her death (panel 4). The injury on the left side (panel 3) is much less than on the right (panel 2), probably in large part due to the further decrease in momentum by the ricochet and the dura stopping any remaining low-speed fragments of bone and bullet from entering the opposite side. The main injury and deficits were all produced on the right side. This emphasizes that the path of missiles in the brain is unpredictable, and extensive searching for fragments is necessary in order to treat such patients.

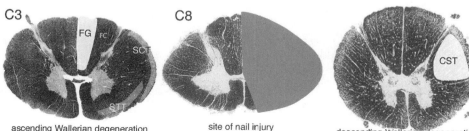

ascending Wallerian degeneration   site of nail injury   descending Wallerian degeneration

FIGURE 17.6. *Brown-Sequard syndrome spinal cord injury. The site of injury is demarcated in gray, while the subsequent Wallerian degeneration is shown in white.*

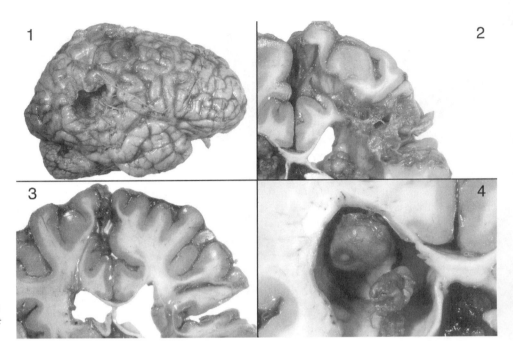

FIGURE 17.7. *Brain from a woman who survived ten years after being shot in the back of the head.*

CONTUSIONS

Q17.9. Figure 17.8 shows a brain from an unhelmeted young man who struck a car while riding his bicycle. He was thrown over the car and struck his head. He remained unconscious at the scene, and died shortly after the emergency medical technicians arrived. At autopsy, he had a linear (not comminuted or fractured like an egg) occipital bone fracture that extended several centimeters. What type of injury is this called? Where, specifically, are the injuries in the figure? Where would you predict he struck his head? Considering their surrounding structures, postulate how they formed? Do you wear your helmet?

A17.9. *The massive contrecoup contusion involves the orbitofrontal surfaces of the frontal lobe, the frontal poles, the temporal poles, and the superior bank of the temporal lobe abutting the lateral fissure. It is greater on the left-hand side, and true to the contrecoup process, he had a right occipital bone fracture.*

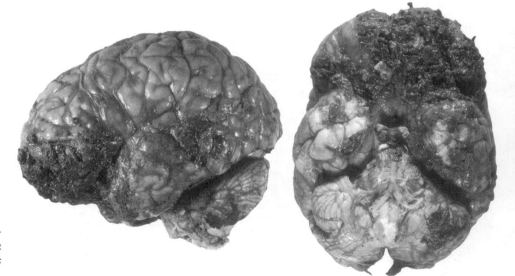

FIGURE 17.8. *Brain from an unhelmeted young man who was struck and thrown by a car while riding his bicycle.*

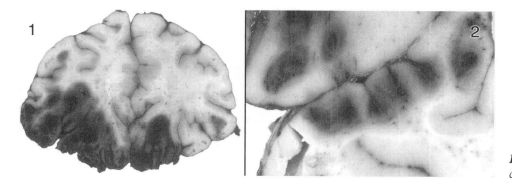

FIGURE 17.9. *Coronal section and close-up from the brain in Figure 17.8.*

Contrecoup contusions remain somewhat of a mystery. While the orbital shelf supporting the frontal lobes is rough and could act like a food grater, the frontal and temporal poles and the lateral fissure are not so irregular. Some have postulated that the brain suddenly pulling backward, away from these sites, may produce a local vacuum between the brain and bone that induces the injury. Although a complete mechanism remains a mystery, the pattern of injury is typical.

Anyone with a brain should wear a helmet while bicycling.

Q17.10. Examine the close-up photograph of the contusions from the temporal lobe (see Fig. 17.9). Describe the general appearance of the hemorrhages. Are they generally deep in the sulci or on the gyral surfaces? Why do they not represent a vascular infarct? Hypothesize how they formed.

A17.10. *These multiple thin fingers of blood are known as splinter hemorrhages. Brain contusions usually involve the surface more than the sulcal depths, since this is the site of actual contact. Contusions often bridge from gyrus to gyrus, sparing the sulci, while infarcts invariably involve the sulci. Avulsion of the small arteries feeding the cortex from the meninges and the subsequent bleeding that tracts around them is the probable origin of splinter hemorrhages. Where there is blood, the oxygen delivery has stopped, and the involved brain is dead.*

HEMORRHAGES

Q17.11. Examine Figure 17.10 showing the CT head scan of man who was involved in an altercation. During the fight, he fell to the ground and banged the side of his head. What do you see on the scan? Where is the lesion? What is its shape and distribution? What else do you see around the head? Your goal here is to determine where the hemorrhage is. You need to determine its placement in the coverings of the brain, as well as its anatomic location in relationship to the brain and regional structures.

A17.11. *The scan shows a dense, lens-shaped lesion over the right lateral temporal area. The mass compresses the underlying brain and produces a significant mass effect. The entire right hemisphere is shifted to the left, and the right lateral ventricle is compressed.*

In addition to the intracranial findings, the soft tissues on both sides of the skull also show extensive edema and evidence of hemorrhage. This suggests he may have been struck while his head was on a hard surface, such as the ground.

This hyperdensity represents hemorrhage between the overlying bone and the dura. Since the dura has great tensile strength, it confines the hemorrhage to the epidural space. However, the dura is not firmly attached to the skull table, especially in younger individuals, and so can be dissected away by blood under arterial pressure. At the sutures, the dura is firmly tacked down, so epidural hemorrhages usually do not extend beyond these sites. All of these aspects tend to produce a lens-shaped collection of epidural blood.

Q17.12. Now examine the brain in Figure 17.11 from a 14 year old who fell from a roof while intoxicated. After the accident he was able to walk home. He was found dead in his bed the next morning. At autopsy, his skull had a left temporal fracture, and when opened, about 200 ml of blood poured out. What is wrong with his brain? Where is the damage? Look for any asymmetry. How was he able to walk home?

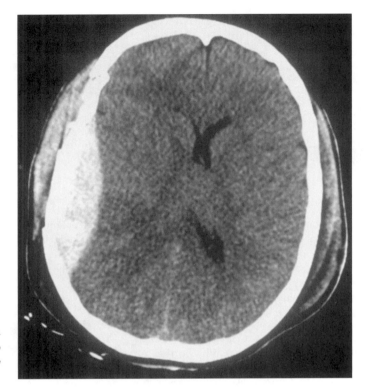

FIGURE 17.10. *Head CT scan from a man who was knocked to the ground in a fight and reportedly struck his head.*

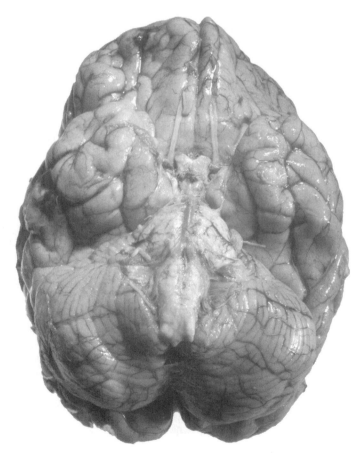

FIGURE 17.11. *Brain from a 14-year-old boy who fell from a roof while intoxicated.*

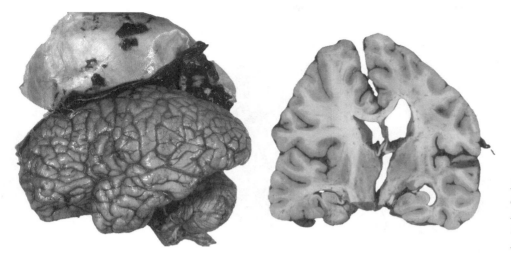

FIGURE 17.12. Brain from an elderly patient who fell in the hospital. About a week later, he was found on the floor. A head CT scan showed a subdural hematoma.

A17.12 The brain has a left frontal lobe indentation, which is where the epidural hematoma compressed his brain. No blood is on the brain, since it was confined to the epidural space. Although the boy fractured his skull and lacerated his middle meningeal artery at the time of impact, the blood required time to dissect between the dura and bone. The delayed mass effect allowed the boy time to walk home and go to bed (presumably with a severe headache) before he perished.

A patient who remains lucid after major head trauma, but later becomes increasing confused and lethargic, should be considered a surgical emergency. You do not want to miss a treatable epidural hematoma.

Q17.13. Review Figure 17.12. The patient had a past medical history of coronary artery disease, acute renal failure due to cholesterol emboli, and hypertension. He fell in the hospital. About a week later he was found on the floor in his feces. A CT scan demonstrated subdural blood. Where is the blood? What evidence does the brain have for this hemorrhage? How do these changes differ from those seen in epidural hematomas?

A17.13. Most of the blood has leaked away at autopsy, indicating either it was very recent or that the patient was unable to clot well. The latter is typical of individuals with liver failure, blood dyscrasias, and who are being treated with anticoagulants. Nevertheless, the brain has evidence of a subdural bleed, since the left hemisphere is indented, but retains its knobby surface. Unlike an epidural hematoma, in which the flat dura compresses the brain, blood in a subdural hemorrhage coats the brain surface, and applies pressure around the gyri rather than just on their tops. Note the right cortex is smooth which indicates compression from the left hematoma.

While the results of an epidural and subdural hemorrhage may appear similar, the mechanisms are different. Epidural hematomas are most often the result of an arterial rupture, and are created by arterial pressure dissecting the dura off the skull. The process typically occurs over hours. In contrast, subdural hematomas most often arise from rupture of bridging veins connecting to the dura. These are low-pressure hemorrhages, usually occurring over a more extended period of time, and are often clinically more insidious than epidural hematomas.

Q17.14. Figure 17.13 is from a patient who had prior head trauma. He had a subdural hematoma evacuated several times. How has the blood become adherent to the dura? What happened to the blood on the right brain surface?

A17.14. The blood is brownish orange, rather than red, since it is partially organized and contains blood breakdown product (hemosiderin). Such hemorrhages organize from the dural surface, not from the meninges. Hence, as fibroblasts and blood vessels become incorporated into the clot, it becomes adherent to the dura, and not to the underlying brain. If they don't enlarge, the brain may be remarkably spared by such hemorrhages.

This case emphasizes that such hemorrhages have a propensity to rebleed and may be difficult to treat successfully.

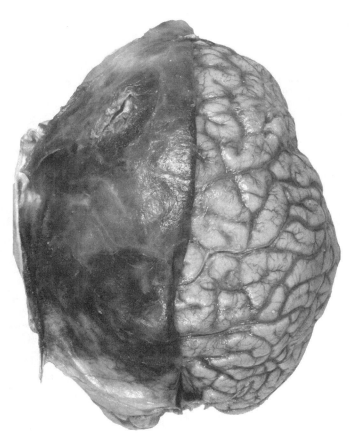

FIGURE 17.13. Chronic subdural hematoma. The dura covering the right hemisphere has been reflected over onto the left to show the underlying brain and the color of the hematoma.

Q17.15. Finally, examine Figure 17.14. How could the brain get like this? What happened to the blood that produced this defect?

A17.15. *The left cerebral hemisphere has been markedly indented. Had this happened rapidly, it would have resulted in extensive hemorrhage, necrosis, herniation, and death. Such massive remodeling of brain tissue can only happen by slowly growing masses, such as low grade meningiomas, or as in this case, chronic, recurrent, subdural hemorrhages. As in the last case, this patient*

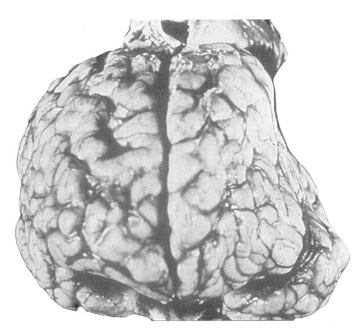

FIGURE 17.14. Brain from a patient with a chronic subdural hematoma. From slide files at Harvard Medical School.

bled, organized, and rebled multiple times into the subdural space. This scenario is unfortunately too common in elderly patients, whose increasing confusion may be misinterpreted as dementia.

HERNIATION

Q17.16. In the next case, the patient developed a large subdural hematoma over the right cerebrum after he was emergently given tissue plasminogen activator for a large pulmonary embolus. Examine Figure 17.15 showing a coronal section of his brain at autopsy. On which side was the blood (assume right is on right)? Describe what you see. First, focus on the subfalcine herniation. What has happened to the brain tissue? What important vascular structure was compromised by this mass effect? What is its territory, and what brain functions lie in this region? Predict the sequelae you might see from this compromise. Second, scrutinize the uncal herniation. Describe the uncus itself. How did these changes develop? What important structures lie near the uncus? Use the intact brain for reference. What are the neurologic sequelae? The midbrain and upper pons also developed so-called Duret hemorrhages secondary to the uncal herniation. What important neuroanatomic sites live in this region, and what would be the resulting neurologic deficits?

A17.16. *The patient had been anticoagulated, so the large amount of blood washed away at autopsy. The massive right-sided subdural hematoma has compressed the brain and produced a massive right to left shift.*

On the coronal section, the right cingulate gyrus has been shifted to the left, underneath the falx. The right uncus is necrotic and the left has a hemorrhage. The anterior cerebral arteries feeding much of the medial brain travel just underneath the cingulate gyri. When an evolving hemispheric mass extrudes the cingulate gyrus beneath the falx, it may compromise the blood flow through one or both arteries, leading to acute infarcts of the medial brain. As in this case, even brief reestablishment of blood flow may create tissue hemorrhages. In the medial brain lives the motor region serving the legs; its destruction would lead to lower limb paralysis. Important limbic structures also lie in the medial brain, including the cingulate gyrus, the cingulum, and portions of the frontal lobe involved in motivation.

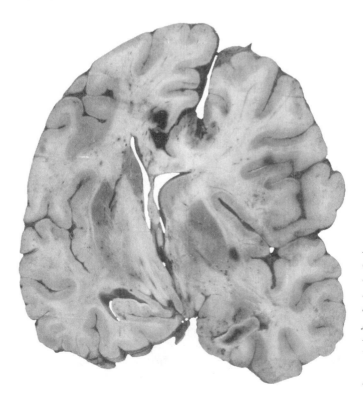

FIGURE 17.15. *Subfalcine and uncal herniation. The patient had recently undergone a brain biopsy. He later became acutely short of breath after he embolized a large blood clot from his leg to his pulmonary arteries. In a desperate attempt to save him, he was given tissue plasminogen activator. As his respiratory status improved, he suddenly became comatose.*

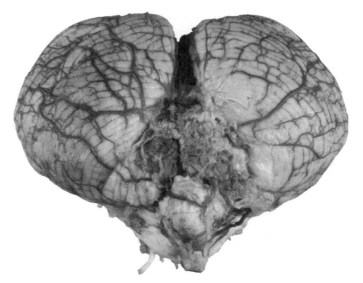

FIGURE 17.16. *Tonsilar herniation. A patient with a primary central nervous system lymphoma fell and rapidly became comatose. At presentation in the hospital, she had "blown pupils."*

The uncus, along with the anterior hippocampus, has undergone hemorrhagic necrosis as it was squeezed over the tentorium. Medial to the uncus lives the cerebral peduncle, and between these two lies the pulsating posterior cerebral artery. Wedged closely between the posterior cerebral artery and the superior cerebellar artery lies the vulnerable third nerve. Lateral to the uncus is the anterior portion of the hippocampus. Obviously uncal herniation may have major sequelae, including third-nerve palsies and their accompanying "blown pupils" (Why would this happen?), posterior cerebral artery territory infarcts (What would be the major deficit?), hemiparesis from compression of the peduncle, and possibly impairment of memory.

An even more ominous sequelae is the frequent development of hemorrhages in the midbrain and upper pons, as they are compressed caudally and have their vessels avulsed from their roots. As discussed in the diffuse projection system laboratory, this region of the brain is home to the reticular activating system, the raphe nuclei, locus ceruleus, and ventral tegmental area. The loss of these areas would produce coma and would be incompatible with life. The diminutive aqueduct also courses through the region; its compression would add acute hydrocephalus to the many other insults.

Q17.17. Inspect Figure 17.16 from base of the brainstem and cerebellum. First orient yourself. Which side is dorsal, and which side is ventral? Describe the findings. What has happened to the cerebellar tonsils? What important structure has been compromised? What essential neuroanatomic loci live in this region? List as many as you can. Guess the clinical sequelae.

A17.17. *Dorsal, as always, is up. The medulla is the round structure in the center of the picture, which is surrounded by necrotic cerebellar tonsils. The patient had swelling in the posterior fossa that compressed the cerebellum and brainstem, which lead to herniation of the cerebellar tonsils through the foramen magnum. During the process they compressed and destroyed the medulla, especially the posterior medulla. The lower medulla is the home of such essential elements as the reticular formation controlling the autonomic nervous system, the cardiovascular input*

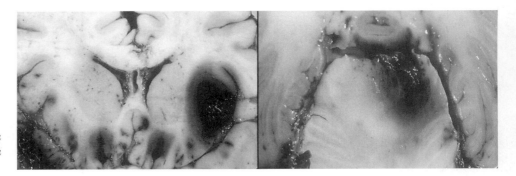

FIGURE 17.17. *Two views of a brain from a patient involved in a motorcycle accident.*

portion of the solitary nucleus and tract, the parasympathetic output to the body from the dorsal motor nucleus of the vagus, the swallowing centers and their ambiguus motor nuclei, and the descending control fibers projecting to the preganglionic sympathetic neurons in the intermediolateral spinal cord. The relatively less important pyramids and ascending sensory tracts, of course, also travel through here. As you may have guessed, such a lesion is compatible only with death.

DIFFUSE AXONAL INJURY

Q17.18. The two images in Figure 17.17 come from the brain of a young man who had a motorcycle accident. He had no lucid interval following the trauma. List all of the different injuries you can find. What has happened to the corpus callosum? What great white matter tract is involved in the second photograph? Hypothesize why this man was immediately comatose.

A17.18. *The microscopic pathology of diffuse axonal injury requires days to develop and cannot be seen when patients such as this motorcycle driver die rapidly. The gross correlate of the microscopic axonal spheroids are the midline or paramedian tears of the corpus callosum and superior cerebellar peduncle. Why these structures, in particular, are sheared probably has to do with several factors, including their proximity to major dural structures (falx and tentorial notch), the large bodies of gray matter they connect, and the rotational changes of the peripheral brain around these more central structures. The macroscopic changes are merely a reflection of the much more extensive damage to the axons, especially in the paramedian centrum semiovale. Damage to the axons is immediate, and essentially inactivates their ionic transmission capabilities. Thus coma is immediate, rather than delayed.*

In less severe brain injury, as in cases of concussion, the damage to axons may only temporarily inhibit their function. The greater the degree of injury, the more permanent the axonal damage. While tabloids periodically run stories of people who awaken after years of coma, these "articles" never describe the neuropsychiatric testing results that demonstrate how debilitated the victims remain. Generally, the longer the coma, the worse the final clinical outcome.

Chapter 18—REVIEW

You have reached the final laboratory. You have learned the nervous system from the tips of your fingers to your neocortex. Time to consolidate all of that information.

The exercises in this chapter will reinforce the knowledge you have. Use this time to fill in the gaps. Refresh those synapses that are still a little weak. Potentiate those long-term memories.

LEARNING OBJECTIVE

- Review salient aspects of neuroanatomy, including anatomic, systemic, and functional anatomy.

    Schedule (2.5 hours)
    60 Anatomic review
    50 System review
    40 Functional anatomy

ANATOMIC REVIEW

Q18.1. Identify the following structures in Figure 18.1:
- Olfactory bulbs
- Olfactory tracts
- Optic nerves
- Optic chiasm
- Gyrus rectus
- Mammillary bodies
- Internal carotid artery
- Basilar artery
- Vertebral artery
- Uncus
- Frontal lobe
- Temporal lobe
- Cerebral peduncles

Functional Neuroanatomy: An Interactive Text and Manual, by Jeffrey T. Joseph and David L. Cardozo
ISBN 0-471-44437-5 Copyright © 2004 John Wiley & Sons, Inc.

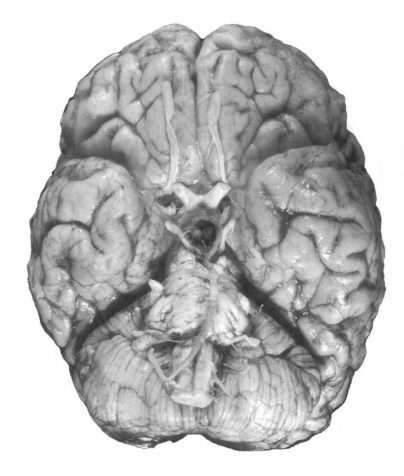

FIGURE 18.1. *Base of brain.*

- Oculomotor nerve (III)
- Trigeminal nerve (V)
- Cerebellum
- Flocculus
- Medulla
- Pontine base

A18.1. *See Figure 18.2.*

Q18.2. Identify these structures on the coronal section in Figure 18.3:
- Anterior cerebral arteries
- Middle cerebral arteries
- Septum pellucidum
- Nucleus accumbens
- Gyrus rectus
- Internal capsule
- Claustrum
- Corona radiata
- Cingulate gyrus

A18.2. *See Figure 18.4.*

Q18.3. Identify these structures in the coronal section in Figure 18.5:
- Globus pallidus internus
- Globus pallidus externus
- Amygdala
- Hippocampus
- Fornix columns
- Hypothalamus

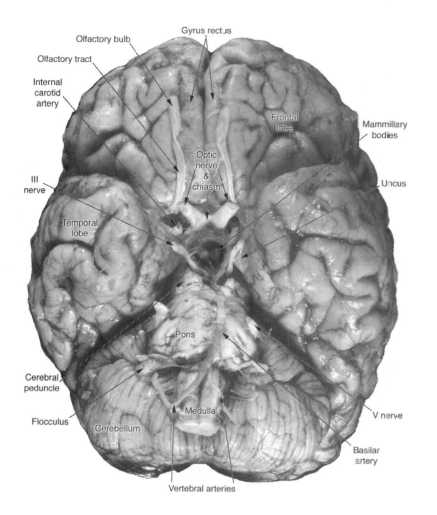

FIGURE 18.2. *Salient structures on the base of brain.*

- Temporal horn of lateral ventricle
- Optic tract
- External capsule
- Extreme capsule

A18.3. See Figure 18.6.

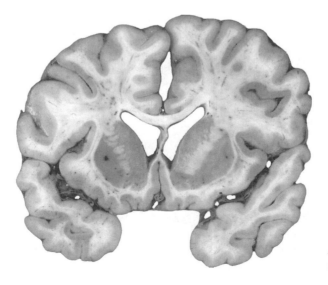

FIGURE 18.3. *Coronal section at the level of the nucleus accumbens.*

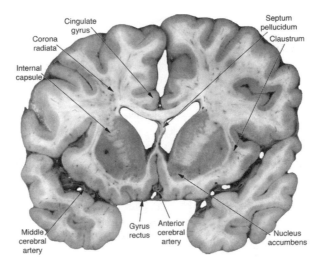

FIGURE 18.4. Salient structures at nucleus accumbens level.

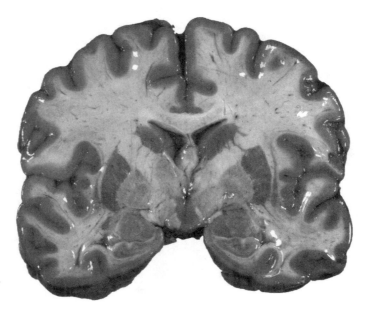

FIGURE 18.5. Coronal section at the level of the amygdala.

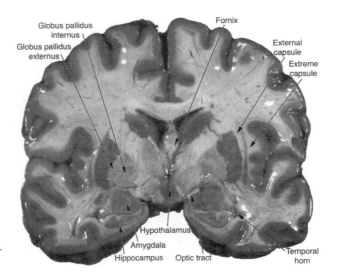

FIGURE 18.6. Salient structures coronal section.

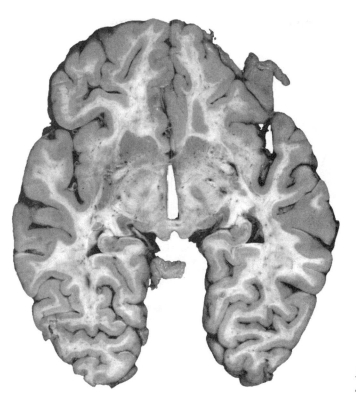

FIGURE 18.7. *Horizontal section at level of lateral geniculate nucleus.*

Q18.4. Identify the following in the low horizontal section in Figure 18.7:
- Ventral striatum (nucleus accumbens)
- Anterior commissure (it's lateral on this section)
- Putamen
- Internal capsule
- Superior colliculus
- Lateral geniculate nucleus
- Medial geniculate nucleus
- Hippocampus
- Tail of caudate nucleus
- Posterior commissure

A18.4. *See Figure 18.8.*

Q18.5. In Figure 18.9 showing a close-up coronal section of the brain with the brainstem still attached, identify:
- Base of pons
- Cerebral peduncles
- Internal capsule
- Substantia nigra
- Red nucleus
- Subthalamic nucleus
- Third ventricle (iii)
- Anterior nucleus thalamus
- Fornix
- Interpeduncular cistern (icis)
- Posterior cerebral artery
- Medial dorsal nucleus
- Ventral lateral thalamus

A18.5. *See Figure 18.10.*

Q18.6. By looking only at the histology in Figure 18.11, what can you say clinically about the patient? Identify these structures in the midbrain histologic section in Figure 18.11:
- Red nucleus
- Cerebral peduncle
- Medial lemniscus

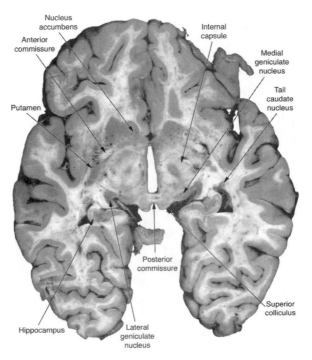

FIGURE 18.8. *Salient structures in low horizontal section.*

- Periaqueductal gray
- Oculomotor nucleus
- Superior colliculus
- Medial geniculate body

A18.6. *The middle of the cerebral peduncle on one side is degenerate, having undergone Wallerian degeneration from an internal capsule infarct in the distant past. The patient had a dense hemiplegia. See Figure 18.12.*

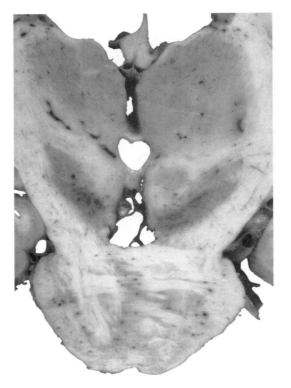

FIGURE 18.9. *Close-up coronal section, brainstem intact.*

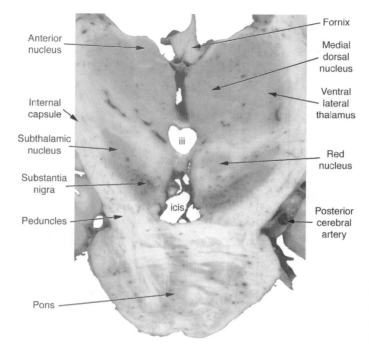

Anterior
nucleus

Internal
capsule

Subthalamic
nucleus

Substantia
nigra

Peduncles

Pons

Fornix

Medial
dorsal
nucleus

Ventral
lateral
thalamus

Red
nucleus

Posterior
cerebral
artery

iii

icis

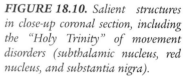

FIGURE 18.10. *Salient structures in close-up coronal section, including the "Holy Trinity" of movement disorders (subthalamic nucleus, red nucleus, and substantia nigra).*

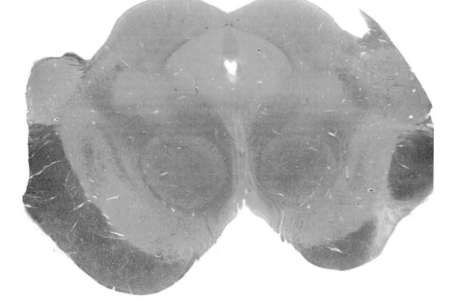

FIGURE 18.11. *Histologic section of the midbrain.*

Medial
geniculate
nucleus

Medial
lemniscus

Superior colliculus

Periaqueductal
gray

Medial
longitudinal
fasciculus

Cerebral
peduncle

Red
nucleus

Oculomotor
nucleus

III fibers

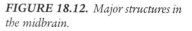

FIGURE 18.12. *Major structures in the midbrain.*

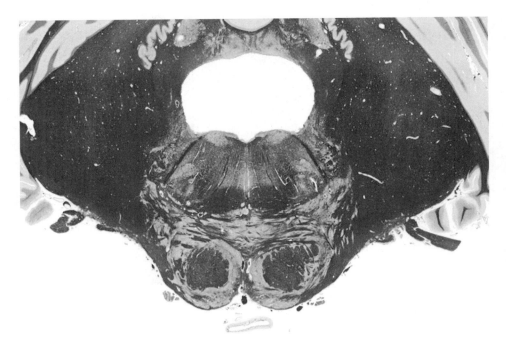

FIGURE 18.13. *Histologic section of lower pons.*

Q18.7. Many systems intersect at the lower level of the pons. In Figure 18.13 identify:
- Abducens nucleus
- Abducens nerve (VI)
- Facial nerve (VII)
- Vestibulocochlear nerve (VIII)
- Facial nucleus
- Superior olivary nucleus
- Fastigial nucleus
- Emboliform nucleus
- Globus nucleus
- Dentate nucleus

A18.7. *See Figure 18.14.*

Q18.8. The medulla is a mine field of structures. Identify the follow in Figure 18.15:
- Corticospinal tracts
- Inferior olivary nucleus
- Hypoglossal nucleus and nerve fibers

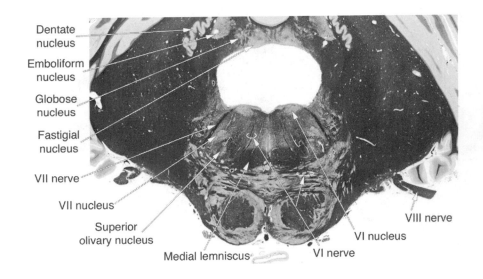

FIGURE 18.14. *Salient structures at the lower pontine level.*

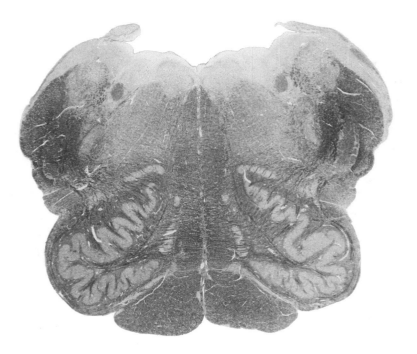

FIGURE 18.15. *Histologic section of the medulla at the level of the hypoglossal nucleus.*

- Medial lemniscus
- Solitary tract
- Nucleus of solitary tract
- Dorsal motor nucleus of vagus
- Inferior cerebellar peduncle
- Spinal trigeminal nucleus and tract

A18.8. *See Figure 18.16.*

Q18.9. What general level of the spinal cord is shown in Figure 18.17? Identify these structures:

- Intermediolateral cell column
- Clarke's column
- Gracilis tract
- Corticospinal tract
- Anterior white commissure

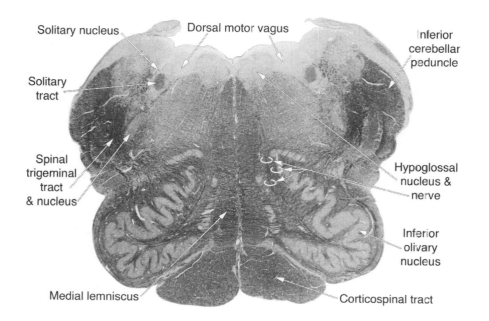

FIGURE 18.16. *A few structures in the middle medulla.*

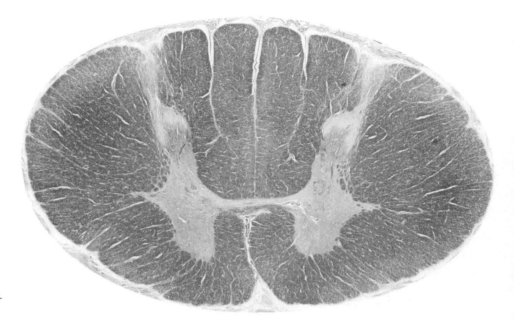

FIGURE 18.17. *Spinal cord histology.*

- Lissauer's tract
- Spinothalamic tract
- Dorsal spinocerebellar tract

A18.9. Since this figure contains the intermediolateral cell column and has small ventral horns, it must be from somewhere in the thoracic spinal cord. See Figure 18.18.

SYSTEM REVIEW

INST Below are listed several major neural systems, each accompanied by a schematic diagram of brain regions. Some of the regions are enhanced histologic sections, while others are derived from slices of brain cut in various directions. For each of the "diagrams" below, trace the pathway(s) of the specified systems from their origin to their termination. Label appropriate nuclei and tracts and indicate sites of decussation. You may find it helpful to determine the type of material (e.g., histology or gross brain), the plane of section of each image, and its orientation. Beware: the orientation of many levels is not standard!

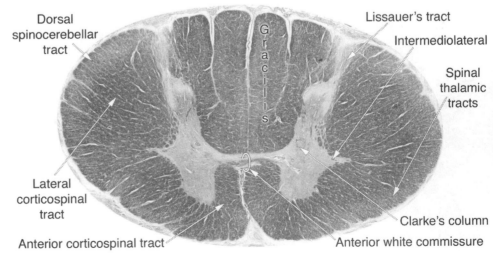

FIGURE 18.18. *Some major structures in the spinal cord.*

Ascending Spinothalamic System

Q18.10. Trace the spinothalamic system in Figure 18.19. Notice the two sections of spinal cord. Indicate the sites of the neuron cell bodies and synapses. Be cognizant of the sides. They may switch!

A18.10. *The information travels a short distance in the cord and then crosses over to the opposite side. Note that signals are transmitted to multiple levels of the brainstem, in sites involved with processing pain and temperature information. See Figure 18.20.*

Ascending Somatosensory System

Q18.11. Trace the posterior column–medial lemniscal system in Figure 18.21. Note the two levels of medulla. Indicate the sites of the neuron cell bodies, synapses, decussations, and final projection.

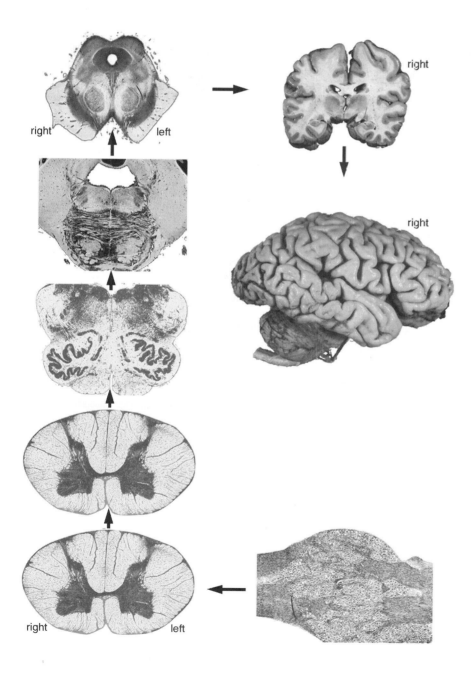

FIGURE 18.19. Spinothalamic worksheet.

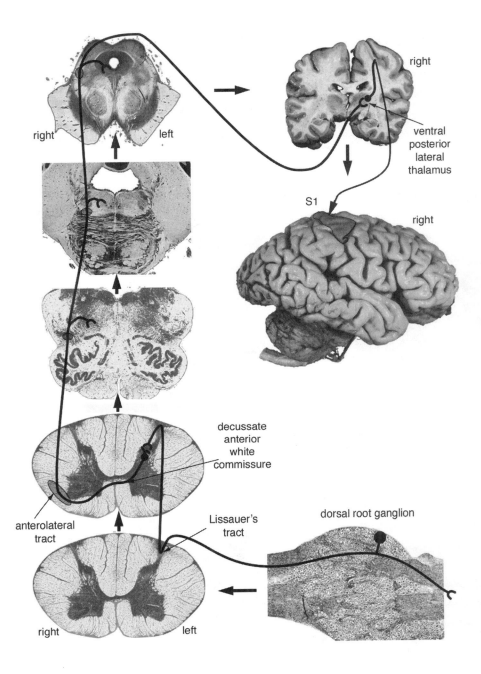

FIGURE 18.20. *Ascending spinoth-alamic fiber pathways.*

A18.11. Somatosensory information ascends ipsilaterally in the cord and crosses in the lower medulla. The medial lemniscus moves progressively more lateral up through the brain stem to the ventral posterior lateral thalamic nucleus. See Figure 18.22.

Trigeminothalamic System

Q18.12. Trace the trigeminal pain and temperature system in Figure 18.23. Note the several levels of medulla; use these to differentiate the tract, nucleus, and rostral projection.

A18.12. Pain and temperature information from the face has its "dorsal root ganglion" neuron cell bodies in the trigeminal ganglion. The signals enter the brain in the middle of the pons, then descend ipsilaterally into the medulla and upper most spinal cord, where they synapse in the spinal trigeminal nucleus. From there the impulses cross to the opposite side, join up with the spinothalamic fibers from the body, and ascend in the lateral medulla. More rostrally, they become juxtaposed to the medial lemniscus prior to entering the thalamus. See Figure 18.24.

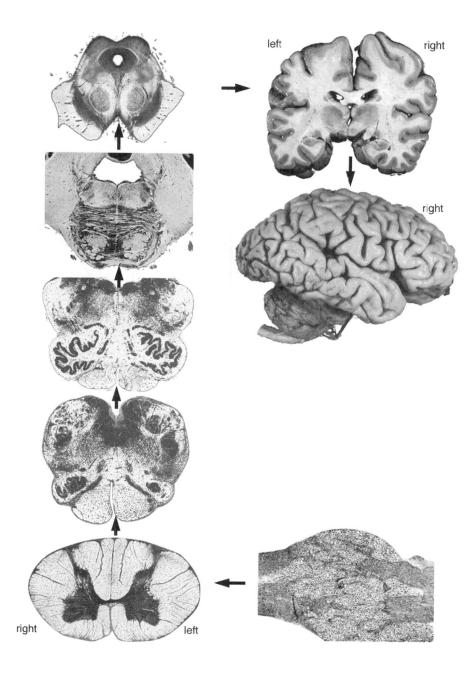

FIGURE 18.21. *Posterior column–medial lemniscal system worksheet.*

Trigeminal Somatosensory System

Q18.13. Indicate the pathways and nuclei of the trigeminal lemniscal system in Figure 18.25. Be cognizant of the side and orientation.

A18.13. The decussation of facial somatosensory information occurs in the pons, near the level of the principal trigeminal sensory nucleus. This information joins up with the medial lemniscus but still maintains its somatotopy. From the upper pons to the thalamus, the sensory homunculus is a person lying down, with their feet pointed lateral and head medial. See Figure 18.26.

Visual System

Q18.14. In Figure 18.27, trace the visual pathway from the left visual field (horizontal view from above) to the primary visual cortex. Indicate the proper input layer of cortex. Note that the lower part of the figure is a split view of occipital cortex, showing both a sagittal (left) and a coronal (right) view. Trace the pathway to each view.

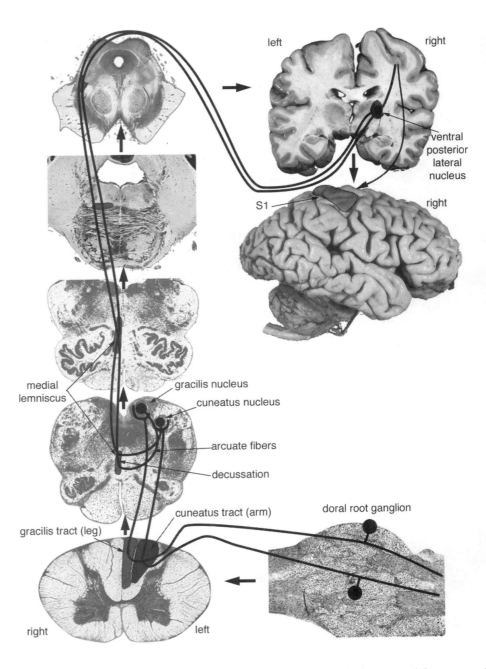

left   right

ventral
posterior
lateral
nucleus

S1   right

medial lemniscus   gracilis nucleus

cuneatus nucleus

arcuate fibers

decussation

doral root ganglion

cuneatus tract (arm)

gracilis tract (leg)

right   left

FIGURE 18.22. Posterior column–medial lemniscal fiber pathways.

A18.14. The homonymous fields project to the contralateral sides of the both retina and thence onward to the ipsilateral lateral geniculate nucleus and primary visual cortex. The upper visual field projects to the lower retina, which later passes through the optic radiations in the temporal lobe. In contrast, the lower visual field takes the "high road" through the parietal lobe. See Figure 18.28.

Auditory System

Q18.15. In Figure 18.29, start from the left external ear (viewed from below) and trace the pathway to the primary auditory cortex. Be cognizant of the sides. Indicate whether the pathways are ipsilateral, contralateral, or bilateral. Name the pertinent sites of synapses.

A18.15. Hearing has extensive bilateral projections, only a few of which are shown here. For this reason unilateral lesions to the auditory system beyond the cochlear nucleus do not produce deafness. See Figure 18.30. Also, most sounds reach both ears, so patients may not even recognize a unilateral loss.

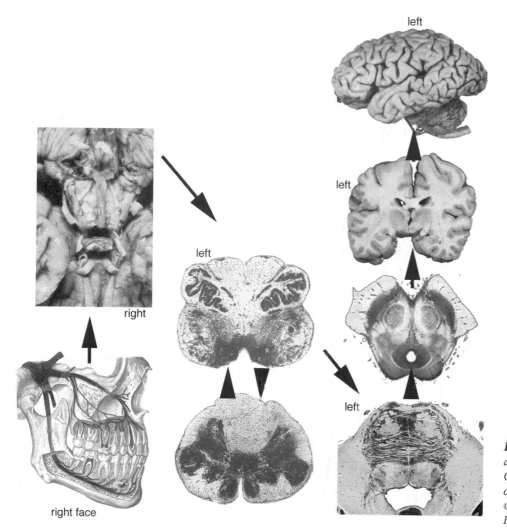

FIGURE 18.23. (Trigeminal nerve diagram modified from C. D. Clemente, Anatomy A Regional Atlas of the Human Body, 3rd edition, © 1987, Urban & Schwarzenberg, Baltimore and Munich, figure 696.)

Corticospinal System

Q18.16. Trace the corticospinal pathway from the cortex to the lower motor neurons in Figure 18.31. Indicate sides, sites of decussation, and locations of synapses. Pay attention to the orientation of the images.

A18.16. These long fibers originate in the motor cortex of the frontal lobes. Most of the fibers cross at the cervicomedullary junction. Uncrossed fibers project bilaterally to more medial muscle groups, while the lateral, crossed fibers project to lateral groups. See Figure 18.32.

Cerebellar Systems

Q18.17. Draw the main cerebellar connections from the dorsal root ganglion to the cerebral cortex in Figure 18.33. Separately superimpose the corticospinal tracts from the previous exercise. Pay attention to the sides and the orientations of the specimens. Use separate colors for ascending and descending tracts. Let the dentate nucleus represent all of the deep nuclei.

A18.17. The cerebellar system has several "double cross" subsystems. The main one indicated here is the spino-cerebellar-dentate-thalamus-cortex-pyramidal tract-lower motor neuron pathway. Many details; understand the general principle of the double cross. Others double crossed systems also exist but are not covered here. The ascending tracts are thick while the descending tracts are thin. See Figure 18.34.

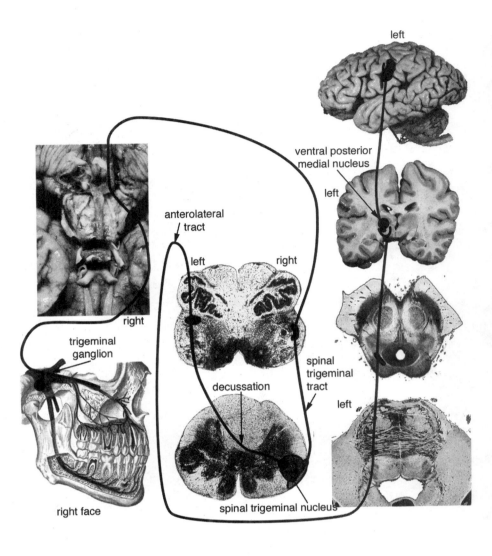

left

ventral posterior
medial nucleus

left

anterolateral
tract

left   right

trigeminal
ganglion

spinal
trigeminal
tract

decussation

left

right

spinal trigeminal nucleus

right face

FIGURE 18.24. (*Trigeminal nerve diagram modified from C. D. Clemente, Anatomy A Regional Atlas of the Human Body, 3rd edition, © 1987, Urban & Schwarzenberg, Baltimore and Munich, figure 696.*)

Basal Ganglia Circuits

Q18.18. In Figure 18.35 use one side to label the main nuclei. On the other side, draw a simplified "wiring diagram" for the basal ganglia. Indicate whether the connections are inhibitory or excitatory and the main transmitters used.

A18.18. *Glutamate is the principal excitatory neurotransmitter while GABA is the inhibitory one. Dopamine (DA) both facilitates and inhibits transmission in target neurons via their D1 and D2 receptors, respectively. The main inputs (cortex) and outputs (thalamus) of the system are excitatory, but among the deep nuclei only the subthalamic output is excitatory. See Figure 18.36.*

Any diagram such as this one must, of necessity, be inaccurate and only roughly models the true complexity of nature.

Cortical Integration

Q18.19. Label the major functional cortical areas (unimodal, etc.) delineated in Figure 18.37. Indicate the major functions of the selected areas (vision, motor, etc.). (Abbreviations: tp: temporal pole; ins: insula; ph: parahippocampal gyrus; of: olfactory area; hip: hippocampus.)

A18.19. *See Figure 18.38. Primary cortical areas are primary visual (v1), primary somatosensory (s1), primary auditory (a1), and primary motor (m1). Unimodal association cortices are the visual (va), somatosensory (sa), motor (ma), and auditory (aa). Other functional cortical types are multimodal cortices (Mul), paralimbic (PL), and limbic (L).*

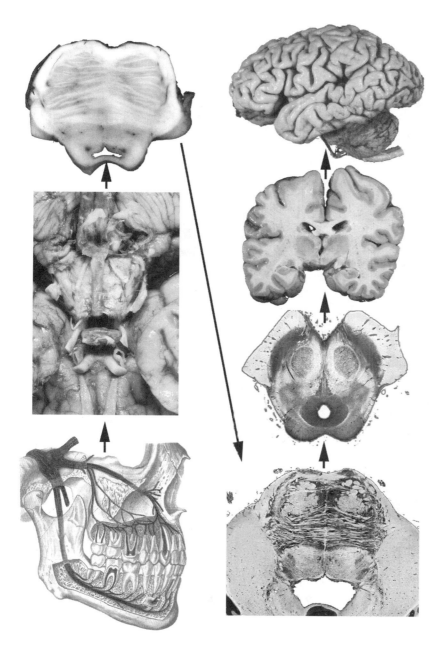

FUNCTIONAL ANATOMY REVIEW

Q18.20. Examine Figure 18.39. In what plane has the brain been dissected? Name some nearby anatomic sites. Where it the pathology? In what vascular territory?

A18.20. This is a coronal section. The patient underwent a falcine meningioma resection but developed vasospasm as a complication. This produced a bilateral, but not precisely symmetric hemorrhagic infarction in both anterior cerebral artery territories. Nearby anatomic sites include the corpus callosum, both cingulate gyri and the cingulum bundle, as well as the corona radiata (involving some of the internal capsule fibers).

Q18.21. What may have been some of the patient's clinical symptomatology?

A18.21. This patient became abulic, and showed a total disinterest in his environment. The patient also had bilateral leg weakness, due to the more posterior extension of this infarction into the medial leg motor areas. He also seemed unconcerned about his poor bladder control.

Review the anterior cerebral vascular territories and the limbic system. Select lesions of only the anterior circulation are uncommon.

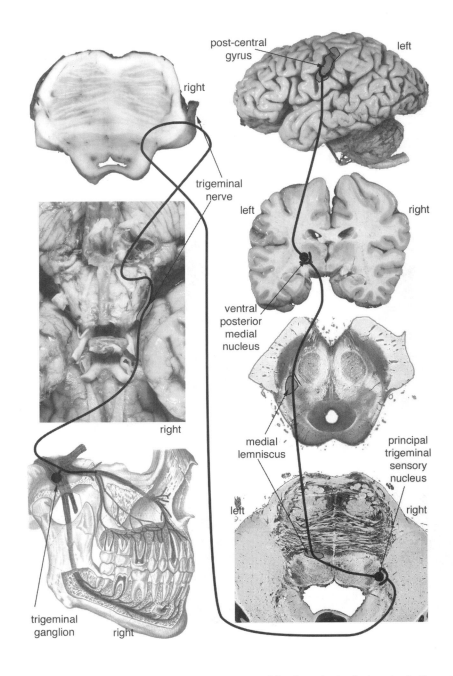

FIGURE 18.26. (Trigeminal nerve diagram modified from C. D. Clemente, Anatomy A Regional Atlas of the Human Body, 3rd edition, © 1987, Urban & Schwarzenberg, Baltimore and Munich, figure 696.)

Q18.22. Examine closely Figure 18.40. Orient yourself. Where is the lesion, including side? Can you tell what level this is? Does the lesion "fit" a vascular territory? Is it well-circumscribed?

A18.22. *The metastatic tumor occupies most of the patient's left midbrain but spares the cerebral peduncle. The level of this slice is ambiguous (but not ambiguus!), but it seems to be above the superior cerebellar peduncle decussation and just below the red nucleus.*

Q18.23. Name several of this patient's clinical findings.

A18.23. *The third nerve exits at this level, so you would expect the patient to have at least a left oculomotor palsy (left eye abducted and rotated). In addition, since the cerebellar output from at least the right cerebellum (it's above the decussation) has been interrupted, you would expect right cerebellar findings (right ataxia, dysmetria).*

Given the size of this mass, it is likely that it impinged on additional structures and produced other symptomatology, including right-sided weakness (due to compression of the left cerebral peduncle) and probably coma (due to interruption of the ascending diffuse system fibers from the locus ceruleus, raphe nucleus, substantia nigra, and lateral midbrain cholinergic fibers).

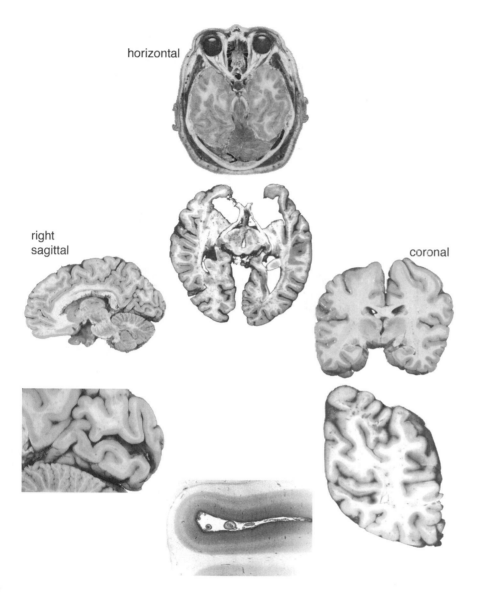

horizontal

right
sagittal

coronal

FIGURE 18.27. Visual system worksheet. (Upper image adapted from the Visible Human Project at the National Library of Medicine (http://www.nlm.nih.gov/research/visible/visible_human.html) using the Head Browser designed at the University of Michigan.)

Review the vascular distribution at the top of the basilar artery. At the midbrain the basilar artery essentially splits into four vessels: the two posterior cerebral arteries and the two superior cerebellar arteries. Tiny vessels branch off the top of the basilar and the early portion of the posterior cerebral artery to supply the midbrain. Also review some of the important anatomic structures in and around the midbrain, including the substantia nigra, the "reticular activating system," the dentatorubro- and dentatothalamic fibers, and the pathways of the ascending and descending fiber bundles.

Q18.24. This next patient had several neurologic complications from trauma. However, just examining the slice in Figure 18.41, what do you see? Where is the lesion (right is on the right)? Given just this slice, what would have been his major deficit?

A18.24. *While the slice shows two major areas of pathology, the lower lesion is in the right primary visual cortex, and so would have produced a left homonymous hemianopsia. The upper pathologic area is in secondary visual processing areas, but in the absence of primary information, this lesion could not be clinically evaluated.*

Review the visual pathway, from the object in space, through the lens, and through the brain.

Q18.25. Note the location of this mass lesion in Figure 18.42. Assuming its pressure effect blocks signaling (both electrical and humoral), detail what the patient's deficits and gains could have been.

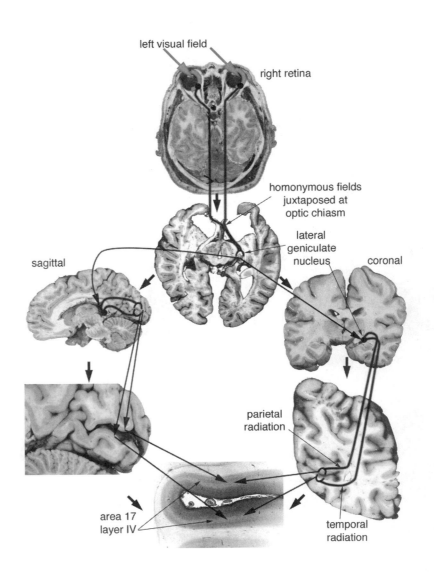

left visual field

right retina

homonymous fields
juxtaposed at
optic chiasm

lateral
geniculate
nucleus

coronal

sagittal

parietal
radiation

area 17
layer IV

temporal
radiation

FIGURE 18.28. *Visual system worksheet. (Upper image adapted from the Visible Human Project at the National Library of Medicine (http:// www.nlm.nih.gov/research/visible/ visible_human.html) using the Head Browser designed at the University of Michigan.)*

A18.25. *This tumor occupies and impinges on the pituitary stalk (it is a hypothalamic granular cell tumor). Its mass effect would block transport of vasopressin and oxytocin, and so would lead to diabetes insipidus. In addition most of the anterior pituitary function would be lost, due to disruption of the hypothalamic-pituitary portal system. This would lead to deficits in growth hormone (GH), thyroid-stimulating hormone (TSH), follicle-stimulating hormone (FSH), luteinizing hormone (LH), and adrenocorticotropin (ACTH). The patient's prolactin level would be slightly elevated, due to blockage of dopamine from the hypothalamus, and hence disinhibition of prolactin secretion.*

While it may seem mundane (unless you plan to be an endocrinologist), review the clinically important hypothalamic-pituitary axis. Specifically review:

- *The adenohypophysis, its portal system, and the role of the hypothalamus in pituitary hormone secretion*
- *How prolactin secretion differs from other pituitary hormones (dopamine inhibition)*
- *The neurohypophysis, its neurotransmitters, and how its control differs from the adenohypophysis*
- *The regional anatomy around the hypothalamus, including the chiasm and vessels*

Q18.26. Examine Figure 18.43 (left is on right). Where is the lesion? What is it? Described the involved structures.

A18.26. *The pontine hemorrhage has obliterated the patient's left pontine tegmentum and smaller portions of the base. It has destroyed this patient's left medial lemniscus and left spinothalamic fibers, as well as the left trigeminal primary sensory nucleus. This patient previously suffered from uncontrolled hypertension.*

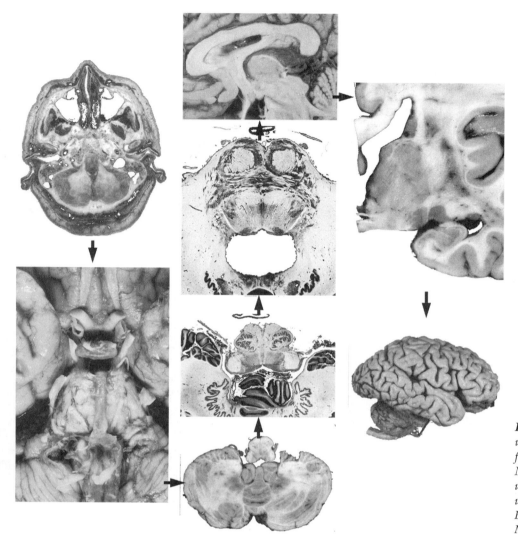

FIGURE 18.29. *Auditory system worksheet. (Upper left image adapted from the Visible Human Project at the National Library of Medicine (http://www.nlm.nih.gov/research/visible/visible_human.html) using the Head Browser designed at the University of Michigan.)*

Q18.27. Assuming you could give this person an accurate sensory examination, what would you find? Be specific to side. What might you expect on motor testing?

A18.27. *The patient would have lost both pain and temperature as well as proprioceptive and vibration sensation from the contralateral or right side of the body, since both of these tracts cross below this level (spinothalamic fibers in the cord and posterior column fibers in the medulla). In addition sensation from the ipsilateral or left face would have been eliminated. Since the left trigeminal motor nucleus lies in this area, the patient would be unable to produce force for chewing on the left side (ipsilateral).*

    Other more minor motor findings might include a right partial paralysis (involvement of descending corticospinal fibers), perhaps left face weakness (left seventh nerve nucleus, below this level) and perhaps an intranuclear ophthalmoplegia from involvement of the left medial longitudinal fasciculus. Clinically the patient had a rapid onset of coma and was obtunded by the time he reached the emergency ward.

    This is a good time to review the sensory pathways in the brainstem. The two major ascending pathways, the spinothalamic and medial lemniscal pathways, become juxtaposed to each other in the pons, which means that the dissociated sensory deficits that are characteristic of focal lesions in the spinal cord and medulla would now be extremely rare. The primary sensory and motor nuclei of the trigeminal system also lie in the pontine tegmentum about a third of the way up the pons, while the pain and temperature spinotrigeminal nucleus lies mostly in the medulla.

Q18.28. Examine the pair of images in Figure 18.44. What type of scan are they? How can you tell if they are enhanced or not? Where is the lesion? Describe as accurately as

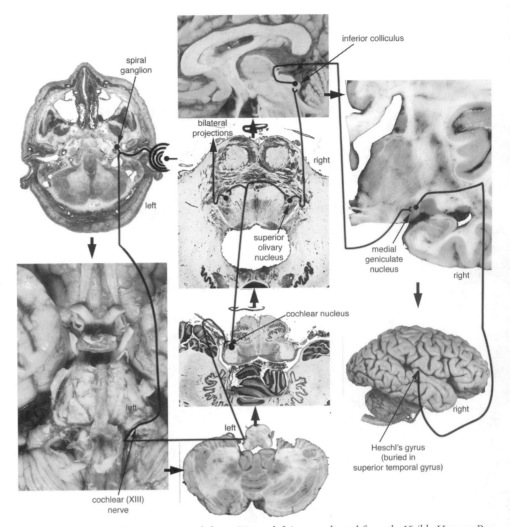

FIGURE 18.30. *Auditory system worksheet. (Upper left image adapted from the Visible Human Project at the National Library of Medicine (http://www.nlm.nih.gov/research/visible/visible_human.html) using the Head Browser designed at the University of Michigan.)*

you can the involved structures and brain regions. What would be the most likely tumor?

A18.28. These are contrast-enhanced CT scans. With CT scans, contrast can be near the same apparent density as bone, so it is important to compare them with nonenhanced images. In this case small vessels in the brain, especially along the meningeal surface, show signal, indicating they are enhanced with contrast.

The lesion is in the left parietal white matter and extends across the corpus callosum to the contralateral deep white matter. While most such tumors crossing the corpus callosum and showing ring-enhancement would be glioblastoma (a high-grade astroglial tumor), this case was a primary central nervous system lymphoma. Only glial tumors and primary lymphoma show such extensive infiltration of brain parenchyma.

Q18.29. Describe several deficits you might predict, based on these scans.

A18.29. The massive amount of tumor in the left parietal lobe impinged on the optic radiation between the lateral geniculate nucleus and the primary visual cortex, which produced a right homonymous hemianopsia. The patient also had impaired stereognosis on the right, from the tumor's effect on the primary and supplementary somatosensory cortex on the left. More interestingly, he was unable to read or name faces, although he could write letters and spell words. The tumor destroyed the patient's splenium of the corpus callosum, so information from his left visual field in his right visual cortex could not transmit to the left speech area. Since he had a right hemianopsia, no visual information about language could reach his speech area, and he was thus unable to read. Although the mass did not reach to his fusiform gyrus, his ability

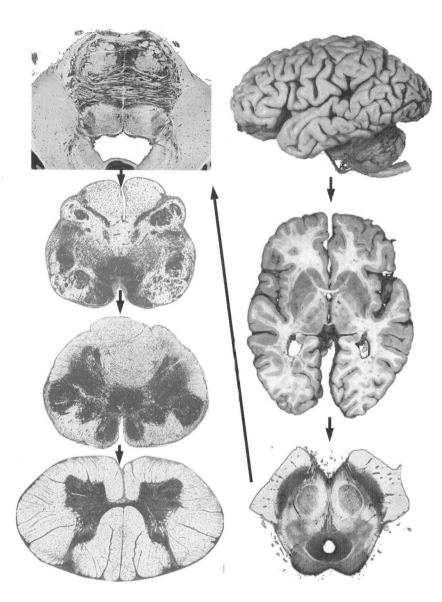

FIGURE 18.31. *Corticospinal pathway worksheet.*

to name faces was also impaired by the same mechanisms (no right visual information from left-sided mass, inability to send crossing information from right fusiform gyrus through the involved corpus callosum). Other languages functions were relatively preserved. Make some simple diagrams to try to illustrate to yourself the pathways involved and the reasons for his deficits.

Q18.30. Examine the scans in Figure 18.45. Indicate their type and orientation. Where is the lesion? Upon what structures does it impact? This patient's deficits evolved over several months. Predict the patient's neurologic presentation.

A18.30. *The left scan is a horizontal T1, while the right is an enhanced coronal (T1 plus gadolinium). Look at the vessels to determine if it is enhanced. A person could not have such a mass grow rapidly; it would be incompatible with life. While the tumor shows a great deal of mass effect, including shifting the midline to the right, it produced remarkably few symptoms. The patient developed "speech difficulties" about three months prior to evaluation, including paraphasic errors. These deficits were most certainly due to impingement on the speech areas in the left hemisphere, especially Wernicke's area. He also developed a more rapidly progressive right-sided weakness, from the tumor's compression of the descending motor tracts on the left.*

To see how the tumor produced changes further from the lesion than indicated on the Figure 18.45 scans, examine his FLAIR image in Figure 18.46. The sequence of pulses in these scans

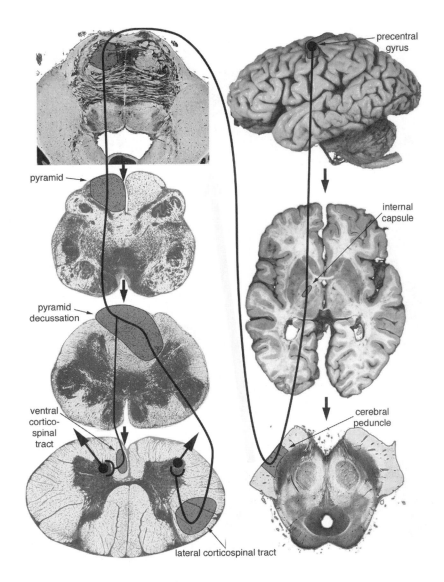

precentral gyrus

pyramid

internal capsule

pyramid decussation

ventral cortico-spinal tract

cerebral peduncle

lateral corticospinal tract

FIGURE 18.32. *Corticospinal tract pathways.*

enhances edematous tissue. You can see that the area of FLAIR abnormality is significantly greater than that of the tumor proper.

It is probable that this tumor developed edema relatively recently, and hence produced this patient's more rapid onset of weakness than of language deficits. Of note, after resection, almost all of his neurologic deficits resolved. He remains tumor-free after four years.

Two points are of note. First the brain has a surprising, but not infinite, capacity to accommodate to slowly growing masses. Most meningiomas grow slowly. However, secondary factors may precipitate a rapid onset of symptoms in an otherwise slowly growing neoplasm. For example, if the tumor slowly compresses and then obstructs a vessel, the neurologic deficit may appear relatively rapidly. Second, usually the initial neurologic symptoms and signs are greater than in subsequent follow-up after medically decreasing the edema. Most types of lesions produce some surrounding edema, which itself can block transmission of signals and produce deficits.

Q18.31. The scans in Figure 18.47 are from a 16-year-old girl with a known history of Gorlin's syndrome. What type of scans are they? Orientations? Where is the lesion?

A18.31. *The left scan is an enhanced horizontal T1 MRI, while the right is a similar type but in a sagittal orientation. The lesion is in the cerebellum, mostly in the vermis, but it also involves a bit of the medial left hemisphere.*

Q18.32. Why is the ventricular system dilated? Predict what would have been her presenting deficits. What is the most likely tumor type?

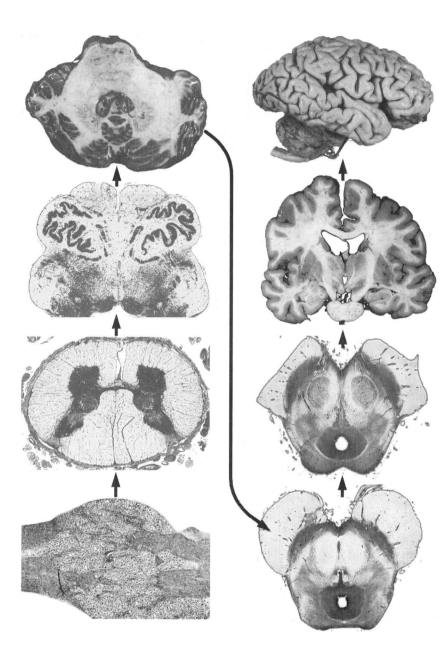

FIGURE 18.33. *Cerebellar system worksheet.*

A18.32. *Note the dilatation of both her temporal horns and her fourth ventricle. This implies that the exit from the fourth ventricle through the foramina of Magendie and Luschka are obstructed. The aqueduct appears in the sagittal view. You would predict that she would be ataxic and have demonstrable dysmetria on examination. However, these were not elicited. Her main complaints were headache, nausea, and vomiting, presumably due to her acute hydrocephalus.*

You may never see a patient with Gorlin's syndrome. Another name for this syndrome is multiple basal cell carcinoma syndrome. The patient had already had several basal cell "nevi" removed. This syndrome is associated with medulloblastoma, which was the type of tumor she had in her vermis. Although this syndrome is rare, you will certainly encounter patients with other rare syndromes, including those associated with cancer.

This is a good time to review the flow of the cerebral spinal fluid and the sites that can produce hydrocephalus.

Q18.33. Figure 18.48 is a histologic image of the spinal cord from a man who had metastatic breast carcinoma to the spine. It has been stained for myelin (black). From what level was this section taken? Where is the pathology? Be as specific as possible.

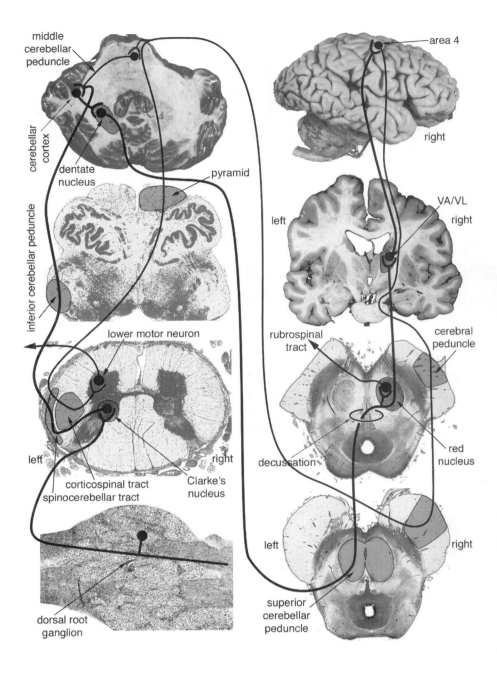

FIGURE 18.34. Cerebellar systems.

A18.33. This lumbar section of cord shows myelin pallor in both lateral corticospinal tracts and some pallor in the posterior columns, especially the medial aspects.

Q18.34. How can you explain the loss of the lateral corticospinal tracts? The loss in the posterior columns? Predict this patient's neurologic deficits.

A18.34. The patient had a pathologic fracture of a thoracic vertebral body, which lead to a spinal cord compression injury. The loss in the lateral cortical spinal tracts represents Wallerian degeneration of these fibers distal to the lesion. He developed paraplegia after this fracture. The pallor in the posterior columns cannot be explained by his thoracic fracture, since this is proximal to the lesion. This latter Wallerian degeneration is most likely due to a peripheral neuropathy, since it involves the medial fibers more than the lateral. It is these medial fibers that have the longest path in the body. The type of neuropathy is undetermined; it is typical of diabetic neuropathy or a chemotherapeutic toxic axonal neuropathy. In any case, the loss of fibers in the posterior columns would produce a loss of proprioceptive, light touch, and vibration sense in the lower limbs.

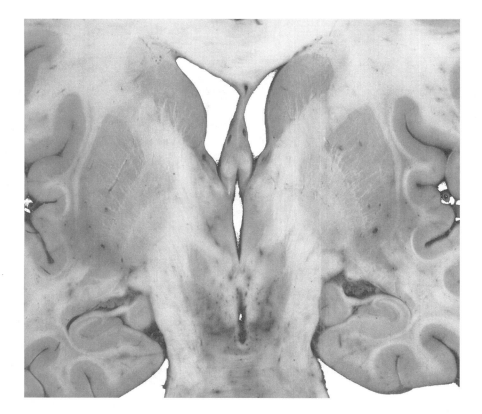

FIGURE 18.35. *Basal ganglia circuit worksheet.*

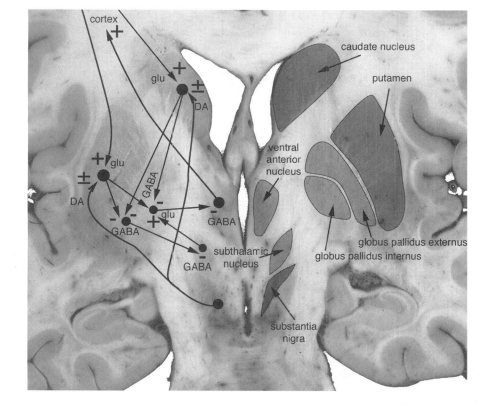

FIGURE 18.36. *"Simplified" version of the basal ganglia circuitry.*

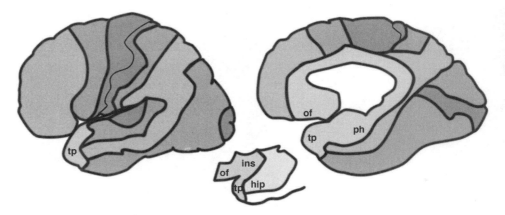

FIGURE 18.37. *Functional cortical division worksheet.*

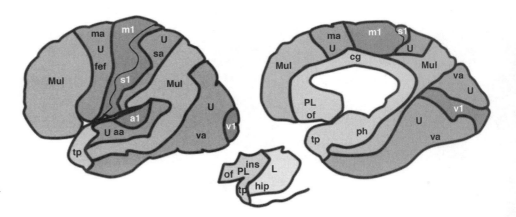

FIGURE 18.38. *Functional divisions of the cerebral cortex.*

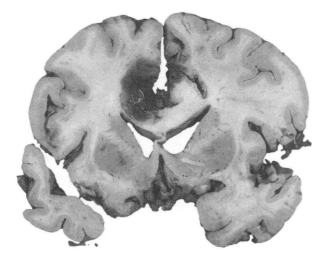

FIGURE 18.39. *Complications from falcine meningioma removal.*

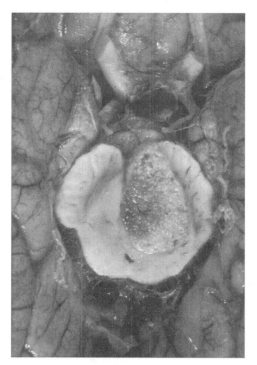

FIGURE 18.40. Mass lesion.

    The pathology of this cord is complex, since it involves two separate processes. Remember that Wallerian degeneration is distal to the lesion. This is a good time to review the structure of the spinal cord. Review the pathways and information content of the posterior columns, the corticospinal tracts, the spinothalamic tracts, and the spinocerebellar tracts. Remember how the various levels of the spinal cord differ, both histologically and functionally.

Q18.35. The pair of images in Figure 18.49 are from a patient who had fractured his spine. At what level is the spinal cord injury? Using the radiology images, draw a diagram of the anatomic distribution of his spinal cord pathology on the section of spinal cord in Figure 18.50. Beware of dorsal and ventral!

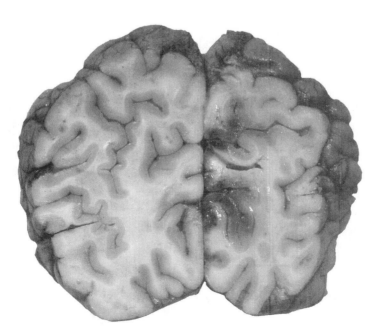

FIGURE 18.41. Trauma.

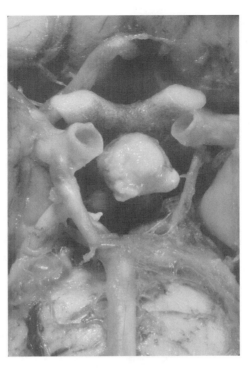

FIGURE 18.42. *Mass lesion in the base of the brain.*

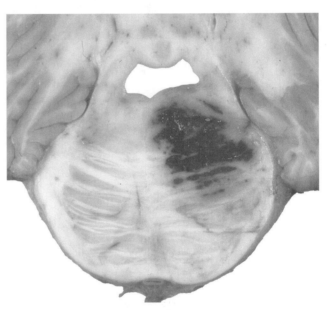

FIGURE 18.43. *Intraparenchymal hemorrhage.*

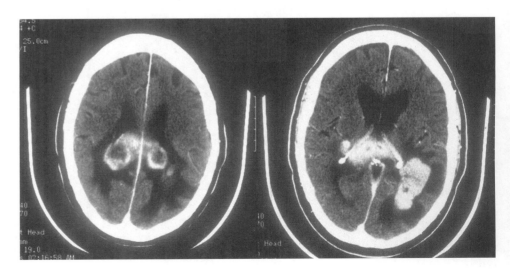

FIGURE 18.44. *Brain tumor.*

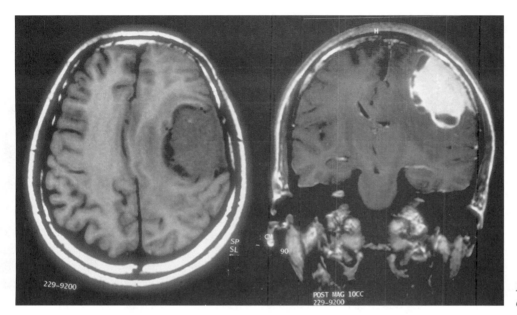

FIGURE 18.45. Tumor on surface of brain.

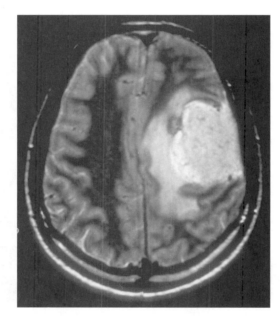

FIGURE 18.46. FLAIR sequence MRI from same patient as in Figure 18.45.

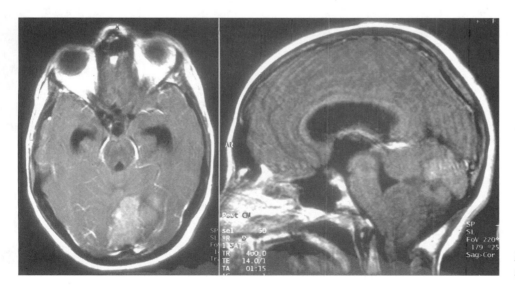

FIGURE 18.47. Tumor in Gorlin's syndrome.

487

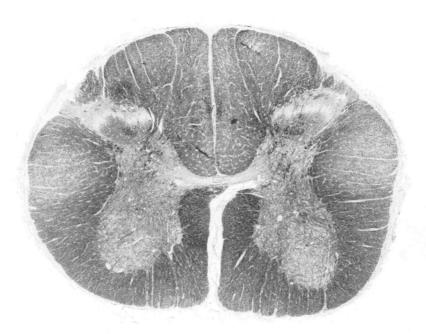

FIGURE 18.48. *Spinal cord histology from man with an aggressive breast carcinoma.*

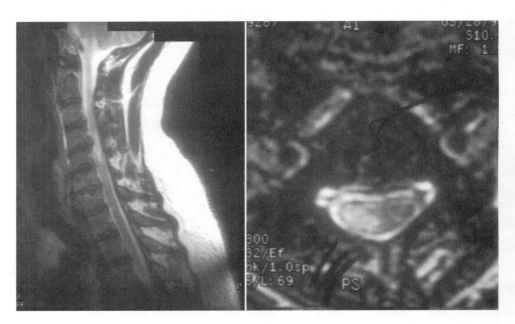

FIGURE 18.49. *Spinal cord trauma. (Kindly provided by Dr. Julian Wu, Beth Israel Deaconess Medical Center, Boston)*

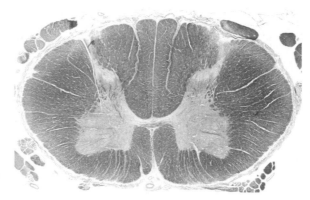

FIGURE 18.50. *Spinal cord trauma worksheet. See Figure 18.51.*

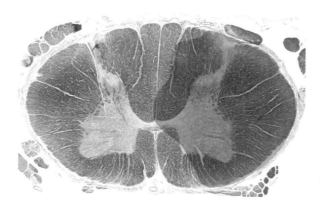

FIGURE 18.51. *Approximate distribution of spinal cord injury in Figure 18.49.*

A18.35. *The first elongated vertebrae on the left side of the cord in the sagittal image is the axis, or C2. The major cord lesion is at the lower edge of C4, so the exiting nerves would be at the C4 level. The lesion is on the right side of the patient, more or less hemisecting the C4 cord.*

  Remember that in the radiology, the cord is both upside-down and left-right inverted.

Q18.36. Detail the long tracts involved. Describe what you would expect to find on sensory and motor testing.

A18.36. *This is basically a Brown-Sequard syndrome at around the C4–C5 level. Acutely you may expect to see no function through this region of cord, due to edema from the injury. Assuming no further secondary injury occurs, the main tracts involved are on the right side and include the descending lateral corticospinal tract, the cuneatus and most of the gracilis, most of the spinothalamic tracts, a portion of the anterior white commissure, and the spinocerebellar fibers. The patient would have no right C4 sensation or movement (loss of sensation to the upper chest and back and paralysis of the trapezius and rhomboids). The patient would also be hemiplegic on the right. He would have a dissociated sensory loss below C4, with a right-sided somatosensory loss and a left-sided loss of pain and temperature sensation. The cerebellar tract symptomatology would be obscured by his hemiparesis.*

Q18.37. Examine the giant sections in Figure 18.52. The right image is a close-up from the left. First orient yourself. Which was is dorsal, which ventral, and how can you tell? Try to identify as many structures as you can. Predict the life this young man led.

A18.37. *Dorsal is up. To figure this out, look at the right side and identify the midbrain. You should be able to identify the red nucleus (R), the cerebral peduncle (CP), where the substantia nigra is (SN, not pigmented in this young man), and the lateral geniculate nucleus (LGN). Others structures you may be able to identify include the hippocampus (Hip), thalamus, and the pineal (Pin). The material labeled "Hetero" is heterotopic gray matter. Although most of this probably represents heterotopic or incompletely migrated cortex, some portions may also be basal ganglia; you would need a microscope to tell. See Figure 18.53.*

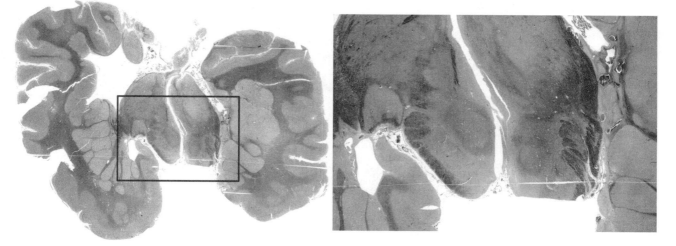

FIGURE 18.52. *Giant histologic sections from a 20-year-old institutionalized man.*

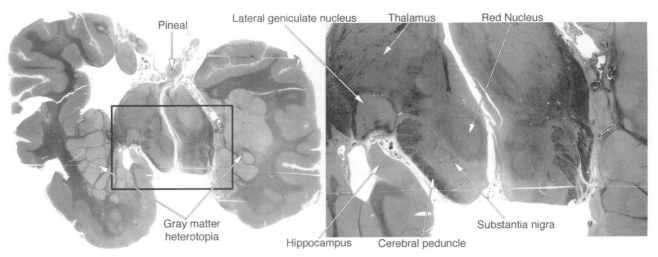

Pineal   Lateral geniculate nucleus   Thalamus   Red Nucleus

Gray matter heterotopia

Hippocampus   Cerebral peduncle   Substantia nigra

FIGURE 18.53. *Some recognizable structures in the brain from Figure 18.52.*

This patient spent most of his 20 years in an institution, unable to speak or understand language. Surprisingly, he did not have seizures. He was unable to walk but was able to travel around in a wheelchair. Although he couldn't speak, he was able to communicate his basic needs, like eating. The cause of his malformation remains unknown, but given the poorly formed dorsal areas, you may guess he lacked an early dorsalizing factor.

Q18.38. The images in Figure 18.54 and Figure 18.55 are from a 71-year-old diabetic patient who had an artificial valve replacement for a rheumatic mitral valve several years prior to her death. She was using warfarin. While in the hospital for evaluation of her nausea, she had a rapid deterioration in her neurologic condition. Where is the lesion? Be specific as to the level and the side. What fiber tracts and nuclei would have been destroyed by this lesion?

A18.38. *The hemorrhagic infarct is in the caudal left pontine base (see the external photograph to see the rostro-caudal extent). The descending corticospinal tracts pass perpendicular through this portion of the base. In addition the sixth nerve fibers pass medially from dorsal to ventral before passing out of the brainstem between the pons and the medulla. These fibers would have been interrupted by the most medial part of the lesion. The pontine base neurons projecting to the cerebellum would have been destroyed on the left side, and the vestibular and cochlear fibers and nuclei on the left would have been at least partially involved.*

Q18.39. Predict the salient features on her neurologic examination.

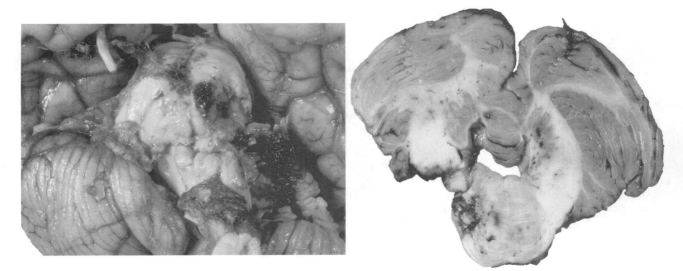

FIGURE 18.54. *Complications of diabetes and an artificial mitral valve.*

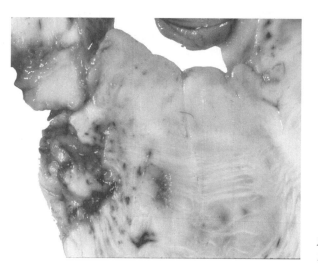

FIGURE 18.55. *Close-up of Figure 18.54.*

A18.39. *Her chart recorded that she had a right-sided upper extremity paralysis, a left sixth nerve palsy, and a Babinski sign on the left (and later on the right). She had been admitted to the hospital for nausea, which may have been secondary to a sudden loss of vestibular input on the left. From the extent of the lesion, you may also have predicted that she had lost her hearing on the left from involvement of her cochlear nuclei as well as a right-sided cerebellar ataxia (which would have been more difficult to test, given her partial right-sided paralysis).*

Q18.40. A patient had a major complication from a surgical repair of an abdominal aortic aneurysm. See Figure 18.56 for a histologic section through his spinal cord. Review the circulation to the spinal cord at this level. How could the major artery feeding the cord at this level been affected by the operation? What would have been the patient's initial symptoms?

A18.40. *This section is taken from the thoracic spinal cord (not easy to tell, except it lacks much gray matter). The lower spinal cord receives much of its blood from a single major artery. (During development most of the radicular arteries that feed the spinal cord regress, leaving only a few dominant vessels. This artery is the main vessel that feeds the lumbar and thoracic spinal cord.) Since the artery originates from the abdominal aorta, it may be injured during repairs of aneurysms in this region.*

The patient came out of anesthesia with a complete paraparesis. While you may not predict this based just on the shown pathology, an acute infarct would have produced significant edema, giving a clinically greater territory than that produced by just the infarcted tissue.

Q18.41. Describe the area involved by the infarct. What long tracts are involved? Which seemed to be spared? Given just this extent of pathology shown here, predict what would have been his long-term neurologic deficits.

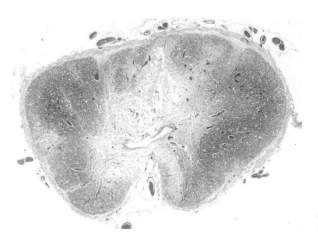

FIGURE 18.56. *Complications from an abdominal aortic aneurysm repair.*

A18.41. *The posterior columns seem to have been severely affected, at least more medially. From this you would predict that he would be unable to perceive somatosensory information below the middle thoracic level. Notice the central cord has also been destroyed. It is in this region that the spinothalamic fibers cross, so you may also anticipate a loss of pain and temperature fibers at the involved levels of the cord (thoracic), but preserved sensation both below and above the lesion. The corticospinal tract in this section is not involved, and so the patient's motor function would probably have partially returned.*

Congratulations! You're reached the end of both the chapter and the text. Good luck on your future contacts with the brain.

Appendix I—NORMAL NEUROIMAGING

The appendix contains "normal" CT and MRI scans. These represent the basics of neuroimaging; no advanced techniques are presented. Use these reference scans to compare with the various pathologic scans throughout the text.

Functional Neuroanatomy: An Interactive Text and Manual, by Jeffrey T. Joseph and David L. Cardozo
ISBN 0-471-44437-5 Copyright © 2004 John Wiley & Sons, Inc.

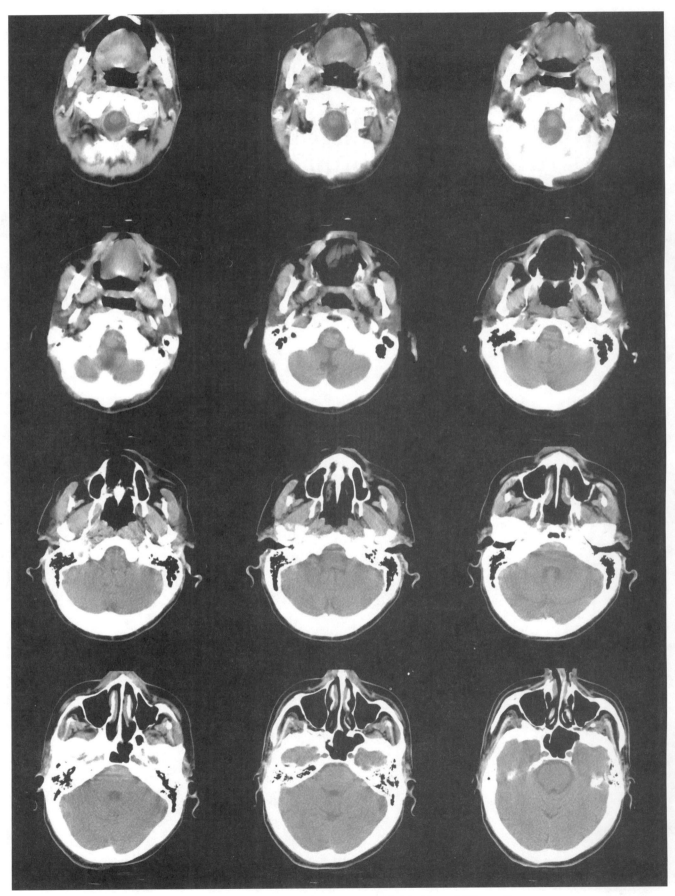

FIGURE I.1. *Normal CT, part I.*

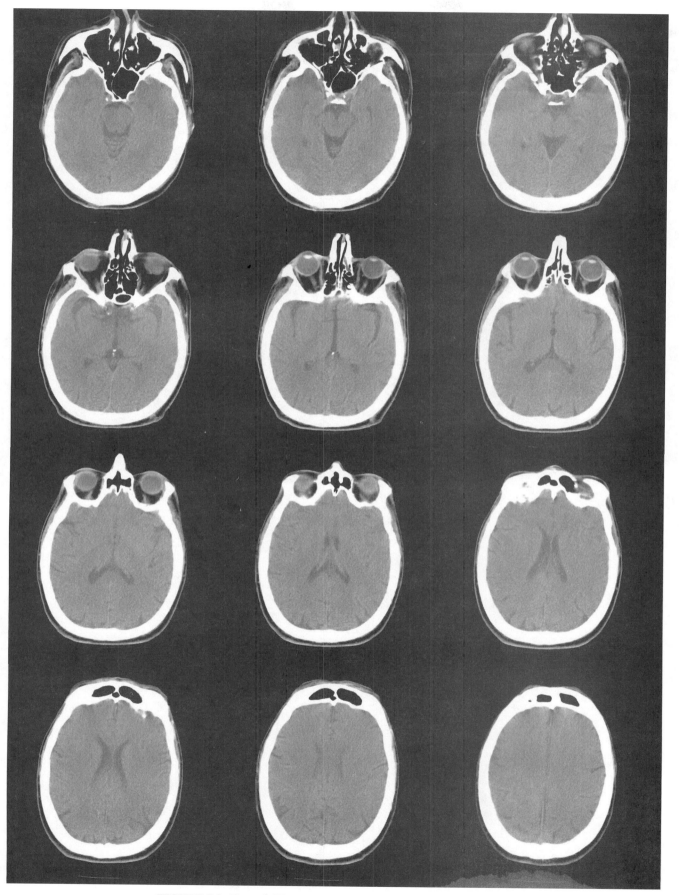

FIGURE I.2. *Normal CT, part II.*

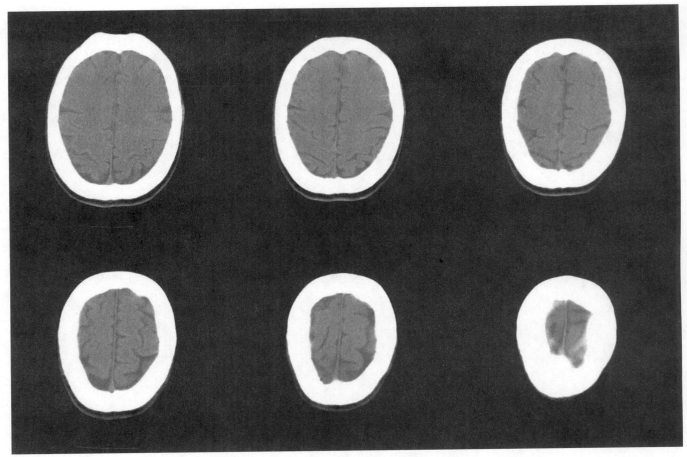

FIGURE I.3. Normal CT, part III.

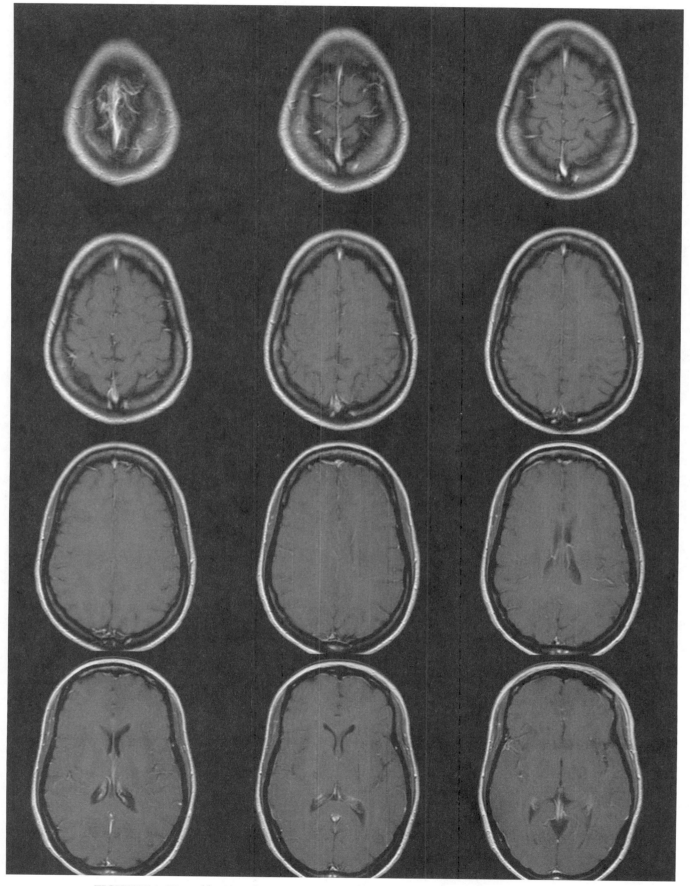

FIGURE I.4. *Normal horizontal T1 MRI (enhanced), part I.*

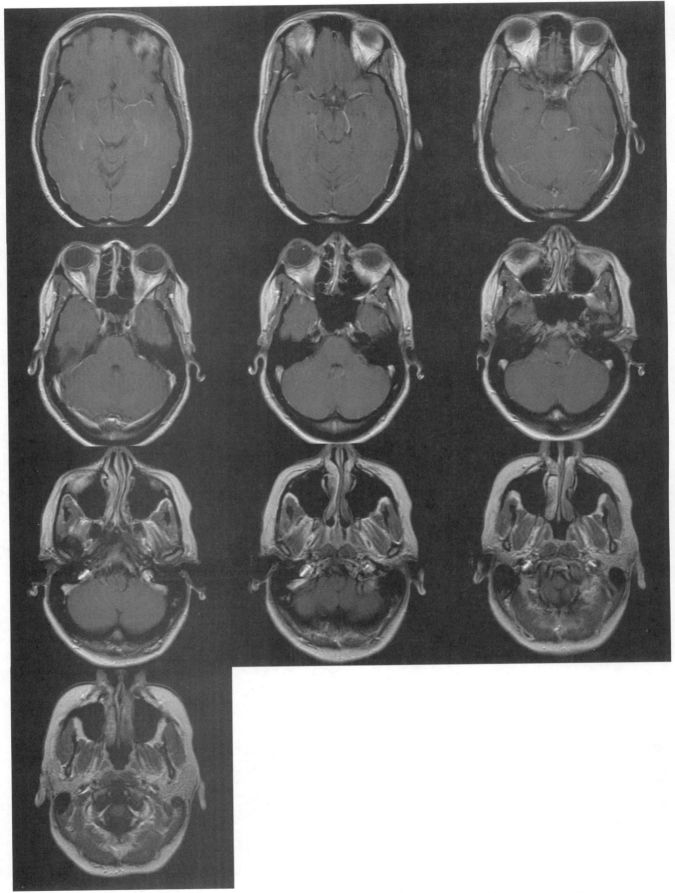

FIGURE I.5. *Normal horizontal T1 MRI (enhanced), part II.*

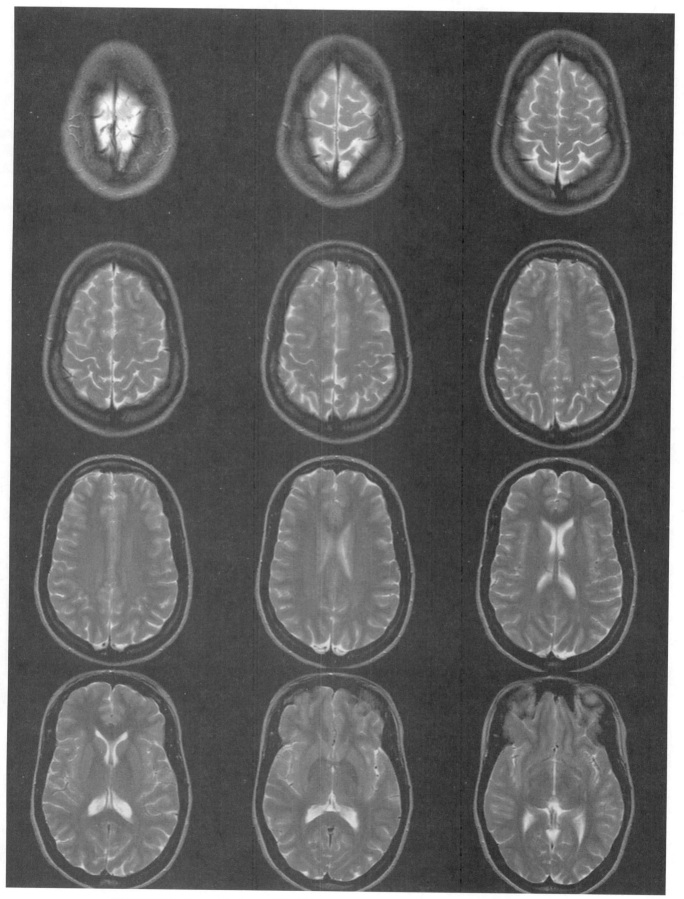

FIGURE I.6. *Normal horizontal T2 MRI scan, part I.*

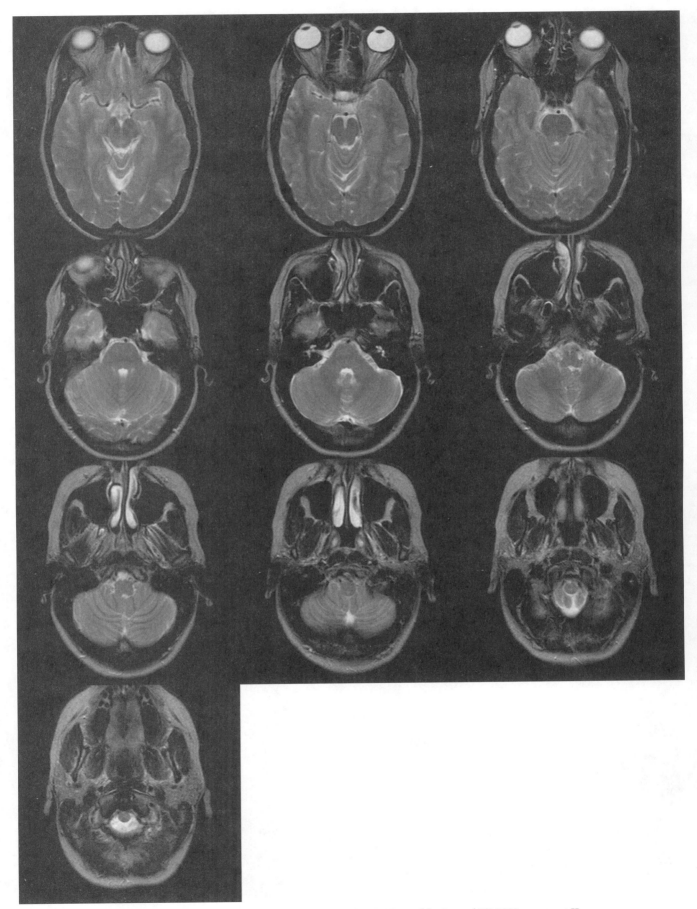

FIGURE I.7. *Normal horizontal T2 MRI scan, part II.*

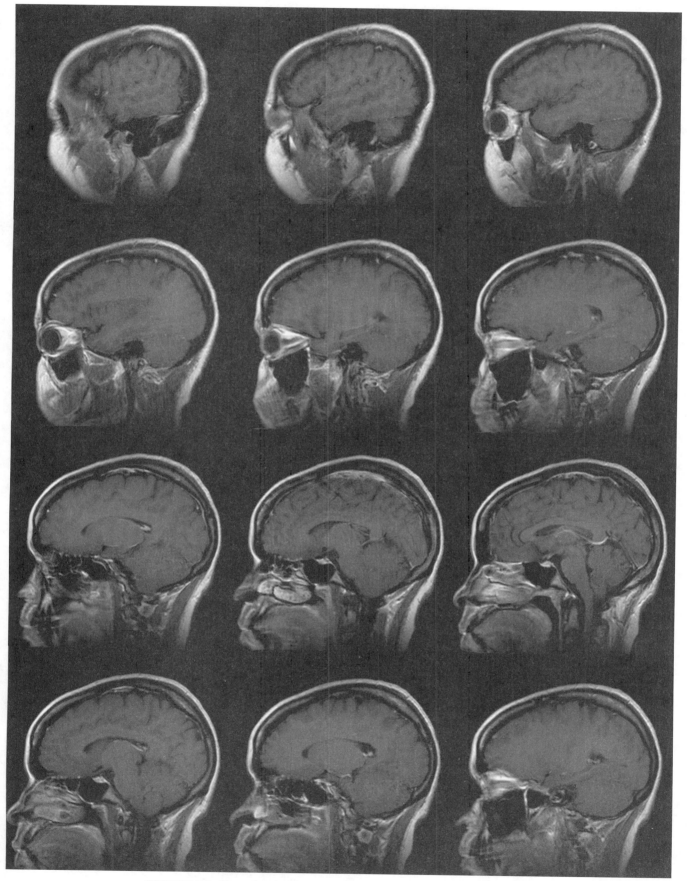

FIGURE I.8. *Normal sagittal T1 MRI.*

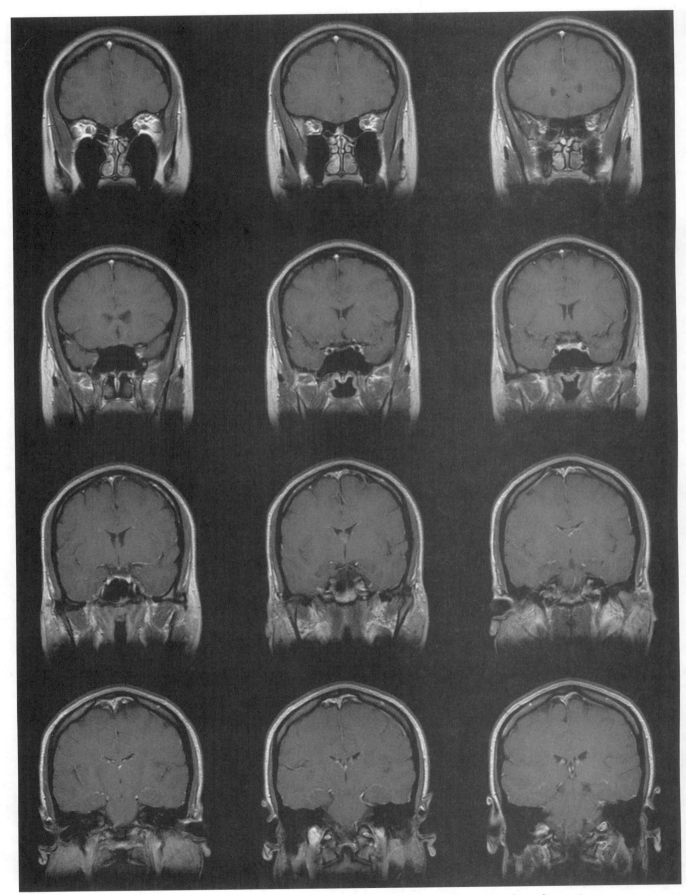

FIGURE I.9. Normal coronal T1 MRI (enhanced), part I.

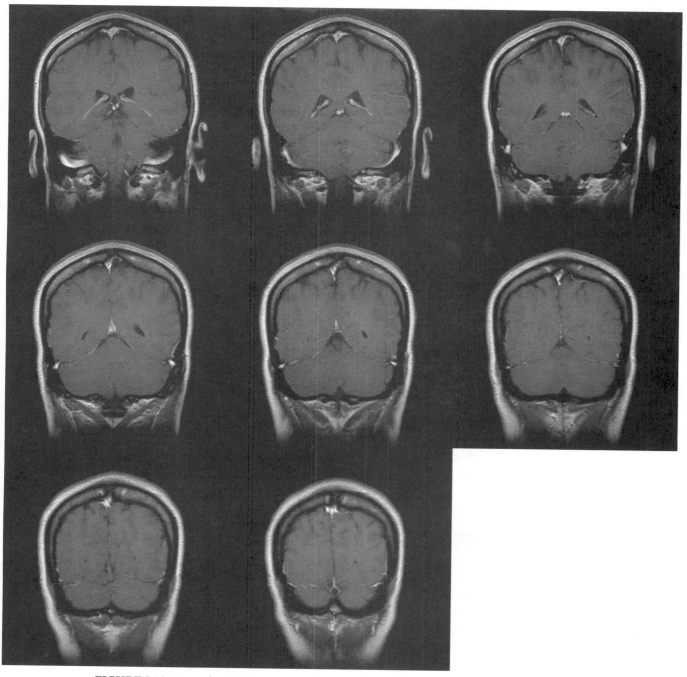

FIGURE I.10. *Normal coronal T1 MRI (enhanced), part II.*

Appendix II—BRAIN ATLAS

This appendix is a guide only for the laboratories of this text. It makes no attempt to be complete. For further neuroanatomic questions, consult more detailed atlases.

Functional Neuroanatomy: An Interactive Text and Manual, by Jeffrey T. Joseph and David L. Cardozo
ISBN 0-471-44437-5 Copyright © 2004 John Wiley & Sons, Inc.

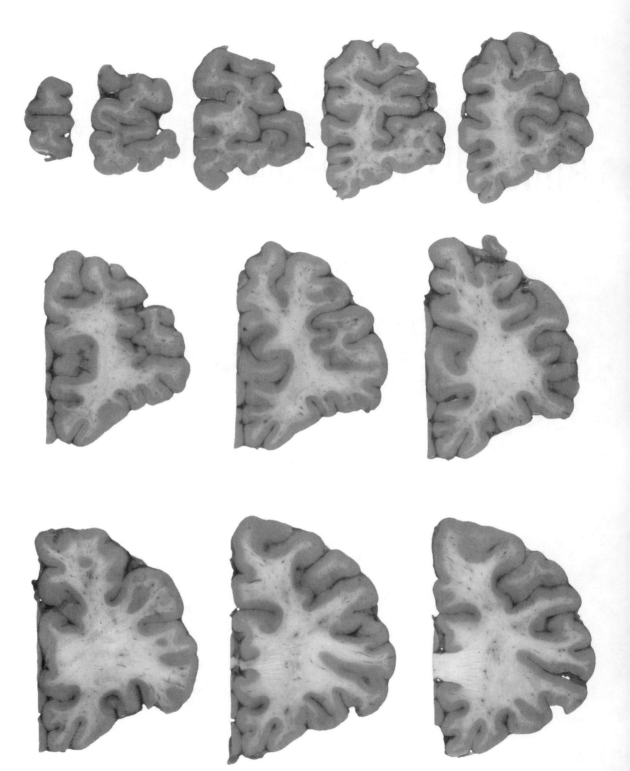

FIGURE II.1. *Coronal 1.*

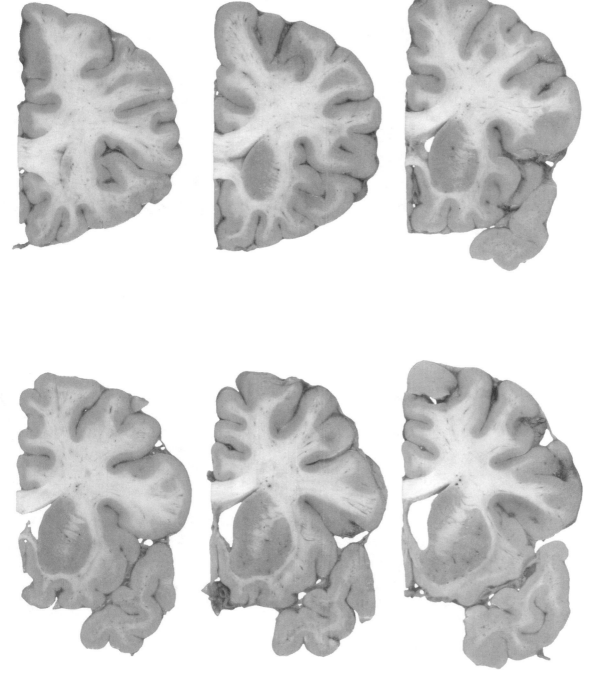

FIGURE II.2. *Coronal 2.*

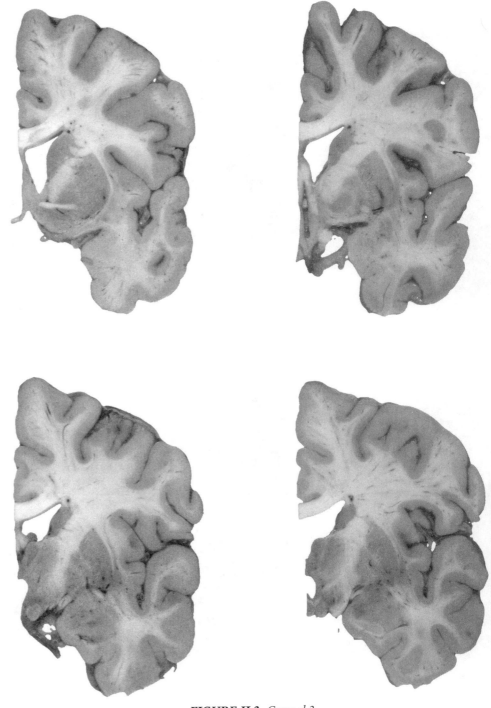

FIGURE II.3. *Coronal 3.*

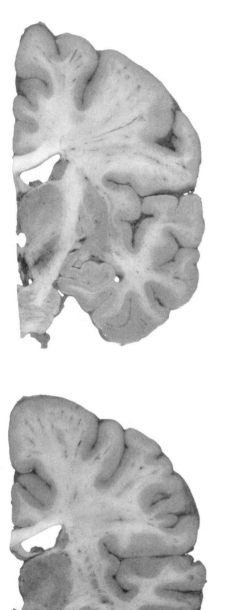
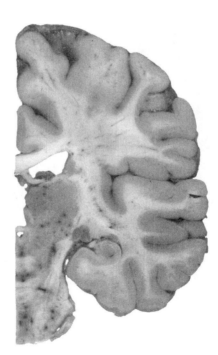

FIGURE II.4. Coronal 4.

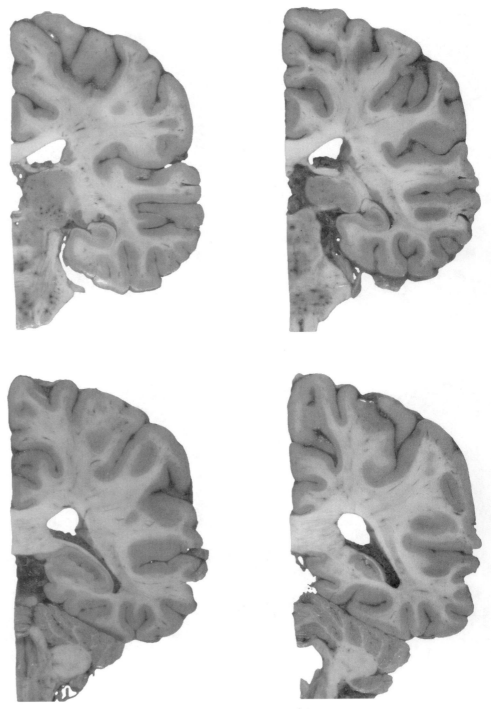

FIGURE II.5. *Coronal 5.*

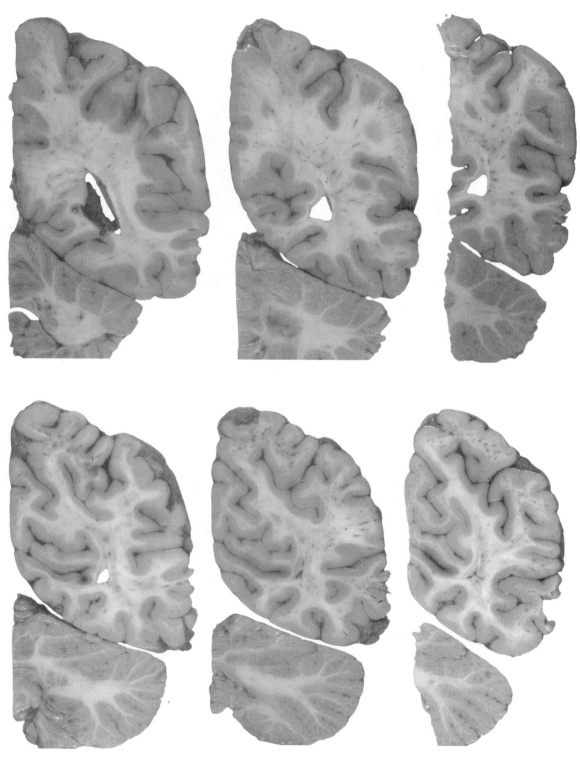

FIGURE II.6. *Coronal 6.*

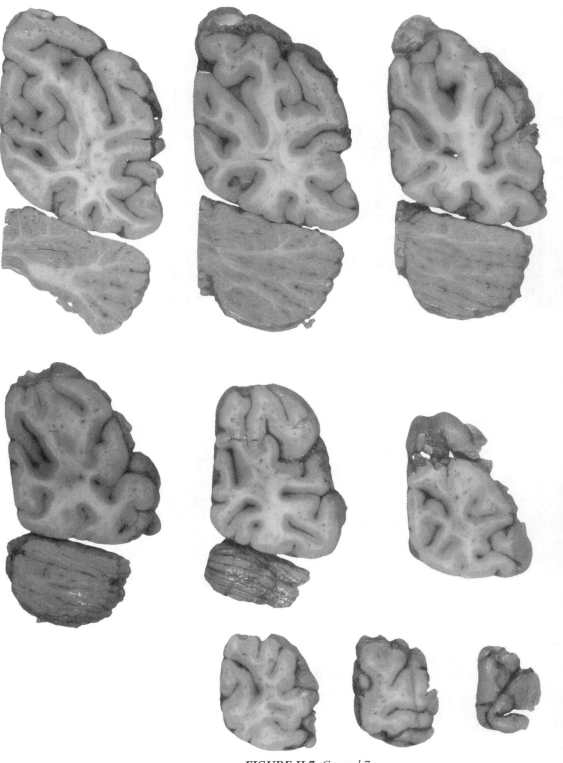

FIGURE II.7. *Coronal 7.*

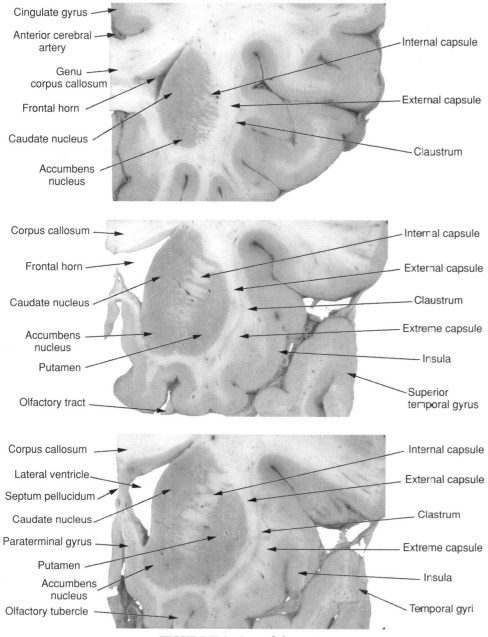

Cingulate gyrus

Anterior cerebral artery

Genu corpus callosum

Frontal horn

Caudate nucleus

Accumbens nucleus

Internal capsule

External capsule

Claustrum

Corpus callosum

Frontal horn

Caudate nucleus

Accumbens nucleus

Putamen

Olfactory tract

Internal capsule

External capsule

Claustrum

Extreme capsule

Insula

Superior temporal gyrus

Corpus callosum

Lateral ventricle

Septum pellucidum

Caudate nucleus

Paraterminal gyrus

Putamen

Accumbens nucleus

Olfactory tubercle

Internal capsule

External capsule

Clastrum

Extreme capsule

Insula

Temporal gyri

FIGURE II.8. *Coronal close-up 1.*

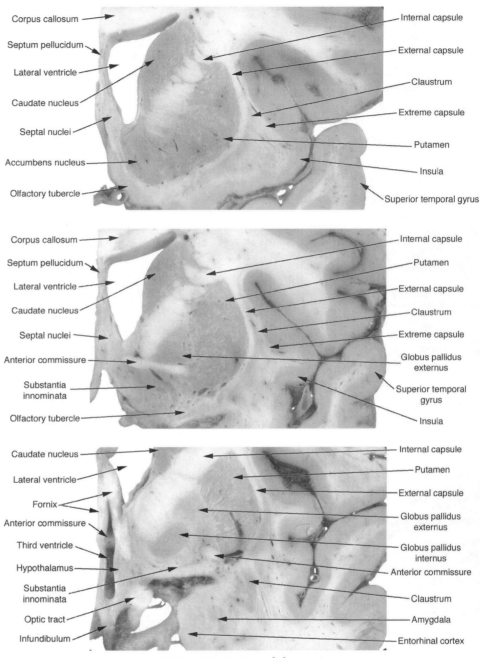

FIGURE II.9. *Coronal close-up 2.*

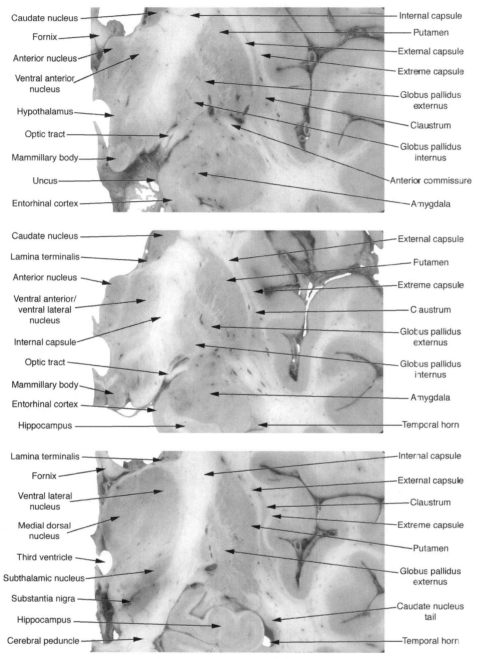

Caudate nucleus — Internal capsule
Fornix — Putamen
Anterior nucleus — External capsule
Ventral anterior nucleus — Extreme capsule
Hypothalamus — Globus pallidus externus
Optic tract — Claustrum
Mammillary body — Globus pallidus internus
Uncus — Anterior commissure
Entorhinal cortex — Amygdala

Caudate nucleus — External capsule
Lamina terminalis — Putamen
Anterior nucleus — Extreme capsule
Ventral anterior/ventral lateral nucleus — Claustrum
Internal capsule — Globus pallidus externus
Optic tract — Globus pallidus internus
Mammillary body — Amygdala
Entorhinal cortex —
Hippocampus — Temporal horn

Lamina terminalis — Internal capsule
Fornix — External capsule
Ventral lateral nucleus — Claustrum
Medial dorsal nucleus — Extreme capsule
Third ventricle — Putamen
Subthalamic nucleus — Globus pallidus externus
Substantia nigra —
Hippocampus — Caudate nucleus tail
Cerebral peduncle — Temporal horn

FIGURE II.10. *Coronal close-up 3.*

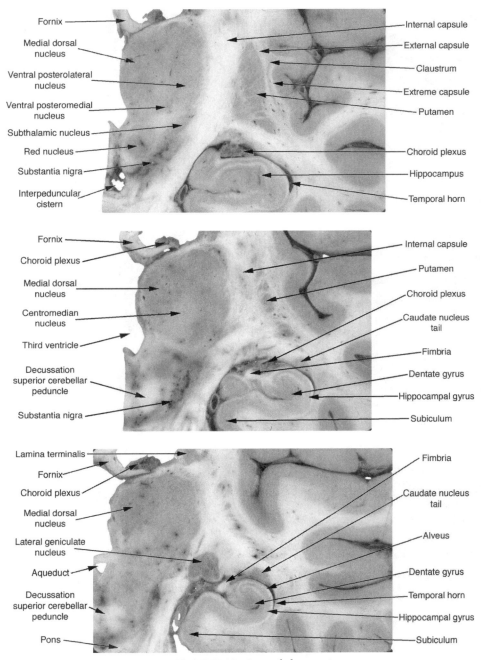

Fornix

Medial dorsal
nucleus

Ventral posterolateral
nucleus

Ventral posteromedial
nucleus

Subthalamic nucleus

Red nucleus

Substantia nigra

Interpeduncular
cistern

Internal capsule

External capsule

Claustrum

Extreme capsule

Putamen

Choroid plexus

Hippocampus

Temporal horn

Fornix

Choroid plexus

Medial dorsal
nucleus

Centromedian
nucleus

Third ventricle

Decussation
superior cerebellar
peduncle

Substantia nigra

Internal capsule

Putamen

Choroid plexus

Caudate nucleus
tail

Fimbria

Dentate gyrus

Hippocampal gyrus

Subiculum

Lamina terminalis

Fornix

Choroid plexus

Medial dorsal
nucleus

Lateral geniculate
nucleus

Aqueduct

Decussation
superior cerebellar
peduncle

Pons

Fimbria

Caudate nucleus
tail

Alveus

Dentate gyrus

Temporal horn

Hippocampal gyrus

Subiculum

FIGURE II.11. *Coronal close-up 4.*

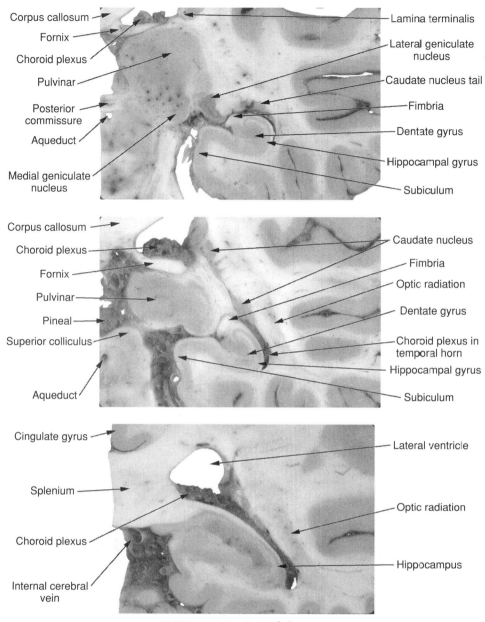

Corpus callosum

Fornix

Choroid plexus

Pulvinar

Posterior
commissure

Aqueduct

Medial geniculate
nucleus

Lamina terminalis

Lateral geniculate
nucleus

Caudate nucleus tail

Fimbria

Dentate gyrus

Hippocampal gyrus

Subiculum

Corpus callosum

Choroid plexus

Fornix

Pulvinar

Pineal

Superior colliculus

Aqueduct

Caudate nucleus

Fimbria

Optic radiation

Dentate gyrus

Choroid plexus in
temporal horn

Hippocampal gyrus

Subiculum

Cingulate gyrus

Splenium

Choroid plexus

Internal cerebral
vein

Lateral ventricle

Optic radiation

Hippocampus

FIGURE II.12. Coronal close-up 5.

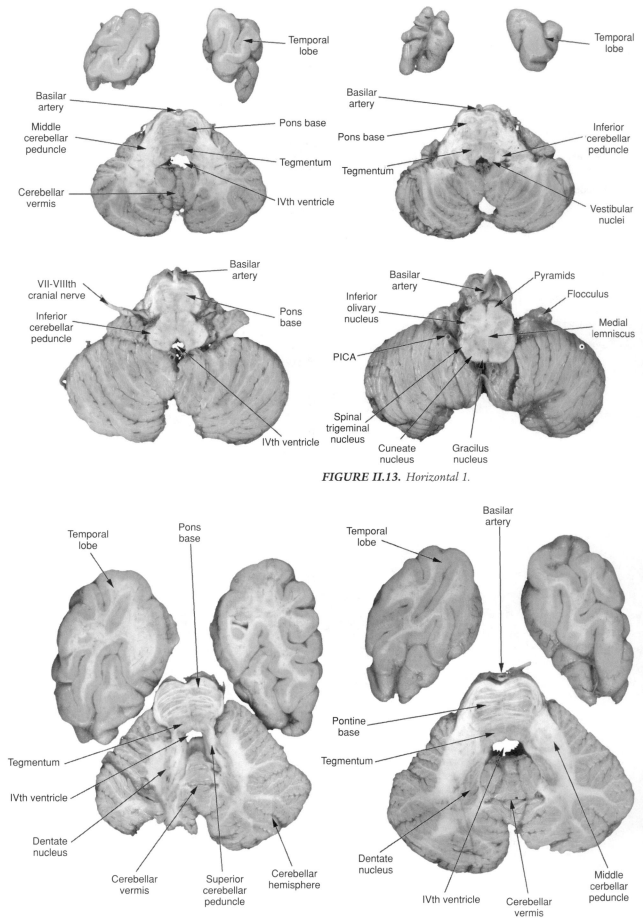

FIGURE II.13. *Horizontal 1.*

FIGURE II.14. *Horizontal 2.*

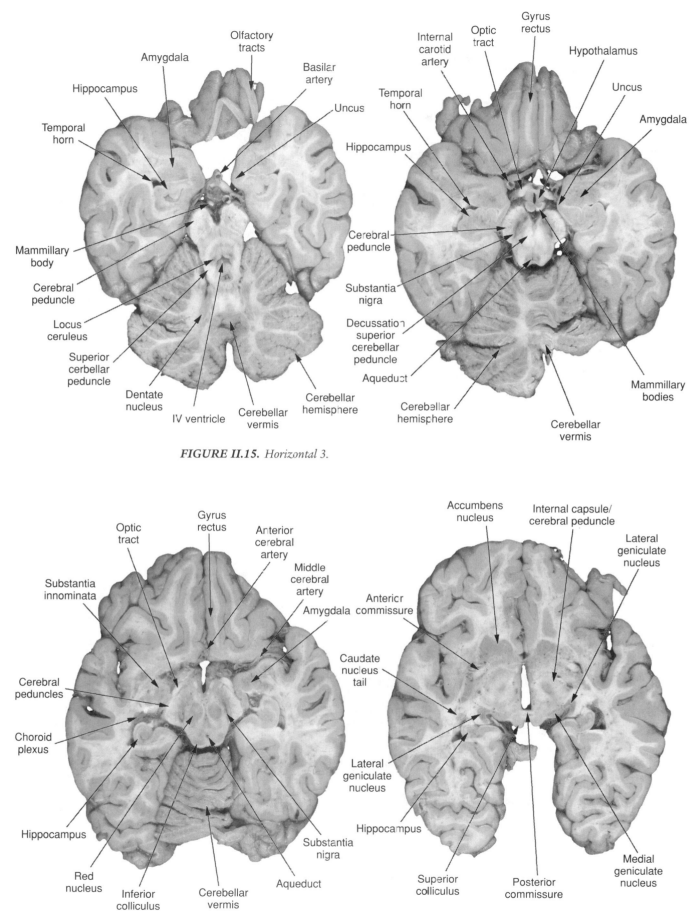

FIGURE II.15. *Horizontal 3.*

FIGURE II.16. *Horizontal 4.*

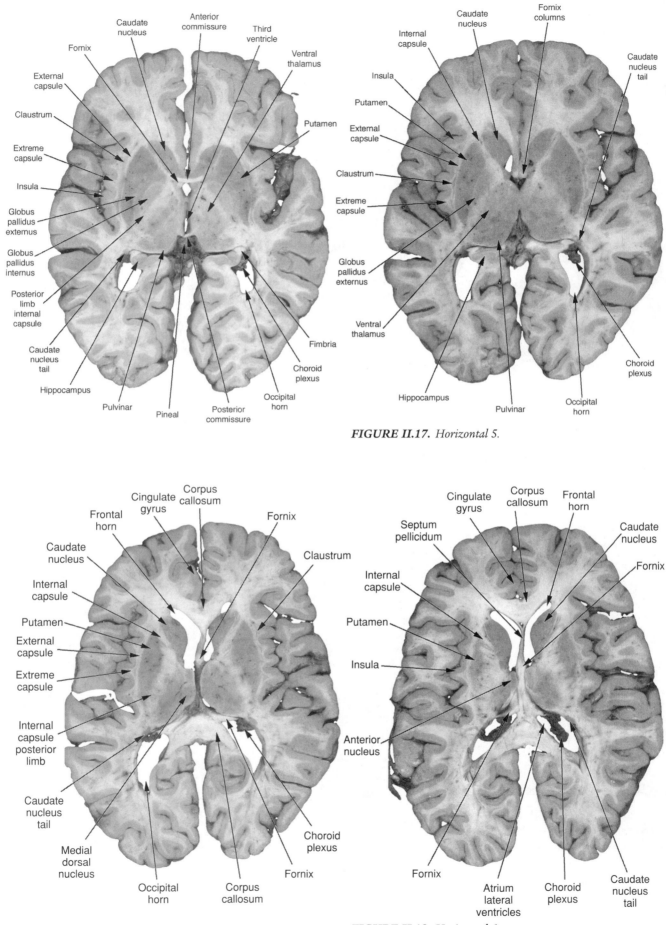

FIGURE II.17. *Horizontal 5.*

FIGURE II.18. *Horizontal 6.*

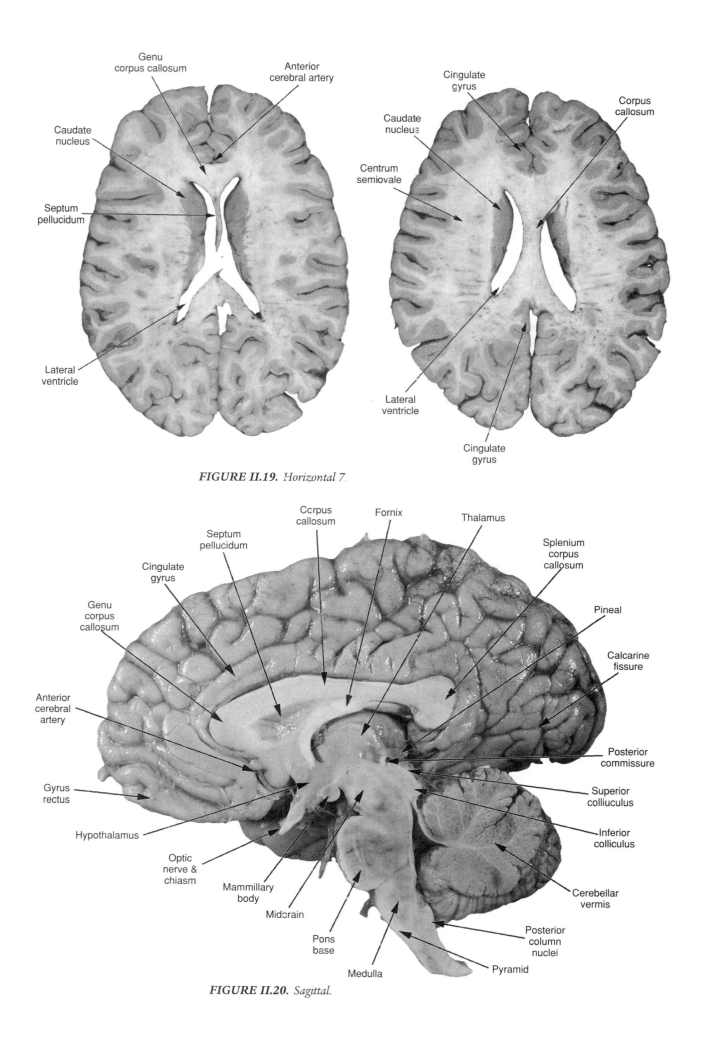

FIGURE II.19. *Horizontal 7.*

FIGURE II.20. *Sagittal.*

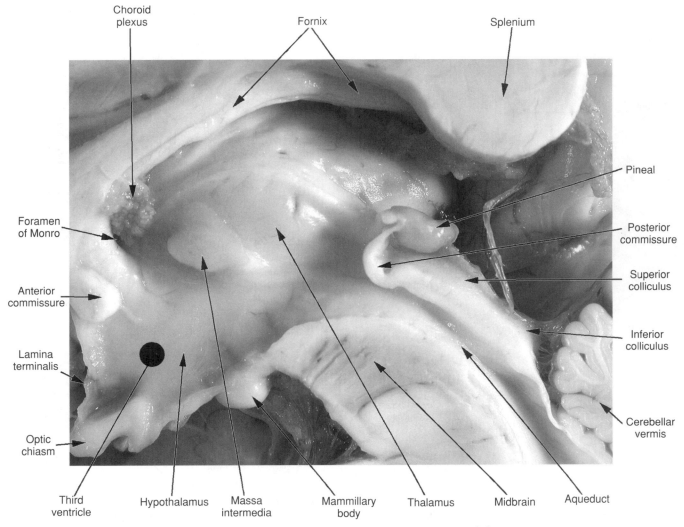

Choroid plexus

Fornix

Splenium

Pineal

Foramen of Monro

Posterior commissure

Anterior commissure

Superior colliculus

Inferior colliculus

Lamina terminalis

Optic chiasm

Cerebellar vermis

Third ventricle

Hypothalamus

Massa intermedia

Mammillary body

Thalamus

Midbrain

Aqueduct

FIGURE II.21. *Sagittal close-up.*

Appendix III—SHEEP BRAIN DISSECTION

SHEEP BRAIN "TEAR"

You may find the following material instructive as a demonstration of how white matter tracts travel in bundles. The procedure is messy but will illustrate subcortical "U" fibers, the corpus callosum, and its radiation into the centrum semiovale.

INST Take the sheep brain from which you dissected the dura. Spend a few minutes identifying the surface features and relating them to the human brain. Specifically try to find the olfactory bulbs, the optic nerve, and the trigeminal nerve.

INST Cut the sheep brain in half. Using the whole human brain specimen, appreciate how you are different from a sheep. Specifically compare the size of the cerebrum and cerebellum in both species. Which is more developed in humans?

INST You are now going to embark on a gruesome but instructive digression. As you saw earlier, determining the path of the white matter tracts in the cerebrum is difficult on cut sections. Here you will follow these paths more mechanically, by stripping portions of the brain along the underlying white matter bundles.

INST The main tool is a scalpel, a Popsicle stick and your fingers. First, cut a groove around the outer rim of the lateral cortex, about a half centimeter deep (see Fig. III. 1).

INST Next jam the Popsicle stick into the groove in the cortex around the middle of the brain, hold onto the cortex, and tear the tissue forward, away from the brain. If you are lucky, the gray matter will tear away, along with some underlying white matter. Since the tracts do form bundles over short distances, it should rip along these fibers and you should be able to follow some of the tracts. Use this technique both forward and backward. You may want to try different depths of dissection. See Figure III.2. Notice that in deeper dissections, the white matter tracts travel downward (projection fibers), while at shallower depths, more association fibers are visible.

Functional Neuroanatomy: An Interactive Text and Manual, by Jeffrey T. Joseph and David L. Cardozo
ISBN 0-471-44437-5 Copyright © 2004 John Wiley & Sons, Inc.

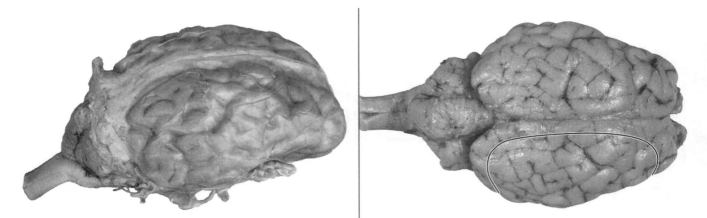

FIGURE III.1. *Sheep brain with dura intact* (left) *and removed* (right). *The scalpel line is shown on the right.*

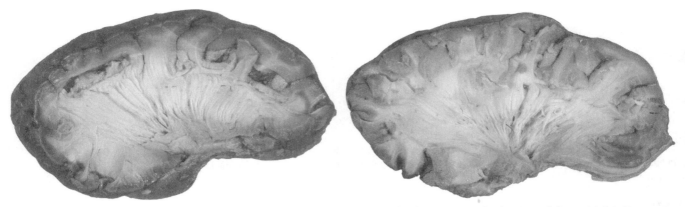

FIGURE III.2. *White matter tear at two levels, more superficial* (left) *and deeper* (right). *Deeper projection fibers are present on the right.*

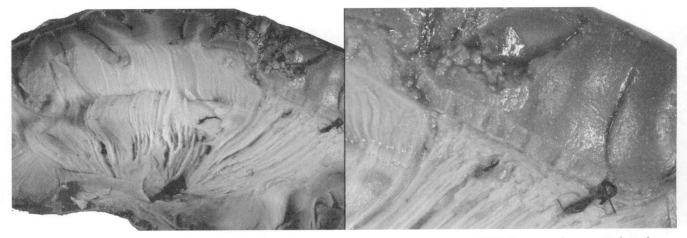

FIGURE III.3. *Close-ups of dissections. Some subcortical "U" fibers may be seen on the right, just underneath and perpendicular to the more vertical rips in cortex.*

INST Notice the subcortical "U" fibers connecting nearby regions of cortex (see the right-hand close-up in Fig. III.3). In the middle of the brain you should be able to trace the fibers diving down into the corona radiata and either crossing the corpus callosum or entering the internal capsule. As you dissect deeper and deeper into the occipital lobes (don't do it all at once), you will eventually encounter the optic radiations. These are the same fibers you saw on the coronal slices in the occipital lobes. Can you identify any other tracts? Try to identify the three major types of white matter tracts:

- Commissural fibers
- Cortico-cortical fibers
- Ascending/descending tracts

Appendix IV—
NEUROIMAGING PRINCIPLES*

ecent developments in neuroimaging have revolutionized brain research and the care of patients with neurological disorders. Ongoing work promises to provide even greater advances in the near future. This appendix summarizes the most common techniques that are used currently to image the human central nervous system.

Many of the methods described below are similar to those used to image other parts of the body. Therefore, this appendix may serve two purposes: first, to introduce or help explain techniques that you will see used in imaging all organ systems, and second, to describe some of the special challenges and opportunities of neuroimaging in particular.

As you read, it will be useful to keep in mind the fundamental radiological concept of image contrast. Most imaging techniques depict tissues in monochromatic, two-dimensional pictures. Structures can be recognized because they appear "lighter" or "darker" in the image, depending on some particular physical property. Understanding which physical property forms the basis of contrast in a particular image can help you to interpret the image.

PLAIN RADIOGRAPHY

How It Works

This is the familiar technique sometimes called simply "X-ray." A source of nearly parallel X-rays is directed at a detector, either a sheet of X-ray sensitive film or an electronic device. The body part to be imaged is placed between the source and the film. The X-ray source is turned on briefly, and as the radiation passes through the head, it is absorbed to varying degrees by bone, CSF, soft tissue, and anything else through which it passes on the way to the detector. After the film is developed, or the data from the detector are converted to a viewable image, portions that were more heavily exposed appear darker, and portions that were less exposed are lighter. The resulting image is a shadow or projection of the head onto a flat surface, in which image contrast is based on relative X-ray attenuation, also known as radiodensity or radio-opacity. Different tissues in the body have characteristically different

---

* This appendix was contributed by William A. Copen, Massachusetts General Hospital, Department of Radiology, 55 Fruit Street, Boston, Massachusetts 02114

Functional Neuroanatomy: An Interactive Text and Manual, by Jeffrey T. Joseph and David L. Cardozo

radiodensities. Calcium (such as is found in bones) is very radiodense and so it appears nearly white in plain radiographs. Soft tissues, such as brain tissue, the spinal cord, muscle, or parenchymal organs like the liver are somewhat lower in density. Fat is less dense than soft tissue, and air is the least dense of all of these materials, appearing black in plain radiographs.

Applications

Unfortunately, the brain and spinal cord are both enclosed on all sides by thick layers of bone, through which X-rays must pass on the way into and out of the body. This bone blocks so much radiation that the relatively subtle difference in density between, say, a brain tumor and normal brain is imperceptible in a plain radiograph. Plain radiographs can detect many kinds of vertebral pathology, such as fractures or bone tumors, but they cannot visualize the spinal cord, or determine the effects of bony pathology on the cord. Before the advent of cross-sectional imaging techniques that are capable of imaging the brain directly (see below), plain radiographs were sometimes used to infer the presence of intracranial pathology from indirect signs, such as the presence or displacement of calcified intracranial structures. However, plain radiographs currently have virtually no application in imaging the brain. For example, even when a skull fracture is present and visible in plain radiographs, a CT scan is necessary to assess its effect on the brain.

CONVENTIONAL ANGIOGRAPHY

How It Works

This technique is used to visualize the blood vessels of the brain (and less commonly the spinal cord), and to investigate qualitatively the direction and velocity of blood flow in those vessels. As in plain radiography, X-ray attenuation forms the basis of image contrast.

Neuroangiography is performed in a special angiography suite, with all involved personnel wearing masks, gowns, gloves, and lead aprons to protect them from scattered radiation. The angiographer, usually a neuroradiologist, first inserts a sterile catheter into a peripheral blood vessel, usually a femoral or brachial artery. The angiographer then advances the catheter through the vasculature until it reaches a desired vessel close to the body part of interest. In cerebral angiography, the catheter is usually advanced into a vertebral or carotid artery. As the catheter is being advanced, its progress is followed using a fluoroscope. This device consists of two components: an X-ray emitter and an electronic detection device called an image intensifier. The image intensifier works like the tube inside a television camera, except that it detects X-rays instead of visible light. This tube is connected to a computer, which displays images to look like moving plain radiographs that can either be viewed in real time or recorded. While advancing the catheter, the angiographer periodically injects small quantities of a radio-opaque contrast agent in order to visualize nearby vascular anatomy and ensure that the catheter is following the proper course.

When the catheter reaches the desired target, the angiographer injects a larger bolus of contrast material in order to acquire higher quality images that are used for diagnostic interpretation. These images typically have higher spatial resolution than the fluoroscopic images and require higher doses of X-rays. After it has been injected, the contrast agent stays within the vessels, rather than diffusing out into the brain, because it cannot cross the blood–brain barrier. Therefore, as it passes through the vasculature, the vessels transiently become more radiodense and then return to normal density as the contrast agent is washed away. A typical rate of image acquisition during contrast injection is two or three images per second. This is sufficient to depict the vessels containing the contrast agent as it passes through arteries (arterial phase) and into draining veins (venous phase).

Images can be recorded in two different ways. The older method uses conventional X-ray film, which is loaded into a rapid film cassette changer so that sequential image exposures can be obtained quickly. The filmed images obtained in this manner are called cut films. In cut films, vessels with radio-opaque contrast agent in them appear white. The radio-opaque bones of the skull also appear white.

In modern techniques, images are recorded digitally by the computer connected to the fluoroscope. The digital images are composed of many tiny squares or pixels ("picture element"). Each pixel is colored black, white, or a shade of gray in between, depending on the quantity of X-rays detected at the corresponding spot on the detector. To provide an appearance that is consistent with that of traditional cut films, the computer assigns darker colors to regions where there is little attenuation, and lighter colors to regions where many X-rays are attenuated (see Fig. IV.1).

Using a computer instead of film to record angiographic images makes possible a process called digital subtraction angiography (DSA), in which the computer digitally subtracts the radiodensity in

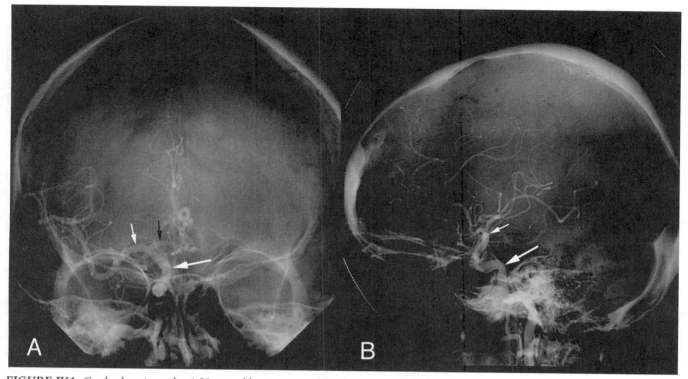

FIGURE IV.1. *Cerebral angiography. A 59-year-old woman complained of a severe headache of 10 days duration. Lumbar puncture demonstrated subarachnoid blood and xanthochromia, but CT angiography was not revealing. Therefore, conventional angiography was performed to search for an aneurysm. However, that study, including these frontal (A) and lateral (B) views obtained during injection of the right internal carotid artery, was unremarkable. The right internal carotid artery (large white arrows), middle cerebral artery (small white arrows), and anterior cerebral artery (small black arrows) are labeled. Note that the middle cerebral artery is not well seen in the lateral image, as it courses perpendicular to the plane of the image. Note also that the left anterior cerebral artery is opacified with contrast via the anterior communicating artery.*

each pixel from the density of the corresponding pixel in a precontrast image that was acquired earlier. In the subtracted image, the attenuating effects of surrounding bones and soft tissue are "cancelled out," leaving a clear picture of the contrast agent alone (see Fig. IV.2).

Many angiography suites have two emitter-detector pairs, so that both anterior-posterior and lateral images can be acquired during the same injection. It is also common to acquire oblique views, to enhance visualization of certain vessels.

Applications

Cerebral angiography is the gold standard for evaluating vascular occlusion, stenosis, aneurysm, dissection, or malformation, and for documenting delayed, collateral, or retrograde flow in cerebral vessels. Because angiographic images are acquired over time, delayed flow or retrograde flow via collateral vessels can be appreciated. With modern equipment, a skilled angiographer can visualize vessels with diameters as small as 0.1 mm. Furthermore, while the intra-arterial catheter is in position, it can be used to deliver various therapies. For example, a thrombolytic agent can be applied directly at the site of a thromboembolic occlusion and emboli can be mechanically disrupted to restore vascular patency. Coils can be deployed within aneurysms to promote thrombogenesis and healing. Occlusive glue can be injected into arteriovenous malformations.

Unfortunately, even purely diagnostic brain angiography is somewhat risky. As the catheter is advanced into the brain, emboli may be dislodged from vessel walls or released from clots that form on the catheter tip. Sometimes, high concentrations of contrast agent may cause transient or even permanent renal failure. Overall morbidity from the procedure is about 2.5%, high enough that angiography is reserved for cases in which important clinical questions cannot be answered by less invasive means.

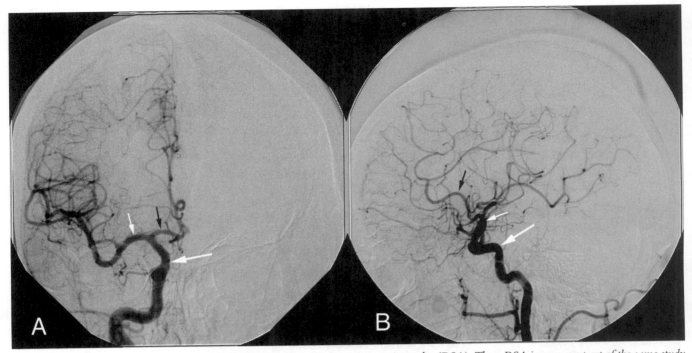

FIGURE IV.2. *Digital subtraction angiography (DSA). These DSA images are part of the same study shown in Figure IV.1. Note that they were obtained slightly later during the right internal carotid injection, so that additional smaller arteries are visible. The right internal carotid artery (large white arrows), middle cerebral artery (small white arrows), and anterior cerebral artery (small black arrows) are again labeled. Again, the middle cerebral artery is not well seen in the lateral image. Several branches of the external carotid artery are visible inferiorly, especially in the lateral image, having filled via retrograde flow of contrast through the carotid bifurcation.*

COMPUTED TOMOGRAPHY (CT)

How It Works

This technique was once known popularly as "CAT scan" (computed axial tomography). Nowadays, the word "axial" is usually omitted, because images may be acquired or reconstructed in planes other than the axial plane. In CT, as in plain radiography or conventional angiography, image contrast is based on differences in X-ray attenuation. However, CT, as well as the remainder of the techniques that will be presented subsequently, are different in that they produce cross-sectional rather than projectional images.

A CT scanner, like other devices that measure X-ray attenuation, requires an X-ray emitter as well as some means of quantifying the intensity of X-rays that have passed through the patient's body. In a CT scanner, both the emitter and the X-ray detectors are housed in the "gantry," a large, ring-shaped housing about 7 ft in its outer diameter, 3 ft in its inner diameter, and a little over a foot thick. The patient to be scanned lies on a table that is slid into the gantry, to bring the body part to be imaged into the center of the ring. A large number of X-ray detectors are arranged in a single plane around the inner perimeter of the ring. A single X-ray emitter is also located in the inside of the ring. It is positioned so as to emit a fan of X-rays that passes through the patient's head, to be measured by the detectors that are diametrically opposed to the emitter. The emitter physically moves around the inside of the ring while emitting radiation, thus generating X-ray attenuation data at multiple angles. After the emitter has traversed the circle, a computer processes the hundreds of thousands of X-ray measurements thus acquired to construct a two-dimensional image of that section or "slice" of the patient's body that lies within the plane of the scanner (see Fig. IV.3). This image is made up of thousands of tiny pixels, each of which represents the radiodensity of a particular small brick-shaped region of tissue in the head, called a voxel. To be consistent with plain radiography, pixels that are more radiodense are depicted in lighter shades of gray, and more radiolucent pixels are darker shades of gray. By convention, axial CT images (like axial images in other modalities such as MRI and PET)

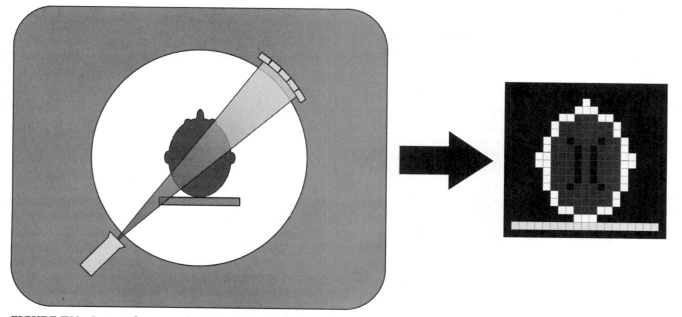

FIGURE IV.3. *Computed tomography (CT). Schematic diagram of a CT scanner's gantry with a patient's head positioned in its center (left). The X-ray tube (lower left) emits a fan of X-rays, which pass through the patient's head, and are absorbed by detectors on the other side of the gantry (upper right). The tube continues to emit X-rays while it rotates around the inner diameter of the scanner. The X-ray absorption measurements obtained by the detectors are processed by a computer to yield a CT image (right). A real CT image is composed of many more pixels than are shown here, so that the spatial resolution of the image is much higher.*

are displayed with the patient's right side on the left side of the image, as though one were looking up at the imaged section from below.

In older CT scanners, after a single image slice has been processed, the table on which the patient is lying slides a little farther into the scanner, so that a more superior or inferior slice of the body can be imaged in the same manner. In today's more sophisticated scanners, the table usually moves continuously as the emitter revolves around the circumference of the scanner. These newer scanners are called "spiral" or "helical" scanners, because of the shape that the X-ray beam describes as it passes through the patient. Many modern scanners are "multislice" scanners, which are helical scanners that are capable of acquiring several image slices simultaneously, because they have several adjacent rows of detectors. Multislice scanners work much more rapidly than single-slice scanners, and can image the entire brain in approximately 30 s.

CT images may be viewed on computer workstations, or printed on sheets of film to be viewed on light boxes. Using a workstation confers many advantages, such as the ability to improve lesion detection by altering brightness and contrast (see below) or enlarging areas of interest.

Image Terminology

A lesion that is darker than surrounding brain tissue on a CT image is called hypodense or less attenuating. Similarly, a lesion that is "brighter" is called hyperdense or more attenuating. For example, a small acute lobar hemorrhage will appear as a hyperdense lesion in the affected lobe. A subacute infarct will appear as a hypodense region.

Windowing

It will be useful at this point to introduce the concept of windowing. Substances with an extremely wide variety of radiodensities can be found normally or pathologically in the human body. Radiodensity in CT images is measured in Hounsfield Units (HU), which is named after Sir Godfrey Hounsfield, a British pioneer in the development of CT technology. The range of radiodensities is illustrated in Figure IV.4. The CT scanner is capable of measuring radiodensities throughout this entire range accurately (as long as it is kept calibrated). However, it is not possible to represent the entire range

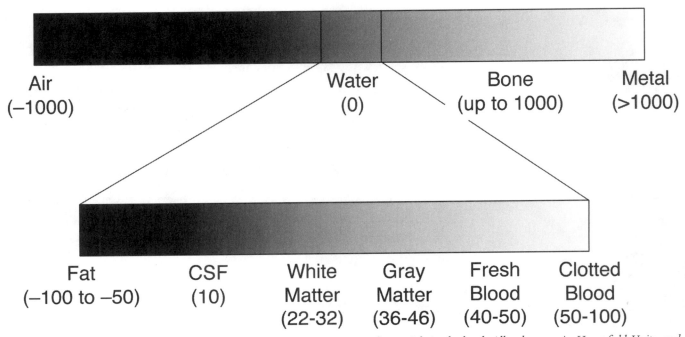

FIGURE IV.4. *X-ray attenuation of materials in the head. All values are in Hounsfield Units, and are approximate except for the values for air and water, which are by definition −1000 and 0, respectively.*

simultaneously on a single computer screen, film, or sheet of paper without sacrificing some contrast between tissues of similar density. For example, one could represent air density as black, bone as white, and everything in between as shades of gray. But in that case, gray matter, white matter, edematous or infarcted brain, and tumors would be indistinguishable, at the same apparent gray level.

Therefore, when displaying CT images on a computer screen or printing them on film, it is necessary to choose an appropriate window: a range of densities that will be distinguishable from one another as shades of gray. Everything less dense than that range will appear uniformly black, and everything more dense will appear uniformly white. The window can be defined by two values: the minimum and maximum densities that will be distinguishable as shades of gray. More often, the window is defined by a different pair of numbers: the level, which is the density at the middle of the range, and the width or window (the latter is an unfortunately ambiguous term), which is the difference between the highest and lowest densities represented. Window and level values are often displayed along with CT images, or printed with them on film. For example, "W 200, L 50" would mean that pixels with attenuation between −150 and 250 HU appear as shades of gray, while those with attenuation less than −150 HU appear black, and those with attenuation over 250 HU appear white. Note that increases in level and window are exactly equivalent to decreases in brightness and contrast, respectively, in a black-and-white television image.

Although a great many window and level settings are possible, there are two basic window and level settings that are most often used for interpreting CT scans of the head: bone windows and brain windows (see Fig. IV.5). Bone windows allow good visualization of different bone densities, but make all soft tissues, including the brain, appear a single shade of gray. On the other hand, brain windows provide good contrast between normal and abnormal brain tissue, but make all bones look uniformly white, so that fractures, tumors, or other bone problems cannot be easily appreciated. Bone windows and brain windows are just two ways of looking at the same digital data, like watching the same videotape with different brightness and contrast settings on your television.

In certain situations, customized window settings can help to increase the conspicuity of a lesion with a density very similar to that of normal brain tissue, such as a very early infarct or a chronic subdural hematoma. To make these lesions more conspicuous, one could choose a level directly between the two densities of interest, and a very narrow window.

Contrast Enhancement

The same kind of radio-opaque contrast agent described in the section on angiography (above) can also be used in CT. In CT, however, it is not necessary to perform the risky and time-consuming

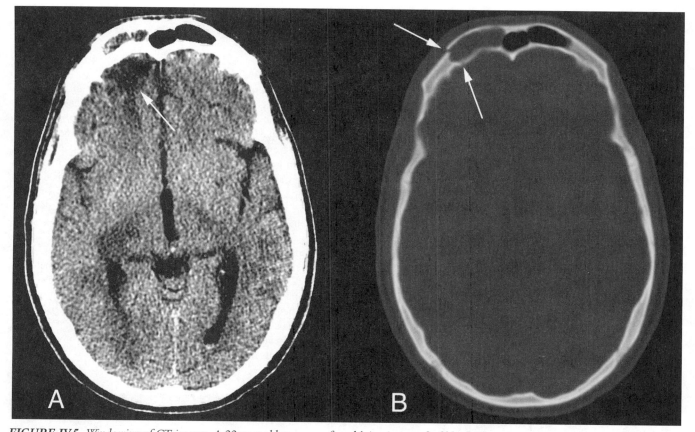

FIGURE IV.5. *Windowing of CT images. A 22-year-old man was found lying in a pool of blood following an assault. A noncontrast axial CT image viewed using brain windows (A) shows an area of hypodensity in the right frontal lobe (arrow) likely representing contusion. The nearby right frontal sinus is opacified, possibly with blood. Another hypodense region lies near the posterior limb of the right internal capsule, which probably represents another contusion. Hyperdense blood layers in the occipital horn of the left lateral ventricle. The same image viewed using bone windows (B) shows fractures of the anterior and posterior walls of the right frontal sinus (arrows) that were not appreciated with brain windows.*

procedure of advancing an intra-arterial catheter into the brain. Instead, the contrast agent is delivered through an ordinary intravenous catheter. After injection, the material washes through the systemic circulation and in minutes distributes within the interstitial spaces according to each tissue's relative perfusion. For example, a CT image of the liver acquired a minute or two after injection would show increased radiodensity, because of the presence of contrast material in the vasculature and extracellular space in the parenchyma. Over minutes to hours, the contrast agent is excreted in the urine.

The brain and spinal cord are important exceptions. The contrast agent cannot cross the blood–brain barrier, so that in a CT image acquired several minutes after contrast injection, most regions of the brain and spinal cord will demonstrate only very minimally increased radiodensity, as a result of the small fraction of contrast that remains within the vasculature. Significantly increased density following contrast injection, or contrast enhancement, is abnormal and signifies locally increased permeability of the blood–brain barrier. This can be an important clinical sign, which is seen in many kinds of neoplasm, as well as infection, hemorrhage, subacute infarction, and other conditions. Contrast enhancement may identify a lesion, especially a tumor, that otherwise would be inapparent on CT. It should be noted that contrast enhancement is a normal finding in portions of the brain and spinal cord that do not have a blood–brain barrier, such as the choroid plexus, pituitary gland, pineal gland, and area postrema.

Any center that has a CT scanner should be able to perform a scan with contrast. The decision whether a CT scan should be performed with contrast (or whether pre- and postcontrast scans should be done) can be made by the referring physician. More commonly, this decision is made by a radiologist on the basis of clinical history provided by the referring physician. It is important that this history include any potential contraindications to contrast administration, such as a contrast allergy or renal failure.

CT Angiography

Several new and specialized CT techniques that utilize intravenously administered contrast agents deserve mention. In one, CT angiography or CTA, CT images are acquired rapidly during the intravenous administration of a bolus of contrast agent as the contrast agent passes through the arteries of the brain (see Fig. IV.6A). Less commonly, in a technique called CT venography or CTV, images are acquired as the contrast agent drains from the brain's veins. Whether the vessels of interest are arteries or veins, they appear very dense in images acquired while they are filled with contrast. Therefore, alterations in vessel caliber can be detected, such as atherosclerotic or vasospastic narrowing, or aneurysmal dilatation. Vasculitis often produces an appearance of alternating narrowing and dilatation. An artery occluded by an embolus will not become opacified with contrast; it will abruptly appear less dense from its point of occlusion to a point where it receives collateral flow from some other vessels (see Fig. IV.6).

Individual CTA or CTV images often undergo additional analysis by a computer that can assemble them into a three-dimensional model of the blood vessels. The computer can then mathematically eliminate the tissues surrounding the vessels, which are less dense because they do not contain contrast material, to produce a three-dimensional model of the vessels alone. This model may be used to create various kinds of three-dimensional renderings of the contrast-opacified vessels (see Fig. IV.6B). The ability to create three-dimensional spatial models of vascular anatomy represents an advantage of CTA over conventional catheter angiography. However, CTA is capable of imaging only larger vessels, down to about 1–2 mm in diameter.

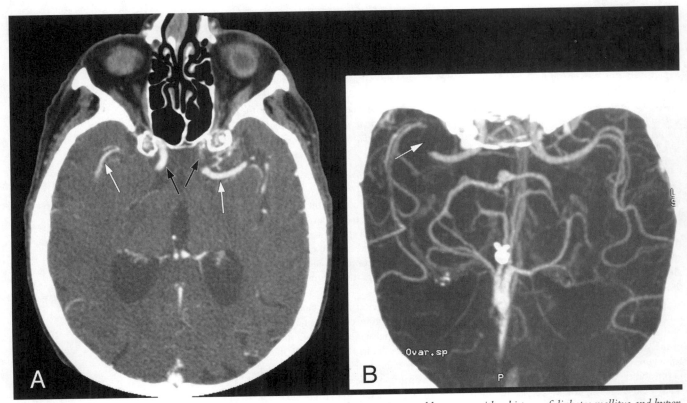

FIGURE IV.6. *CT angiography. An 80 year-old woman with a history of diabetes mellitus and hypertension awoke from a nap with dysarthria and difficulty moving her left arm. Conventional CT obtained about 2 h later appeared normal. A single axial image obtained as part of a CT angiogram (A) shows portions of the internal carotid (black arrows) and middle cerebral (white arrows) arteries. Other portions are not seen, possibly because they are out of the plane of this image. A computer-generated projection of all of the CTA data (B) shows a filling defect in the proximal right middle cerebral artery (arrow), consistent with embolic occlusion.*

CT Perfusion Imaging

CT perfusion imaging is a less widely available technique that depicts cerebral perfusion at the capillary level. This provides information about how much blood is actually reaching the cells in various regions of the brain.

As in CTA or CTV, images are acquired as the contrast agent passes through the brain. However, in this case, images are acquired not at one time point but at multiple time points, as the contrast passes into the brain, through the capillary bed, and out again through the veins. The vessels of interest are microscopic, rather than larger vessels that can be visualized directly. The small region of brain parenchyma that is represented by each image pixel transiently becomes more dense as contrast material enters it, then becomes less dense again as the contrast material washes out. For each image pixel, a density-versus-time curve is plotted, and various kinds of mathematical manipulations convert this curve into measurements of perfusion in the corresponding brain tissue (see Fig. IV.7). These are most useful in acute stroke, when tissue can be identified that is at risk of inclusion into a growing infarct.

Applications of CT

CT is the method most often used for imaging the brain clinically. In the United States, CT scanners are available at nearly every large and medium-sized hospital, and a head CT scan can usually be obtained on an emergent basis with very little delay. In most cases in which brain imaging is clinically indicated, a decision must be made whether to order a CT scan or MRI. The advantages and disadvantages of these two techniques will be compared in the section on applications of MRI below.

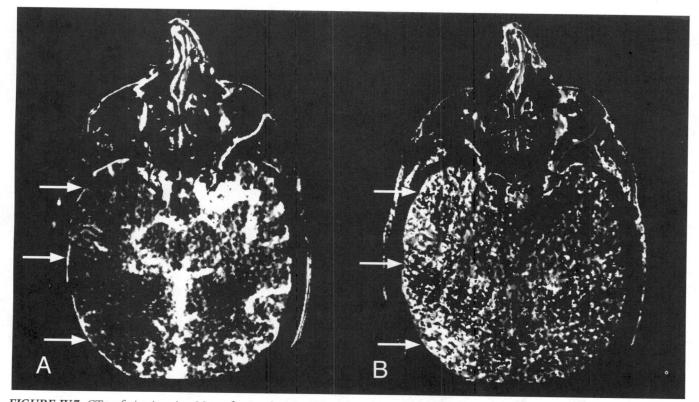

FIGURE IV.7. *CT perfusion imaging. Maps of regional cerebral blood flow (A) and mean intravascular transit time (B) generated during the same CT examination that was shown in Figure IV.6 demonstrate altered perfusion in the entire right middle cerebral artery territory (arrows). This region is dark in the cerebral blood flow map, signifying reduced blood flow, and bright in the mean transit time map, signifying prolonged intravascular transit of blood. These findings suggest that the entire MCA territory is at risk of infarction because of the embolic occlusion of the MCA that is shown in the CTA images in Figure IV.6.*

MAGNETIC RESONANCE IMAGING (MRI)

How It Works

Unlike the other modalities mentioned so far, in which image contrast is based on differential X-ray attenuation, MRI produces contrast based on chemical differences in the tissue. X-rays are altered or absorbed by the electric clouds around atomic nuclei. Contrast in an X-ray image comes from the differential penetration of X-rays through various tissues. An MRI, however, is based on a quantum mechanical property of an atom's nucleus known as its spin. For this reason, MRI is conceptually more complex than other techniques based on X-rays. The following as is a simplified discussion of how MR images are produced.

An Introduction to MR Physics

To detect the spin of a nucleus, it is first lined up in a magnetic field, then bumped from its alignment by adding energy as a brief electromagnetic pulse, and finally, detecting the equivalent energy it gives up as it realigns with the original magnetic field. The energies involved in detecting spin of an individual nucleus are incredibly small, and so large numbers of nuclei must be sampled to get any signal. To align many nuclei all together, MRI scanners utilize extremely powerful magnetic fields (commonly at 1.5 T; compare with the Earth's puny 0.00005 T field).

All atomic nuclei are charged; those with an odd number of protons and neutrons together have the property of "spin." Nuclei with spin are like tiny bar magnets (dipoles) which are affected by an external magnetic field. Each nuclear spin is a vector, having its own direction and magnitude. When a patient's atoms are placed inside the large magnet of an MR scanner, many of the nuclei will align themselves with the magnetic field. Because these nuclei are "spinning" they behave in a magnetic field much like a spinning toy top does in a gravitational field; they "precess" (see Fig. IV.8). These nuclei all precess at a known frequency, called their "Larmor frequency," which is directly related to the magnetic field strength:

$$\nu = \lambda B_0$$

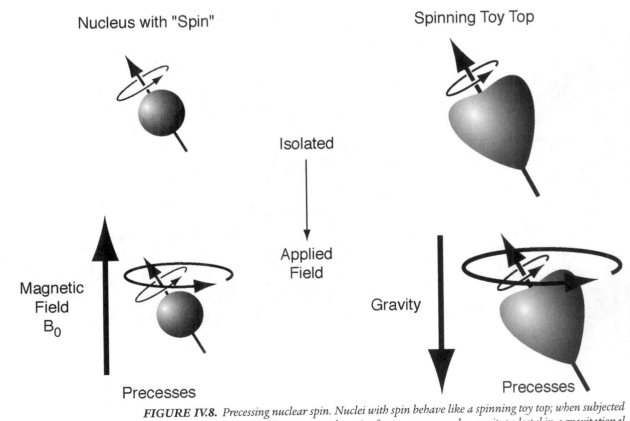

FIGURE IV.8. *Precessing nuclear spin. Nuclei with spin behave like a spinning toy top; when subjected to an external field, both will precess. As the axis of a top precesses when on its pedestal in a gravitational field, so will a nucleus with spin precess in a magnetic field.*

where ν (nu) is the Larmor frequency, B_0 is the strength of the external magnetic field, and λ (lambda) is a constant whose value depends on the identity of the nucleus (e.g., ^{1}H, ^{13}C). For most imaging, especially clinical imaging, the main nucleus examined is the most abundant one in the body, ^{1}H (the hydrogen nucleus, otherwise known as a proton).

Like other vectors, dipole spin vectors can be separated into two components. The "longitudinal" component lies parallel to the external magnetic field, while the "transverse" component is perpendicular to this field. Once placed in the external field, all of the individual spin vectors precess at the same frequency, but are out of phase with one another. What this means mathematically is that all of their "longitudinal" component are in the same direction, but their "transverse" components are randomly oriented. Summing all the millions of individual spin vectors will form a single vector representing the total or net nuclear magnetic moment at a particular instant in time. Since all of the longitudinal components point in the same direction, their sum is one big vector. However, all of the transverse components are randomly oriented, so when added up they sum to zero. The resulting net vector points in the direction of the external field and does not precess (see Fig. IV.9).

So, how do you get spin information out of the tissues when all of the little arrows add up to form one large arrow? The trick is to jolt them out of their position and then watch them return to baseline. Nuclei in each tissue have their own signature way of returning to their starting orientation.

The initial step in producing an MR image is to perturb the spinning nuclei by pulsing them with another magnetic field perpendicular to the main field. In a scanner a short pulse of radio frequency is used to induce a second magnetic field B_1. As the nuclei return to their initial orientation, they give up their added energy in a tissue-specific way, which is used to produce an image.

The radio frequency pulse is given at exactly the Larmor frequency, which forces the nuclei to resonate. This causes two important things to happen: the individual spins become locked in phase with one another and their net vector is knocked away from its axis (see Fig. IV.10). The "longitudinal component" of the net vector parallel to the main magnetic field (B_0) becomes smaller and the "transverse component" perpendicular to the main field is no longer zero (see Fig. IV.10).

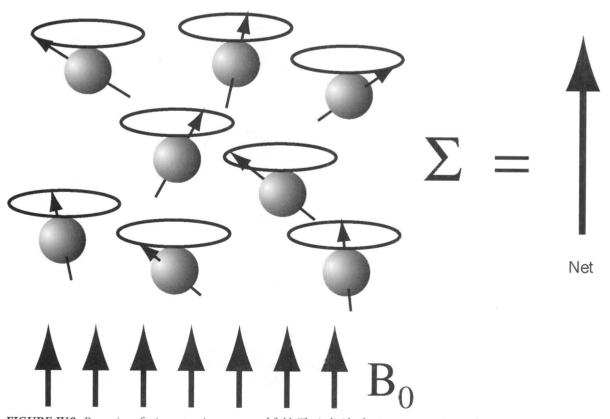

FIGURE IV.9. *Precession of spin vectors in an external field. The individual spins are precessing at the same angular frequency, but with random phase. Therefore, the sum of all of the individual spin vectors is a net magnetization vector that is parallel to the external field B_0 and does not precess.*

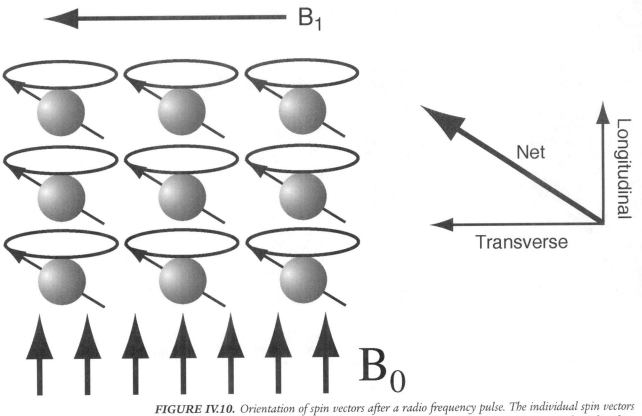

FIGURE IV.10. *Orientation of spin vectors after a radio frequency pulse. The individual spin vectors have been "knocked over" by the radio frequency pulse and are now in phase with one another. Therefore, the net magnetization vector is knocked over as well and it begins to precess about the external field B_0. The net magnetization vector now has both longitudinal (parallel to B_0) and transverse (perpendicular to B_0) components. As the individual spins relax back to their original state, the longitudinal component of the net vector grows back to its original magnitude (with time constant T_1), and the transverse component shrinks back to zero (with time constant T_2). The tissue emits a radio frequency signal whose amplitude is proportional to the magnitude of the transverse component.*

Both of these changes represent a higher energy state of the system, in effect an absorption of the applied radio frequency energy, and hence magnetic energy. After the radio frequency pulse is complete, the spins will relax back to their original state. This relaxation is accompanied by a release of energy in the form of additional radio frequency radiation, again at the Larmor frequency. The released energy is the signal that gets measured and used to prepare the image. Like an antenna on your radio, the signal is detected by a coil that is placed near the patient's head.

During relaxation, the individual spins spiral back toward their initial alignment with the external field, and in the process will lose their phase coherence with each other. The effect on the net magnetization vector is that it will also spiral back up to its original position and stop precessing. Its longitudinal component will grow back to its original size and its rotating transverse component will shrink back to zero. The regrowth of the longitudinal component is called T_1-relaxation. It is a first-order process that occurs with time constant T_1 (in time T_1 it will have grown to within one "e-th" or $(1 - \frac{1}{e})$ or 63% of its original value). This means that the longitudinal component exponentially regrows toward its original value: $L = L_0 \times [1 - e^{-(\text{time}/T_1)}]$. To realign with the main magnetic field, the nuclei transfer their additional energy to the local surroundings or "lattice"; the greater the tissue's lattice structure, the faster the energy is transferred and the shorter the T_1 parameter. Nuclear spins also experience variations in the local magnetic fields in the tissue. Such variations cause these spins to precess at different rates and hence become incoherent or dephased. The disappearance of the transverse component is called T_2-relaxation. It is also a first-order process, and it occurs with time constant T_2: $e^{-(\text{time}/T_2)}$. The T_2 term represents the rate at which the spins become dephased because of local magnetic field inhomogeneties. The more inhomogeneous the fields, the shorter the T_2 term.

The above simplified discussion leaves us with some magnetic resonance information about the bulk tissue. Producing an anatomic image requires getting that information from small voxels of tissue.

To obtain the tissue's positional data, various other magnetic fields are applied as gradients in different orientations. All of the different signals from the person are received as radio frequency energy from the coils. A series of mathematical calculations, requiring high-speed computers, transforms these signals into images. Each two-dimensional pixel on a computer screen represents a corresponding three-dimensional voxel of tissue.

Images are not formed simply by applying one radio frequency pulse and then measuring emitted energy. Instead, various additional magnets must be turned on and off, with precise timing, so as to superimpose smaller magnetic field gradients upon the larger B_0 field. At the same time, radio frequency pulses of carefully controlled frequencies, durations, and bandwidths must also be applied at precise intervals and durations. Radio frequency energy emitted from the tissue must be sampled at precise times. These actions are controlled by a computer according to a set of instructions called a pulse sequence, which enables the intensity of the signal arising from each voxel to be independently measured. The exact instructions in the pulse sequence also determine whether the slices are sagittal, coronal, axial, or oblique, and determine the spatial resolution of the image, its contrast-to-noise ratio, and the amount of time it will take to acquire the image. It is these pulse sequences that produce the specific types of images (e.g., T_1- or T_2-weighted scans) you see on the monitor. These pulse sequences allow neuroradiologist to perform all sorts of wonderful tricks to obtain biological information.

Clinical MR Imaging
T_1- and T_2-Weighted Images

Different bodily tissues have characteristically different T_1 and T_2 parameters, the exact values of which depend on the strength of the main magnetic field B_0. As mentioned above, the T_1-relaxation is fastest in the most structured tissue, which in the brain is white matter. White matter has the shortest T_1 value (around 510 ms at 1.5 Tesla), gray matter is intermediate (760 ms), and CSF the longest (2650 ms). In contrast, the T_2 value relates to the local magnetic field homogeneity. CSF is the most homogeneous tissue in the brain and so has the slowest dephasing and hence the longest T_2 value (280 ms); gray matter is intermediate (77 ms) and white matter the least homogeneous (67 ms).

The most common pulse sequence in use today is called the "spin–echo (SE) sequence," which is used to produce T_1- and T_2-weighted scans. The spin–echo sequence refers to the particular order in which various radio frequency pulses are applied and signals from the tissue are measured. The signal intensity S is a function of two timing parameters and one density parameter: TR ("time to repeat"), TE ("time to echo"), and N_H (total number of hydrogen nuclei producing the signal). Using the two relations above for T_1 and T_2, the signal intensity of a pixel in a spin–echo image is determined by the following equation:

$$S\,(\text{TR, TE}) = N_H e^{-\text{TE}/T_2}(1 - e^{-\text{TR}/T_1})$$

where T_1 and T_2 refer to the intrinsic T_1 and T_2 times of the tissue in the voxel corresponding to the pixel and N_H is the number of hydrogen nuclei in the voxel. Varying these parameters in the spin–echo sequence produces different kinds of images. Note that TR in the above equation appears in conjunction with T_1, and TE in conjunction with T_2. In a spin–echo image, the TR determines the degree of T_1-weighting and the TE determines the degree of T_2-weighting. A short TR (in the range of the tissue's T_1) results in a large degree of T_1-weighting, while a long TR results in very little T_1-weighting. A short TE (in comparison with the tissue's T_2) results in very little T_2-weighting, whereas a long TE (comparable to the tissue's T_2) results in a great deal of T_2-weighting. Therefore, a T_1-weighted image will be acquired with short TR and short TE, and a T_2-weighted image will be acquired with long TR and long TE. An image with very long TR and very short TE will have very little T_1- or T_2-weighting, so the N_H term will predominantly determine image contrast; such images are termed "proton-density-weighted."

In a T_1-weighted image, tissue with longer T_1-relaxation produces less signal (directly from the equation above) and will appear darker, while the tissue with shorter T_1 will produce a larger signal and appear brighter (see Fig. IV.11A). In these images, T_2 has very little effect on the image. Similarly, in a T_2-weighted image, tissue with longer T_2 will appear brighter and tissue with shorter T_2 will appear darker (see Fig. IV.11B). T_1 has little effect on a T_2-weighted image. In a proton-density-weighted image, more accurately known as a spin-density-weighted image, the basis for image contrast is simply the number of spins within each pixel, and neither T_1 nor T_2 has much effect on the image.

While the above discussion is complex and a bit arcane, a few simple points may help you to interpret these images. Based on their T_1- and T_2-values and effects of spin–echo imaging, the

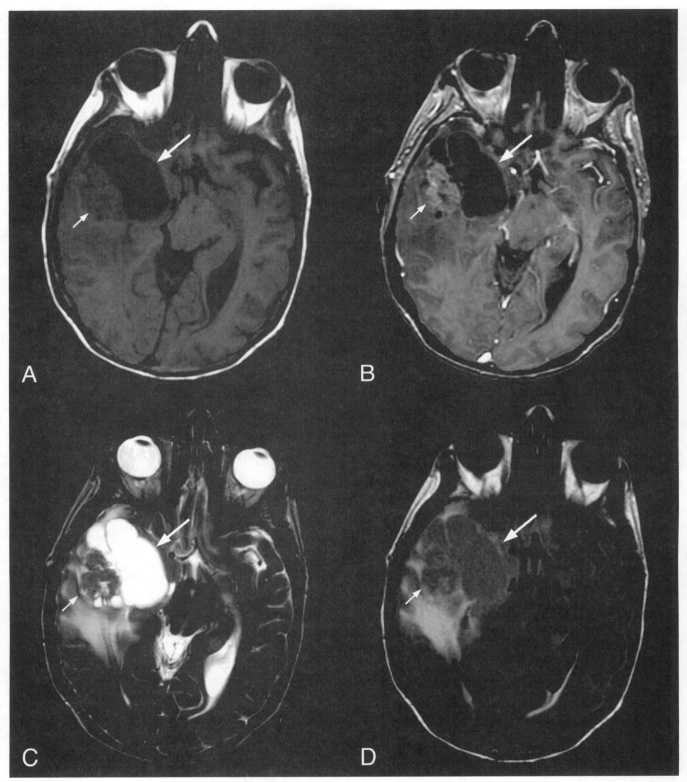

FIGURE IV.11. *Conventional MR images. A 56-year-old woman with ovarian cancer complained of new right-sided headache, right eye pain, and dizziness. MRI shows a large mass in the right temporal lobe, with both cystic and solid components. The cystic component (large white arrows) is hypointense in T_1-weighted images (A), and demonstrates no contrast enhancement in post-gadolinium T_1-weighted images (B). It is very hyperintense in T_2-weighted images (C), but only slightly hyperintense in FLAIR images (D) because of its water content. However, it is not black like CSF, so it must contain more protein than the ventricular fluid. The solid component of the mass (small white arrows) is isointense to normal brain in T_1-weighted images (A), enhances heterogeneously after contrast administration (B), and is slightly hyperintense in T_2-weighted images (C). T_2-weighted and FLAIR images show a surrounding region of hyperintensity reflecting vasogenic edema (black arrows).*

relative signal intensities or brightness of various tissues in T_1- and T_2-weighted images are as follows (at 1.5 T):

$$T_1\text{-weighted image: White matter} > \text{Gray matter} >> \text{CSF}$$

$$T_2\text{-weighted image: CSF} >> \text{Gray matter} \geq \text{White matter}$$

Note that the brightness of each pixel in an MR image is determined by the intensity of the signal emanating from the voxel of tissue corresponding to that pixel. Therefore, when looking at an MR image, it is appropriate to call a lesion hyperintense if it is brighter than surrounding tissue, hypointense if it is darker, and isointense if it is of the same brightness. These terms are more technically descriptive than the informal "brighter" or "darker." X-ray-related words like "hypodense," "hyperdense," "lucent," and "opacity" are incorrect in this context.

Fluid-Attenuated Images (FLAIR Images)

Many pathological processes increase the water content of brain tissue and hence give an increased T_2 signal on imaging. However, these areas of pathology may be difficult to distinguish from simple CSF spaces. A special pulse sequence designed to specifically suppress the free water signal, termed a FLAIR (fluid-attenuated inversion recovery) image, can better differentiate these tissues (compare Fig. IV.11C with IV.11D). A FLAIR image is basically a T_2-weighted image in which signals emanating from simple free fluids is suppressed. In these scans, water appears black ("attenuated") instead of white. FLAIR imaging increases the conspicuity of T_2-hyperintense lesions by suppressing the overpowering effects of CSF. Diseases accompanied by brain edema, including most areas with tissue damage, will be hyperintense on FLAIR images, while the surrounding CSF will be black. Chronic lacunar infarcts and prominent perivascular (Virchow–Robbins) spaces both look like small, round, bright lesions in T_2-weighted images. However, the former also appear bright in FLAIR images, whereas the latter are filled with CSF, and will therefore appear black in FLAIR images.

Contrast-Enhanced Images

Like X-ray imaging, contrast agents are available for MRI. However, in MRI the effect of the contrast agent is determined not by its X-ray attenuation, but by its magnetic properties. All currently approved MRI contrast agents are based upon the gadolinium ion, which is highly paramagnetic because of its seven unpaired electrons. Because the gadolinium ion alone is toxic, the contrast agent is a gadolinium chelate, in which a large protein is bound to the ion. This not only reduces toxicity, but helps prevent the contrast agent from crossing the blood–brain barrier. (This is the same approach used for iodinated contrast agents.) As with CT, contrast enhancement of brain or spinal cord parenchyma, obtained several minutes after administration, signifies abnormally increased permeability of the blood–brain barrier.

The effect of gadolinium or other paramagnetic contrast agents is to greatly shorten the T_1 characteristics of the tissue, which produces hyperintensity in T_1-weighted images. At high concentrations these agents produce hypointensity in T_2-weighted images. In practice, postcontrast MR images are almost always T_1-weighted, so that contrast enhancement is evidenced by hyperintensity. Such images are often marked "+C," "post-gado," simply "post," or with the name of the contrast agent used (see Fig. IV.11B).

Distinguishing Different Scans

Different pathologies have characteristically different appearances in T_1-weighted images, T_2-weighted images, and the many other kinds of MR images that are be generated. To more easily interpret these lesions on an MR study, you need to identify the type of image as you look at it. Often MR images are marked with a description such as "sagittal T_1" that explains the type of image. However, these descriptions may be absent or in a form that is difficult to understand. It will be helpful if you can identify different MR scans merely by looking at the images, rather than reading their descriptions.

Start by looking at the CSF in the ventricles and subarachnoid spaces. If the CSF looks very bright, the image is almost certainly T_2-weighted (see Fig. IV.11B). T_2-weighted images are acquired with a long TR ("time to repeat," see above) and a long TE ("time to echo," see above). The TR and TE values are often displayed along with the image and can be helpful in determining the type of scan. Generally, tissues containing abundant water appear bright in T_2-weighted images. This is why

CSF and fluid-containing cysts appear very bright in these images. Vasogenic edema accompanies a wide variety of pathologic processes. It releases additional water into the affected areas and causes the brain or spinal cord to appear hyperintense in T_2-weighted images.

T_1-weighted images are particularly well suited for defining anatomic detail. Tissues with high water content, such as CSF or fluid-filled cysts, are very dark in T_1-weighted images. A limited number of materials display very high signal intensity in T_1-weighted images. These include fat, paramagnetic contrast agents, extravasated blood at certain stages of posthemorrhagic evolution, highly proteinaceous material such as proteinaceous cysts, and most melanoma metastases. Because fat and contrast enhancement both result in hyperintensity on T_1-weighted images, a technique called fat suppression is sometimes used to eliminate the signal from fat and enable more definite identification of enhancing structures.

On an MRI, if CSF appears very dark, the scan is probably a T_1-weighted or FLAIR image (compare Fig. IV.11A and IV.11D). Distinguishing between T_1-weighted and FLAIR images may take a few extra moments until you have some experience. T_1-weighted images are obtained with short TR and short TE (about 500 ms and 20 ms, respectively). Although T_1-weighted images of both the brain and spinal cord are routinely acquired, FLAIR imaging is usually used only for the brain. FLAIR images sometimes appear slightly more grainy than T_1-weighted images. Especially in older patients, FLAIR images, but not T_1-weighted images, often show a hyperintense rim immediately surrounding the lateral ventricles. FLAIR images are created using a third major imaging parameter, TI ("time of inversion"), which is sometimes displayed along with TR and TE.

To determine if a scan is enhanced, first be sure it is T_1-weighted. Then look at the vessels. If many of them "light-up," especially meningeal vessels, a contrast agent has most likely been given. Remember that contrast enhancement within the brain parenchyma indicates breakdown of the blood–brain barrier. Except for a few small sites (e.g., choroid plexus, pineal gland) this indicates brain pathology.

Practical Points
Patient Eligibility and Scanning Logistics

An MR scanner looks like a large, hollow tube, with outer diameter of about 6 ft and inner diameter of about 2 ft. The most important component of the scanner is an extremely powerful magnet, formed by many coils of wire wrapped within the tube, which creates a powerful magnetic field within its bore. Nowadays, most MR magnets are superconducting, which means that their cores are filled with liquid helium to keep them cold. The scanner (sometimes informally called the "magnet") must be enclosed in a special room whose construction limits the penetration of external radio frequency energy and magnetic fields, and also limits the effects of the magnet outside of the room. You should exercise caution when entering a magnet room. The magnetic field will erase your credit cards, may destroy your beeper and your digital watch, and may even tear small ferromagnetic objects from your person and send them hurtling through the air toward the magnet. A steel IV pole, crash cart, or gurney wheeled into a magnet room may launch itself toward the scanner with enough force to cause major damage or serious injury. Patients and staff members have been killed in such unfortunate accidents.

Needless to say, patients with mobile iron or steel objects in their bodies are not candidates for MRI. Before scanning, a careful history must be taken to ensure that the patient's body does not contain a pacemaker, shrapnel, or metal fragments that sometimes lodge in machine workers' eyes without their even knowing it. If there is any doubt, a plain radiograph of the orbits may be obtained to rule out the presence of any metal. Many aneurysm clips and prosthetic heart valves are MR-compatible, but some older devices are not. Dental fillings may cause artifacts that degrade the quality of MR images, but they do not constitute a safety hazard. Hip replacements and other artificial joints, inferior vena cava filters, and orthopedic fixation plates typically cause no problems. Lists of which specific medical devices are and are not MR-compatible are usually kept near the MR scanners in most institutions. MR-compatible models of such common hospital machines as ventilators and IV fluid pumps are often available.

Technical Aspects

A typical MR pulse sequence takes from 30 s to several minutes to run. A complete examination includes several pulse sequences. For example, an MR examination of the brain may entail acquiring a set of sagittal T_1-weighted images, axial T_2-weighted and FLAIR images, and a few others. The entire examination may take 30 or 40 min to complete, or even more for detailed examinations of the entire spine. During this time, electrical components within the scanner produce very loud banging and thumping noises, so that the patient must wear earplugs or pneumatic headphones that allow him to listen to music.

MR images are degraded significantly by any patient motion that occurs while a pulse sequence is running. Therefore, children or patients who are uncooperative or in significant distress may not be good MRI candidates unless they are sedated. Claustrophobic patients may not tolerate the very confined space of the scanner unless also sedated. Very obese patients simply will not fit in the scanner. So-called open MRI scanners are less enclosed, and can allow some patients to undergo imaging who might otherwise be too claustrophobic. However, open MRI scanners usually have less powerful magnets, and therefore may produce images that are of lower quality.

Like CT images, MR images are generated digitally. No film is involved in image generation, and in principle it is better to view the images on computer screens. In practice, however, MR images, like CT images, are sometimes printed on film and viewed on light boxes. Also like CT images, MR images must be windowed properly when they are viewed. Practically speaking, however, windowing is a less subjective issue in MRI. This is because the contrast between different tissues in MRI is much greater, and it usually isn't necessary to sacrifice contrast in one part of an image to bring out contrast in another part of the image.

FUNCTIONAL MRI TECHNIQUES

Magnetic Resonance Angiography (MRA)

In conventional MRI, rapidly moving substances such as blood yield no detectable signal. This is because "labeled" protons leave the detection field before their signal is detected. Routine scans show black flow voids in major arteries. In MRA, however, the magnetic properties of flowing blood are exploited intentionally, to produce images of major blood vessels. This is accomplished using the same scanner as other forms of MRI, but with a different pulse sequence. In MRA images, moving blood appears white instead of black (see Fig. IV.12A). Like CTA images, MRA images can be converted by

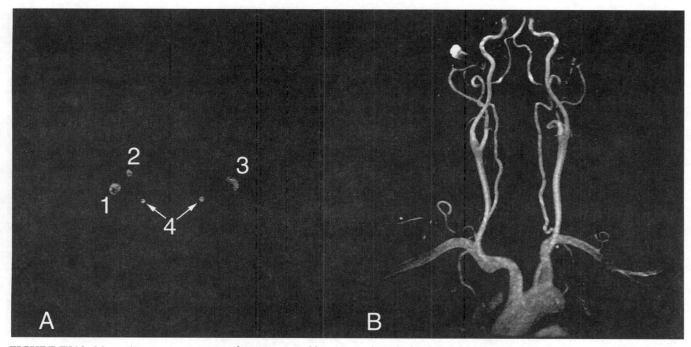

FIGURE IV.12. *Magnetic resonance angiography. A 71-year-old man complained of occasional spells that were thought to represent transient ischemic attacks. Conventional MR images were normal. A representative axial MRA image (A) shows that the right internal (1) and external (2) carotid arteries, left carotid bifurcation (3), and both vertebral arteries (4) are widely patent at this level. Note the paucity of signal arising from all structures that do not contain fast-moving blood. A computer-generated maximum intensity projection of this and all of the other acquired raw axial MRA images (B) shows normal-appearing cervical and cerebral arteries.*

a computer into a spatial model and used to generate three-dimensional renderings that can provide more informative visualization of vascular lesions (see Fig. IV.12B).

Currently, MRA images offer lower resolution compared to conventional X-ray angiograms. MRA can only visualize large vessels (larger than about 1–2 mm in diameter). However, MRA technology is improving rapidly. Since it requires no contrast agent, the technique has the advantage that is completely noninvasive.

Diffusion-Weighted Imaging (DWI)

DWI is a relatively new technique that is used almost exclusively for imaging the brain, although DWI images of the spinal cord and even other body parts have been studied recently. In DWI, the intensity of each pixel is influenced by the mobility of water molecules within the corresponding voxel of tissue. It reflects the extent to which water diffuses freely because of Brownian motion. Most DWI images are both T_2- and diffusion-weighted, so that either a lengthened T_2 or decreased water diffusion (or a combination of the two) will cause hyperintensity. DWI uses basically the same scanner hardware as conventional MRI. Its implementation requires only new pulse sequence programming.

Although it has a number of other important applications, DWI is most important in the setting of acute stroke. An ischemic cell loses its ability to regulate ion flow and hence water content. Interstitial water, which is normally mobile, floods into ischemic cells, where its motion becomes more restricted. Water mobility in brain tissue falls rapidly during ischemia, so that DWI can visualize ischemic damage during the hyperacute period, when other pulse sequences may show little or no abnormality (see Fig. IV.13A). Because current therapies are effective only in the first few hours of ischemia, DWI is a powerful tool in the management of this common and devastating disease.

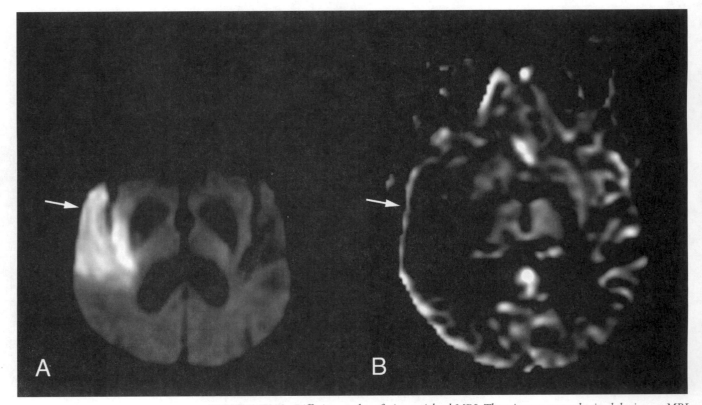

FIGURE IV.13. *Diffusion- and perfusion-weighted MRI. These images were obtained during an MRI examination of the patient introduced in Figures IV.6 and IV.7, performed only slightly later. A diffusion-weighted image (A) shows a hyperintense region in the right temporal lobe, consistent with acute infarction. A map of regional cerebral blood flow (B) shows a dark region, signifying impaired perfusion, that is slightly larger than the diffusion abnormality. This suggests that a small quantity of additional tissue may be at risk of inclusion into the infarct.*

Perfusion-Weighted Imaging (PWI)

In this technique, sequential T_2-weighted images of the brain are acquired rapidly during intravenous administration of a paramagnetic contrast agent, usually containing gadolinium. The signal intensity in each pixel decreases and then returns to normal as the contrast agent passes through the microvasculature of that pixel. A computer calculates the signal intensity in each pixel over time and then mathematically converts the data into a graph of contrast agent concentration versus time. This graph is then used to calculate perfusion parameters for the corresponding tissue voxel, such as regional blood volume or regional blood flow (see Fig. IV.13B). Like CT perfusion imaging, perfusion-weighted MRI is most often used to evaluate acute stroke. This technique can identify the tissue around an infarct having a tenuous blood flow. Such tissue is at risk of ischemia and is the target of current acute stroke therapies. Perfusion-weighted MRI is also used to study the vascularity of brain tumors.

Perfusion-weighted MR images currently are of higher technical quality than CT perfusion images (compare Fig. IV.7 with Fig. IV.13B). They can depict perfusion over the entire brain, while CT perfusion imaging is limited to only a few image slices. However, CT perfusion imaging can be performed rapidly along with a standard CT examination, whereas MRI is logistically more challenging for emergent patients (see below).

Distinguishing and Interpreting Different Types of MR Images

CSF is also dark in DWI images. DWI images have lower spatial resolution than conventional images and may appear more grainy, with little difference in intensity between gray and white matter. Acute ischemic lesions will be easily distinguished as very hyperintense areas (see Fig. IV.13), although the appearance of subacute and chronic infarcts is more variable.

PWI images have a distinctive appearance. Their spatial resolution is generally low, similar to that of DWI images. In some kinds of perfusion-weighted images (exceptions being mean transit time and time-to-peak images), the greater amount of blood flow to the gray matter makes it appear much brighter than white matter. Because many kinds of PWI images look very similar to one another, it is impossible to determine exactly what perfusion parameter is being depicted in a PWI image, and therefore how to interpret the image, without some kind of explicit annotation.

In raw MRA images, large vessels appear bright (unlike in any other kind of MR image). These images are often labeled with the name of one of the two major MRA sequences: PC (phase contrast) or TOF (time of flight).

Activation Mapping or Functional Magnetic Resonance Imaging (fMRI)

Some MRI pulse sequences are able to detect the small changes in regional cerebral blood flow, volume, or oxygenation that accompany local increases in brain activity. Using such sequences, brain areas activated by tasks performed in the MR (e.g., moving a finger, watching a visual pattern) will "light up" on the scan. Originally, this kind of imaging required serial acquisition of images during intravenous administration of a contrast agent. Newer techniques have made exogenous contrast agents unnecessary by using deoxyhemoglobin, which is paramagnetic, as an endogenous contrast agent.

The signal changes detected by these methods are very small. To improve detection of activation, the subject usually starts and stops the task several times while being scanned. The signal acquired during the task is compared to the signal acquired before and after the task, and the changes are taken to represent increased activity specific to that task (see Fig. IV.14).

This kind of MRI is often called functional MRI (fMRI), although this term also includes some other methods as well. As evidenced elsewhere in this text, fMRI has enabled tremendous progress in brain-mapping research. More recently, fMRI has been used clinically, for example in neurosurgical planning. When resecting diseased brain tissue, neurosurgeons wish to preserve "eloquent" tissue that controls important neurological functions. In the past, these areas were localized intraoperatively by having the awake patient perform certain tasks, while electrodes placed directly on the cerebral cortex suppressed the activity beneath them. Some eloquent areas can now be identified on functional studies by having patients perform the same tasks in an MR scanner prior to surgery. These images can then guide the neurosurgeon during the operation.

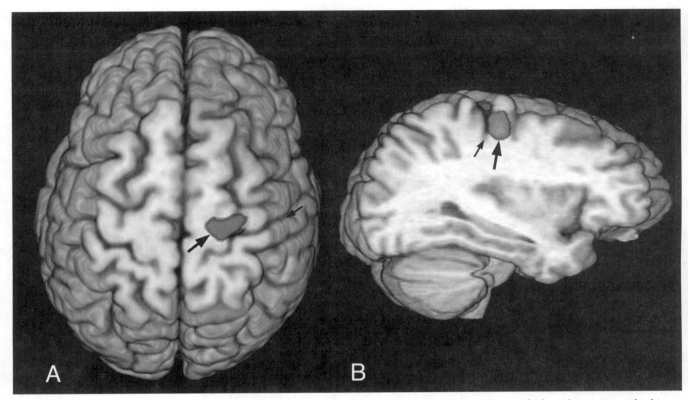

FIGURE IV.14. *MR activation map. A normal subject underwent high-resolution T_1-weighted imaging, and three-dimensional surface renderings of the brain were generated, depicting views of the brain from above (A) and from the right after slicing away part of the right hemisphere in a parasagittal plane (B). The subject performed a left-hand clenching task, while a pulse sequence sensitive to small differences in regional cerebral blood flow identified areas of cortical activation during the task, which have been superimposed on the anatomic images (large arrows). The right central sulcus has been marked for orientation (small arrows). (Figure kindly contributed by Bradley R. Buchbinder.)*

Applications of MRI: Comparison to CT

For most pathological processes affecting the brain, MRI is a more informative imaging tool than CT. MR images can be acquired in sagittal, coronal, or oblique planes in addition to axial planes, which facilitates visualization of lesions. Although CT has better spatial resolution, MRI better resolves contrast between soft tissues of differing composition. In practice, this is usually more important, even in the identification of very small lesions. Furthermore, the basis of image contrast in MR images can be varied (e.g., T_1- and T_2-weighted images), thus allowing greater flexibility in achieving lesion conspicuity. Also, the very high radiodensity of bone creates CT artifacts in tissues surrounded by large quantities of bone. The spinal cord and posterior fossa are poorly visualized on CT scans. MRI is unaffected by such artifacts. CT, but not MRI, exposes the patient to ionizing radiation.

Despite these considerations, in some situations CT is more useful than MRI. For example, acute hemorrhage typically is better detected by CT than MRI. While freshly extravasated blood may be nearly isointense to adjacent brain tissue in most MR images, it is quite dense on CT. For this reason, CT is the method of choice in the many clinical scenarios in which an acute bleed is suspected. In acute trauma, CT also has the advantage that it can better detect skull fractures. Finally, CT is better than MRI at detecting the calcification that can occur in granulomatous disease or some tumors.

The generally greater utility of MRI comes at the expense of significant logistical challenges. MR scanners are more expensive than CT scanners, and as a result they are available in fewer centers. They tend to be more heavily utilized, so that patients must wait longer for access to them. As mentioned above, some patients simply cannot undergo MR imaging because they won't fit in the scanner, won't lie still during imaging, or have metal objects in their bodies. While a CT scan may be completed in a few minutes, a complete MRI examination of the brain may take from 30 min to an hour. Furthermore, it is much more difficult to monitor an unstable patient in an MR scanner than in a CT scanner. These differences, coupled with CT's more immediate availability and superior detection of hemorrhage, makes CT a more frequent choice for emergent patients. Finally, the cost of an individual MRI exam is greater than that of a CT exam.

POSITRON EMISSION TOMOGRAPHY (PET)

How It Works

In PET, the brain itself is not directly imaged. Instead, this technique shows the distribution of an exogenously administered radioactive compound within the brain. For example, by injecting a patient with 6-^{18}F-DOPA, which is taken up by neurons that synthesize dopamine, a PET image would show where the 6-^{18}F-DOPA was distributed and effectively localize dopaminergic neurons.

A variety of radioactive nuclei are used in PET. All have in common that they decay by emitting positrons. Each emitted positron travels up to a centimeter before it collides with an electron, after which both are annihilated. This annihilation releases two photons of exactly the same energy, traveling in exactly opposite directions. The PET scanner must then detect the simultaneously emitted photons and determine their origin.

A PET scanner superficially looks much like a CT scanner, with a ring-shaped gantry and a table on which the patient lies. The scanner contains a circle of photon detectors that are arranged in a ring, much like the X-ray detectors in a CT scanner. The paired photons that are produced by a single positron–electron collision will arrive at two different detectors at nearly the same time, which identifies them as coming from the same collision. Because the photons must exit the point of collision in opposite directions, the point of their origin is known to lie along the straight line that connects the two detectors. The PET scanner generates a planar image composed of many pixels, the brightness of each representing the quantity of photons arising from a corresponding voxel of brain tissue. After each planar image slice has been recorded, the table moves further into the scanner, allowing a different image slice to be generated.

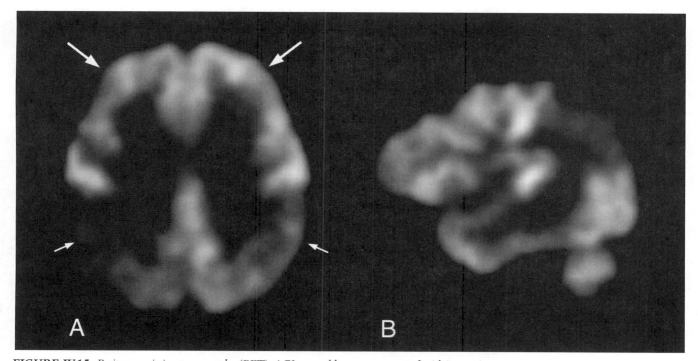

FIGURE IV.15. *Positron emission tomography (PET). A 73-year-old woman presented with increasing forgetfulness. An axial PET image obtained after injection of ^{18}F-deoxyglucose (A) demonstrates symmetrically decreased tracer activity in both parietal lobes (small arrows), in comparison to the normal-appearing frontal lobes (large arrows), signifying decreased metabolic function in the parietal lobes. A left parasagittal image (B), generated by computer from the axial images, shows that metabolism is also somewhat decreased in the temporal lobes. These findings are consistent with Alzheimer's disease. (Figure kindly contributed by Alan J. Fischman.)*

Applications

PET images have much lower spatial resolution compared to CT and MRI. PET requires preparation of radio-labeled compounds with very short half-lives. This often necessitates an on-site cyclotron or other devices of similar expense and logistical challenge. For these and other reasons, PET's clinical use in this country is confined to large academic centers.

Nevertheless, PET remains a useful tool in some clinical settings and especially in research. The strength in PET lies in the wide variety of positron-emitting compounds that can be prepared for measurement of particular biological processes. In essence, its strength is that it images biochemical processes. For example, ^{15}CO inhaled by a patient travels with cerebral blood and its distribution can be used to image regional cerebral blood flow. ^{18}F-deoxyglucose (^{18}FDG) is taken up by metabolically active brain cells and phosphorylated to ^{18}FDG-6-phosphate, which is then trapped in the cell. Subsequent PET imaging provides a map of regional glucose metabolism (see Fig. IV.15).

One of the most immediately intriguing applications of PET was its ability to detect increased neural activity in localized brain regions during particular cognitive tasks. This is possible because more active brain tissue has higher rates of blood flow and glucose metabolism, both of which can be imaged using appropriate radio-labeled molecules. This function of PET has largely been supplanted by functional MRI, which is both easier to use and faster, giving much better temporal resolution.

CONCLUSION

This appendix has discussed briefly the techniques most commonly used to image the brain and spinal cord in clinical settings. The complexity of the central nervous system, and the wide range of disease processes that affect it, give rise to an ever-increasing variety of imaging tools. Understanding some of the links between central nervous system disease and its manifestations as contrast in neuroimages not only provides a helpful adjunct for the care of patients with neurologic disorders, but also presents an opportunity for increasing one's understanding of brain physiology and pathophysiology.

Appendix V—MATERIALS LIST

GENERAL LABORATORY MATERIALS

Anatomic Specimens

Obtaining human anatomic specimens has become extremely difficult, given the declining autopsy rate and physicians fears of lawyers and HIPPA rules. If available, most of the laboratories will work best if an intact whole and half human brain is accessible as a reference. If a brain is not available, brain models and an atlas are the best substitute. Some laboratories also require an intact spinal cord. These are more difficult to substitute, since no good models really exist for spinal cords. Atlases and the photographs in this manual are the only real substitute.

Skulls and skeletons lend themselves to modeling. If the real thing is not available, substitute them with models. Pictures don't do justice to the three-dimensional teaching points of a skull or vertebral column.

Model of Brain and Skull

Many brain models are available, from toy footballs to thousand dollar variants. To teach anatomic relationships, a model of the brain in the skull is best, since students can see the anatomic relationships between the brain and its casing. Many are available at Carolina Biological Supply Company.

Model of Ventricles

We use a model produced by Somso® and available at Carolina Biological Supply Company.

Neuroanatomy Atlas

While this manual has an abbreviated atlas, it is not a substitute for a good comprehensive neuroanatomy atlas. Several are available, including:

- *The Brain Atlas: A Visual Guide to the Human Central Nervous System* by T. A. Woolsey, J. Hanaway, and M. H. Gado (Wiley)
- *Structure of the Human Brain: A Photographic Atlas* by S. J. DeArmond, M. M. Fusco, and M. M. Dewey (Oxford University Press)
- *Atlas of the Human Brain* by J. K. Mai, J. Assheaer, and G. Paxinos (Academic Press)

Functional Neuroanatomy: An Interactive Text and Manual, by Jeffrey T. Joseph and David L. Cardozo
ISBN 0-471-44437-5 Copyright © 2004 John Wiley & Sons, Inc.

Microscopic Slides

Most of the slides used in this text can be prepared from materials received on a general pathology autopsy service. These include select sections of adult brain, skeletal muscle, and peripheral nerve, as well as a fetal brain. Most useful for students are slides stained for myelin (e.g., Luxol fast blue) and counterstained with H&E. Some slides are also prepared with Nissl stains. A few slides utilize more specialized stains. Below is a list of slides that are used in different parts of the textbook. Unless otherwise specified, we suggest an H&E/LFB stain or equivalent myelin brain stain.

- Spinal cord (sacral, lumbar, thoracic, and cervical levels, plus a dorsal root ganglion)
- Medulla (best to use halves to have more levels, including near the cervicomedullary junction, caudal medulla with the hypoglossal nucleus, and rostral medulla with the inferior cerebellar peduncle)
- Pons (caudal and rostral, including locus ceruleus)
- Midbrain (caudal and rostral)
- Cerebellum, including cortex and dentate nucleus
- Hippocampus (myelin stain and a Nissl stain)
- Primary visual cortex (myelin stain and a Nissl stain)
- Primary motor cortex and primary sensory cortex (Nissl stain)
- Skeletal muscle (snap-frozen best)
- Peripheral nerve (Masson trichrome stain)
- Fetal brain at around 20 week gestation, including germinal matrix, cerebellum, and some brainstem (H&E stain)

The following pathologic slides are also extremely helpful, if available:

- Alzheimer's disease hippocampus (Bielschowsky silver stain)
- Lewy body disease or Parkinson's disease midbrain
- Demyelinated plaque from case of progressive multifocal leukoencephalopathy (myelin stain)
- H&E slide of Duchenne muscular dystrophy
- H&E slide of polymyositis
- Huntington's disease, caudate nucleus
- Multiple sclerosis demyelinated plaque; best if plaque involves medial longitudinal fasciculus in pons
- Periventricular heterotopia or another major brain malformation

Animal Specimens

The text uses sheep brains to illustrate the relationship of the dura to the brain and to dissect white matter tracts. Another chapter dissects cow eyes. These materials are available at several sites, including Carolina Biological Supply Company.

CHAPTER 1 EXTERNAL MATERIALS
Anatomic Specimens

- Intact half brain
- Intact whole brain
- Spinal cord
- Skull
- Skeleton
- Sheep's brain with dura intact

Models

- Whole brain and skull model

Miscellaneous

- Dissecting equipment with scissors
- Brain trays
- Neuroanatomy atlas

CHAPTER 2 INTERNAL MATERIALS

Anatomic Specimens

- Intact half brain
- Intact whole brain
- Half brain for dissection
- Spinal cord for transverse dissection

Models

- Ventricle model
- Whole brain and skull model

Miscellaneous

- India ink
- Paper towels to dry India ink
- Dissecting instruments
- Brain knife
- Cutting board
- Brain trays

CHAPTER 3 HISTOLOGY MATERIALS

Microscopic Slides

- Skeletal muscle cross section, snap-frozen tissue
- Peripheral nerve, Masson trichrome stain
- Peripheral nerve teased fiber preparation (these are great but difficult to obtain)
- Spinal cord, cross sections at various levels, H&E/LFB (myelin stain)
- Cerebellum, H&E/LFB (myelin stain)
- Progressive multifocal leukoencephalopathy case, H&E/LFB (myelin stain)

CHAPTER 4 NEURORADIOLOGY MATERIALS

Anatomic Specimens

- Intact half brain
- Intact whole brain
- Coronally dissected brain from laboratory 2
- Spinal cord
- Skull

Miscellaneous

- Brain trays

CHAPTER 5 SOMATOSENSORY MATERIALS

Anatomic Specimens

- Spinal cords, intact specimens
- Skeleton to examine vertebral column

Microscopic Slides

- Spinal cord transverse sections of spinal cord, including dorsal root ganglion, H&E/LFB (myelin stain)
- Medulla, H&E/LFB (myelin stain)
- Pons, H&E/LFB (myelin stain)
- Midbrain, H&E/LFB (myelin stain)

Models

- Whole brain and skull model
- Brainstem model

Miscellaneous

- Neuroanatomy atlas
- Paper clips (for two-point discrimination testing)

CHAPTER 6 CRANIOSENSORY MATERIALS

Anatomic Specimens

- Intact half brain
- Intact whole brain
- Brain hemisphere to horizontally dissect
- Coronally sliced brain from laboratory 2

Microscopic Slides

- Spinal cord, H&E/LFB (myelin stain)
- Medulla, H&E/LFB (myelin stain)
- Pons, H&E/LFB (myelin stain)
- Midbrain, H&E/LFB (myelin stain)
- Coronal section of thalamus, H&E/LFB (myelin stain)

Models

- Ventricular model

Miscellaneous

- India ink
- Paper towels to dry ink
- Dissecting equipment
- Brain knife
- Brain trays
- Dissecting board

CHAPTER 7 VISION AND HEARING MATERIALS

Anatomic Specimens

- Intact half brain
- Intact whole brain
- Skull
- Horizontal slices from laboratory 6
- Coronal slices from laboratory 2
- Fixed cow eyes

Microscopic Sections

- Primary visual cortex, area 17

Models

- Brainstem model

Miscellaneous

- Brain knife
- Dissecting instruments
- Dissecting board
- Brain trays
- Six inch long pen with distinct tip, or red-headed pin for blind spot testing

CHAPTER 8 NEUROMUSCULAR MATERIALS

Anatomic Specimens

- Spinal cord

Microscopic Sections

- Spinal cord transverse sections, H&E/LFB (myelin stain)
- Normal cross section of skeletal muscle, preferably snap-frozen, H&E
- Duchenne muscular dystrophy biopsy, H&E
- Polymyositis muscle biopsy, H&E
- Peripheral nerve, longitudinal and transverse, Masson trichrome stain

Miscellaneous

- Neuroanatomy atlas

CHAPTER 9 BASAL GANGLIA MATERIALS

Anatomic Specimens

- Intact half brain
- Intact whole brain
- Coronal sections from laboratory 2
- Posterior fossa transverse sections from laboratory 2

Microscopic Slides

- Midbrain, H&E/LFB (myelin stain)
- Caudate nucleus or putamen and globus pallidus, H&E/LFB (myelin stain)
- Case of Huntington's disease, H&E/LFB (myelin stain)

Models

- Head and neck model
- Ventricle model

Miscellaneous

- Brain knives
- Dissecting equipment
- Dissecting board

- Brain trays
- Modeling clay, four colors, to build a basal ganglia.

CHAPTER 10 CEREBELLUM MATERIALS
Anatomic Specimens

- Intact half brain
- Intact whole brain
- Posterior fossa transverse sections from laboratory 2
- Intact half brainstem and cerebellum from laboratory 6

Microscopic Slide

- Cerebellum with dentate nucleus, H&E/LFB stain (myelin stain)

Miscellaneous

- Brain knives
- Dissecting instruments, including scalpel and handle
- Dissection board
- Brain trays

CHAPTER 11 CRANIAL NERVES MATERIALS
Anatomic Specimens

- Whole brain, to show relationship with brainstem
- Half brain, to show relationship with brainstem
- Intact half brainstem and cerebellum from laboratory 6, for dissection
- Transverse sections through brainstem (from laboratory 2)
- Skull

Microscopic Slides

- Spinal cord transverse sections, H&E/LFB (myelin stain)
- Medulla, H&E/LFB (myelin stain)
- Pons, including locus ceruleus, H&E/LFB (myelin stain)
- Midbrain, H&E/LFB (myelin stain)

Model

- Brainstem model
- Head and skull model

Miscellaneous

- Colored chalk
- Pipe cleaners
- Neuroanatomy atlas
- Dissecting instruments
- Brain knives
- Dissecting board
- Brain trays

CHAPTER 12 BRAINSTEM SYSTEMS MATERIALS

This laboratory uses a frame that holds files in a file cabinet, along with photocopies on clear transparency acetates (as for an overhead projector) of brainstem slices to teach the various systems in the brainstem. In the major exercise, students will trace each system through a series of nine transparencies hung from the frame, using different colored threads. Corresponding nuclei will be outlined with similarly colored markers. See Figure V.1 for a simplified perspective of how to set up these models.

In addition the laboratory uses a cut-and-paste technique, requiring scissors and glue, to review more brainstem anatomy.

Anatomic Specimens

- Brainstem
- Skull

Microscopic Slides

- Spinal cord, H&E/LFB (myelin stain)
- Medulla, H&E/LFB (myelin stain)
- Pons, H&E/LFB (myelin stain)
- Midbrain, H&E/LFB (myelin stain)
- Multiple sclerosis, with a plaque involving the medial longitudinal fasciculus, H&E/LFB (myelin stain)

Models

- Head and brain model
- Brainstem model

Miscellaneous

- Sets of full-page overhead "acetates" with printed brainstem sections (nine per set) photocopied from the appendix to Chapter 12 (Figs. 12.50 through 12.58)
- Hanging folder frame (normally used in a file cabinet) to hold acetates (available at any office supply store); see Figure V.1
- Rings, 1 inch, hinged to connect acetates to frame (available at any office supply store)
- Hole punch; pass rings through holes in acetates and attach to frame
- Yarn (white, red, green, orange, yellow, blue, brown, purple—available at craft or sewing stores; makes for a nice work-related outing during work hours!)
- Yarn needle (heavy needle that can punch through overhead acetates—available at craft or sewing stores)
- Colored markers to match yarn colors; must be able to write on plastic overhead acetates (available at any office supply store)
- Black marker (rather than white)
- Glue
- Scissors
- Photocopies of brainstem nuclei from end of chapters (Figs. 12.49 and 12.50)
- Neuroanatomy atlas including brainstem

CHAPTER 13 HYPOTHALAMUS MATERIALS

Anatomic Specimens

- Intact whole brain
- Intact sagittal half brain
- Previously dissected coronal slabs

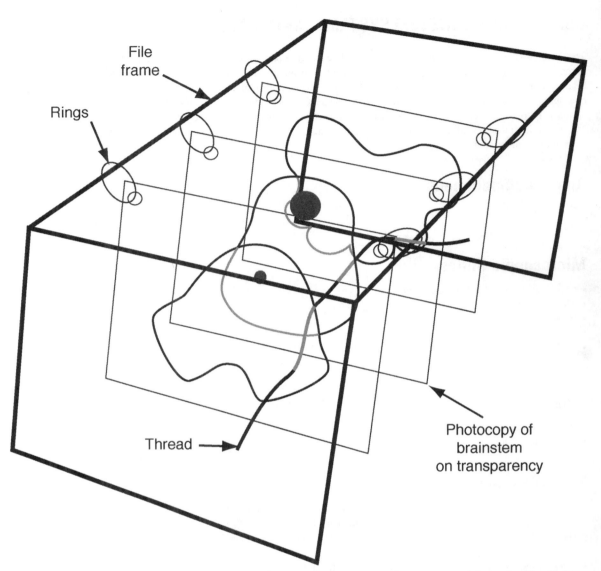

FIGURE V.1. *Diagram showing brainstem model. This model is constructed from a hanging file folder rack, paper rings, and photocopied overhead acetates from the end of the chapter.*

Microscopic Slides

- Hypothalamus, with supraoptic and paraventricular nuclei, H&E/LFB
- Pituitary, including anterior and posterior portions, H&E
- Vasopressin-immunostained section of human hypothalamus, including the supraoptic and paraventricular nuclei
- Medulla, H&E/LFB (myelin stain)
- Pons, H&E/LFB (myelin stain)
- Midbrain from patient with Parkinson's disease, H&E/LFB stain

Miscellaneous

- Brain dissection knife
- Dissecting instruments, including scalpel blade and handle
- Brain trays
- Dissecting boards

CHAPTER 14 LIMBIC MATERIALS
Anatomic Specimens

- Intact whole brain
- Intact sagittal half brain
- Previously dissected coronal slabs
- Previously dissected horizontal slabs

Microscope Slides

- Hippocampus with surrounding parahippocampal gyrus (entorhinal cortex) and temporal neocortex, Nissl stain of 40 micrometer sections
- Hippocampus stained for myelin (H&E/LFB)
- Bielschowsky-stained section from Alzheimer's disease brain (an equivalent would be a β-amyloid and tau-immunostained slides from an Alzheimer's disease brain)

Miscellaneous

- Brain dissection knife
- Dissecting instruments, including scalpel blade and handle
- Brain trays
- Dissecting boards

CHAPTER 15 NEOCORTEX MATERIALS
Anatomic Specimens

- Intact whole brain
- Intact sagittal half brain
- Previously dissected coronal slabs
- Previously dissected horizontal slabs

Microscopic Slides

- Primary somatosensory and motor cortex (banks of central sulcus), Nissl stain
- Association cortex (e.g. anterior middle frontal gyrus), Nissl stain
- Hippocampus and parahippocampal gyrus, Nissl stain (same as the limbic system lab)

Models

- Brain and skull

Miscellaneous

- Brain dissection knife
- Dissecting instruments
- Brain trays
- Dissecting boards

CHAPTER 16 DEVELOPMENT MATERIALS
Anatomic Specimens

- Intact whole brain
- Intact sagittal half brain

Microscopic Slides

- Normal fetus at around 20 weeks gestation, including germinal matrix, cerebellum, and brainstem
- Periventricular nodular heterotopia stained for myelin (LFB and H&E)

CHAPTER 17 TRAUMA MATERIALS

Anatomic Specimens

- Skull
- Intact whole brain
- Skeleton

Models

- Brain with skull

CHAPTER 18 REVIEW MATERIALS

Anatomic Specimens

- Intact half brain
- Intact whole brain
- Previously dissected coronal slabs
- Previously dissected horizontal slabs
- Skull
- Skeleton

Models

- Brain with skull
- Brainstem

APPENDIX III SHEEP BRAIN MATERIALS

Anatomic Specimens

- Sheep brains with dura intact

Miscellaneous

- Popsicle sticks
- Scalpel and blade
- Dissecting board
- Brain tray

KEY TERMS FOR SELF STUDY

Give short definitions of the following terms:

Chapter 1

internal acoustic meatus
angiogram
anterior
anterior cerebral artery
anterior communicating artery
anterior horns
anterior spinal artery
arachnoid
arachnoid granulations
basilar artery
cauda equina
caudal
central canal
central sulcus
cerebellum
cerebral aqueduct of Sylvius
cerebrospinal fluid
cervical spinal cord
cingulate gyrus
circle of Willis
cisterna magna
cisterns
coronal
corpus callosum
Cranial nerve V (trigeminal)
cribriform plate
diencephalon
dorsal
dorsal root ganglion
dorsal spinal roots
dura
epidural space
falx cerebri
foramen magnum
forebrain

fourth ventricle
frontal lobes
great vein of Galen
hindbrain
horizontal
inferior
insular cortex
internal carotid artery
jugular vein
lateral ventricles
lingual gyrus
lumbar spinal cord
mammillary bodies
medulla
meninges
mesencephalon
midbrain
middle cerebral artery
neural tube
occipital lobes
olfactory bulb
olfactory nerve
olive (inferior olivary nucleus)
optic canal
optic chiasm
optic nerve
parasagittal
parietal lobes
parietooccipital sulcus
pia
pons
postcentral gyrus
posterior
posterior cerebral artery
posterior horns

Functional Neuroanatomy: An Interactive Text and Manual, by Jeffrey T. Joseph and David L. Cardozo
ISBN 0-471-44437-5 Copyright © 2004 John Wiley & Sons, Inc.

posterior inferior cerebellar artery
precentral gyrus
preoccipital notch
prosencephalon
pyramidal decussation
pyramids
rostral
sacral spinal cord
sagittal
sigmoid sinus
straight sinus
subarachnoid space
subdural space
superior
superior orbital fissure

superior sagittal sinus
superior temporal gyrus
Sylvian fissure
telencephalon
temporal bone
temporal lobes
tentorium
third ventricle
thoracic spinal cord
transverse fissure
transverse sinus
ventral
ventral spinal roots
vertebral arteries

Chapter 2

amygdala
anterior cerebral artery
anterior commissure
aqueduct
calcarine fissure
caudate nucleus
centrum semiovale
cerebellum
cerebral peduncles
choroid plexus
cingulate gyrus
claustrum
corona radiata
corpus callosum
corticospinal tract
dentate nucleus
dorsal horn
dorsal root ganglia
external capsule
extreme capsule
foramen of Luschka
foramen of Magendie
foramen of Monro
fornix
fourth ventricle
frontal cortex
genu of corpus callosum
globus pallidus
globus pallidus externus
globus pallidus internus
hippocampus
inferior cerebellar peduncle
inferior colliculus
inferior olivary nucleus
insula

lateral geniculate nucleus
lateral ventricle
mammillary bodies
medulla
midbrain
middle cerebellar peduncle
nucleus accumbens
oculomotor nerve
olfactory tract
optic nerve
optic tract
parietooccipital sulcus
pineal
pons
precentral gyrus
putamen
pyramid
pyramidal tract
red nucleus
septum pellucidum
spinal root
splenium of corpus callosum
subcortical "U" fibers
substantia nigra
superior cerebellar peduncle
superior colliculus
temporal lobe
thalamus
third ventricle
uncus
ventral horn
vertebral artery
vertebral body
Wallerian degeneration

Chapter 3

actin
acute bacterial meningitis
alpha actinin
astrocyte
ATPase stain

axon
Betz cell
dendrites
dorsal root ganglion neuron
endoneurium

epineurium
GFAP
glia
glial fibrillary acidic protein
glycogen granules
Golgi
H&E
immunoperoxidase stain
internal granular neuron
interneuron
Luxol fast blue
lymphocyte
macrophage
Masson trichrome stain
microglia
mitochondria
molecular layer
motor neuron
myelin

myelin basic protein
myofiber
myosin
neuropil
neutrophil
Nissl substance
nodes of Ranvier
oligodendrocyte
one slow red ox
perineurium
polymorphonuclear leukocytes
progressive multifocal leukoencephalopathy
Purkinje cell
purulent meningitis
sarcomere
Schwann cell
teased fiber
Z band

Chapter 4

FLAIR-fluid attenuated inversion recovery
caudate nucleus
CT-computerized tomography
DWI-diffusion weighted
glioblastoma multiforme
lentiform nucleus
MRI-magnetic resonance imaging

MRA- magnetic resonance angiography
PET-positron emission tomography
pineal gland
SPECT-single photon emission tomography
striatum
volume averaging

Chapter 5

abducens nucleus
anterior white commissure
basis pontis
cerebral peduncle
cuneate nucleus
dorsal root ganglion
fourth ventricle
gracilis nucleus
intermediolateral column
kinesthetic
Lissauer's tract
oculomotor nucleus
pyramidal decussation
solitary tract
subarachnoid space
substantia nigra
anterior spinal artery
anterolateral system
cauda equina
Clarke's column
dorsal columns
dura
free nerve endings
hypoglossal nucleus

internal arcuate fibers
lamina of Rexed
medial lemniscus
pia mater
pyramids
spinal trigeminal nucleus
subdural space
two point discrimination
anterior white commissure
arachnoid
cerebral aqueduct
cuneate fasciculus
dorsal horn
facial nucleus
gracilis fasciculus
inferior olivary nucleus
intervertebral foramen
lateral (surround) inhibition
nociception
pontine trigeminal nuclei
red nucleus
spinothalamic fibers
substantia gelatinosa
ventral horn

Chapter 6

anterior commissure
anterior nucleus
anterolateral tract

calcarine cortex
caudate nucleus
central sulcus

centrum semiovale
choroid plexus
cingulate gyrus
claustrum
corpus callosum
diencephalon
extreme capsule
fornix
Gasserian ganglion
genu
globus pallidus
herniation
hippocampus
hypothalamus
insula
internal capsule
internal medullary lamina
lateral geniculate nucleus
lateral medullary infarct
Lissauer's tract
mammillary bodies
medial dorsal nucleus
medial geniculate nucleus

PICA
postcentral gyrus
post-central gyrus
posterior inferior cerebellar artery
precentral gyrus
principal trigeminal sensory nucleus
pulvinar
putamen
red nucleus
sensory homunculus
spinal trigeminal nucleus
spinal trigeminal tract
splenium
substantia nigra
subthalamic nucleus
superior colliculus
thalamus
trigeminal ganglion
trigeminal motor nucleus
ventral posterolateral nucleus
ventral posteromedial nucleus
ventral tier nuclei
VPM

Chapter 7

calcarine fissure
Heschl's gyrus
heteronomous hemianopsia
homonymous hemianopsia
inferior colliculus
lateral geniculate body
lateral lemniscus
macula
medial geniculate nucleus

Meyer's loop
oculomotor nerve
optic pit
optic disk
optic radiations
organ of Corti
pituitary adenoma
stripe of Gennari
trapezoid body

Chapter 8

amyotrophic lateral sclerosis
anterior horn cell
compound muscle action potential (CMAP)
dermatome
electromyography (EMG)
endorneurium
epineurium
fascicle
fasciculation
fibrillation
Guillain-Barré syndrome

motor unit
muscular dystrophy
myotome
nerve conduction velocity (NCV)
neuropathy
node of Ranvier
perineurium
poliomyelitis
polymyositis
sensory nerve action potential (SNAP)

Chapter 9

amygdala
anterior commissure
anterograde transport
basal ganglia
caudate nucleus
cingulate gyrus
cocaine
corpus callosum

D1 receptor
D2 receptor
direct pathway
dopamine
external capsule
extrapyramidal
fornix
frontal association cortex

gamma amino butyric acid (GABA)
globus pallidus
globus pallidus externus
globus pallidus internus
glutamate
hippocampus
horse radish peroxidase
Huntington's disease
immunoperoxidase
in situ hybridization
indirect pathway
insular cortex
internal capsule
lateral geniculate nucleus
lectin
lentiform nucleus
medial geniculate nucleus

met-enkephalin
nucleus accumbens
optic chiasm and tract
Parkinson's disease
polyglutamine
putamen
retrograde transport
striatum
substance P
substantia nigra pars compacta
substantia nigra pars reticulata
subthalamic nucleus
triplet repeat
tyrosine hydroxylase
ventral anterior thalamus
ventral lateral thalamus
ventral tegmental area

Chapter 10

cerebrocerebellum
Clarke's column
climbing fiber
dentate nucleus
emboliform nucleus
fastigial nucleus
flocculus
folia
globose nucleus
Golgi cells,
inferior cerebellar peduncle
interposed nuclei
middle cerebellar peduncle

mossy fiber
nodulus
olivocerebellum
nystagmus
PICA
posterior inferior cerebellar artery
Purkinje neuron
spinocerebellum
Superior cerebellar artery
superior cerebellar peduncle
tentorium
vermis
vestibulocerebellum

Chapter 11

basis pontis
abducens nerve
abducens nucleus
AICA
anterior inferior cerebellar artery
cerebellopontine angle
cochlear nerve
cranial nerve
cuneatus nucleus
decussation of superior cerebellar peduncle
dorsal motor nucleus of the vagus
extra ocular muscles
facial nerve
facial nucleus
foramen magnum
foramen ovale
foramen rotundum
glossopharyngeal nerve
gracilis nucleus
hypoglossal nerve
inferior colliculus
inferior olivary nucleus
inferior oblique
inferior olive

inferior rectus
internal auditory meatus
jugular foramen
lateral rectus
locus ceruleus
medial longitudinal fasciculus
medial rectus
MLF
multiple sclerosis
nucleus ambiguous
oculomotor nerve
oculomotor nucleus
optic canal
paramedian pontine reticular formation
pedunculopontine nucleus
raphe nucleus
red nucleus
serotonin
superior colliculus
superior rectus
superior oblique
superior orbital fissure
trigeminal nerve
trochlear nerve

trochlear nucleus
vagus nerve

vestibular nucleus
vestibulocochlear nerve

Chapter 12

abducens nerve
abducens nucleus
accessory cuneate nucleus
acetylcholine
anterolateral system
aqueduct
arcuate fibers
basis pontis
cochlear nerve
cochlear nuclei
corticobulbar tracts
corticospinal tract
cribriform plate
crossed pattern
cuneatus nucleus
decussation of superior cerebellar peduncle
decussation of the pyramids
demyelination
dorsal motor nucleus of the vagus
facial nerve
facial nucleus
foramen magnum
foramen ovale
foramen rotundum
fourth ventricle
glossopharyngeal nerve
gracilis nucleus
hypoglossal foramen
hypoglossal nerve
hypoglossal nucleus
immunoperoxidase
inferior cerebellar peduncle
inferior colliculus
inferior oblique
inferior olivary nucleus
inferior rectus
in-situ hybridization
internal auditory meatus
internuclear ophthalmoplegia
jugular foramen
lateral lemniscus
lateral rectus
locus ceruleus
medial lemniscus

medial longitudinal fasciculus
medial rectus
medulla
midbrain
middle cerebellar peduncle
multiple sclerosis
norepinepherine
nucleus ambiguus
oculomotor nerve
oculomotor nucleus
olfactory bulbs
olfactory nerve
olfactory tract
optic canal
optic chiasm
optic nerve
optic tract
periaqueductal gray
pons
posterior commissure
principal trigeminal sensory nucleus
raphe nuclei
red nucleus
serotonin
spinal trigeminal nucleus
spinal trigeminal tract
substantia nigra
superior cerebellar peduncle
superior colliculus
superior oblique
superior olivary nucleus
superior orbital fissure
superior rectus
supranuclear palsy
tectum
tegmentum
trigeminal motor nucleus
trigeminal nerve
trochlear nerve
trochlear nucleus
vagus nerve
vestibular nerve
vestibular nuclei

Chapter 13

adenohypophysis
adrenocorticotrophic hormone
amygdala
anterior thalamic nucleus
circumventricular organs
diabetes insipidus

dopamine
dorsal motor nucleus of vagus
facial nerve
follicle stimulating hormone
fornix
glossopharyngeal nerve

growth hormone

infundibulum

intermediolateral column

luteinizing hormone

mammillary bodies

narcolepsy

neurohypophysis

optic chiasm

oxytocin

panhypopituitarism

paraventricular nucleus

periaqueductal gray

pituitary

portal system

prolactin

Rathke's cleft

reticular formation of medulla and pons

solitary nucleus

stria terminalis

supraoptic nucleus

thyroid stimulating hormone

vagus nerve

vasopressin

Chapter 14

acetylcholine

acetylcholinesterase

Alzheimer's disease

Ammon's horn

amygdala

amyloid

anterior perforated substance

basal nucleus of Meynert

cingulate cortex

cingulate gyrus

dentate gyrus

diagonal band of Broca

emotion

entorhinal cortex

fimbria

fornix

hippocampus

hypothalamus

insula

limbic system

mammillary body

mammillothalamic tract

memory

olfactory cortex

orbitofrontal cortex

Papez circuit

parahippocampal gyrus

piriform cortex

plaques

septal nuclei

septum

stria terminalis

subiculum

tau protein

uncus

Chapter 15

allocortex

aphasia

association cortex

attention

auditory cortex

border zone

Broca's area

Brodmann

corticocortical connections

corticobulbar fibers

corticopontine fibers

corticospinal fibers

frontotemporal dementia

granular layer

gustatory cortex

language

lateral geniculate nucleus

limbic cortex

medial geniculate nucleus

motor cortex

multimodal association area

neglect syndrome

neocortex

olfactory cortex

orbitofrontal cortex

paralimbic cortex

Pick's disease

prosopagnosia

pyramidal layer

sensory cortex

somatosensory cortex

visual cortex

watershed area

Wernicke's area

Chapter 16

anencephaly

Bergmann radial glia

epilepsy

encephaloclastic lesion

floor plate

germinal matrix

heterotopia

holoprosencephaly

lissencephaly

neural crest

notochord

neural tube

pachygyria

polymicrogyria

subventricular zone

sonic hedgehog

ventricular zone

Chapter 17

aneurysm

Brown-Sequard syndrome

contrecoup contusions

coup contusions

diffuse axonal injury (DAI)

epidural hemorrhage

hematoma

hematomyelia

hemorrhage

mass lesion

meningioma

splinter hemorrhages

subdural

subfalcine herniation

tonsilar herniation

uncus

uncal herniation

Index

Abducens nerve, 263, 292, 307–309
Abducens nucleus, 309
Abductor pollicis brevis, 207
Accumbens nucleus, 459–460, 513, 514, 519
Acetylcholine system, 371–372
Acidophilic dye, 50
Actin filaments, 53, 54
Activation mapping, 545–546. *See also* Functional MRI
    (fMRI)
Adenohypophysis, 343
Aggression, limbic system and, 374–375
AIDS, 73
Alcoholism, 254–255
Alveus, 516
Alzheimer's disease (AD), 50, 375–379, 412, 547
Ammon's horn, 363, 367
Amygdala, 332, 347, 365, 366, 374, 375, 460, 514,
    515, 519
Amygdalofugal pathway, 332
Amygdaloid complex, 356
Amyloid β (Aβ) protein, 376–378
Amyloid precursor protein (APP), 378
Amyotrophic lateral sclerosis (ALS), 191, 203–204,
    205, 208
Anastomoses, 91
Anencephaly, 422–424
Aneurysms, 28
Angiograms, 86–93. *See also* Angiography
  applications for, 91–93
  CT, 85, 534
  postmortem, 17, 19
Angiography, 77. *See also* Angiograms; Magnetic resonance
    angiography (MRA)
  operation of, 528–530
Anterior cerebral artery, 17, 513, 519, 521
Anterior cingulate cortex (CG), 405
Anterior circulation, 5
Anterior commissure, 37, 141, 216, 514, 515, 519, 520, 522
Anterior inferior cerebellar arteries (AICA), 91, 241, 261
Anterior nucleus, thalamus, 216, 357, 515, 520
Anterior structures, 3
Anterior vessels, 14, 15
Anterograde transport, 213
Anterolateral-spinothalamic system, 107–109, 296
  comparison with lemniscal system, 157–159
  fibers, 127, 128, 129, 143, 146

  pathways, 129–131
  trigeminal input into, 135
Aortic aneurysm, 491
Aphasia, 404–405
  global, 409
Apparent diffusion coefficient (ADC), 100
Aqueduct, 516, 517, 519, 522
Arachnoid, 6, 22, 25
Arachnoid granulations, 24, 30, 43, 45
Arcuate fibers, 124
Area postrema, 332
Arhinencephaly, 430
Arteries, overlapping, 104. *See also* Anterior inferior
    cerebellar arteries (AICA); Basilar artery; Carotid
    artery; Cerebral arteries; Posterior inferior cerebellar
    arteries (PICA); Spinal arteries; Superior cerebellar
    arteries (SCA); Vertebral arteries
Aspiny neurons, 219
Association cortices, 383
Association fibers, 30
Astrocytes, 46, 51, 64–65, 73, 75
  cancer of, 83–84
Atomic nuclei, MRI and, 536–539
ATPase, 53, 54
Atrium lateral ventricles, 520
Attention, cortex and, 386, 405–407
Attenuation, with CT, 531–532
Auditory cortex, 179
  receptive fields in, 180–182
Auditory system, 161, 166, 271, 296, 477–478
  anatomy of, 177–179, 269
  deficit, clinical case, 183–184
  nuclei, 179
  pathways, 164–165
  review of, 470
  signals, 310
Autonomic nervous system, 271–273, 297–298, 333, 344–347
Axonal damage, 455
Axonal degeneration, 46
Axonal myelination, 192
Axonal neuropathies, 191
Axons, 50, 62–63
  myelinated and unmyelinated, 201

Back pain, 112
Basal forebrain, 360

Functional Neuroanatomy: An Interactive Text and Manual, by Jeffrey T. Joseph and David L. Cardozo
ISBN 0-471-44437-5 Copyright © 2004 John Wiley & Sons, Inc.

Basal ganglia, 140, 142, 211–232
    circuits, 472, 483
    components of, 217–219
    coronal dissection of, 213–216
    electrophysiology data related to, 228
    histology of, 218–219
    Huntington's disease and, 228–232
    intrinsic connections in, 212, 220–226
    materials related to, 553–554
    movement and, 227
    physiology of, 226–228
    structures around ventricles, 217
    structures of, 211–212
    wiring diagram of, 227
Basal nucleus of Meynert, 356, 360, 371
Basilar artery, 13, 88, 89, 261, 518, 519
"Basket brain," 432–434
Basket neurons, 234
Basophilic dye, 50
Bergmann glial, 421
Betz cells, 51, 61, 398
"Blind spot," 166, 169
Blood, CT scans of, 82–83
Blood-brain barrier, 84, 340
Blood-nerve barrier, 50–51
Blood supply, to the brain and spinal cord, 5–6
Bone windows, 78, 82, 83
Border zones, 389
Bradykinesia, 226
Brain. *See also* Brainstem; Cerebellum; Cerebrum;
        Fetal brain; Half brain; Medulla
    anatomical atlas of, 505–522
    axes of, 4
    blood supply to, 5
    coronal sections of, 171, 506–517
    coverings of, 6, 21–26
    development of, 413–439
    divisions of, 2
    external anatomy of, 4–5, 7–12
    herniation of, 443
    horizontal dissection of, 136–142, 143, 518–521
    internal anatomy of, 29–48
    major arteries of, 17
    major divisions of, 7
    malformations of, 414
    orientation of, 7
    sagittal sections of, 521–522
    sheep, 523–525, 558
    soft tissue coverings of, 24–26
Brain base, 12, 334, 335, 458–459
    features of, 10–11
Brain contusions, 442
Brain hemorrhages, 26–28, 449–453, 454
Brain imaging techniques, 18, 29, 78–79, 527–548
Brain injury. *See* Trauma
Brain slicing, 30
Brainstem, 7, 34, 109, 121–129, 240, 259–288, 462
    anterolateral versus medial lemniscal pathways in, 129–131
    auditory pathways in, 181
    clinical tips concerning, 294
    control systems involving, 273–284
    diffuse projection systems of, 273
    divisions of, 260
    functions of, 261
    histology of, 269–273
    key concepts related to, 290–292
    landmarks in, 40
    long tracts in, 293–294
    macroscopic anatomy of, 265–267
    main tracts in, 164–165
    regional anatomy of, 262–265
    relationship to the skull, 260
    somatosensory pathways through, 130–131

    three-dimensional anatomy of, 294–295
    transverse histology of, 286–288
    transverse sections of, 38–40
    vasculature of, 261–262, 267–269
Brainstem exercises, sections for, 318–329
Brainstem lesions, 285
    case review of, 299
Brainstem nuclei, 290, 346
    motor nuclei, 273–274
Brainstem structures, 11–12, 268
    external, 263–264
    materials related to, 555
Brain structures. *See also* Brainstem structures
    CT imaging of, 81
    identifying, 40–41
Brain tissue, handling, 1
Brain tumor, 486–487
Brain ventricles, 35, 36, 43–45, 518. *See also* Fourth
        ventricle; Third ventricle
Branchial arches, 290, 291
Broca, Pierre Paul, 355
Broca's aphasia, 48
Broca's area, 403–404
Brodmann areas, 382, 384
Brown-Sequard syndrome, 446, 447, 489

Calcarine fissure, 172, 521
Callosal fibers, 30
Capillaries, 68
Carotid artery, 13, 90
    angiogram after injection of, 89
CAT scans. *See* Computed tomography (CT); CT
        entries
Cauda equina, 14
Caudal medulla, 144
Caudal structures, 3
Caudate nucleus, 36, 138, 212, 215, 513, 514, 515, 517,
        520, 521
    histology of, 219, 220
    tail, 515, 516, 517, 519, 520
Central auditory pathways, 164–165
Central nervous system, 105
    development of, 2, 420
Centromedian nucleus, 516
Centrum semiovale, 137, 521
Cerebellar activation, 254
Cerebellar connections, 246–253
    extrinsic, 235–237
Cerebellar cortex, 235, 243
    development of, 420–421
Cerebellar hemorrhage, 255–258
Cerebellar infarct, 242–243, 253
Cerebellar peduncles, 126, 127, 235, 241, 298, 303
Cerebellar systems, 298–299, 481, 482
    review of, 471
Cerebellar vermis, 518, 519, 521, 522
Cerebellopontine angle (CPA), 264
Cerebellum, 7, 13, 38, 233–258, 518, 519. *See also* Cerebellar
        entries
    anatomic divisions of, 234
    brainstem components associated with, 269, 271
    circuitry and function of, 237
    clinical aspects of, 238–239, 239–240, 254–258
    development of, 417
    dissection and regional anatomy of, 240–243
    functional divisions of, 238
    function of, 234, 239
    histology of, 234, 243–245
    input and output structures of, 246–247
    materials related to, 554
    neuronal types in, 244
    transverse sections of, 38–40
    vascular territories of, 242

Cerebral angiograms, 87–88, 529–530
Cerebral arteries, 85, 387–388. *See also* Anterior cerebral
    artery; Middle cerebral artery; Posterior cerebral
    arteries (PCA)
  dissection of, 16
  vascular territories of, 19
Cerebral circulation, 89, 90
Cerebral cortex, 4, 381–412. *See also* Cortex cellular and
    laminar organization of, 395–399
  divisions of, 484
  neural networks in, 407–408
  vascular supply of, 387–389
Cerebral hemispheres, 7–10
  development of, 418–419
Cerebral infarct, embolic, 68
Cerebral peduncles, 40, 47, 263, 519, 515
  atrophy in, 409
Cerebrocerebellum, major components of, 248
Cerebrospinal fluid (CSF), 14, 24, 25, 30
  flow of, 44
  in MRI scans, 93
Cerebrum, 7. *See also* Cerebral entries
  coronal dissection of, 37, 214
Cervical spinal cord, 113, 115, 116, 144
  histology of, 119
Cervicomedullary junction, 121–122
Cholinergic neurons, 357, 371–372
Chorea, 228, 229
Choroid plexus, 30, 35, 44, 66–67, 93, 516, 517, 519,
    520, 522
  in temporal horn, 517
  ventricular flow from, 45
Cingulate gyrus, 356, 360, 513, 517, 520, 521
Circle of Willis, 16, 88
  dissection, 18
Circulation, brainstem, 261–262
Circulation angiograms, 256
Circumventricular organs, 332, 340
Cisterna magna, 26
Cisterns, 6, 26
Clarke's columns, 117, 235
Claustrum, 513, 514, 515, 516, 520
Climbing fibers, 234
Cocaine binding, 221, 222
Cochlear nerve, 264
Cochlear nuclei, 312
Cognitive functions, higher, 253–254
Commissural fibers, 36, 385
Compound action potential, 202, 206
Compound muscle action potential (CMAP), 193–194
Computed tomography (CT). *See also* CT entries angiography
    with, 534
  MRI versus, 543, 546–547
  operation of, 530–535
  PET versus, 548
Concussion, 455
Connectivity, methods related to, 399
Contralateral neglect, 406–407
Contrast, in MRI images, 536, 541
Contrast agent, 94
Contrast enhancement
  with CT, 532–534
  with MRI, 536, 541
Contrast material, in angiography, 528
Contrecoup contusion, 24, 442, 448
Contusions, 448–449. *See also* Contrecoup contusion;
    Coup contusion
Coronal dissection, basal ganglia, 213–216
Coronally dissected brain, comparison with coronal MRI,
    40–42
Coronal plane, 4
Coronal sections, half-brain, 33–37
Coronal T1 MRI, 96

Corpus callosum, 10, 11, 12, 35, 36, 37, 138, 139, 513, 514,
    517, 520, 521
  multiple sclerosis and, 285
Cortex. *See also* Cerebral cortex; Cortical entries; Neocortex;
    Sensory cortex
  development of, 422
  basal ganglia connections with, 222
  classifying, 382
  clinical cases related to, 408–412
  commissural connections to, 403
  connectivity of, 385–386, 399–403
  corticocortical connections to, 401–402
  functional lateralization in, 386
  functional types of, 382–384
  histology of, 384
  thalamocortical and subcortical connections to, 400–401
Cortical afferents/efferents, 401
Cortical areas, functional affiliations of, 403–408
Cortical gyration, 416–418
Cortical layers, 419–420
Cortical neuron, 176
Cortical zones, functionally similar groups of, 390–394
Corticobulbar tracts, 40, 293
Corticospinal system, review of, 471
Corticospinal tracts, 40, 47, 252, 293, 479, 480
  pathways in, 47
Coup contusion, 442
Cranial nerve III, 13. *See also* Oculomotor nerve
Cranial nerve IV, 263. *See also* Trochlear nerve
Cranial nerve V, 13. *See also* Trigeminal nerve
Cranial nerve VI, 513, 514. *See also* Abducens nerve
Cranial nerve VII, 518. *See also* Facial nerve
Cranial nerve VIII, 518. *See also* Vestibulocochlear nerve
Cranial nerve IX, 264. *See also* Glossopharyngeal nerve
Cranial nerve X, 264. *See also* Vagus nerve
Cranial nerve XII, 264. *See also* Hypoglossal nerve
Cranial nerves, 24, 135, 260, 265, 289–328
  building, 302–318
  exits and functions of, 266
  materials related to, 554
  specific, 292–293
Craniopharyngioma, 348–351
Craniosacral system, 333
Craniosensory systems, 133–159
  materials related to, 552
Creatine kinase, 197
Creutzfeldt-Jacob disease (CJD), 1
CT angiography (CTA), 534, 535. *See also* Computed
    tomography (CT)
CT artifacts, 85–86
CT perfusion imaging, 535
CT scans, 27, 28, 78, 80–86, 494–496
  applications for, 81–85
CT venography (CTV), 534, 535
Cuneate nucleus, 518
Cyclopia, 424

"Dawson's fingers," 284, 286
Decussating fibers, 143
Decussation superior cerebellar peduncle, 516, 519
Dementia, frontotemporal, 412
Demyelinating neuropathies, 191
Demyelination, 72
Dendritic tree, 62–63
Dentate gyrus, 358, 516, 517
Dentate nucleus, 234, 245, 518, 519
Dentatorubropallidoluysian atrophy (DRPLA), 212
Dermatomes, 153
Dermatomyositis, 199
Descending sympathetic fibers, 345
Development, materials related to, 557–558
Diabetes, 309, 333–334, 490
Diencephalic herniation, 443

Diencephalon, 5
Diffuse axonal injury (DAI), 442, 455
Diffuse systems, 261, 273
  brainstem, 280–284
Diffusion-weighted imaging (DWI), 100, 544
Digital subtraction angiography (DSA), 528–530
Dipole spin vectors, 537, 538
Dissecting knives, 34
Dissociated sensory loss, 125, 448–449
Distal numbness/weakness, acute onset of, 208–209
DNA sequence analysis, 438
Dopamine, 212, 261
Dopamine neurons, 342
Dopamine system, 220–222
Dorsal column fibers, 117–118
Dorsal column/lemniscal system, 106–107, 108, 120
Dorsal motor nucleus, 344
  of vagus, 316
Dorsal root ganglia (DRG), 15, 110, 187–188
  histology of, 113–114
  neurons of, 51
Dorsal spinocerebellar tract, 236
Dorsal structures, 3
Duchenne's muscular dystrophy, 197–198. *See also* Muscular
    dystrophy
Dura, 6, 21, 22
  folds, 20
  sheep, 24, 25, 523, 524
Duret hemorrhages, 453
Dystrophin, 197

Efferent signals, 302–303
Eggshell fracture, 445
Electromyography (EMG), 195–196
Electron microscopy, 57
Electrophysiology, clinical, 192–196, 206
Embolic infarct, 48
Emitter-detector pairs, 529
Emitters, for CT, 530, 531
Emotions, limbic system and, 359, 373–374
Encephaloclastic lesions, 415, 431–434
Endoneurium, 50
Entorhinal cortex, 363, 364, 514, 515
Environmental agents, holoprosencephaly and,
    429–430
Ependyma, 66
Ependymal cells, 30, 32
Epidural, 6
Epidural hemorrhages and hematoma, 442, 451
Epidural space, 6, 112
Epilepsy, 254, 436, 438
Epineurium, 51
External capsule, 513, 514, 515, 516, 520
External granular cell layer, 421
Extortion, 279
Extraocular muscle system, 272, 273–280
  motor nuclei, 274, 275
  testing, 278–280
Extrapyramidal system, 212
Extreme capsule, 513, 514, 515, 516, 520
Eye
  dissection of, 166
  structures of, 167
Eye movements, 296–297
  brainstem components involved in, 271, 272, 273–280
  cerebellum and, 233, 234
  components controlling, 249, 251
Eye Movement Web site, 280

Face muscles
  brainstem components controlling, 269, 272
  movements of, 297
Face-name association task, 407

Faces
  cells responsive to, 176, 177
  receptive fields for, 152
Facial motor nucleus, 311
Facial nerve, 264, 309–310. *See also* Cranial nerve VII
Falcine meningioma, 484
Fasciculation, 195, 206
6-^{18}F-DOPA, in PET, 547–548
Fetal brain, 416–422
Fiber tracts, 136–137
Fibrillation, 195
Filamin 1, 438–439
Fimbria, 364, 516, 517, 520
First dorsal interosseous, 207
Fissures, cortical, 387
Flocculus, 236, 241, 518
Fluid-attenuated inversion recovery (FLAIR), 78
  images using, 96, 540, 541
Folia, 234
Foramen of Luschka, 43, 44
Foramen of Magendie, 43, 44
Foramen of Monro, 522
Forebrain, 5, 371
Fornix, 340, 357–358, 364, 514, 515, 516, 517, 520, 521, 522
Fourth ventricle, 518, 519
Fractures, skull, 443–445
Frontal eye fields, 278
Frontal horn, 513, 520
Frontal lobe (F), 7, 9, 405
Frontotemporal dementia (FTD), 412
Functional anatomy, review of, 473–492
Functional MRI (fMRI), 152–153, 181, 254, 382, 545–546.
    See also Activation mapping; Magnetic resonance
    imaging (MRI)
  use in neurosurgery, 408

GABAergic Purkinje neurons, 237
Gadolinium, in MRI, 540, 541
Gag reflex, 314
Ganglion cells, 164
Gasserian ganglion, 24, 135, 144, 307
Genu corpus callosum, 513, 521
Germinal matrix, 420, 415
"Giant motor unit," 195
Glial cells, 50
Glial fibers, 65
Glial fibrillary acidic protein (GFAP), 50, 51, 65
Glioblastoma multiforme, 98, 300
Glioma, cortical, 408
Globus pallidus, 216, 219
  externus, 514, 515, 520
  internus, 514, 515, 520
Glossopharyngeal nerve, 264, 292, 313–314
Golgi stain, 62
Gorlin's syndrome, 480, 481, 487
Gracilis fiber, 118
Gracilis nucleus, 122, 124, 518
Granular cortex, 173
Granular neurons, 234, 421
Granulomatous diseases, 69
Gray matter, 15, 29–30, 35. *See also* White matter
  brainstem, 38
  nuclei, 40
  spinal cord, 58–60, 115–116
  structures, 36
Guillain-Barré syndrome, 209
Gyri
  cortical, 387, 389
  functions of, 9–10
Gyrus rectus, 519, 521

Half brain, coronal sections of, 33–37
Hand weakness, 207–208

Head. *See also* Skull
  injuries to, 24
  missile injuries to, 447
  movements of, 297
  muscles of, 310
Head CT scans, 82, 83
Hearing
  evolution of, 292
  materials related to, 552–553
Hearing loss, 183–184, 313
Hematoxylin and eosin (H&E) stain, 50
Hemiplegia, 47
Hemispheric infarction, 408–409
Hemorrhages, 26–28, 46–47, 442, 449–453
Hemosiderin, 69
Herniated disc, 154·
Herniation, 443, 453–455
Herpes encephalitis, 69
Heschl's gyrus, 179, 404
Heteronymous deficit, 182
Heterotopias, 415, 435, 436
Hindbrain, 5
Hippocampal formation, 362–364, 366–368
Hippocampal gyrus, 367, 369, 516, 517
Hippocampus, 356, 515, 516, 517, 519, 520
Histology
  materials related to, 551
  nervous system, 49–75
Holoprosencephaly, 424–427
  environmental agents producing, 429–430
  in older children, 426
  trisomy 13 and, 430–431
Homonymous hemianopsia, 182, 184
Horse radish peroxidase (HRP), 213, 223, 399–400
Hounsfield Units (HU), 531, 532
Huntingtin protein, 232
Huntington's disease, 211, 228–232
  brain and, 230
  histology of, 231–232
Hypoglossal nerve, 264, 316–318
Hypoglossal nucleus, 465
Hypothalamic neurons, 332
Hypothalamic tumor, 348–351
Hypothalamus, 331–353, 514, 519, 521, 522
  circulation supplying, 335–336
  clinical cases related to, 348–353
  diseases affecting, 333
  histology of, 339
  hormones and transmitters associated with, 341–343
  inputs and outputs associated with, 332
  interactions involving, 332
  limbic system and, 356
  materials related to, 555–556
  microscopic anatomy of, 338–341
  regional anatomy of, 332–333, 334–338
Hypoxic-ischemic hemorrhages, 431–432

Image intensifier, 528
Imaging, planes used in, 93. *See also* Brain imaging
      techniques; Magnetic resonance imaging (MRI);
      Neuroimaging
Infarction
  hemispheric, 408–409
  identifying and localizing, 100
  in unimodal association cortex, 410–411
  vascular territory partial, 48
Inferior cerebellar peduncle, 38, 518
Inferior colliculus, 165, 519, 521, 522
Inferior olivary nucleus (ION), 122, 125, 234, 518
Infundibulum, 514
Inheritance, of Huntington's disease, 229
Innervation ratios, 202
Insula, 361, 513, 514, 520

Insular cortex, 9, 333, 361
"Interference pattern," 195
Intermediate hemispheres, 238, 249
Intermediolateral cell column, 346
Internal capsule, 36, 37, 513, 514, 515, 516, 515, 519, 520
  posterior limb, 520
Internal carotid artery, 519
Internal cerebral vein, 517
Internal granular layer, 234
Internuclear ophthalmoplegia, 285–286
Intortion, 279
Intraparenchymal hemorrhages, 442

Kinesthetic information, 106, 107, 117, 150

Laboratory materials, 549–550
Lacunar infarcts, 300–301
Lamina, 60
Lamina terminalis, 515, 516, 517, 522
Laminectomy, 112
Language, cortex and, 386, 403–405
Larmor frequency, 536–537, 538
Lateral cuneate nucleus, 236
Lateral geniculate nucleus (LGN), 170, 172, 384, 461, 516,
      517, 519
Lateral (surround) inhibition, 106–107
Lateral medullary infarct, 154–156
Lateral ventricle, 138, 139, 513, 514, 517, 521
Learning, limbic system and, 359, 372
Lectins, 213
Lemniscal fibers, 126–127
Lemniscal system, 106–107, 135
  comparison with anterolateral system, 157–159
Lentiform nucleus, 83
Leukocytes, polymorphonuclear, 70
Leukoencephalopathy, 71–74
Lewy body disease, 352–353
Limbic cortex, 384, 394, 396
Limbic lobe (LL), 9, 356
  surface components of, 360–361
Limbic system, 355–379
  amygdaloid connections of, 358
  anatomic components of, 356–357, 359–366
  clinical case study related to, 375–379
  cortical connections of, 357
  corticoid components of, 357, 365–366
  functional affiliations of, 359, 372–375
  hippocampal connections of, 358
  internal components of, 361–366
  materials related to, 557
  organization of, 366–371
  septal connections of, 358
Line/stripe of Gennari, 165, 172
Lissauer's tract, 117, 118–119
Lissencephaly, 416
Locus ceruleus, 280–281, 519
Lumbar spinal cord, 115, 116, 120
Lymphocytes, 69–70
  activity of, 199

Macrophages, 68–69, 73
Macular sparing, 174
Magnetic fields, with MRI, 536–537, 538
Magnetic resonance angiography (MRA), 78, 102–104,
      543–544
  scans, 93
Magnetic resonance imaging (MRI), 21, 78, 93–102, 536–547.
      See also Coronal MRI; Functional MRI (fMRI)
  advantages of, 42
  applications for, 98–100
  artifacts, 100–102
  clinical, 539–542
  cost of, 101

Magnetic resonance imaging (MRI) (*Continued*)
    CT versus, 546–547
    imaging techniques in, 542–543, 543–547
    PET versus, 548
    physics of, 536–539
    proton-weighted, 92
    scans, 99, 100, 497–503
Mammillary bodies, 13, 332, 357, 364, 365, 515, 519, 521, 522
Mammillothalamic tract, 332, 337–338, 357, 364, 365
Massa intermedia, 522
Mastication, 297
    muscles of, 307
Materials lists, 549–558
Medial brain surface, 11
Medial dorsal nucleus, 216, 515, 516, 520
Medial forebrain bundle, 332
Medial geniculate nucleus (MGM), 384, 517, 519
Medial lemniscal system, 270
    components of, 269
    fibers, 146
    pathways, 129–131
Medial lemniscus, 46, 125, 126, 128, 295–296, 518
Medial longitudinal fasciculus (MLF), 276, 277, 278, 297
Medulla, 13, 38, 81, 122–125, 277, 465, 521
    function of, 261
    histologic sections of, 123
    structures in, 124
Medullary autonomic centers, 346
Medullary infarct, 154–156, 299–300
Melanin-concentrating hormone (MCH), 343
Memory, limbic system and, 359, 372
Meninges, 21, 25
Meningitis, 70–71
Merosin, 53
Met-enkephalin, 223–225
Meyer's loop, 172
Microglia, 68–69
Microgyria, 434
Microscopes, tips for, 51–52
Midbrain, 5, 7, 13, 38, 144, 145, 463, 521, 522
    function of, 261
    landmarks in, 127–129
    sensory pathways in, 147
Middle cerebellar peduncle, 518
Middle cerebral artery, 519
Middle peduncle, 38
Midsagittal MRI scan, 41, 42
Missile injuries, 447
Molecular layer, 234
Monoradicular syndrome, 153
Mossy fibers, 234, 237
Motion artifacts, 100
Motor activity, 211
Motor gyrus, 33, 35
Motor neurons, 60, 196–197
    loss of, 206
Motor nuclei, brainstem, 273–274
Motor systems, 187–209, 296–297
Motor units, 187, 188, 189, 202–204
    size of, 203
Movement disorders, 463
Multimodal association cortex, 383, 393–394, 397
    atrophy of, 411–412
Multiple sclerosis, clinical case associated with, 284–286
Muscle(s)
    histology of, 52–54, 196
    skeletal, 50
    nerve and muscle fiber counts for, 202
    structure and function of, 188–190

Muscle cells, 50, 52
Muscle fibers
    necrosis of, 199
    types of, 54
Muscle innervation/denervation, 190–192, 199–204
Muscle proteins, 190
Muscular dystrophies, 190, 196. *See also* Duchenne's muscular dystrophy
Myelin, 50, 65, 201
Myelinated axons, 35, 55, 57, 60, 123, 201
Myelination, 421–422
Myelin sheaths, 55, 57
    degeneration of, 46
    destruction of, 191
Myocytes, 50, 521
Myofibers, 50, 52–53
Myofibrillary filaments, 196
Myofibrils, 54
Myopathy, muscular, 197–199

Neck muscles, brainstem components controlling, 269
Neocortex
    layers of, 384
    materials related to, 557
Neostriatum, 212
Nerve conduction recordings, 206
Nerve conduction studies, 192–193
Nerve conduction velocity (NCV), 207
Nerve myotome table, 193
Nerve root, 56
Nerves. *See also* Cranial nerves; Neural entries
    histology of, 200–202
    peripheral, 50
Nervous system. *See also* Central nervous system; Nerve entries; Peripheral nerve
    cells of, 74–75
    histology of, 49–75
    layout of, 5
    orientation of, 3
    principles of differentiation in, 414
    tissues and cell types in, 50–51
    trauma to, 441–455
Nervous tissue, handling, 1
Nervus intermedius, 264
Neural crest, 415
Neural networks, in the cerebral cortex, 407–408
Neural plate, 415
Neural systems, review of, 466–473
Neural tube, 415
    closure of, 422–424
    Sonic hedgehog expression in, 427–428
Neuroanatomy
    anatomical atlases of, 549
    approaches to, 2–3
    terminology for, 3–4
Neuroangiography, 528–530
Neurofibrillary tangles, 377
Neuroimaging, 77–104
    "normal," 493–503
    principles of, 527–548
Neuromuscular system, 187–209
    clinical cases related to, 207–209
    materials related to, 553
Neurons, 51
    functions of, 49
    types of, 60, 61
Neuropil, 60
Neuropil threads, 378
Neurosurgery, functional MRI in, 408
Neurotransmitter networks, diffuse, 261
Neutrophils, 51, 52, 70
Nissl histology, 368
Nissl substance, 51, 61, 114

Nociception, 107
Nociceptive fibers, 117, 118, 150
Nociceptive reflexes, 109
Nociceptive systems, 135, 144
Nodes of Ranvier, 50, 201
Nodulus, 236
Norepinephrine system, 280–281
Notochord, 415, 428
Nuclei, 30, 60. *See also* Atomic nuclei
    oligodendroglial, 64
Nucleus accumbens, 459–460, 513, 514, 519
Nucleus ambiguus, 314, 316
Nystagmus, 239–240, 255

Occipital horn, 520
Occipital lobe, 7, 9
Oculomotor nerve, 263, 292, 302–303
    exiting midbrain, 304
Olfactory bulb, 13
Olfactory nerve, 24, 290
Olfactory tracts, 13, 513, 519
Olfactory tubercle, 513, 514
Oligodendrocytes, 51, 63–64, 75
Olivocerebellar system, 251, 252
"On-center" cell, 169
Ophthalmicus profundus, 292
Optic chiasm, 13, 182, 521, 522
Optic disk, 166
Optic pathways, 171
    nerve, 13, 162–163, 169, 290, 521
    radiation, 517
    tract, 340, 514, 515
Optic pit, 167
Orbitofrontal area, 24
Organ of Corti, 164
Organ vasculosum of the lamina terminalis (OVLT), 332, 340
Otx-2 gene, 428–429
Oxytocin, 342

Pachygyria, 415
Pain
    autonomic responses to, 347
    sensation of, 107–109
Pain and temperature system, anterolateral, 271, 272
Paleostriatum, 212
Pallidoluysian projection, 224
Papez circuit, 357
Papova virus infections, 74
Parabrachial nuclei, 346–347
Parahippocampal gyrus, 356, 361, 363, 364, 369, 370
Paralimbic cortex, 384, 394
    regions of, 395
Paramedian pontine reticular formation (PPRF), 274
Parasympathetic nervous system, 316, 333
Paraterminal gyrus, 513
Parietal eye fields, 278
Parietal lobe, 7, 9
Parkinson's disease, 211, 226, 334
    wiring diagram for, 227
Patellar stretch reflex, 187–188
Peduncles, brainstem, 38, 39
Pedunculopontine nucleus, 371
Pencillary fibers of Wilson, 219
Perfusion-weighted imaging (PWI), 544, 545
Peripheral nerve, 50, 74
    histology of, 52, 55–58, 202–202
Peripheral sensory cells, 50
Periventricular heterotopias, 437
Pharyngeal sensory fibers, 314
"Phase" artifacts, 101
Phase contrast (PC) images, 545
Phenytoin, 254
Pia, 6, 22

Pick's disease, 412
Pineal gland, 24, 517, 520, 521, 522
Piriform olfactory cortex, 356, 359, 361–362, 370–371
Pituitary, 13, 24
    histology of, 338–339
Pituitary fossa, 42
Plaques
    in the cortex, 377
    demyelinated, 285
Poliomyelitis, 190–191, 205, 207
Polymicrogyria, 415, 433
Polymorphonuclear leukocytes, 51, 52, 70
Polymyositis, 198–199
Pons, 13, 38, 464, 516, 518, 518, 521
    landmarks in, 126–127
"Pontine gliomas," 300
Ponto-mesencephalic reticular formation, 109
Porencephaly, 432–434
Positron emission tomography (PET), 547–548
Postcentral gyrus, 151, 153, 398
Posterior cerebral arteries (PCA), 17, 91
Posterior circulation, 5, 257, 269
    main vessels in, 91
Posterior column deficit, 156–157
Posterior column nuclei, 521
Posterior commissure, 141, 517, 519, 520, 521, 522
    eye movements and, 403
Posterior fossa, 39
Posterior inferior cerebellar arteries (PICA), 91, 154, 241, 257, 261, 518
Posterior parietal cortex (P), 405
Potential spaces, 6
Precentral gyrus, 33, 35, 151, 153, 398
    motor neurons of, 47
Primary motor cortex, 41, 382–383
Primary olfactory cortex, 356
Primary sensory cortex, 382–383
Primary sensory-motor cortex, 390–392
Primary somatosensory cortex, 399
Primary visual cortex, 172, 407
    blood supply to, 174
    cell physiology in, 175–177
Progressive multifocal leukoencephalopathy (PML), 71–74
Projection fibers, 30, 36, 385
Projection neurons, 223
Prolactin, 342
Prosopagnosia, 410–411
Proton-density-weighted images, 539
Pulvinar, 517, 520
Pupillary constriction, 274–276
Purkinje cells, 61, 62, 63, 234, 237, 243, 244, 421
Putamen, 215–216, 222, 513, 514, 515, 516, 520
    histology of, 219
Pyramidal neuron, 75
Pyramidal tracts, 46–47, 296
    decussation of, 121
Pyramids, 518, 521

Radial glial fibers, 415
Radicular, 153
Radiofrequency pulse, with MRI, 537, 538, 539
Radiography, operation of, 527–528
Raphe nuclei, 281–283
Rapid-eye movement (REM) sleep, 371
"Rathke's cleft," 339
Receptive fields, 107, 167, 168, 169, 175
    in auditory cortex, 180–182
    oriented, 176
Receptors. *See also* Receptive field entries
    pain and temperature, 109
    peripheral touch and tactile, 107
Red nucleus, 298–299, 516, 519
Reticular formation, 109

Retina, 164
  histology of, 167, 168
  topography of, 174
Retinal ganglion cells, 168
  physiology of, 167–169
Retrograde transport, 213
Rexed layers, 117
Root entry zone, 117–120
Rostral pons, 282
Rostral structures, 3

Sarcomere, 53
Scalp, 21, 22
Scanners
  for CT, 530–531, 531–532, 533–534, 535
  for PET, 547
Schwann cells, 50, 57
Schwannomas, 310, 313
Sciatic nerve, 201
Sections, microscopic, 553
Seizures, 435–439
Sensory action potential, 194
Sensory cerebellar tracts, 236
Sensory cortex, 134, 150–153
Sensory fibers, 146, 149
Sensory homunculus, 134, 151, 152
Sensory receptors, peripheral touch and tactile, 107
Sensory systems, 295–296
Septal area, 356
Septal nuclei, 514
Septum pellucidum, 513, 514, 520, 521
Serotonin receptors, 283–284
Serotonin system, 281–284
Sheep brain
  dissection of, 523–525
  materials related to, 558
Sinuses, 20–21, 91
Skeletal muscle, *see* muscle
Skull, 21, 22–24. *See also* Head
  auditory orifices in, 179
  base structures of, 23
  fractures of, 443–445
  models of, 549, 550, 551, 552, 557, 558
  plain film of, 79–80
  thickness of, 83
Soft tissue coverings, of the brain, 24–26
Solitary nucleus, 314, 316, 333, 344
Solitary tract, 297
Somatosensory nuclei, 125
Somatosensory system, 105–131, 295–296
  review of, 467–468
Sonic hedgehog, 414
  expression in neural tube, 427–428
Sonic hedgehog knock-out mouse, phenotype of, 428–429
Spin, of atomic nuclei, 536–539
Spinal arteries, 19
Spinal cord, 113–121. *See also* Spinal nerve(s)
  anatomy of, 114–117
  blood supply to, 5–6
  dissection of, 14–15, 31–33
  external anatomy of, 4–5, 12–16
  histology of, 58–61, 204–205, 466
  injury to, 446–447
  major divisions of, 14, 115
  MRI landmarks of, 110–112
  relationship of vertebral column to, 110
  root entry zone of, 117–120
  structure of, 205, 485
  tracts and gray matter in, 32
  trauma to, 488–489
  vessels in, 67
Spinal epidural space, 112
Spinal MRI, 112

Spinal muscular atrophy (SMA), 205
Spinal nerve(s), 110. *See also* Spinal cord
  functional divisions of, 292
  injury to, 192
Spinal sensory roots, 112, 113–114
Spinal trigeminal nucleus, 142, 307, 308, 345, 518
Spinal trigeminal tract, 296
Spin-echo (SE) sequence, 539
Spinocerebellar tracts, 236
Spinocerebellum, 238, 250
  subdivisions of, 249
Spinothalamic system, 107–109, 119
  fibers, 122, 125, 293
  review of, 467
  tracts, 122, 296
Spiny neurons, 219
Splenium corpus callosum, 517, 521, 522
Splinter hemorrhages, 449
"Split brain" cases, 10
Stellate neurons, 234
Stria terminalis, 30, 332, 358
Striatum, 83, 212
Stripe/line of Gennari, 165, 172
Stroke, embolic, 48
Subarachnoid hemorrhages, 28, 442
Subarachnoid space, 6
Subdural hemorrhages or hematoma, 442, 451, 452
Subfalcine herniation, 443, 453
Subfornical organ, 340, 341
Subiculum, 332, 516, 517
Substance P staining, 223–225
Substantia gelatinosa, 117
Substantia innominata, 514, 519
Substantia nigra, 216, 220, 353, 515, 516,
    519
  histology of, 221
Subthalamic nucleus, 216, 515, 516
Subventricular zone, 420
Sulci, cortical, 387, 389
Superior cerebellar arteries (SCA), 91, 241
Superior cerebellar peduncle, 38, 243, 518, 519
Superior colliculus, 517, 519, 521, 522
Superior olivary nucleus, 165
Superior peduncle, 38
Superior sagittal sinus, 24
Superior temporal gyrus, 513, 514
Suprachiasmatic nucleus, 332
Surround (lateral) inhibition, 106–107
Sylvian fissure, 7, 9, 138
Syrinx, 156

T1 MRI scans, 40, 41, 497–498, 501–503
T_1- and T_2-weighted images with MRI, 539–541,
    541–542
T2 MRI scans, 98, 499–500
Taste sensations, 310, 315
Tau protein, 378
T cells, 73
Tectum, 109
Tegmentum, 518
Telencephalon, 5
Temperature control, 349
Temporal gyri, 513
Temporal horn, 515, 516, 517, 519
Temporal lobe, 7, 9, 518
  capillary network in, 20
Tentorium, 24, 25, 240
Terminology, neuroanatomical, 3–4
Thalamocortical circuits, 134
Thalamus, 129, 138, 140, 146–160, 521, 522
  anatomic divisions of, 147
  connection to the cortex, 400–401
  nuclei, 400–401

sensory relay nuclei in, 148
sensory traffic in, 134
structures, 147, 148, 384
ventral anterior and ventral lateral, 216
Third ventricle, 514, 515, 516, 520, 522
Thoracic spinal cord, 115
Time of flight (TOF) images, 545
Time to echo (TE) parameter, 539, 541–542
Time to repeat (TR) parameter, 539, 541–542
Timing tasks, cerebellar activation during, 254
Tissue imaging, 77–79
Tongue
    innervation of, 318
    movements of, 297
Tonic-clonic seizures, 435–439
Tonsilar herniation, 443, 454
"Top of the basilar" infarct, 301
Tracing studies, 224, 225
Transmitters, 213
Transmitter systems, 261
Transverse gyrus of Heschl. *See* Heschl's gyrus
Transverse plane, 4
Trapezoid body, 165
Trauma, 441–455
    materials related to, 558
Trigeminal ganglion, 24
Trigeminal lemniscal system, 474
Trigeminal nerve, 142, 292, 306–307
Trigeminal nuclei, 145
Trigeminal primary sensory nucleus, 296
Trigeminal somatosensory system, review of, 469
Trigeminal system, 133, 135, 142–146
Trigeminothalamic system, review of, 468
Trisomy 13, holoprosencephaly and, 430–431
Trochlear nerve, 263, 303, 304
Trochlear nucleus, 305
Two-point discrimination test, 121
Type I and II muscle fibers, 196
Tyrosine hydroxylase (TH), 213, 220, 221, 342

"U" fibers, of sheep brain, 523, 524, 525
Ulnar nerve, 200
Uncal herniation, 443, 453
Uncus, 356, 360–361, 515, 519
Unimodal association areas, 393
Unimodal association cortex, 383
    infarction in, 410–411
Unmyelinated fibers, 58

Vagus nerve, 264, 292, 314–316, 344
Vagus nucleus, 297–298
Vascular anatomy, imaging, 92–93
Vascular territory infarction, 48
Vasculature, nervous tissue, 18
Vasopressin, 342
Venogram, 21
Venous sinuses, 6
Venous structures, 91
Ventral anterior nucleus, 515

Ventral anterior thalamic nucleus, 216
Ventral lateral nucleus, 515
Ventral lateral thalamic nucleus, 216
Ventral posterior-lateral (VPL) nucleus, 134, 148, 384, 516
Ventral posterior-medial (VPM) nucleus, 135, 148, 384
Ventral spinocerebellar tract, 246
Ventral tegmental area (VTA), 220
Ventral thalamus, 520
Ventricles, model of, 549, 551, 552, 553. *See also* Brain
        ventricles
Ventricular system, 43–44
Ventricular zone, 420
Vermis, 238, 249
Vessels, histology of, 67–68
Vertebral arteries, 88, 268–269
Vertebral column, 110–112. *See also* Spinal cord MRI
    landmarks of, 110–112
Vestibular nerve, 264, 277
Vestibular system, 249, 251
    nuclear complex, 276, 312
    nuclei, 518
Vestibulocerebellum, 238, 239
Vestibulocochlear nerve, 310–313
Virchow-Robin space, 51, 69, 70
Vision and hearing materials, 552–553
Visual cortex, 172
    histology of, 165–166
    topography of, 174
Visual cortical areas, higher, 177
Visual deficit clinical cases, 182–183, 184–185
Visual fields, 178
    deficits in, 163, 177
    cortical representation of, 173–174
Visual field testing, 184
Visual pathways, 162, 169–172
Visual system, 161, 475–476
    dissection of the eye, 166
    optic nerve, 162–163
    retina, 164
    review of, 469–470
    topography of, 163
Volume averaging, 81

Wallerian degeneration, 46, 47, 191, 462, 482
Wernicke's aphasia, 404
Wernicke's area, 386
White matter, 15, 30, 35, 64. *See also* Gray matter
    brainstem, 38
    bundles in, 30
    fibers in, 12
    injury to, 71
    plaques in, 285
    sheep brain, 523, 524, 525
    spinal cord, 58–59, 115–116
    structures in, 36
Windowing, with CT, 531–532, 533

X-ray imaging, 78, 79–80, 527–535
    MRI versus, 536